Risk Assessme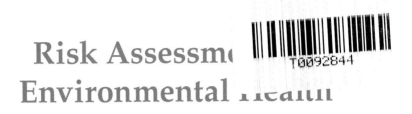 Environmental Health

Understanding risk to humans is one of the most important problems in environmental public health. Risk assessment is constantly changing with the advent of new exposure assessment tools, more sophisticated models, and a better understanding of disease processes. Risk assessment is also gaining greater acceptance in the developing world where major environmental problems exist.

Developed in partnership with the Association of Schools of Public Health, this comprehensive text offers a thorough survey of risk assessment, management, and communications as these practices apply to public health.

Features

- Provides a practical overview of environmental risk assessment and its application by discussing the process and providing case studies and examples.

- Focuses on tools and approaches used for humans in an environment involving potential chemical hazards.

- Fully updated, the first part introduces the underlying principles and techniques of the field, and the second examines case studies in terms of different risk assessment scenarios.

- Useful "stories" suitable for case studies.

Risk Assessment for Environmental Health

Second Edition

Edited by

Mark G. Robson

Distinguished Professor, Rutgers University, New Brunswick, NJ, United States

William A. Toscano

University of Minnesota School of Public Health, Minneapolis, MN, United States

Qingyu Meng

California Department of Toxic Substances Control, Sacramento, CA, United States
Desert Research Institute, Reno, NV, United States

Debra A. Kaden

Principal Consultant at Ramboll US Consulting, Inc., Boston, MA, United States

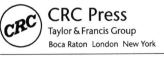

CRC Press
Taylor & Francis Group
Boca Raton London New York

CRC Press is an imprint of the
Taylor & Francis Group, an **informa** business

First edition published 2023
by CRC Press
6000 Broken Sound Parkway NW, Suite 300, Boca Raton, FL 33487-2742

and by CRC Press
4 Park Square, Milton Park, Abingdon, Oxon, OX14 4RN

© 2023 Taylor & Francis Group, LLC

CRC Press is an imprint of Taylor & Francis Group, LLC

Library of Congress Cataloging-in-Publication Data
Names: Robson, Mark G., 1955- editor. | Toscano, William, 1945- editor. |
Meng, Qingyu (Professor of public health), editor. | Kaden, Debra Ann, editor.
Title: Risk assessment for environmental health / edited by Mark G. Robson,
Board of Governors Distinguished Service Professor, Rutgers University,
William Toscano, PhD, Professor Emeritus, Division of Environmental Health Sciences,
University of Minnesota School of Public Health, Qingyu Meng, Adjunct Research Professor,
Desert Research Institute, Debra Kaden, Principal Consultant at Ramboll US Consulting, Inc.
Description: Second edition. | Boca Raton, FL : CRC Press, 2023. |
Revised edition of: Risk assessment for environmental health / Mark Robson, William Toscano,
editors. c2007. | Includes bibliographical references and index. | Identifiers: LCCN 2022032401 (print) |
LCCN 2022032402 (ebook) | ISBN 9780367261511 (HB) | ISBN 9780367261443 (PB) |
ISBN 9780429291722 (EB) Subjects: LCSH: Health risk assessment. | Environmental health. |
Public health. Classification: LCC RA427.3 .R569 2023 (print) | LCC RA427.3 (ebook) |
DDC 362.1--dc23/eng/20220729 LC record available at https://lccn.loc.gov/2022032401LC
ebook record available at https://lccn.loc.gov/2022032402

ISBN: 978-0-367-26151-1 (hbk)
ISBN: 978-0-367-26144-3 (pbk)
ISBN: 978-0-429-29172-2 (ebk)

DOI: 10.1201/9780429291722

Typeset in Palatino
by SPi Technologies India Pvt Ltd (Straive)

"Follow The Risk"
By Junfeng Zhang (2021)

Around the globe rises the cooking smoke
Fire glares the face of a giant
as vivid as in my dream last night
Telling us to "follow the risk"

For over forty years, never has he ceased
to wake up the world
There is a huge health risk from the cooking smoke
for those who had to burn dirty fuels
they can only afford

In the fairy tale, only a giant can wake up the world
But not magically he did
With endless effort to follow the risk
Inhaling the very same smoke
that even shortened his biological life
Could I suspect

I love to watch fires in my kitchen
Smokeless, soothing, and beautiful
I know they are from a clean fuel
This is the type of fires he's lived through
I once wondered
Living in an affluent world
Why he cares about
those smoke-impacted souls underprivileged
Then his voice started to thunder
"Follow the risk"

Around the globe he's followed the cooking smoke
Showing the world
Things can be done
From improved stoves to cleaner fuels
As clean air is a right
for every man, woman, and child

When I miss him, I'd close the eyes
Then I see smoking fires
where his face appears
I hear a sonorous voice
"Follow the risk"
This is the voice of a humble man, yet a giant
Who's made the world a better place

Contents

List of Boxes ix

Foreword xi

Preface xiii

Editors xv

Contributors xvii

1. Introduction to Risk Assessment 1
   Mark G. Robson, William A. Toscano, Qingyu Meng, and Debra A. Kaden

2. The Risk Assessment–Risk Management Paradigm 15
   Gilbert S. Omenn and David L. Eaton

3. Risk Assessment and Regulatory Decision-Making in Environmental Health 39
   Felicia Wu and Joseph V. Rodricks

4. Exposure Assessment: The Ways We Measure Exposure and Its Application to Risk Assessment 57
   Donghai Liang

5. Biological Monitoring of Exposure to Environmental Chemicals throughout the Life Stages: Requirements and Issues to Consider for Birth Cohort Studies 73
   Parinya Panuwet, P. Barry Ryan, Dana Boyd Barr, and Warangkana Naksen

6. Role of Epidemiology in Environmental Health Research 99
   Wil Lieberman-Cribbin and Emanuela Taioli

7. Toxicological Basis for Risk Assessment 111
   Mark G. Robson and William A. Toscano

8. The Application of Physiologically Based Pharmacokinetic (PBPK) Modeling to Risk Assessment 153
   Raymond S. H. Yang, Yasong Lu, and Zhoumeng Lin

9. Adverse Outcomes Pathways (AOPs) 179
   Elizabeth V. Wattenberg

10. Epigenetics in Risk Assessment 187
    Carmen Marsit and Jinze Li

11. Probabilistic Models for Characterizing Aggregate and Cumulative Risk 199
    Qingyu Meng

12. Occupational Risk Assessment 225
    Adam M. Finkel, Douglas O. Johns, and Christine Whittaker

13. Children's Environmental Health Risk Assessment 267
    Rebecca C. Dzubow and Ruth A. Etzel

14. Addressing the Limits of Risk Assessment by Focusing on Safer Alternatives
    Risk Assessment for Environmental Health 279
    Joel Tickner, Molly Jacobs, and Margaret H. Whittaker

15. How European Countries Approach Regulatory Risk Assessment 317
    Helmut Greim

16. Envirome Disorganization and Ecological Riskscapes: The Algal Bloom Epitome 327
    Matteo Convertino and Haojiong Wang

17. Risk Communication 347
    Elaine M. Faustman, Jill C. Falman, and Susan L. Santos

Index 367

List of Boxes

Box 1.1 Built Environment (as well as Careers in Environmental Public Health) 3

Richard J. Jackson

Box 1.2 Polyhalogenated Aryl Hydrocarbon Receptor Ligands 5

Charles Miller

Box 1.3 Health Risks of PCBs and PCDFs...10

Matthew Berens

Box 1.4 Health Effects of TCE...11

Adel Soroush

Box 1.5 Risk Assessment of Nanomaterials and Other Advanced Materials and Technologies......12

James Ede

Box 2.1 Context 23

Box 3.1 Risk of Pesticides in the Environment...51

Wattasit Siriwong

Box 3.2 Roundup 52

Suren Bandara

Box 4.1 Stress..70

Nancy Fiedler

Box 4.2 Air Pollution Exposure Assessment 70

Junfeng Zhang

Box 7.1 The Comparative Toxicogenomics Database (CTD)..122

Carolyn Mattingly

Box 7.2 Heavy Metals, Lead, and Mercury..126

Robert Rottersman, Michael Gochfeld and Joanna Burger, Joanna Burger and Michael Gochfeld

Box 7.3 Health Effects of Arsenic 135

Paul Tchounwou

Box 7.4 Environmental Justice 141

Angele White

Box 7.5 Geographic Information Systems (GIS) 143

Yannis Vassilopoulos

Box 8.1 Bioavailability: An Independent Variable in Risk Assessment.................................171

Michael Gallo

Box 10.1 Endocrine-Disrupting Compounds (EDCs) and Epigenetics 189

John A. McLachlan and Christopher A.B. McLachlan

Box 12.1 Assessing Trends in Workplace Population Risk...227

Adam M. Finkel

Box 12.2 Occupational Safety *or* Health? Resource Allocation at OSHA 232

Adam M. Finkel

Box 12.3 Asbestos in the Workplace...234
Jeffery Mandel

Box 12.4 More Risk-Risk Trade-Offs in Occupational Health and Safety.......................252
Adam M. Finkel

Box 12.5 Controls, Profit, Employment, and Health..256
Adam M. Finkel

Box 12.6 Information Disclosure: An Important and Free-Standing Part of the Hierarchy..........257
Adam M. Finkel

Box 12.7 Repeated Head Trauma..259
Adam M. Finkel

Box 12.8 Night Shift Work and Breast Cancer Risk..260
Mingzhu Fang

Box 14.1 Bisphenol A (BPA) – A Case of the Challenges of a Risk-Based System 282
Joel Tickner, Molly Jacobs, and Margaret H. Whittaker

Box 14.2 A Risk Assessment Challenge: How Do We Manage Thousands
of Extremely Persistent and Ubiquitous Chemicals?..284
Simona Andreea Bălan

Box 14.3 Example: A Solutions-Approach to Trichloroethylene in Massachusetts 289
Joel Tickner, Molly Jacobs, and Margaret H. Whittaker

Box 14.4 The Commons Principles for Alternatives Assessment.......................................291
Joel Tickner, Molly Jacobs, and Margaret H. Whittaker

Box 17.1 Typology of Risk Communication Objectives...351
Elaine Faustman, Jill Falman, and Susan Santos

Box 17.2 Examples of Tailoring Messages / Tools for Specific Audiences 352
Elaine Faustman, Jill Falman, and Susan Santos

Box 17.3 Questions to Consider 359
Elaine Faustman, Jill Falman, and Susan Santos

Box 17.4 Checklist to Aid in Audience Identification...360
Elaine Faustman, Jill Falman, and Susan Santos

Box 17.5 Primary Risk Perception Factors...361
Elaine Faustman, Jill Falman, and Susan Santos

Box 17.6 Acceptability of Risk Comparison...363
Elaine Faustman, Jill Falman, and Susan Santos

Foreword

Risk Assessment in Context

Bernard D. Goldstein, MD

Risk analysis can be viewed as the second of three historical phases of the almost century-long modern attempt to meet the challenges of protecting our environment and ourselves. The first phase was marked by "Command and Control." Public disgust with dirty air and water, and with chemicals littering our landscapes, resulted in new laws and new local, national, and international agencies. The driving forces were sensory. But we soon found that scientific evidence was needed to control what we could see and smell.

Inevitably, advances in the measurement of compounds in air, water, soil, and food, and in analysis of their effects, led to the recognition that many agents that we could not see, smell or taste were responsible for adverse effects in ecosystems and humans. Risk assessment was developed as a means to better identify and understand the effects of external agents, thereby allowing orderly and consistent approaches to risk management.

The concepts underlying risk assessment were long in use, although defined and practiced in widely different ways until the field was in essence codified in 1983 by a US National Academies of Science Committee and then adopted for use by the United States Environmental Protection Agency (USEPA) and other national and international agencies. The development of a formal basis for assessing risk was a major turning point in environmental protection. It provided a conceptual basis for writing laws and regulations aimed specifically at reducing risk, a measure useful for setting priorities, and a yardstick for measuring results. The adoption of risk assessment also spurred major scientific advances, not the least of which was the development of the field of exposure assessment far beyond its roots in industrial hygiene. The first graduate programs focusing on assessing exposure in the general population, and the establishment of the International Society of Exposure Science, occurred within a few years after the publication of the Red Book. Importantly, the development of exposure science has led to better linkage between epidemiology and toxicology: the two existing core disciplines underlying the initial development of the risk paradigm.

Sustainability can be considered the third historical phase of environmental control. Like risk assessment when it was first adopted, the sustainability paradigm is not new. Its major components include a recognition of the need to consider future generations, the development of broader approaches to environmental control that cut across the silos often imposed by media-specific laws and by geography, and a focus on primary prevention rather than cleaning up afterward. In speaking to those involved in environmental protection, I often summarize sustainability as requiring them to consider not only how to minimize risk but also how to maximize benefit. Unfortunately, the challenges to human well-being within a sustainable planet seem to be increasing with a list that includes manifestation of the problems long predicted to result from global climate change and continuing population growth, and new challenges caused by a global pandemic and by war.

Responding to the many challenges of sustainability is complicated by our inability to consider risk-related issues in a broader context. Two current examples are our failure to optimize nuclear power due to concerns about radioactive waste disposal and the return to wars of conquest by countries that through accidents of geography or geology control fossil fuels. Nuclear waste control challenges have been a major impediment to nuclear power, at least in the United States. The Yucca Mountain nuclear storage alternative was halted by Congress in large part because of a National Academy of Sciences (NAS) analysis that starting 100 years from now, there could be breakthrough to groundwater that might lead to cancer risk in the local population. Yet any reasonable risk assessment would indicate that radiation breakthrough at the waste depository would lead to perhaps one additional case of cancer in the 23rd century, while by then mortality due to global climate change that could have been avoided by nuclear power would almost certainly be in the millions.

The second example begins with recognition that war is the antithesis to sustainability. Many observers have pointed to a role for Russia's near stranglehold on natural gas supplies for Germany and other European Union countries as a reason for Russia's belief it could attack Ukraine with impunity. Would it have made a difference if Germany had not changed its mind to drill for its own shale gas because of environmental concerns? And would it have made a difference to understanding the extent of this risk if fossil fuel interests in the United States had not blocked risk-related research when large-scale unconventional shale gas development began more than a decade ago in the United States?

Obviously, the risk assessment paradigm will not by itself be the answer to these and other major challenges to sustainability. Yet risk science is broader than risk assessment, as is evident from this book. By providing accurate descriptions of risk, including its temporal component, risk analysis is a central component of many of the needed trade-off analyses within and across the three legs of sustainability, as well as providing the information required for a dispassionate cross-silo analysis of existing and future risks.

Risk assessment as described in the chapters of *Introduction to Risk Assessment* provides a very timely analysis pertinent to the ongoing use of risk assessment/risk management to appropriately prevent and control environmental threats. These chapters also provide ample evidence of how risk science is reaching out to deal with issues of central concern to developing and maintaining a sustainable planet.

Preface

PREFACE FROM THE FIRST EDITION

Understanding risk to humans is one of the most important challenges in environmental public health. Over the past 25 years, schools of public health have developed courses to meet the growing needs of environmental health students as well as other public health disciplines to understand the risk assessment process used by government, industry, and academic researchers.

Courses in risk assessment in schools of public health vary in approaches taken. In discussion with colleagues, it became apparent to us that there is no appropriate text that covers environmental health risk assessment and meets the needs of public health students. Because of the importance of risk assessment in environmental and occupational health sciences, the Environmental and Occupational Health Council of the Association of Schools of Public Health selected risk assessment as a topic for their annual summer meeting held in 2004 at the University of Minnesota. We organized and chaired the meeting and used it as the framework on which to build a risk assessment textbook. This textbook is the deliverable of the 2004 Minneapolis meeting. It is written primarily by faculty colleagues at the member school of the Association of Schools of Public Health. The chapters and topics in this volume were identified at the meeting as the most relevant for textbook use in a graduate-level introduction to the risk assessment process. In addition, case studies used by faculty for illustrative purposes in their own courses are included.

This book should be considered a useful primary resource for students in public health, environmental since, environmental engineering, and other related disciplines. There are many other important references used by faculty: the classic "Red Book," *Issues in Risk Assessment* (1993) from the National Academy of Sciences, the WHO document *Human Exposure Assessment: An Introduction* (2001), and the EPA Superfund document *Volume 1: Human Health Evaluation Manual, Part A* (1989).

Risk assessment is constantly changing with the advent of new exposure assessment tools, more sophisticated models, and a better understanding of disease processes. Risk assessment is also gaining greater acceptance in the developing world, where major environmental problems exist.

We hope that you find this textbook of value in your teaching, and we welcome your comments on improving chapters, adding case studies, and expanding the topics contained in the text.

Mark G. Robson and William A. Toscano

PREFACE FOR THIS EDITION

Fifteen years after the first edition was published, we were encouraged to revise and update the textbook. We expanded our editorial team to include two additional scientists, one from the private sector and one from government, to broaden our perspective on environmental risks. During the time that we started on the second edition, an entirely new risk emerged, COVID-19, a novel coronavirus, SARS-CoV-2, which had not previously been reported in humans. Based on that fact, there are places in the text that specifically reference the COVID-19 risk.

Our publisher, Taylor & Francis, has encouraged us to design this as an interactive textbook with online updates and expanded resource information. Since the first edition, many tools that have improved the science underlying risk assessment were developed. These include big data, machine learning and new computational tools, advances in genomics and molecular biology, epigenetics, exposure science, and analytical chemistry to assess mixtures exposome. Many of the new advances have not yet come into common use by risk assessors but show great promise in better describing and assessing risk.

This new edition of *Risk Assessment for Environmental Health* has 16 chapters covering the basic information that public health students need to know for their daily responsibilities. The new additional also provides an overview of the risk process, it explains the risk paradigm and the application of risk assessment to regulatory decision-making. Exposure assessment, biomonitoring, and the application of epidemiology in the risk assessment process are introduced. Toxicological principles, which are the underpinning to most risks are described. Exposure pathways, risk models, workplace risks, and the integration of risks into human impact assessment are discussed.

We felt it was important to evaluate and distinguish the application of risk assessment as a tool across federal agencies in the United States, as well as globally, through comparing and contrasting the regulatory approaches taken in different countries and the reasons for the differences.

There are a number of information boxes included in the chapters that provide snapshots of important topics and current issues as related to risk. These boxes are supplemental and will continue to be added to the dynamic online version of the textbook.

We are hopeful that this new textbook will be seen as a useful and informative resource for public health students and serve as an introduction to risk assessment as part of their graduate training.

Mark G. Robson, William A. Toscano, Qingyu Meng, and Debra A. Kaden

Editors

Professor Mark G. Robson earned his PhD in plant science from Rutgers University in 1988 and his MPH in environmental health from the University of Medicine and Dentistry of New Jersey (UMDNJ) in 1995. He is currently Distinguished Professor of Plant Biology at Rutgers School of Environmental and Biological Sciences and also is Visiting Professor and Senior Academic Advisor at Chulalongkorn University in Bangkok Thailand.

Professor William A. Toscan earned his PhD in biochemistry at the University of Illinois, Urbana-Champaign, in 1978. He was a Postdoctoral Fellow in Pharmacology at the University of Washington Medical School, Seattle, from 1978 to 1980, after which he joined the toxicology faculty at the Harvard School of Public Health. In 1989, he moved to the University of Minnesota School of Public Health as Associate Professor and in 1993 to the Tulane School of Public Health and Tropical Medicine, where he was Professor and Chair of Environmental Health Sciences. In 1999, he returned to the University of Minnesota School of Public Health, where he is Professor Emeritus of Environmental Health, University of Minnesota School of Public Health.

Dr. Qingyu Meng is an Adjunct Research Professor at Desert Research Institute and a Staff Toxicologist at Department of Toxic Substances Control, California Environmental Protection Agency. His research focuses on air pollution exposure assessment and chemical exposures in consumer products. He contributed to multiple Integrated Science Assessments, which serve as the scientific basis for setting National Ambient Air Quality Standards for criteria pollutants. He has authored and co-authored more than 70 peer-reviewed publications in exposure science. He is a member of the Society of Toxicology and the Society for Risk Analysis, and was President of the Tri-state Chapter of the International Society for Exposure Science. He is an associate editor of *Human and Ecological Risk Assessment – An International Journal.*

Dr. Debra A. Kaden has more than 30 years of experience in toxicology and environmental health sciences, with an emphasis in the area of air toxics. She is a senior practitioner in the Ramboll's Health Science practice. Dr. Kaden is a member of the Society for Risk Analysis (SRA) – where she sits on several committees and is a past president of the New England chapter. She is also a member of the Society of Toxicology (SOT) and the International Society for Exposure Science (ISES). Dr. Kaden has authored more than 25 peer-reviewed publications in toxicology and environmental health sciences. She has spearheaded critical reviews of the state of science to identify research priorities for understanding exposure and health effects of mobile source air toxics, diesel exhaust, and electric and magnetic fields. She has also organized and convened workshops and conferences on scientific topics relevant to air pollution. She earned her MS and PhD degrees in toxicology from the Massachusetts Institute of Technology.

Contributors

Simona Andreea Bălan
Senior Environmental Scientist,
    California Department of Toxic Substances
    Control

Suren Bandara
Amgen
San Francisco, CA

Dana Boyd Barr
Department of Environmental Health Rollins
    School of Public Health
Emory University
Atlanta, GA

P. Barry Ryan
Department of Environmental Health at Rollins
    School of Public Health
Emory University
Atlanta, GA

Matthew Berens
Postdoctoral Associate in the Natural Resources,
    Research Institute at the University of
    Minnesota

Joanna Burger
Professor at the Environmental and
    Occupational Health Sciences Institute at
    Rutgers University

Matteo Convertino
Tsinghua Shenzhen International Graduate
    School
University Town of Shenzhen
Tsinghua Park, Nanshan District, Shenzhen,
    P.R. China

Rebecca C. Dzubow
US Environmental Protection Agency

David L. Eaton
Department of Environmental & Occupational
    Health Sciences
University of Washington School of Public Health
Seattle, WA

James Ede
Vireo Advisors, LLC

Ruth A. Etzel
Department of Environmental and
    Occupational Health, George Washington
    University School of Public Health
Washington, DC

Jill C. Falman
Institute for Risk Analysis and Risk
    Communication (IRARC), Department of
    Environmental and Occupational Health
    Sciences
University of Washington School of Public
    Health
Seattle, WA

Mingzhu Fang
Chief, Bureau of Risk Analysis, Division
    of Science and Research, New Jersey
    Department of Environmental Protection

Elaine M. Faustman
Department of Environmental and
    Occupational Health
University of Washington School of Public Health
Seattle, WA

Nancy Fiedler
Professor and Deputy Director, Environmental
    and Occupational Health Sciences Institute,
    Rutgers University

Adam M. Finkel
Health Science at the University of Michigan
Ann Arbor, MI

Michael Gallo
Professor Emeritus of Toxicology, Rutgers
    University

Michael Gochfeld
Professor Emeritus of Environmental and
    Occupational Health Sciences, Rutgers
    University

Bernard D. Goldstein
Professor Emeritus, Former Dean,
    University of Pittsburgh Graduate School of
    Public Health

Helmut Greim
Technical University of Munich
München, Germany

Richard Jackson
Professor Emeritus, Environmental Health,
    School of Public Health, University of
    California Los Angeles

Molly Jacobs
University of Massachusetts, Lowell Center for
    Sustainable Production
Lowell, MA

Douglas O. Johns
Spokane Mining Research Division
National Institute for Occupational Safety and
    Health, Centers for Disease Control and
    Prevention
Spokane, WA

Debra A. Kaden
Ramboll US Consulting, Inc.
Boston, MA

Donghai Liang
Gangarosa Department of Environmental Health
Emory University Rollins School of Public
    Health
Atlanta, GA

Wil Lieberman-Cribbin
Icahn School of Medicine at Mount Sinai
New York, NY

Jinze Li
Environmental Health
Emory University Rollins School of Public Health
Atlanta, GA

Zhoumeng Lin
Center for Environmental and Human
    Toxicology, Department of Environmental
    and Global Health, College of Public Health
    and Health Professions
University of Florida
Gainesville, FL

Yasong Lu
Quantitative Clinical Pharmacology, Daiichi
    Sankyo, Inc.
Basking Ridge, NJ

Jeffery Mandel
Associate Professor Emeritus, Division of
    Environmental Health Sciences at the
    University of Minnesota School of Public
    Health

Carmen Marsit
Environmental Health
Emory University Rollins School of Public Health
Atlanta, GA

Carolyn Mattingly
Professor and Chair, Department of Biological
    Sciences,
North Carolina State University

Christopher McLachlan
Freelance Editor

John A. McLachlan
Professor of Pharmacology at the Tulane
    Medical School

Qingyu Meng
California Department of Toxic Substances
    Control
California Environmental Protection
    Agency
Sacramento, CA
Desert Research Institute
Reno, NV

Charles Miller
Professor, Department of Global
    Environmental
Health Sciences at the Tulane School of Global
Public Health and Tropical Medicine

Warangkana Naksen
Faculty of Public Health
Chiang Mai University
Chiang Mai, Thailand

Gilbert S. Omenn
University of Michigan
Ann Arbor, MI

Parinya Panuwet
Gangarosa Department of Environment Health,
    Rollins School of Public Health
Emory University
Atlanta, GA

Mark G. Robson
Board of Governors Distinguished Service
    Professor
Rutgers University
New Brunswick, NJ

Joseph V. Rodricks
Ramboll US Consulting, Inc.
Arlington, VA

Robert Rottersman
Risk Assessor, Ramboll Group A/S, Industrial
    Hygiene

Susan L. Santos
FOCUS GROUP
New Orleans, LA

Wattasit Siriwong
Chulalongkorn University

Adel Soroush
Postdoctoral, Chemical Engineering,
    University of Illinois, Chicago

Emanuela Taioli
Institute for Translational Epidemiology,
   Population Health Science and Policy, Mount
   Sinai Hospital
New York, NY

Paul Tchounwou
Professor at the Jackson State University,
   College of Engineering and Science

Joel Tickner
University of Massachusetts, Lowell School
   of Health, Head of the Lowell Center for
   Sustainable Production
Lowell, MA

William A. Toscano
Division of Environmental Health Sciences
University of Minnesota School of Public Health
Minneapolis, MN, USA

Yannis Vassilopoulos
Partner and CIO, IatroDesign, LLC

Haojiong Wang
Laboratory of Information Communication
   Networks, Graduate School of Information
   Science and Technology, Hokkaido
   University, Sapporo, Japan

Elizabeth V. Wattenberg
Division of Environmental Health Sciences
School of Public Health University of Minnesota
Minneapolis

Angele White
Coordinator of Environmental Justice,
   Georgetown University

Christine Whittaker
Division of Science Integration
National Institute for Occupational Safety and
   Health, Centers for Disease Control and
   Prevention
Cincinnati, OH

Margaret H. Whittaker
ToxServices, LLC
Washington, DC

Felicia Wu
Department of Food Science and Human
   Nutrition and Department of Agricultural,
   Food, and Resource Economics
Michigan State University
East Lansing, MI

Raymond S. H. Yang
Toxicology and Cancer Biology, Colorado State
   University and Ray Yang Consulting, LLC,
   Fort Collins
Fort Collins, CO

Junfeng (Jim) Zhang
Professor of Global and Environmental Health,
   Nichols School of the Environment at Duke
   University

1 Introduction to Risk Assessment

Mark G. Robson
Rutgers University, New Brunswick, NJ, USA

William A. Toscano
University of Minnesota School of Public Health, Minneapolis, MN, USA

Qingyu Meng
California Department of Toxic Substances Control, Sacramento, CA, USA
Desert Research Institute, Reno, NV, USA

Debra A. Kaden
Ramboll US Consulting, Inc.Arlington, VA, USA

CONTENT

Literatures Cited..13

The environment we are living in is full of uncertainties, unknowns, and risks. Since early 2020, a risk reemerged – the pandemic of COVID-19, caused by SARS-CoV-2, a novel coronavirus that had not previously been reported in humans. The risks induced by COVID-19 brought the concept of risk assessment and risk communications squarely into the public eye, including fundamental concepts such as exposure pathways, susceptible populations, and public health.

The COVID-19 pandemic brought the terminology of risk assessment into the popular press. Exposure pathways were discussed, and people began to use terms such as ventilation, inhalation, ingestion, and dermal absorption. These were terms that had been mostly confined to the engineering, scientific, and biomedical community until COVID-19. Network news anchors regularly spoke about personal protective equipment (PPE) and the types of PPE (e.g., face masks) and efficiency of one type of mask over another. Furthermore, much was learned about the populations who are at risk in a short time. The risk of death is greatest for adults who are 65 years of age and older and in individuals with comorbidities (CDC 2021). The risk of severe illness and death is higher in populations of people of color and brought to light issues of poverty and access to care as risk factors when examining the prevalence and treatment of particular health problems. We also saw that people who smoke are at higher risk, as well as persons with cardiovascular disease and diabetes, lifestyle influences risk.

Those highlighted fundamental issues and terminologies during the COVID-19 pandemic are cornerstones of environmental risk assessment. Environmental risk assessment, which was first utilized for public health protection in the middle of the last century, is a relatively new science in environmental public health.

In the mid-20th century, many environmental events were presented in the popular press or on television documentaries – a deadly smog in Donora Pennsylvania in 1948 was associated with the death of 20 people (Jacobs et al. 2018); the Cuyahoga River caught fire. Overuse of dichlorodiphenyltrichloroethane (DDT) prompted Rachel Carson to publish *Silent Spring* in 1962 (Carson 1962). Because of these and other high-profile environmental events, pressure was exerted on the federal government to act. The National Environmental Protection Act (NEPA) was signed into law in 1970. The US Environmental Protection Agency (US EPA) came into existence on December 2, 1970, but risk assessment did not become a part of the American regulatory process until 1975 when the first official risk assessment on polyvinylchloride was published (Kuzmack and McGaughy 1975).

In the early days of risk assessment, there was no standardized methodology on how to assess the actions of environmental agents on human health, and the need for a codified process was apparent. The National Research Council called for the formation of a committee in 1983 to codify the process. The committee developed a document, titled *Risk Assessment in the Federal Government: Managing the Process*. This document is known as *The Red Book* simply because the cover of the document was red (Figure 1.1). Most risk assessments performed since then have been following the recommendations from *The Red Book*.

DOI: 10.1201/9780429291722-1

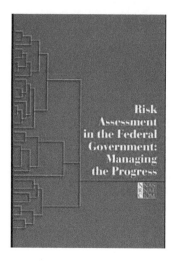

Figure 1.1 The "Red Book" published in 1983 by the National Academies Press first codified the risk assessment process in the United States.

Risk assessment is defined in many ways, but one of the most practical definitions for human health risk assessment is in Paustenbach (1989) as the scientific evaluation of the human health impacts posed by a particular substance or mixture of substances.

The importance of environmental risk assessment to public health is that the data produced by a risk assessment are used to establish policies and regulations on the use of environmental agents. In the development of regulations, many questions are encountered frequently: What is to be regulated? How serious are the problems? What is the cost-effectiveness of the regulation? Is the regulatory approach affordable? How many lives are theoretically saved or how many premature deaths, cancers, birth defects, and other noncommunicable diseases are theoretically prevented? With regulation comes costs and with costs come trade-offs. With so many issues to address and a finite number of resources to address these problems, where does the government start? And how do agencies assess the issues in a uniform, credible, and logical way? All of these issues and many others helped define and shape the risk assessment process still in use after 50 years of defining and refining.

Most risk assessments are made using the four-step process, documented in *The Red Book*:

Step 1 – Hazard Identification
Examines whether a stressor has the potential to cause harm to humans and/or ecological systems and if so, under what circumstances.

Step 2 – Dose-Response Assessment
Examines the numerical relationship between exposure and effects.

Step 3 – Exposure Assessment
Examines what is known about the frequency, timing, and levels of contact with a stressor.

Step 4 – Risk Characterization
Examines how well the data support conclusions about the nature and extent of the risk from exposure to environmental stressors.

This four-step process has been repeatedly presented in multiple risk assessment documents published by the National Research Council, with minor modifications. For example, a "problem formulation" step is emphasized in *Science and Decisions Advancing Risk Assessment* (NRC 2009). Some people also like to include a fifth and sixth step in this sequence, risk management and risk communication. We will cover these two in Chapters 17 and 18 of the textbook.

A few classic examples of environmental risk assessment include auxins (e.g., 2,4–dichlorophenoxyacetic acid), DDT, and some other persistent organic pollutants (e.g., aldrin). Prior to World War II, chemicals that stimulate plant growth called auxins were discovered (Thimann and Koepfli 1935; Weijers et al. 2018). Indole-3-acetic is the most abundant naturally occurring auxin. It was soon discovered that polychlorinated compounds, such as 2,4–dichlorophenoxyacetic acid (2,4-D), 2,4,5–trichlorophenoxyacetic acid (2,4,5–T) (Figure 1.2) could also act as auxins. These compounds were widely marketed as herbicides because of their effectiveness at killing weeds (Quareshy et al. 2018).

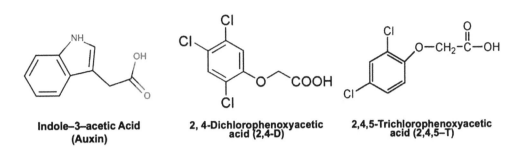

Indole–3–acetic Acid (Auxin)　　2, 4-Dichlorophenoxyacetic acid (2,4-D)　　2,4,5-Trichlorophenoxyacetic acid (2,4,5–T)

Figure 1.2　Examples of polychlorinated compounds used as herbicides. 2,4,5–T was commonly known as Agent Orange, widely used in Vietnam as a defoliant contained dioxin as a contaminant (see Boxes 1.2 and 1.3).

BOX 1.1　BUILT ENVIRONMENT (AS WELL AS CAREERS IN ENVIRONMENTAL PUBLIC HEALTH)

Richard J. Jackson

Each one of us who tries to assess risks must avoid one of life's greatest risks, a risk to our own lives, that is the failure to spend our lives in meaningful and self-fulfilling ways.

The most vivid time in my own career was at the Centers for Disease Control and Prevention (CDC). The primary focus was of course epidemiology, and for much of CDC's history it had focused on infectious diseases – originally its name was the US "Communicable Disease Center." I was fortunate to be asked in 1994 to lead CDC's National Center for Environmental Health. This was a powerful opportunity to advance the field of environmental public health.

Of the many environmental threats that the Center dealt with, a critical one was an old one – namely, childhood lead poisoning. I found that often our investigations brought us to the homes, and the paint, that were putting children at greatest risk. But these homes conveyed far greater harms than a single element like lead. Most often these were the homes of poor families: they had failing heating and ventilation systems, dangerous windows and stairs, water intrusion and mold, insect and vermin infestation, and often the children's caregivers confronted long dangerous travel to schools, work, and medical care. They very often depended upon unreliable and infrequent public transportation. We found that the rates of asthma in children in these homes were higher than in the homes of the less poor, and while the nation had a program for preventing childhood lead poisoning, there was no epidemiology for asthma.

Not only did atoms like lead present risks, but at that time, we were increasingly learning about hormonally active chemicals in the environment. The National Center for Environmental Health (NCEH) was fortunate to have the world's most advanced laboratory for measuring chemicals in people (biomonitoring), and this was made even more robust by its work in supporting the largest population sample of the American people, the National Health and Nutrition Examination Survey (NHANES). The survey employed physical examinations and collection of biological specimens, including urine and blood. The tests included routine sampling but in addition very refined and intensive analysis of chemicals and their degradation products. CDC increasingly was examining levels of many chemicals, not just lead and other metals, but pesticides, solvents, cotinine, plasticizers, and hormonally active chemicals. These data demonstrated widespread body burdens of chemicals and identified which age groups, locales, and occupations experienced higher exposures. Also important was documenting the average chemical body burden levels in the US population – data that are essential in epidemiologic studies, including cancer and birth defect clusters. As an example, by working with our Birth Defects Monitoring Program, we documented increased rates of hypospadias, a disorder where the urinary meatus of an infant boy's penis is mislocated, a change well-documented in test animals exposed to estrogen-like chemicals *in utero*.

Repeatedly, our examination of a panorama of illnesses and disorders led us to the same issue: *where people lived* was often driving the disease rates. This finding was true for lead and asthma, but also for air and water pollution, vehicle-and violent deaths, heat-related deaths, inactivity and obesity, cardiac, and other chronic diseases like depression. Much of this was occurring against the background of massive increases in CO_2 in the atmosphere and average global temperatures. People were suffering as much from where they lived as they were from income and racial disparities. People forced to live far from school and work, in most cases because of income, were at higher risk than those in more favored circumstances. One narrow but important example was that the absence of trees in very poor neighborhoods, frequently the result of mortgage denial and redlining generations before, led to much higher daytime and summertime temperatures in these neighborhoods. And persons already struggling with challenges related to age or disabilities, race, and poverty, were facing the greatest risks. Most disturbing to me was that our society's decision-makers in housing development, transportation plans, school and utility siting, and investment and construction lacked even the barest insight into how their actions were shaping health. For example, transportation engineers were universally aware of their obligations in regard to safety, and a small group was alert to the environmental impacts of their decisions, but virtually none understood that they were extraordinarily influential shapers of the healthfulness of our environments.

In response, we at CDC assembled a team to confront the built environment as a powerful influencer of health. We received pushback. I was told that a generation before that concern about "place," "where you live and work as a health issue," was brought up but failed to get political and fiscal traction. We then invited CDC leaders in many specialized areas, for example, NASA experts on "heat islands," or researchers documenting "Community Policing through Environmental Design." My first publication on the issue was in 2001 when I wrote for an organization called "Sprawlwatch"; this thought piece generated political pushback from the American Homebuilders; they even demanded through congressional complaints that CDC fire me.

With Howard Frumkin and Andrew Dannenberg, we developed the seminal special issue on the Built Environment and Health for the *American Journal of Public Health*, the first time the journal embraced the issue in a century. The book, *Urban Sprawl and Public Health*, led by Dr. Frumkin, was life changing for many young urban planners and health scientists. After CDC, I went on to become the California State Public Health Officer, and to develop a PBS series where I visited a dozen cities looking at where the built environment promotes health, e.g., Boulder Colorado, and where it brought serious harm, for example, cities ruined by the highway robbery of social capital, the destruction of fine downtowns by condemning large areas where people of color in the poor resided, for example, Atlanta, Georgia, and Syracuse, New York.

I have offered these brief reflections in the hope that they inform the career decisions of young risk assessors, health researchers, urban planners, and policy leaders. I suggest that one's early training (in my case pediatrics and epidemiology) **does not need to be our career terminus**; it can be the first station on a longer, often deeper, but sometimes far wider journey, enriching the learning and variety of our lives. My next reflection is that **service to the public** brings an immense variety of experiences with profound and meaningful learning. For me, the best part of public service was that I was never bored; I met brilliant and generous people, and the opportunities to be creative are abundant – so if your job does not bring you this, find a different one.

We shape the places we live in – the buildings, neighborhoods roads, and parks – **and they shape us**, including our enjoyment of life and our health. We humans require, like an essential vitamin, contact with loved ones and with nature. Well-designed healthy places help provide this to everyone.

REFERENCES

Dannenberg, A., Frumkin, H., Jackson, R. J. (2011). *Making Healthy Places: Designing and Building for Health, Well-Being, and Sustainability*. Island Press, Washington, DC.

Dannenberg, A. L., Jackson, R.J., Frumkin, H., Schieber, R.A., Pratt, M., Kochtitzky, C., Tilson, H.H. (September 2003). The Impact of Community Design and Land-Use Choices on Public Health: A Scientific Research Agenda. *American Journal of Public Health*, 93(9), 1500–1508.

Designing Healthy Communities. (2012). Media policy Center Four Hour PBS Television Series. http://designinghealthycommunities.org/

Frumkin, H., Frank, L., Jackson, R.J. (2004). *Urban Sprawl and Public Health: Designing, Planning, and Building for Healthy Communities*. Island Press, Washington DC, 338 pages.

Jackson, R. J., Kochtitzky, C. (November 2001). *Creating A Healthy Environment: The Impact of the Built Environment on Public Health*. SprawlWatch Clearinghouse Monograph Series.

Jackson, R. J. with Sinclair, S. (October 2011). *Designing Healthy Communities*. Jossey Bass, Wiley & Sons Publishing, Hardcover 366 pages. http://www.josseybass.com/WileyCDA/WileyTitle/productCd-1118033663.html

Polychlorinated biphenyls (PCBs) were manufactured by a company known as Halowax, which marketed polychlorinated for many applications ranging from floor polish to transformer oils. Occasionally, workers would present with a condition called chloracne, a skin disease resembling severe acne, In the mid-1930s, three workers died, which led the corporation to fund researchers to find the possible cause. Through their experiments, it was discovered that the compounds, chlorinated biphenyls, and chlorinated naphthalenes had systemic actions and could be the possible workplace hazards (Drinker et al. 1937). Still, the polychlorinated compounds were thought to be ideal because they were relatively nontoxic, unreactive, fire retardant, and apparently safe in the environment. Major concern arose as a result of a PCB contamination in Yoshu Japan and ten years later in Taiwan (Chen et al. 1994; Kuratsune et al. 1972). Dioxins can be formed from other halogenated compounds, Originally, 2,3,7,8 tetrachlorodibenzo-p-dioxin was a contaminant of the herbicide, 2,4,5-trichlorophenoxyacetic acid 2,4,5–T, or Agent Orange). Now, dioxins are found as contaminants in streams polluted by trichloroethylene (TCE).

BOX 1.2   POLYHALOGENATED ARYL HYDROCARBON RECEPTOR LIGANDS

Charles Miller

Halogenated aryl hydrocarbon receptor ligands (HAHRLs) are produced by specific geological processes, incomplete combustion reactions (both natural and anthropogenic), and industrial processes (both intentional and unintentional). Chlorine and bromine are the typical halogens on the aromatic rings of HAHRLs. Halogenated dioxins, dibenzofurans, biphenyls, and diphenyl ethers are among the major members of this ligand family. Multiple positions for halogenation on the aromatic rings lead to numerous congeners of these chemicals that vary in their effects on the aryl hydrocarbon receptor (AhR). Most congeners are inactive or weakly effective in binding and activating AhR. AhR-activating HAHRLs typically contain a planar complex of two to three aromatic rings with multiple halogens extending from the wider (equatorial) dimension of the structure. For example, the affinity of polychlorinated biphenyl congeners for AhR is associated with increased chlorine at positions that increase molecular planarity by constraining rotation around the C-C bond between the biphenyl groups.

Studies with transgenic mice that lack the AhR show that the toxicity of HARLs is receptor dependent. HAHRLs interact with the AhR to induce a common gene expression profile; however, each ligand may have unique transcriptional signaling features as well. Specific cytochrome P450 1 (CYP1) gene family members serve as canonical transcriptional, proteomic, and enzymatic biomarkers in response to HARLs, although other AhR ligands also induce this response. CYP1 enzymes participate in the metabolic degradation of endogenous and xenobiotic compounds and are variably effective in metabolizing HARLs. Halogen position on the HARLs determines their metabolic reactivity and their potential for bioaccumulation. Metabolism and bioaccumulation of HARLs can also vary widely both within and across different species. For example, the half-life of 2,3,7,8-tetrachlorodibenzo-p-dioxin (TCDD) in the mouse is approximately ten days but is several years in humans. Toxicity of the HARLs varies broadly within and across different species. Some of this variation is explained by differences in the AhR, such as the alanine to valine (A375V) substitution in some strains of mice that reduces the affinity and toxicity of TCDD by approximately tenfold. Differences in the transactivation domain and other regions of AhR also influence toxic responses to HAHRLs. The species-specific variations in AhR affinity, signaling, and toxicity of HAHRLs complicate the use of animal models for extrapolation of risk assessments to humans. Human diversity in response to HAHRLs is not well described but may be significant as well.

Health effects associated with exposure to HAHRLs are reported for most of the organ and tissue types of the body, which is not surprising since the AhR is widely expressed in most cell types. Exposures from environmental contamination, industrial accidents, and Operation Ranch Hand in Vietnam provide insight into the human health effects of these agents. Reproductive, developmental, endocrine, immunological, and neurological effects of HAHRLs are well described, especially in rodent model systems with controlled exposures. Populations that were more heavily exposed to HAHRLs are at risk for soft tissue sarcomas, Hodgkin's and Non-Hodgkin's lymphomas, multiple myeloma, chronic B-cell leukemia, and pulmonary cancers. Dermal effects in humans include chloracne, hyperkeratosis, and pigmentation. HAHRLs may mediate these effects by changing both gene transcriptional and epigenetic programs in cells. Epigenetic reprogramming of gametes by HAHRLs may provide a mechanism for their transgenerational effects (see Chapter 10). Since HAHRLs primarily act through AhR occupancy, their toxic effects are based on receptor occupancy and should follow threshold-based dose-response models.

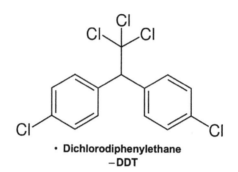

• **Dichlorodiphenylethane**
–DDT

Figure 1.3 Structure of DDT, used in World War II to kill mosquitoes; after the war, DDT was widely used until 1972, when it was banned in the United States and Canada. DDT is still used in some countries to control mosquitoes. The EPA lists DDT as a probable carcinogen and its use was banned 50 years ago; it is still found as a contaminant in some lakes.

DDT, a chlorinated pesticide invented in 1889 (Figure 1.3) was widely used in the Italian campaign because of its effective use as a mosquitocide and was instrumental in controlling malaria that was endemic in the swamps of Southern Italy (Knipling 1945).

After the end of World War II, DDT became the most commonly used insecticide globally, and resistance was starting to appear in 1959 (see https://archive.epa.gov/epa/aboutepa/ddt-regulatory-history-brief-survey-1975.html; accessed August 5, 2021). In the 1960s, DDT was appearing in the human food chain; a Swedish scientist who was looking for DDT in food first observed that PCBs were accumulating in the food supply (Jensen 1972). Today, DDT still has profound and long-lasting impacts on the third generation of an exposed population.

In 1972, the Governing Council of the United Nations Environment Program (UNEP) held a conference in Stockholm to address environmental contaminants and human health. The reason for concern was based on the observation that many of the chemicals in common use remained in the environment long after application and posed an ongoing threat to ecological and human health. A number of principles were adopted calling for global actions on the environment (UNEP 1972). One important outcome of the Stockholm Declaration on the Human Environment was the declaration, "Humans have a fundamental right to freedom, equality and adequate conditions of life, in an environment of a quality that permits a life of dignity and well-being, and bear a solemn responsibility to protect and improve the environment for present and future generations." The Stockholm Convention defined persistent organic pollutants (POPs) (Alharbi et al. 2018) as chemical substances that persist in the environment, bioaccumulate through the food web, and pose a risk of causing adverse effects to human health and the environment. In the United States,

Table 1.1: **The Dirty Dozen**

Aldrin	Endrin
Chlordane	Heptachlor
DDT and metabolites	Hexachlorobenzene
Dieldrin	Myrex
Chlordecone (Kepone)	PCBs
Dioxins & Polychlorinated furans	Toxaphene

these compounds were called persistent, bioaccumulative, and toxic chemicals (PBTs) (Hutzinger et al. 1976). A major outcome of the meeting was a list of 12 compounds of particular concern. The initial list of compounds was called the dirty dozen (Table 1.1). Compounds on the initial list include pesticides and industrial and agricultural chemicals. Many of the compounds are chlorinated, are present in small concentrations, and exert their actions via receptors. The diseases caused by some of the compounds occur *in utero* and present later in life. Risk assessment of the actions of POPs is not straightforward. The exact number of POPs in commerce is not known, posing another layer of difficulty in assessing the risk to human health of this group of compounds. The United States signed on to the convention on May 23, 2001, but the treaty has not been ratified. The convention came into force on May 17, 2004, after 152 countries ratified the declaration. Compounds can be added to the Stockholm Convention list, but, by law, the number is fixed at 12 in the United States.

In the 50 years since the formation of the US EPA, the agency has issued hundreds of documents describing the risks, assessing the risks, offering ways to mitigate the risks, suggesting substitutions for the chemicals or processes of concern, and in many instances making the case that a particular chemical or process be banned or discontinued or regulated in a way to very tightly restrict how it is used.

A comprehensive and up-to-date list with links for the guidance documents on hundreds of chemicals can be found at this link on the US EPA website: https://www.epa.gov/risk/risk-assessment-guidance.

Using pesticides as an example, the US EPA has a list of over 700 pesticide products that are considered to be restricted use pesticides (RUP). These are pesticide products that are not available to the general public in the United States. The "restricted use" classification restricts a product, or its uses, to use by a certificated pesticide applicator or under the direct supervision of a certified applicator. This means that a license is required to purchase and apply the product. Certification programs are administered by the federal government, individual states, and by company policies that vary from state to state.

The reasons for the restrictions and the training required for the individual using a RUP are specified in the Federal Insecticide, Fungicide, and Rodenticide Act (FIFRA). While FIFRA was first authorized in 1947, there were considerable revisions to the act in 1972 when the responsibility for the regulation of pesticide products was transferred from the United States Department of Agriculture to the newly formed US EPA. The revisions to FIFRA and the restrictions that make RUPs are, in effect, a form of risk management based on risk assessment. The pesticides are still available to farmers and they can be used to control pests, but based on the risks that have been identified, users must apply these compounds in a way to reduce the risk and potential harm to humans, wildlife, and the environment.

Protecting susceptible populations is always emphasized in environmental risk assessment. Knowing that children are a vulnerable population, additional guidelines that are more conservative are applied when assessing the risk for children. Generally speaking, we apply additional protective factors or safety factors for children, individuals with comorbidities, elderly, and other high-risk groups. The original risk assessment process was fairly generic, looking at the risks of an average person. Time and experience have taught all of us that there are very few average persons or typical individuals in the population.

As time progressed and more environmental chemicals and scenarios were identified and additional guidance was developed by the federal agencies that were charged with enforcing the regulations and characterizing the risks, the concept of risk benefit also came into being. Pesticides, for example, are purposeful poisons; they are designed to kill pests – namely, insects, or fungi or bacteria or unwanted plants or rodents, they are by their very nature and design toxic chemicals, but they also confer a benefit; they protect the food supply, control vector-borne diseases by controlling the actual vectors, save people from starvation and hunger by preserving the food, etc. So, when we do a risk assessment associated with a pesticide, we not only consider the potential risk to humans, but we also must take into account the lives saved from the application of these pesticides to protect millions from a deadly disease like malaria or making sure the almost one billion people in the world who are undernourished can in fact have access to wholesome and safe food. There are trade-offs and there are risks. But by using risk assessment, we can identify the risks and intervene in the process to mitigate and hopefully eliminate if not substantially reduce the associated risks. Based on all of this, there is available a process of environmental health risk assessment; it is constantly being evaluated, revised, and refined based on new information on exposures and health effects that are added to the databases. However, generally speaking, the original 1983 paradigm is still applicable (Figures 1.4 and 1.5).

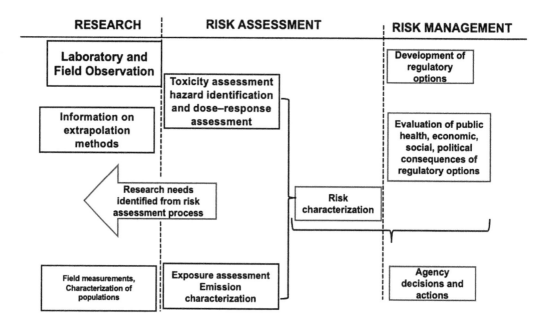

Figure 1.4 Elements of risk assessment and risk management as outlined in the "Red Book".

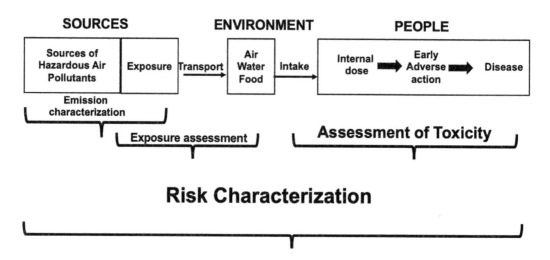

Figure 1.5 Components of risk characterization.

In the 1970s, the battle against infectious disease was declared over by the surgeon general of the United States, and since that time, risk assessment has focused on chronic conditions from exposure to biological agents. In the early 1990s, infectious diseases made a comeback with the outbreak of HIV/AIDs, plague in India, cholera in Peru, Ebola, SARS, MERS. And now a global pandemic of COVID Nowadays, we are facing new challenges and opportunities in environmental risk assessment. Modern risk assessment must deal with both biologic and biotic risks. Today, there are about 100,000 chemicals in commerce – most were developed since World War II, and some of those have become chemicals of emerging concern (e.g., per- and polyfluoroalkyl substances, PFAS). Approximately 2,900 chemicals are produced or imported in quantities of one million pounds or more per year. These are called high production volume (HPV) chemicals. For about half of the HPVs, no basic toxicity or risk data are publicly available (Lawton 2021); for 80% of HPVs, there is no information on developmental or pediatric toxicity. Biomonitoring surveys from CDC have found body burdens of HPVs are widespread in Americans: https://www.cdc.gov/biomonitoring/index.html (accessed July 30, 2021).

To address these concerns, chemical regulations have been modernized. In the European Union, the Registration, Evaluation, Authorization and Restriction of Chemicals (REACH) program, which took effect in 2007, regulates chemical use and production. In the United States, the Frank R. Lautenberg Chemical Safety for the 21st Century Act requires the USEPA to quickly assess chemical safety for many of these chemicals.

Risk assessment methods have also evolved. A large volume of toxicity and exposure data have been generated through new approach methodologies (NAMs). New models and analytical approaches have been developed and applied in toxicity testing and exposure assessment.

Since the publication of the first edition of this textbook (Robson and Toscano 2007), the National Research Council published a series of books documenting the vision of environmental risk assessment for the 21st century. These publications include *Toxicity Testing in the 21st Century: A Vision and a Strategy* (NRC 2007), which promotes the -omics approach and NAMs; *Science and Decisions Advancing Risk Assessment* (NRC 2009), which addresses problem formulation and uncertainties in risk assessment; *Exposure Science in the 21st Century: A Vision and a Strategy* (NRC 2012), which documents the advancement and needs of data and model for exposure science; and *Using 21st Century Science to Improve Risk-Related Evaluations* (NRC 2017), which provides a vision for risk assessment in the future. These publications present the vision, challenges, and opportunities of applying environmental risk assessment for public health protection in the 21st century.

The science of risk assessment continues to evolve, leading to the development of many new tools. These include big data, machine learning and new computational tools (Paltrinieri et al. 2019), advances in genomics and molecular biology, epigenetics, exposure science, and analytical chemistry (Xu et al. 2013) to assess mixtures exposome and to screen the safety of a large number of chemicals. Many of the new advances have not yet come into common use by risk assessors but show great promise in better describing and assessing risk.

This second edition of *Risk Assessment for Environmental Health* has 17 chapters covering the basic information that public health students need to know for their daily responsibilities; it provides an overview of the risk process; it explains the risk paradigm and the application of risk assessment to regulatory decision-making. Exposure assessment, biomonitoring, and the application of epidemiology into the risk assessment process are introduced. Toxicological principles, which are the underpinning to most risks are described. Exposure pathways, risk models, and workplace risks are discussed. Last, we review the application of risk assessment as a tool across federal agencies in the United States as well as globally through comparison and contrast of the regulatory approaches taken in different countries and the reasons for the differences. The final chapter aims at providing some insight into effectively communicating environmental risk to the scientific community and to the public.

The aim of the present edition is to have a useful and practical textbook for an upper-level undergraduate or graduate-level course in risk assessment aimed at master's and doctoral-level students in schools of public health and related professions.

The first edition of this textbook was a complication of chapters from the common themes in the syllabi written by faculty who were experts in these areas. There were also case studies contained in the text for further illustration. The level of material presented was targeted at a master's level student who had some biology and chemistry background and basic quantitative skills.

After ten years, we were approached about updating the textbook; the original text was not as comprehensive as we would like; there were areas that were out of date or less relevant than they had been, and there were newly emerging areas of risk assessment that needed to be addressed. After some discussion, the current version of the textbook is reconfigured as an online and inter-active text that can be updated and regularly refreshed, as well as a printed version. The chapters have been scaled back to areas that we feel are most relevant to a student studying risk assessment in a public health program. In addition, we have added a series of 23 text boxes scattered through-out the chapters. These boxes provide case studies and examples, as well as other considerations for the risk assessment field. These boxes are additional learning material assigned to each chapter according to their topics solely by the editors and not necessarily authored by chapter authors.

BOX 1.3   HEALTH RISKS OF PCBS AND PCDFS

Matthew Berens

PCBs and polychlorinated dibenzofurans (PCDFs) are two classes of structurally similar POPs, several of which are highly toxic to humans and animals. Their level of toxicity varies significantly depending on the individual chemical structure. PCBs and PCDFs are released to the environment primarily as unintended by-products of industrial processes and the unregulated burning of waste. The chemical and physical properties of PCBs and PCDFs cause them to be highly persistent in the environment and to strongly associate with organic matter and animal lipids. This leads to their bioaccumulation and biomagnification in the food chain and promotes the risk of accidental exposure through contaminated water, soil, and sediments.

PCBs were manufactured in the United States from 1929–1979 as components of hydraulic fluids, electrical equipment, plastics, paints, and heat exchangers. Despite a ban on produc-tion set by the US EPA in 1979, residual amounts of PCBs are still detectable on many prod-ucts and continue to end up in the environment. PCDFs were never synthesized commercially but formed as side products during PCBs synthesis and the combustion of other chlorine-containing chemicals. Both PCBs and PCDFs are listed substances under the 2001 Stockholm Convention on Persistent Organic Pollutants.

PCBs and PCDFs cause a wide range of adverse health effects in humans at concentrations as low as 1 ng/kg of body weight. When present in mixtures, these compounds can cause toxic effects that are equal to or greater than the individual compounds. The most important sources of human exposure are through consumption of fatty foods, such as fish, and occupa-tional exposure during the production of chlorinated organic chemicals. However, outdated infrastructure containing PCB-based components (e.g., water pump hydraulic fluids, fluores-cent lights, paint) can still cause small amounts of PCBs and PCDFs to contaminate exposed surfaces, air, and water.

Some of the most notable symptoms of PCB and PCDF exposure include rashes, chloracne, lesions, fatigue, and headaches. Among the most concerning, however, are disturbances to the immune, nervous, endocrine, and reproductive systems. Not only do PCBs and PCDFs sup-press the immune response and decrease thyroid function, but they have also been shown to cause developmental effects such as reduced birth weight and live birth rate. Developmental delays and learning deficits have also been observed in the children of mothers who work in factories and in fishing communities. Many of the compounds are known carcinogens, but it remains unclear whether they all present similar carcinogenic risks. However, the compounds with the highest carcinogenic potential tend to be those that readily partition to organic materi-als and bioaccumulate in the environment.

Avoiding potentially contaminated soils and sediments is the best way to reduce exposure to PCBs and PCDFs. It is also important to follow proper cooking and cleaning guidelines to minimize the risk of accidental consumption. If you suspect that your home or workplace uses equipment that contains PCBs, the equipment should be replaced and discarded as soon as possible before the equipment fails. Contact your local department of health to ensure proper removal and disposal.

BOX 1.4   HEALTH EFFECTS OF TCE

Adel Soroush

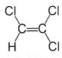

TCE (CAS No. 79-01-6) is an important industrial solvent that is primarily used for degreasing metal parts in automotive, electronic, and metal machining industries. TCE is also found in household products, such as paint removers, adhesives, and carpet cleaning fluids, and it is a chemical intermediate in various chemical manufacturing processes. Because it has been used for nearly 100 years, TCE is a common environmental contaminant. TCE is released into the atmosphere from vapor degreaser operations. It reaches surface water by direct discharge and enters groundwater via leaching from improper disposal practices. TCE is also present in soils and groundwater aquifers as a by-product of the degradation of other chlorinated hydrocarbons. The biodegradation of tetrachloroethylene (also known as perchloroethene, PCE) under anaerobic conditions leads to the formation of TCE, and if the reaction continues, vinyl chloride, a known carcinogen, will be formed. The presence of TCE in the indoor air is a result of its use in consumer products and also vapor intrusion from contaminated groundwater.

The low solubility of TCE in water (1.1 g/L), in addition to its higher density (1.462 g/mL) and lower viscosity (0.59 cP) than water, leads to TCE being transported downwards (with the possibility of lateral spreading) through soils and aquifers as a separate dense non-aqueous phase liquid (DNAPL). Because of non-linear adsorption to the solids, the DNAPL TCE leaves films and droplets behind during its movement through pores and fissures. TCE as a dissolved aqueous constituent shows weak sorption to soils and aquifer solids. Because of its low hydrophobicity (log K_{OW} = 2.29), the presence of natural organic matter, such as humic acid, can suppress TCE adsorption even on sorbents that are considered highly effective, like activated carbon. Thus, dissolved TCE is readily transported through soil to groundwater. Because of its high Henry's law constant (1.18 kPa m³/mol) and high vapor pressure (8 kPa), TCE is volatile. In unsaturated zones, however, when a gas phase also is present, vapor-phase TCE can be adsorbed by a solid phase, resulting in hindered flux by the diffusion through air-filled pores.

TCE is degraded under anaerobic conditions via biotic and abiotic processes to intermediates and products that are more toxic or more resistant to degradation, such as dichloroethylene (DCE) isomers and vinyl chloride. The traditional remediation technique for removing TCE from groundwater is a pump and treat system in which the contaminated water is treated above the ground by air-stripping or activated carbon filtration. Both techniques are also being used to treat drinking water contaminated by TCE. Permeable reactive barriers filled with zero-valent iron particles can also be installed underground to treat and contain TCE plumes. Other novel techniques such as in situ oxidation using potassium permanganate, thermal remediation by electrodes, and steam or enhanced biodegradation are being investigated.

TCE has adverse effects on humans and has been listed as a specific constituent of concern (COC). The California Department of Public Health (CPDH) has regulated TCE as a drinking water contaminant and the federal maximum contaminant level (MCL) is set to 5 µg/L. Acute exposure to TCE vapor can cause central nervous system effects (light-headedness, drowsiness, and headache). Adverse effects on the liver, kidneys, and immune and endocrine systems have been reported in humans with chronic exposure to TCE in the air or in drinking water. A known human carcinogen, TCE causes cancer of the kidneys and may be associated with an increased risk of non-Hodgkin lymphoma and liver cancer.

REFERENCES

National Toxicology Program. 2016. *Trichloroethylene, Report on Carcinogens*, 14th ed.. Research Triangle Park, NC: U.S. Department of Health and Human Services, Public Health Service Available online: https://ntp.niehs.nih.gov/ntp/roc/content/profiles/trichloroethylene.pdf, last accessed March 1, 2021.

Rusyn, I., W. A. Chiu, L. H. Lash, H. Kromhout, J. Hansen, and K. Z. Guyton. 2014. Trichloroethylene: Mechanistic, Epidemiologic and Other Supporting Evidence of Carcinogenic Hazard. *Pharmacol Ther* 141(1): 55–66.

BOX 1.5   RISK ASSESSMENT OF NANOMATERIALS AND OTHER ADVANCED MATERIALS AND TECHNOLOGIES

James Ede

While there is no internationally harmonized definition, nanomaterials (NMs) are generally acknowledged as materials with overall dimensions in the nanoscale (1–100 nanometers). 'Engineered' nanoscale materials are often distinguished from incidental or naturally occurring nanoparticles to acknowledge unique optical, mechanical, electrical, thermal, or magnetic properties that are driving their development and adoption in a multitude of sectors.

Given this broad definition, NMs encompass classes of materials as diverse as the term 'chemicals.' This breadth and diversity bring numerous challenges in assessing their risks including (1) difficulty characterizing materials at the nanoscale, (2) challenges with detecting and quantifying NMs to evaluate exposures, and (3) an inability to predict health and environmental hazards from their physical and chemical properties. Significant strides have been made in addressing these challenges over the last decade, although a number remain. Next, critical elements unique to NM risk assessment are highlighted.

1. *Physicochemical Characterization.* This is a key component of NM risk assessment as the physical and chemical properties of an NM can affect both key determinants of risk: hazard and exposure. Accurate selection, measurement, and reporting of physicochemical properties are essential. Critical elements include the following:
   - *Selecting appropriate characterization parameters.* The full suite of parameters required for meaningful physicochemical characterization will depend on the specific NM and its intended use. The product life cycle must also be considered when developing a testing plan, as NMs may undergo transformations while they proceed from cradle to grave. Recently, guidance on selecting appropriate parameters for risk characterization has been released.
   - *Selecting suitable characterization methods.* Selecting appropriate methods is difficult, as every approach has strengths and weaknesses; comprehensive characterization requires the use of multiple methods. Additional challenges include lack of validated methods or standards, access to specialized equipment or trained personnel, or prohibitively high costs.

2. *Hazard Assessment.* Critical elements for evaluating the hazards of NMs include the following:
   - *Selecting suitable toxicity testing methods.* Many existing toxicity testing methods are suitable for testing NMs. However, some challenges include the need to evaluate health effects under realistic dosing, account for or mitigate assay interference, adjust methods to account for size or other unique properties of NMs, and create realistic approximations of exposure. Testing issues specific to NMs have led to the development of guidance and test guidelines designed or modified for NMs.
   - *Conducting toxicity testing under realistic exposure conditions.* A critical consideration for hazard testing is that exposures must be representative of real-world human or environmental exposures. Unfortunately, this is not always possible and needs to be factored in when evaluating results. Because of these considerations, it is critical that sample preparation be reported, along with toxicity testing results.
   - *Using grouping, categorization, and read-across strategies.* It is not feasible to test the many forms of NMs coming to market on a case-by-case basis as is current practice. Most NM grouping frameworks attempt to form categories based on physical and chemical properties. Such an approach seeks to allow novel NMs to be evaluated for risk by characterizing their physicochemical properties, categorizing them, and using read-across to quickly ascertain hazards. However, as previously discussed, the relationships between physical and chemical properties and toxicological outcomes are complex, and despite significant progress over the last decade, scientists are still working to understand these relationships.

3. *Exposure Assessment.* Critical elements for assessing NM exposures include the following:

- *Developing reliable methods for nanomaterial detection and quantification.* Quantitative exposure assessment for NMs relies on the ability to accurately detect the presence of sub-micron particles, whether in environmental media, occupational settings, or consumer products. The small size, coupled with the low concentrations typical of NM releases and complex environmental matrices, makes detecting NMs in realistic exposure situations challenging, particularly for carbon-based NMs.
- *Accounting for exposure across the product life cycle.* A key consideration in evaluating the risks of NMs is to determine potential exposures across the product life cycle, specifically due to potential release and exposure from products. A key challenge is determining which consumer products use NMs and in what quantities. New nano-labeling laws and mandatory nano-registries are helping to address this.
- *Characterizing release potential.* Determining exposure levels to NMs in products is critical to assessing risk. This requires the development of methods and techniques to evaluate (1) if NMs are released from the various matrices they are incorporated into as part of product development (*e.g.*, solid matrices such as polymers, textiles, or electronics) and (2) in what form (*i.e.*, are pristine NMs released, or are they released as part of larger aggregates with matrix material). Research has shown release potential is modulated by the type of NM, its physicochemical properties, and the matrix material. Accurate assessment of release potential as part of an exposure assessment is essential for NM risk assessment.

4. **Risk Characterization.** While classical chemical risk assessment paradigms are generally applicable, NM risk assessment frameworks incorporate considerations unique to this class of material including aspects of physicochemical characterization, exposure, and hazard assessment, as previously described. NM risk assessment frameworks also incorporate many of the recent tools, test protocols, and guidelines developed to aid in risk characterization, including state-of-the-art hazard and exposure characterization techniques and methods; grouping, categorization, and read-across frameworks; integrated approaches to testing and assessment that incorporate alternative testing strategies (*i.e.*, non-animal testing); and others.

There are many quantitative texts that describe the modeling tools used in risk assessment, in this text we introduce these tools so that a reader can have a basic understanding, and he or she can pursue these topics in more detail if they would like.

Many people will argue that risk assessment is, at its core common sense. But as the French philosopher Voltaire stated in 1764, common sense is not so common.

LITERATURES CITED

Alharbi, O. M. L., A. A. Basheer, and I. Ali. 2018. Health and Environmental Effects of Persistent Organic Pollutants. *J Mol Liq* 263: 442–453. 10.1016/j.molliq.2018.05.029.

Carson, R. 1962. *Silent Spring.* Houghton Mifflin.

CDC. 2021. Coronavirus Disease 2019 (COVID-19). https://www.cdc.gov/dotw/covid-19/index.html

Chen, Y. C., M. L. Yu, W. J. Rogan, B. C. Gladen, and Chen-Chin Hsu. 1994. A 6–Year Follow–Up of Behavior and Activity Disorders in the Taiwan Yu–cheng Children. *Am J Public Health* 84: 415–421.

Drinker, C. K., M. F. Warren, and G. A. Bennett. 1937. The Problem of Possible Systemic Effects from Certain Chlorinated Hydrocarbons. *J Industrial Hygiene Toxicol* 19: 283–311

Greenberg, M., B. D. Goldstein, E. Anderson, M. Dourson, W. Landis, and D. W. North. 2015. Whither Risk Assessment: New Challenges and Opportunities a Third of a Century After the Red Book. *Risk Analysis* 35 (11 November): 1959–1968

Hutzinger, G., G. Sunderstrom, and S. Safe. 1976. Environmental Chemistry of Flame Retardants Part I. Introduction and Principles. *Chemosphere* 5: 3–10.

Jacobs, E. T., J. L. Burgess, and M. B. Abbott. 2018. The Donora Smog Revisited: 70 Years After the Event That Inspired the Clean Air Act. *Am J Public Health* 108: S85–S88.

Jensen, S. 1972. The PCB Story. *Ambio* 1: 123–131.

Knipling, E. F. 1945. The Development and Use of DDT for the Control of Mosquitoes. *J Natl Malaria Soc* 4 (2): 77–92.

Kuratsune, M., T. Yoshimura, J. Matsuzuka, and A. Yamaguchi. 1972. Epidemiologic Study on Yusho, a Poisoning by Ingestion of Rice Oil Contaminated with a Commercial Brand of Polychlorinated Biphenyls. *Environ Health Perspect* 1: 119–128.

Kuzmack, A. M., and R. E. McGaughy. 1975. *Quantitative Risk Assessment for Community Exposure to Vinyl Chloride* EPA.

Lawton, G. 2021. Why Chemical Pollution Is Turning Into a Third Great Planetary Crisis. *New Scientist* 2021: 1–13. https://www.newscientist.com/article/mg25133440-700-why-chemical-pollution-is-turning-into-a-third-great-planetary-crisis/.

Paltrinieri, N., L. Comfort, and G. Reniers. 2019. Learning About Risk: Machine Learning for Risk Assessment. *Safety Sci* 118: 475–486.

Paustenbach. 1989. The Risk Assessment of Environmental Hazards

Quareshy, M., J. Prusinska, J. H. Li, and R. Napier. 2018. A Cheminformatics Review of Auxins as Herbicides. *J Exp Bot* 69: 265–275. 10.1093/jxb/erx258.

Robson, M. G., and W. A. Toscano. 2007. *Risk Assessment for Environmental Health*. New York, NY: Josey–Bass.

Science and Judgment in Risk Assessment. 1994. *National Research Council (US) Committee on Risk Assessment of Hazardous Air Pollutants*. Washington, D.C.: National Academies Press (US).

Thimann, K. V., and J. B. Koepfli. 1935. Identity of the Growth-Promoting and Root-Forming Substances of Plants. *Nature (London)* 135: 101–102.

UNEP. 1972. *Report of the United Nations Conference on the Human Environment*. United Nations (Stockholm).

Weijers, D., J. Nemhauser, and Z. Yang. 2018. Auxin: Small Molecule, Big Impact. *J Exp Bot* 69: 133–136.

Xu, W., X. Wang, and Z. Cai. 2013. Analytical Chemistry of the Persistent Organic Pollutants Identified in the Stockholm Convention: A Review. *Anal Chim Acta* 790: 1–13. 10.1016/j.aca.2013.04.026.

2 The Risk Assessment–Risk Management Paradigm

Gilbert S. Omenn
University of Michigan, Ann Arbor, MI, USA

David L. Eaton
University of Washington School of Public Health, Seattle, WA, USA

CONTENTS

Definition of Risk 15
Historical Perspectives 15
    The Red Book 17
The Objectives of Risk Assessment: Statutes and Programs...18
Biological End Points...19
A Framework for Regulatory Decision-Making..20
Adding Context for Risk Assessments...21
The Risk Commission...21
Special Challenges for Risk Assessment of Chemicals 23
    Data and Testing..23
    Extrapolation...24
    Variation and Uncertainty...25
Emerging Areas in Chemical Risk Assessment 26
Contributions from All Public Health Sciences to Eco-Genetics and Risk Assessment 26
Risk Management–Risk Communication Approaches (See Chapter 17)............................33
Thought Questions 35
Note..35
References...35

LEARNING OBJECTIVES

Students who complete this chapter will be able to

1. Understand the fundamental concept of risk,
2. Recognize the many roles of public health scientists and public health practitioners in analyzing and communicating with the public about risks,
3. Adopt a useful framework for organizing and evaluating scientific inputs about risks,
4. Learn about the major specific statutes that govern the activities of federal regulatory agencies and their state and local counterparts, and
5. Appreciate the particular contributions of toxicologists, exposure assessors, epidemiologists, biostatisticians, geneticists, and behavioral scientists.

DEFINITION OF RISK

Risk is a fundamental concept in environmental health. *Environmental health risk assessment* has been defined as the "systematic scientific characterization of potential adverse health effects resulting from human exposures to hazardous agents or situations" (Faustman 2019; Omenn and Faustman 2002). The short version is that risk is the probability of an adverse health effect from specified exposures.

HISTORICAL PERSPECTIVES

Over the past 45+ years, public health scientists and policymakers have developed and applied systematic approaches to understanding and evaluating the extent of exposures to environmental agents, the nature of potential hazards to health, the variation in susceptibility to such adverse effects, and the probability and magnitude of such impacts on populations. Concurrently, we have come to recognize the importance of risk perception and respectful two-way communication

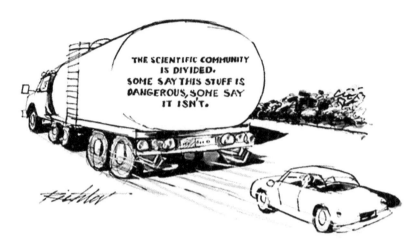

Figure 2.1 Why the public is often confused about the differing views of scientists about potential hazards and health risks.

Source: **Mischa Richter,** *The New Yorker,* **March 21, 1988.**

about risks in proactive interactions with potentially or already affected communities. The goal is to achieve feasible and cost-effective means of reducing such risks, actions acceptable to the public.

At the heart of such analyses and communication are probabilities. Most people, including most physicians and many scientists, are uncomfortable in evaluating probabilities, especially low probabilities with high consequences. Students and practitioners of public health are often called upon to interpret the conclusions, as well as make scientific evaluations. The task is complicated by the fact that well-credentialed scientists, considered experts by the media and the public, may draw different conclusions or make different recommendations. Disclosure of such disagreements leads to confusion or even bewilderment among those who expect science to be about observable facts on which scientists should agree (see Figure 2.1).

In this context, David Bazelon, the widely admired longtime chief judge of the US District Court for the District of Columbia, spoke in 1979 of "the perils of wizardry." He advised technical experts, both inside and outside regulatory agencies, to stay away from the ultimate policy decisions, which are not their charge or specific expertise. He urged us instead to delineate particular elements of the risk to be characterized, focus on those elements, and build a clear record of what is known, what is not yet known but feasibly could be learned, and what is beyond current methods of detection or evaluation. He advised us to expect to be asked again since public health hazards and regulatory responses to them tend to recur. We hope our society will be better prepared each subsequent time (Bazelon 1974).

The situation seemed simpler 60 years ago. In 1958, Congress enacted the Delaney Clause, which instructed the Food and Drug Administration (FDA) to prohibit the addition to the food supply of any substance ("food additive") found to cause cancer in humans or animals. In 1962, Rachel Carson published *Silent Spring*, decrying chemical contamination of streams and waterways. Air pollution in industrial cities and water pollution in such places as Lake Cuyahoga, Ohio, were all too visible. In response to Earth Day on April 1970, President Nixon and Congress created the Environmental Protection Agency (EPA) and then the Occupational Safety and Health Administration (OSHA). Multiple statutes (see Exhibit 2.1) required technical judgments about risks and remedies. Experimental protocols for testing chemicals in animals and schemes for extrapolating the findings to humans stimulated the emergence of risk assessment at the EPA (Albert 1994; Anderson 1983) and the formation of high-level federal working groups among the regulatory agencies and within the executive office of the president (Calkins et al. 1980; Omenn 2003).

Since the boom of environmental regulations in the 1970s, most of the federal legislation controlling hazardous substances has remained in effect, although substantial modifications have occurred. For example, in 2016, after extensive debate and negotiations among public interest groups, affected industries, and regulatory authorities, the Toxic Substances Control Act was

EXHIBIT 2.1   MAJOR HAZARDOUS CHEMICAL LAWS IN THE UNITED STATES

EPA
> Air Pollutants – Clean Air Act, 1970, 1977, 1990
> Water Pollutants – Federal WP Control Act, 1972, 1977 Safe Drinking Water Act, 1974, 1996
> Federal Insecticide, Fungicide and Rodenticide Act (FIFRA), 1972
> Food Quality and Protection Act (FQPA), 1996 Ocean Dumping Marine Protection Act, 1995
> Toxic Substances Control Act (TSCA), 1976; revised as The Frank R. Lautenberg Chemical Safety for the 21st Century Act, 2016
> Hazardous Wastes Act (RCRA), 1976; revised as the Superfund Reauthorization Act, 1986

FDA
> Foods, Drugs, Cosmetics (FDC) Acts, 1906, 1938, 1962, 1977, 1997, 2007

Council for Environmental Quality (CEQ; now Office of Environment Policy)
> Environmental Impacts Act (NEPA), 1972

OSHA
> Workplace Act (OSH Act), 1970

Consumer Product Safety Commission (CPSC)
> Dangerous Consumer Products Act, 1972

Department of Transportation (DOT)
> Hazardous Materials Transportation Act (HMTA), 1975–1979, 1984, 1990

substantially revised as the Frank R. Lautenberg Chemical Safety Act for the 21st Century. One of the new requirements in this act states that EPA must *"make an affirmative finding on the safety of a new chemical or significant new use of an existing chemical before it is allowed into the marketplace."* It explicitly states that initial 'risk evaluations' must be performed on new chemicals. High-priority designation triggers a requirement and deadline for EPA to complete a risk evaluation on that chemical to determine its safety. Low-priority designation does not require further action, although the chemical can move to high priority based on new information. Thus, the process of risk assessment for chemical hazards continues to play a critical role in public health decision-making in the 21st century.

The Red Book

A landmark in this field was the publication in 1983 by the National Academy of Sciences of *Risk Assessment in the Federal Government: Managing the Process*, popularly known as *The Red Book* (NRC 1983). The opening statement captured the challenge:

> This report explores the intricate relations between science and policy,…the assessment of the risk of cancer and other adverse health effects associated with exposure of humans to toxic substances,…a search for the institutional mechanisms that best foster a constructive partnership between science and government, mechanisms to ensure that government regulation rests on the best available scientific knowledge and to preserve the integrity of scientific data and judgments in the unavoidable collision of the contending interests that accompany most important regulatory decisions.

The roots of the controversy lie in improvements in scientific and technologic capability to detect potentially hazardous chemicals, in changes in public expectations and concerns about health protection, and in the fact that the costs and benefits of regulatory policies fall unequally on different groups within American society.

The Red Book was commissioned by Congress after controversial assessments of the risks of saccharin as a nonnutritive sweetener (by FDA), of formaldehyde in home insulation (Consumer Product Safety Commission), of nitrites as preservatives in foods (FDA and US Department of Agriculture), of asbestos removal from schools and homes (OSHA and EPA), of invisible air pollutants, and of many other chemicals in the general environment (primarily EPA). All of these

EXHIBIT 2.2

Key National Academies Reports on Improving the State of the Science in Human Health Risk Assessment of Chemical Hazards (Hyperlinks Provided):

- *Risk Assessment in the Federal Government: Managing the Process (1983; The Red Book)*
- *Science and Judgment in Risk Assessment (1994)*
- *Human Biomonitoring for Environmental Chemicals (2006)*
- *Applications of Toxicogenomic Technologies to Predictive Toxicology and Risk Assessment (2007)*
- *Strengthening Science at the U.S. Environmental Protection Agency: Research-Management and Peer-Review Practices (2000)*
- *Scientific Frontiers in Developmental Toxicology and Risk Assessment (2000)*
- *Toxicity Testing in the Twenty-First Century: A Vision and a Strategy (2007)*
- *Science and Decisions: Advancing the Science (2009)*
- *Toxicity-Pathway-Based Risk Assessment: Preparing for Paradigm Change (2010)*
- *Science for Environmental Protection: The Road Ahead (2012)*
- *Exposure Science in the 21st Century: A Vision and a Strategy (2012)*
- *Review of the Environmental Protection Agency's State-of-the-Science Evaluation of Nonmonotonic Dose-Response Relationships as they Apply to Endocrine Disruptors (2014)*
- *Review of EPA's Integrated Risk Information System (IRIS) Process (2014)*
- *Application of Systematic Review Methods in an Overall Strategy for Evaluating Low-Dose Toxicity from Endocrine Active Chemicals (2017)*
- *Using 21st Century Science to Improve Risk-Related Evaluations (2017)*
- *Understanding Pathways to a Paradigm Shift in Toxicity Testing and Decision-Making: Proceedings of a Workshop – in Brief (2018)*

issues were salient while one of us (GSO) served in the Office of Science and Technology Policy in the Carter White House (1977–1980), as associate director of the Office of Management and Budget (1980–1981), and on the Interagency Regulatory Liaison Group and the Regulatory Analysis Review Group. There was quite a struggle between those who insisted on "zero risk" and those who proposed methods of risk assessment to identify what Lowrance [Lowrance, 1976 #831] called "acceptable risk" and others called "negligible risk," realizing that such a conclusion lies in the eyes of the beholder (see Omenn 2003).

Since the time of the publication of *The Red Book* in 2003, the National Academies of Sciences, Engineering and Medicine (NASEM) has assisted the US EPA and other regulatory agencies in providing new guidance on risk assessment practices to ensure that state-of-the-art science is being used in the risk assessment process (Exhibit 2.2). For example, the incorporation of mechanistic data made available by recent advances in genomics tools and technologies was addressed in a 2007 report on *Applications of Toxicogenomics Technologies to Predictive Toxicology and Risk Assessment* and the 2017 report titled "Using 21st Century Science to Improve Risk-Related Evaluations" (NRC 2017b).

In more recent years, the use of a rigorous evaluative process referred to as 'systematic review' has been championed for data evaluation and 'weight of evidence' decisions in chemical risk assessment. *Systematic review* was defined by the Institute of Medicine (IOM; now the National Academy of Medicine) in 2011 as follows: "Systematic reviews identify, select, assess, and synthesize the findings of similar but separate studies and can help clarify what is known and not known about the potential benefits and harms of drugs, devices, and other healthcare services." Its original applications focused largely on epidemiological data and clinical trials for therapeutics and medical procedures, but more recent efforts have begun to include the concepts of systematic review into the evaluation of animal studies in hazard assessment. The US EPA's program for evaluating chemical risks under the Frank R. Lautenberg Chemical Safety in the 21st Century act is now using systematic review approaches for all steps in the risk assessment process [EPA, 2021 #515].

THE OBJECTIVES OF RISK ASSESSMENT: STATUTES AND PROGRAMS

Exhibit 2.3 outlines the statutory and programmatic objectives for the use of risk assessment in decision-making by regulatory agencies, manufacturers, environmental organizations, and public health departments. The laws governing pharmaceutical approvals and pesticide approvals

EXHIBIT 2.3   OBJECTIVES OF RISK ASSESSMENT

1. Balance risks and benefits.
   - Drugs
   - Pesticides
2. Set target levels of risk.
   - Food contaminants
   - Water pollutants
   - Cleanup levels at polluted (e.g., Superfund) sites
   - Occupational exposures (e.g., Threshold Limit Values and Permissible Exposure Limits, TLVs and PELs, respectively)
3. Set priorities for program activities.
   - Regulatory agencies
   - Manufacturers of new and existing chemicals
   - Environmental and consumer organizations
4. Estimate residual risks and extent of risk reduction after steps are taken to reduce risks.

recognize that these chemicals are designed to kill living cells or microbes; thus, a benefit/risk assessment is essential, and care in their use is mandated. In contrast, the Clean Air Act requires national ambient air quality standards – for sulfur oxides, nitrogen oxides, hydrocarbons, carbon monoxide, particles, photochemical oxidants, and lead – to be set without regard to costs and to protect, with an adequate margin of safety, the most susceptible subgroups in the population. For contaminants in food and water, as opposed to deliberate additives, the statutes recognize that assurance of safety may be associated with some residual level of aflatoxin from a fungus that grows on peanut and corn crops or of by-products from the chlorination of water. Not so well-recognized are objectives 3 and 4 (Exhibit 2.3). All parties have limited staff and financial resources, so deciding in a logical way which risks are most important, for various reasons, is necessary. Finally, the courts, which play a major role in contested regulatory decisions, have supported well-documented claims by agencies that it is time to turn their attention to more pressing remaining risks after taking actions that they consider to be adequate. But critics disagree on other risks. The classic case, decided by the US Supreme Court, involved vinyl chloride (N.v. EPA 1987).

BIOLOGICAL END POINTS

Regulatory controls on chemicals started with a preoccupation about risks of cancer. Now we address multiple biological end points, as shown in Exhibit 2.4. The lowest concentration at which a given chemical may cause each of several adverse effects may vary quite a lot, so characterization of the dose-response relationship for each effect is necessary to guide the focus of risk management.

EXHIBIT 2.4   BIOLOGICAL END POINTS

- Cancers
- Mutations
- Birth defects
- Reproductive toxicity
- Immunological toxicity
- Neurobehavioral toxicity (including neurodevelopmental effects)
- Organ-specific effects
- Endocrine modulation or disruption
- Ecosystem effects

A FRAMEWORK FOR REGULATORY DECISION-MAKING

An elaborate scheme has evolved for the evaluation of individual hazards and risks, as shown in Figure 2.2 from the Office of Science and Technology Policy (Calkins et al. 1980). The first step, hazard identification, seems to generate a yes/no decision about whether the agent, generally a chemical, has the potential to cause adverse effects. In fact, however, epidemiological studies of humans exposed at work or in the general environment, toxicological studies of animals or cells exposed to controlled concentrations of the agent, and structure-activity analysis of the chemical nature of the agent and its relationship to other known chemical hazards all generate quantitative data that must be evaluated with statistical criteria to determine whether a statistically significant excess occurrence of adverse events has been observed (Breslow and Day 1980, 1987; Faustman 2019). These scientific studies lead into the second step, very importantly called risk characterization. This term supplanted *risk assessment* at a time when risk assessment had come to be synonymous with quantitative risk assessment, generating a number, sometimes an excessively precise number, for the potential risks from a given hazard under specified exposure conditions. It is essential to characterize the nature of the adverse effects, including their severity, reversibility, or prevention; the reasonableness of the exposure scenarios; the variation in susceptibility among people exposed or potentially exposed; and the quality of the evidence. Such risk characterization requires substantial narrative, which provides context for the point estimate(s) of risk and for various ways of expressing the uncertainty around that risk estimate.

Finally, the third step is about how the information is used to manage the risk(s). Even before definitive regulatory decisions and actions are taken, the release of information through advisories by public health or environmental agencies and through media coverage is often a powerful influence, however objective. Manufacturers may pull a product or modify its uses; end users, from companies to physicians to pesticide applicators to consumers, may modify their practices or behaviors. Ironically, prohibition or phaseout of one chemical and replacement by a designated substitute has often proved of little value – illustrated by the cases of red dye 2, which was replaced by red dye 40; the flame retardant TRIS in infants' clothes, which was replaced by son and grandson of TRIS; the sweetener cyclamate, which was replaced by saccharin; and the detergent nitrilotriacetic aci, NTA, which was replaced by phosphates. Phosphates led to vast algal overgrowth in lakes, while all of the other replacements mentioned produced cancers in test animals.

More recently, the issue of 'risk trade-offs' with replacement chemicals has been highlighted by the on-going controversy over the widely used fluorinated industrial chemicals, referred to

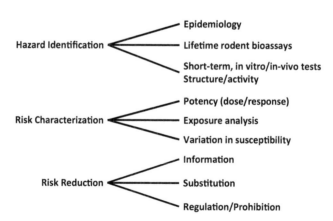

Figure 2.2   Framework for regulatory decision-making.

Source: **Calkins et al. (1980).**

collectively as 'PFAS' ("**P**er and poly **F**luoro **A**lkyl **S**ubstances"). Because of the relatively low acute and subchronic toxicity in traditional laboratory animal studies and the lack of evident health effects in workers with relatively high levels of exposure, PFAS chemicals found widespread use in common consumer products such as fabric stain repellants, nonstick coatings on cookware, and even in firefighting foam. Further, they were relatively water soluble and presumed not to bioaccumulate in the environment. However, in recent years, the surprising environmental persistence, coupled with increasing animal toxicology studies suggesting the potential for long-term health effects, has led to a different – and controversial – public health perspective on PFAS chemicals. Extensive efforts to ban, or at least phase out, the use of the three main PFAS chemicals (PFOA, PFOS, and PfHxA) have led to the proposed use of numerous 'short chain' PFAS molecules as substitutes (IPEN 2019). But we may be seeing history repeat itself, as the 'safety' of these proposed substitutes has not been adequately demonstrated in the eyes of consumer groups and state and federal health regulators charged with protecting public health.

The primary reason substitutes must be viewed with caution is that we always know more about the toxicological or ecological consequences of an agent so well studied as to be removed from commerce than about the proposed substitute.

The original risk assessment framework shown in Figure 2.2 was modified by *The Red Book* to have four parts, by breaking risk characterization into dose-response assessment and exposure assessment components, thereby emphasizing the need to greatly improve the data and response base for exposure assessments. The basic tenants provided in the 1983 Red Book were subsequently included in a broader, three-step process that considers the landscape in which risk assessments are conducted – that of risk-based decision-making in its broadest context (Figure 2.3). The three phases involve (1) problem formulation and scoping, (2) planning and conducting the risk assessment, and (3) incorporating stakeholder input and other considerations necessary for managing the process. Figure 2.3 lays out this approach with the important three-step process of 'risk assessment' (Hazard Identification, Exposure Assessment, and Risk Characterization) clearly center stage in the decision-making/risk management paradigm.

ADDING CONTEXT FOR RISK ASSESSMENTS

One of the biggest problems in the risk assessment/risk management paradigm noted earlier is the long-standing approach of analyzing one chemical at a time, usually for one predominant adverse effect and via one source of exposure. This approach was mandated in most of the statutes in Exhibit 2.1. In contrast, laypeople complain very logically that we are exposed to a sea of chemicals in the air we breathe, the water we drink, the foods we eat, the products we touch, and the soil and dust that contaminate all of the other sources. Thus, an analysis that builds information about the *context* of the exposure under analysis is critical. As outlined in Exhibit 2.5, this process begins by identifying multiple sources of the particular agent under review and the multiple media of contamination and pathways of exposure. Then multiple potential effects should be considered, along with other agents that can cause the same effects. Sometimes people are exposed to several of these agents simultaneously or over time.

Then there are broader public health dimensions, like the overall incidence of cancers, birth defects, asthma, or other end points. Since health is dependent on a sustainable environment, ecological effects should be considered.

Finally, and very importantly, exposures and interventions are very unevenly experienced across the population, with lower-income economic groups and minority ethnic and racial groups at higher risk of exposure and less likely to benefit from risk-reduction action.

THE RISK COMMISSION

This focus on context (see Box 2.1) was developed explicitly during the 1990s by the Presidential/Congressional Commission on Risk Assessment and Risk Management, mandated by the Clean Air Act Amendments of 1990 (Management 1997a, 1997b; Omenn 1996). That commission created the more elaborate framework in Figure 2.4. Putting any new or current risk into the public health (and ecologic) context is right at the top in step 1. An additional innovation is the emphasis, in the center of the hexagon, on proactive identification and engagement of stakeholders. Way too often elaborate risk assessments are performed and decisions made by regulatory agencies before they then go to the public to present the decision and seek support for implementation. However, thoughtful and practical questions are often neglected.

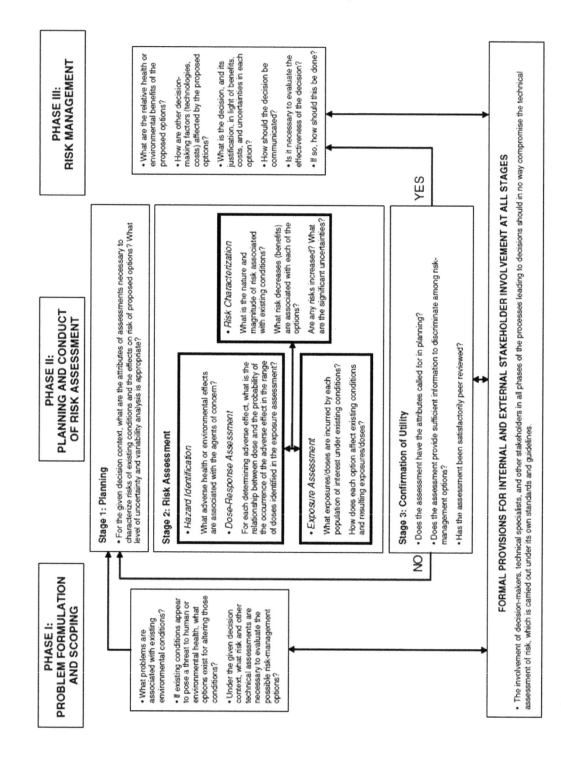

Figure 2.3 A framework for risk-based decision-making that maximizes the utility of risk assessment.

Source: NRC (2009).

EXHIBIT 2.5   BUILDING INFORMATION ABOUT CONTEXT

- Multiple sources of the same agent
- Multiple media or pathways of exposure
- Multiple risks and effects of the same agent
- Multiple agents causing the same effects
- Public health: status and trends
- Ecological health
- Social, cultural, and environmental justice considerations

BOX 2.1   CONTEXT

Moving beyond one chemical, one environmental medium (air, water, soil, or food), or one health effect (cancer or birth defect) at a time in risk assessment and risk management requires a comprehensive public health view.

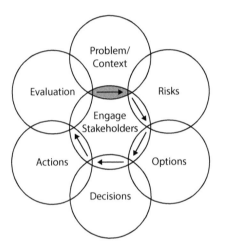

Figure 2.4   Hexagon showing framework for environmental health risk management.

Source: **Management (1997a).**

For example, in a dramatic case involving expensive additional controls on sulfur oxide and arsenic emissions from a copper smelter in Tacoma, Washington, EPA administrator William Ruckelshaus called for public meetings to discuss risk assessment findings and build public understanding. At a televised local meeting, the EPA experts spoke of risk estimates and extrapolations from occupational exposures, including the most important study done with workers at that very smelter. The citizens asked practical questions about whether it was safe to eat vegetables from their gardens, whether their children could safely play outdoors, whether the death of a dog might be due to the arsenic emissions, how they could possibly survive emissions of tons of arsenic per year when "a thimbleful can kill you." The questions and responses passed in the night. Such questions surely could have been addressed under the characterization of risks. Ruckelshaus proudly drew upon *The Red Book* for his decisions and commentaries (Ruckelshaus 1985).

SPECIAL CHALLENGES FOR RISK ASSESSMENT OF CHEMICALS
Data and Testing

A basic problem is the lack of data on potential toxicity. When evaluated in the early 1980s, of approximately 28,000 chemicals used as pesticides, cosmetics, drugs, food additives, and 'high production volume' industrial chemicals, only 6% had adequate toxicity data to allow for a

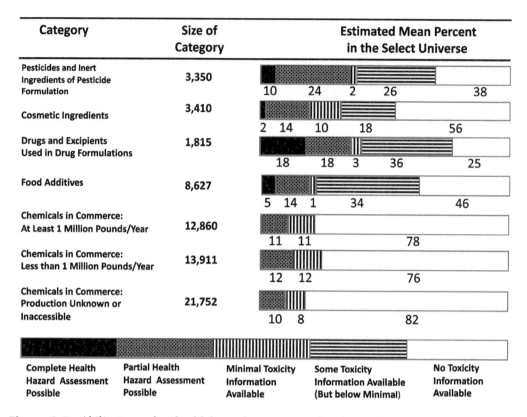

Category	Size of Category	Estimated Mean Percent in the Select Universe
Pesticides and Inert Ingredients of Pesticide Formulation	3,350	10 24 2 26 38
Cosmetic Ingredients	3,410	2 14 10 18 56
Drugs and Excipients Used in Drug Formulations	1,815	18 18 3 36 25
Food Additives	8,627	5 14 1 34 46
Chemicals in Commerce: At Least 1 Million Pounds/Year	12,860	11 11 78
Chemicals in Commerce: Less than 1 Million Pounds/Year	13,911	12 12 76
Chemicals in Commerce: Production Unknown or Inaccessible	21,752	10 8 82

Complete Health Hazard Assessment Possible   Partial Health Hazard Assessment Possible   Minimal Toxicity Information Available   Some Toxicity Information Available (But below Minimal)   No Toxicity Information Available

Figure 2.5 Ability to conduct health hazard assessment of various substance categories.

complete health hazard assessment. For the nearly 13,000 high production volume industrial chemicals (not used as pesticides, food additive, drugs, or cosmetics), 78% had little to no publicly available toxicity data (Figure 2.5; NRC 1984).

Some 35 years later, the number of chemicals in commerce in the United States, and throughout the world, has continued to grow. As of June 2020, the US EPA Toxic Substances inventory contained 86,405 chemicals of which 41,587 are in use in some way.[1] For the vast majority of these chemicals, relatively little toxicity information is available. However, most of these substances are either not widely used or are used in 'closed systems' as chemical intermediates, with little public health exposure. Nevertheless, the level of toxicity testing for many important industrial chemicals for which potential public exposures are possible is seldom adequate to complete a thorough assessment of potential public health impacts. Furthermore, as discussed later in this chapter, the standard toxicological protocols for assessing human health impacts rely upon animal models. There remain many challenges in interpreting the relevance to human health of results obtained from 'high-dose' animal testing.

Alternative strategies for testing chemicals have been examined by modeling the social costs of testing and the consequences of false positives (declaring chemicals hazardous when they are not) – and especially of false negatives (not recognizing health hazards and thereby not avoiding exposures) (Lave et al. 1988; Lave and Omenn 1986). Explicit efforts to deduce which chemicals will be carcinogenic in animal tests on the basis of chemical structure and preliminary in vitro assays were initially disappointing (Omenn et al. 1995; Tennant et al. 1990). However, more recent developments in exposure science, coupled with new molecular approaches in biology, toxicology, and epidemiology in the 21st century, are providing novel approaches to address many of these challenges (NRC 2017a; Zhang et al. 2018).

Extrapolation

Many researchers have struggled with the challenge of extrapolation of the dose-response relationship. First, we must determine the critical health effect, an adverse effect at the lowest dose, together with the strength of the evidence. Numerous "default assumptions" must be applied to go from high-dose exposures (typically 20% to 100% of 50 rodents affected) to acceptable low-dose exposures (low enough that less than 1 person in 10,000 or 1 person in 1,000,000 hypothetically exposed for a lifetime at the maximally permitted dose would be affected). Confidence limits are used in linear or linearized multi-stage models, generating what is recognized to be a (nearly) worst-case scenario of potential risk. Less well-recognized is the need to utilize, generally, the most strikingly positive dataset, to better fit the extrapolation models (Faustman 2019; Omenn and Faustman 2002).

The step from potential hazard to estimated risk depends on the scenarios of exposure – ambient concentrations, portals of entry into the body, time course over a period of years, and dose actually delivered to target organs with variables of absorption, distribution, metabolism, and excretion. A lot of modeling is usually required.

As noted in Box 2.1, real-world exposures often involve mixtures. Examples that have been studied extensively include diesel exhaust, urban smog, industrial effluents, pesticide combinations, and workplaces. On top of these chemical mixtures are exposures to microbial agents prevalent in our environments and to radiation of various kinds. With modern databases, we may be able to link unusual exposures and occupational disease states.

Variation and Uncertainty

The risk of any specific adverse effects from particular exposures to a single agent or a combination of potentially hazardous agents varies among individuals exposed. In addition, the extrapolation of the risk from observable events in test animals or in highly exposed workers to individuals in the general population with much lower exposures depends upon dose-response modeling and undescribed variation in metabolism and sites of action of the agent. These companion problems were called "variation and uncertainty" in a National Research Council report (NRC 1994) *Science and Judgment in Risk Assessment*. This report joins *The Red Book* and the later Risk Commission Report as landmarks.

The hazard identification step has been dominated by results from animal tests. Epidemiology is limited to observations of health conditions in relation to existing or past exposures. For new chemicals or for questions about risks from chemicals at levels below concentrations associated with observable effects in humans, it is essential to test animals and use cell assays for clues to mechanisms. The general presumption – reflecting the precautionary approach inherent in public health – is that a chemical that can produce cancers (or even benign tumors that have some likelihood of progressing to cancers) in animals should be considered capable of causing cancers in humans. The same applies to toxicity to the brain or liver or other organs. In a very few cases, careful and extensive scientific studies have shown definitive evidence that the mechanism mediating the adverse effects in rodents is not at play in humans (see Presidential/Congressional Commission on Risk Assessment and Risk Management, 1997b, pp. 65–68). The classic example is the emergence of kidney tumors in male rats (not mice or monkeys or female rats) from exposures to D-limonene or unleaded gasoline extract; they cause a very unusual accumulation of an alpha-2 mu globulin protein in the kidney tubules of male rats. This biochemical change can lead to cell death, sustained proliferation of remaining cells, and tumor formation. Both the International Agency for Research on Cancer, a unit of the World Health Organization, and the EPA in the United States now recognize a category of agents that are carcinogenic in rodents but not a risk to humans. For example, both the US EPA and International Agency for Research on Cancer (IARC)/WHO classifies agents (or mixtures) as (1) Known to be carcinogenic for humans (2) probably or possibly carcinogenic to humans, or (3) not classifiable as to its carcinogenicity to humans (Table 2.1).

Table 2.1

Extent of Knowledge	IARC	US EPA
Known to be carcinogenic to humans	1	Group A
Probably carcinogenic to humans	2A	Group B1, B2*
Possibly carcinogenic to humans	2B	Group C
Not classifiable as to carcinogenicity to humans	3	Group D
Evidence of noncarcinogenicity to humans	NA	Group E

*Group B2 is distinguished from B1 by the absence of significant human data.

EMERGING AREAS IN CHEMICAL RISK ASSESSMENT

A. Gene-Environment Interactions

There are many reasons to be interested in individual variation in susceptibility. In the practice of occupational medicine, we often encounter patients who are told that a particular set of symptoms may be due to exposures on the job and who then ask, "Why me, Doc? I'm no less careful that the next person." The Occupational Safety and Health Act requires that health standards be set "so that no worker ... shall suffer adverse effects" even if exposed at the maximally permit- ted level for a full working lifetime. The Clean Air Act requires that ambient air standards be set to protect the "most susceptible subgroups" in the population. In the case of the air lead standard, the most susceptible subgroup was determined to be young children; in the case of photochemical oxidants (ozone), adults and children with asthma, chronic bronchitis, or emphysema were identified as such subgroups.

In the postgenomic era informed by the near completion of the human genome sequence for 22,000 genes coding for proteins, we can ask many more questions about the genetic predispositions to susceptibility or resistance to adverse effects from chemical, microbial, and physical agents. We can examine DNA and proteins for "molecular signatures" or "biomarkers" of exposure, early effects (genetic toxicology), and mechanisms of differential susceptibility.

This period should be a golden age for the public health sciences. Sequencing the human genome has generated an avalanche of genetic information to be linked with information about nutrition and metabolism, lifestyle behaviors, diseases and medications, and microbial, chemical, and physical agent exposures (G. S. Omenn 2002; Collins 2004). Both genetics and public health focus on populations. Both fields seek information about heterogeneity of predispositions, environmental exposures, disease risks, and responses to public health and medical interventions. Both explicitly recognize cultural, societal, ethnic, and racial contexts and are sensitive to risks of discrimination.

CONTRIBUTIONS FROM ALL PUBLIC HEALTH SCIENCES TO ECO-GENETICS AND RISK ASSESSMENT

The public health sciences all bring essential capabilities. Epidemiology aims to identify and explain all the factors that influence risk of disease; with biomarkers, we have greatly enhanced power to link qualitative and quantitative findings in test animals and humans. Biostatistics and bioinformatics provide the methods, platforms, and databases for designing studies and analyzing huge, complex datasets. Environmental health can apply molecular signatures to understanding host variation in host-agent interactions for risk assessment and risk management. Pathobiology focuses specifically on the host-pathogen genomic and environmental interactions; polymorphisms in genes controlling receptors essential to penetration of infectious agents (such as malaria-causing plasmodium vivax or AIDS-causing HIV) greatly influence the risk of infection and, hence, appearance of disease symptoms. Behavioral sciences can examine genetic predispositions to various aspects of cigarette smoking behavior and other unhealthful behaviors, which often interact with environmental chemical exposures. And health services researchers are active in designing and assessing well-targeted, cost-effective clinical and preventive genetic services that improve quality of life.

Epigenetics in Risk Assessment: (see Chapter 10 for an extensive discussion).

B. 'Mode of Action' Data to Inform Human Relevance and Animal to Human Extrapolation ("Adverse Outcome Pathways," See Chapter 9)

Over the past 15+ years, there has been a growing appreciation of the value of understanding the 'mode of action' of toxic substances as a key component of understanding risk. The term 'mode of action' (MOA) reflects the molecular, biochemical, and cellular changes that are responsible for the observed toxic response(s). There are two primary reasons for understanding the MOA of a chemical that causes specific toxic effects (adverse outcomes): (1) understanding the dose-response relationship for key molecular events that are responsible for toxic responses allows for better understanding of risk in exposed populations, and (2) MOA may differ substantially between species, which could result in either underestimation or overestimation of risk when extrapolating toxicological data in animal models to humans.

Indeed, the importance of using MOA in cancer risk assessment was recognized in the US EPA's Cancer Risk Assessment Guidelines in 2005:

> The use of mode of action in the assessment of potential carcinogens is a main focus of these cancer guidelines. This area of emphasis arose because of the significant scientific advances that have developed concerning the causes of cancer induction. Elucidation of a mode of action for a particular cancer response in animals or humans is a data-rich determination. Significant information should be developed to ensure that a scientifically justifiable mode of action underlies the process leading to cancer at a given site.
>
> (EPA 2005a, 2005b)

Since that time, numerous workshops and scientific meetings have focused on improving chemical risk assessment by incorporating MOA data into the process. A framework for doing this, referred to as 'Adverse Outcomes Pathways' (AOP) assessment has taken center stage in risk assessment in the 21st century. The AOP is a conceptual framework that utilizes existing knowledge of molecular and cellular changes that result in illness or injury to possible exposures to that substance by an individual or population. AOPs are made up of specific biological elements, described at the molecular level, in a sequence of subsequent biological events (Ankley et al. 2010; Carusi et al. 2018a; Kleinstreuer et al. 2016) Figure 2.6 provides an overview of the AOP framework.

The primary goal of the AOP framework is to compile and synthesize existing biological information at the molecular and cellular levels, such that it can be transparently and efficiently incorporated into a risk assessment paradigm that is critical to scientifically based decision-making (Carusi et al. 2018a) The initial interaction of a chemical with a biological system is depicted as the molecular initiating event (MIE), such as binding to a protein (e.g., receptors, enzymes) or DNA, or interactions with membrane lipids. These MIEs can cause subsequent perturbations at higher biological levels of organization, depicted as intermediate key events (KEs) along an AOP, which ultimately may result in adverse apical responses, such as effects on survival, reproduction, and carcinogenesis (Carusi et al. 2018b).

This approach is useful for both human health and ecological risk assessments. The concept behind the AOP approach is that the potential adverse outcomes associated with

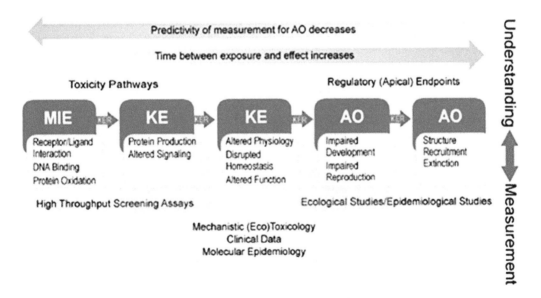

Figure 2.6 Depiction of the role of the AOP framework in linking various data streams to outcomes relevant to regulatory decision-making for chemicals. MIE – molecular initiating event, KE – key event, KER – key event relationship, AO – adverse outcome.

Source: **Ankley and Edwards (2018), as published in Carusi et al. (2018b).**

a specific biological pathway are dependent upon the MIE, which is the ability of the toxic substance to initiate a key molecular event that is necessary, but usually not sufficient by itself, to cause an adverse effect. For example, certain dioxins, dibenzofurans, and co-planar polychlorinated biphenyls, PCBs, can bind to and activate the aryl hydrocarbon receptor (AhR) with varying degrees of affinity (potency) and efficacy (magnitude). In this example of an AOP, activation of the AhR by its cognate ligand (Dioxins, or DL-PCBs) is the MIE, or key initiating event, KIE) (Table A3.7).

A workshop on the AOP approach, sponsored by the US EPA and the National Institute of Environmental Health Sciences, NIEHS, in 2016, noted the following about the utility of AOPs for regulatory decision-making in toxicology:

> An AOP is a framework that allows the placement of available information on biological pathways into an organized, usable, testable format. .... Information in an AOP could be used for assessing chemical risks in a number of ways, including prioritization of chemicals for future evaluation, development of predictive models and IATAs, qualitative or quantitative hazard characterization, and ultimately risk assessment. The utility of an AOP depends on the completeness and maturity of the knowledge underpinning the AOP, the extent to which the links between each KE are understood, and how easily the KEs can be queried. ... At its most basic level, a useful AOP links a MIE convincingly and qualitatively to an (adverse outcome) AO. Adding information about the linkages between the intermediate KEs along a pathway expands the usefulness further, perhaps to the level where evidence provided by mechanistic tests querying particular KEs can characterize chemical hazards. However, for maximal utility, these linkages, or KERs, must be understood quantitatively. Beyond characterizing the pathway, it is important to understand the dose that activates the pathway, and if it is relevant to human or ecological exposure scenarios.
>
> (Kleinstreuer et al. 2016)

For a more detailed discussion of the AOP approach to quantitative risk assessment, see Chapter 9.

C. Computational Toxicology: Physiologically Based Toxicokinetic Modeling, Molecular Structural Analysis, *in Silico* Toxicology and 'Read-Across' Interpolations

The remarkable progress made simultaneously over the past 30 years in both "omics" technologies (genomics, transcriptomics, proteomics, metabolomics) and computational sciences (e.g., computing technology, bioinformatics and artificial intelligence, AI) has led to a 'rethinking' about how predictive toxicology for chemical risk assessments can be done.

It has been recognized for decades that the toxicity of many – indeed most – chemicals is dependent upon the way the chemical is metabolized (biotransformed) in the body. This process of 'biotransformation' is dictated by literally hundreds of different gene products, expressed at varying levels in different tissues. For any given chemical, it is not unusual for it to be converted to a dozen or more different chemical forms – most of them less toxic than the 'parent' compound, but a few that may be much more toxic. It is the balance of 'activation' (formation of the toxic form) to 'detoxification' that ultimately determines the nature and extent of toxic response to a given dose of a chemical. The rate at which each activation and detoxification pathway converts a substance to its toxic or nontoxic product is a major determinant of overall toxic response. The study of these processes is referred to as 'toxicokinetics' ('pharmacokinetics,' if one is discussing drugs). An area of great importance to chemical risk assessment is referred to as 'physiologically based pharmacokinetic(or toxicokinetic'), or PBP(T)K modeling. PBPK modeling "computes and predicts the concentrations of a chemical (and its metabolites) within the body over time from a given external exposure. PBPK models describe the processes of chemical absorption, distribution, metabolism, and excretion (ADME) based on physiological and biochemical mechanisms" (Tan et al. 2020). Figure 2.7 illustrates the conceptual basis of how PBPK modeling can be used to predict concentrations of specific metabolites of a toxic substance at different 'target tissues' in the body. Rate constants for both uptake and elimination are calculated, and mathematical modeling is then used to predict target tissue concentrations at specific doses following exposure.

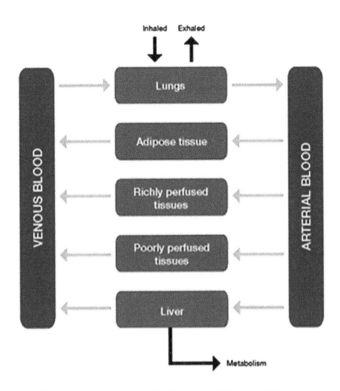

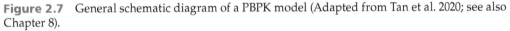

Figure 2.7 General schematic diagram of a PBPK model (Adapted from Tan et al. 2020; see also Chapter 8).

PBPK modeling of environmental chemicals is of great value in extrapolating experimental animal data across routes of administration, different species and/or life stages, and exposure duration (Tan et al. 2020). The incorporation of PBPK modeling into risk assessments has become standard practice and represents a significant improvement in estimating 'target dose' of toxic substances. Genomic differences in the expression of drug-metabolizing enzymes is an important contributor to interindividual differences in response to toxic substances, and PBPK tools can help to address the magnitude of population variability that might occur due to difference in metabolism. There are currently available 'templates' for incorporating PBPK modeling into risk assessments to make such computational approaches more accessible to regulatory toxicologists (Tan et al. 2020).

In silico toxicology (IST) refers to "computational approaches that analyze, simulate, visualize, or predict the toxicity of chemicals" (Myatt et al. 2018). IST utilizes methodologies that determine both biological and chemical properties of an existing or new chemical based largely on a chemical structure. Although *in silico* approaches have been in place for decades (e.g., modeling of structure-activity relationships, SAR), they generally have been used in combination with more traditional *in vivo* and *in vitro* toxicity tests. Capturing a chemical's physico-chemical properties, bioactivity, and safety profiles or toxicity within databases is becoming a key focus of research programs in many industrial sectors such as pharmaceuticals, personal care products, petrochemicals, and biocides. Indeed, the growth in this area of chemical risk assessment has seen astronomical growth in the past decade. Pawar et al. (2020) identified over 900 different publicly available databases of chemical, biological, and toxicological data and resources of potential use for *in silico* chemical risk assessment (Figure 2.8).

But the extraordinary growth in computational sciences and artificial intelligence, coupled with enhanced understanding of key molecular events that may serve as 'triggers' for toxicological responses, now allows for much more sophisticated 'SAR' analyses, including predicting toxic responses for new chemical entities. Such approaches are beginning to be used to generate toxicity assessment information with less need to perform any *in vitro* or *in*

DATABASES

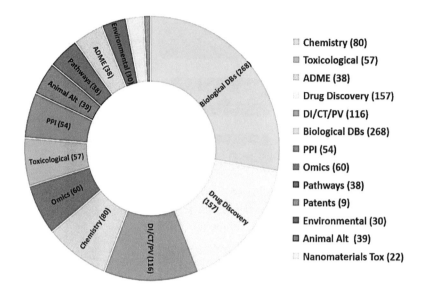

Figure 2.8 Chart showing the number of databases within each group. DI, drug information; CT, clinical trials; PV, pharmacovigilance; PPI, protein-protein interactions; Animal Alt, animal alternatives (Adapted from Pawar et al. 2020).

vivo studies. IST uses molecular models and software tools to predict the potential toxicity of a chemical and in some situations to quantitatively predict the toxic dose or potency. These models are based on experimental data from previous studies of similar molecules, SARs, and other molecular and scientific knowledge (such as structural alerts reported in the literature and predicted metabolism).

A growing area in regulatory risk assessment that relies almost exclusively on computational toxicology approaches is the so-called read-across approach. "Read across" is the process of using known information from one or more source substances to predict the same property for a (data-poor) target substance (Patlewicz et al. 2019). The main purpose of the 'read-across' approach to risk assessment is to make early judgments about the potential toxicity of a new chemical, usually a structural analog of an existing chemical(s) with significant toxicological information available, for which little toxicity information is known. Quantitative structure-activity relationships (QSAR), which rely upon specific chemical features within a molecule, are often the mainstay of read-across approaches. With the greatly expanded knowledge and understanding of how certain functional groups (e.g., a primary or secondary amine group, or double bonds in certain locations) within a complex molecule contribute to the ultimate toxicity of a compound, read across allows reasoned judgments about the potential of a similar molecule to possess, or not, the toxic feature (e.g., DNA damage/mutagenicity or activation of a particular biological receptor) of the model molecule. Read-across approach to chemical hazard assessment is widely used by several European chemical safety organizations, such as the Organisation of Economic Co-operation and Development (OECD) and the *Registration Evaluation Authorisation and Restriction of Chemicals (REACH)* regulation overseen by the European Commission (EC). The US EPA, particularly the Office of Pesticides, Pollutants and Toxic Substances (OPPT), also used read-across approaches in some of its hazard assessment activities, particularly in screening for potential hazards of limited numbers of substances within a tight time line. It is also extensively used internally by many pharmaceutical and chemical manufacturers in assessing the potential toxicity of new chemical entities under consideration for development and production.

Although there is little question that computational toxicology in its various forms holds great promise for furthering regulatory safety of chemical hazards, especially for new chemical entities, it is unlikely to fully replace the need for fundamental toxicological studies, including in some instances the use of laboratory animals in long-term exposures. Following an international workshop on this topic, Andrew Worth, an expert in computational toxicology at the European Union, wrote,

> However, it is still possible, and I believe likely, that some kinds of toxicity will effectively be unpredictable (by computational toxicology approaches). In particular, the repeat-dose and long-term toxicities, as well as the multi-generation effects, may pose an intractable problem. This is not because the Laws of Toxicology break down over such timescales, but because the pathway from insult-to-injury is a long one, and hides multiple uncertainties, with the consequence that small changes in the initial conditions result in large differences in the final outcome. This kind of toxicological behaviour is the biological equivalent of a double (or multiple) pendulum, which exhibits rich dynamic behaviour with a strong sensitivity to initial conditions…. Chaos, in other words.

He and other colleagues have proposed a method-agnostic set of credibility factors that could be used to compare different types of predictive toxicology approaches, which they hope will facilitate communication and cross-disciplinarity among method developers and users, with the ultimate aim of increasing the acceptance and use of predictive approaches in toxicology (Patterson, Whelan, and Worth 2021).

D. **Exposure Assessment Approaches That Consider 'Total Exposures' (Exposome Analyses)**

As we have discussed previously, seldom are humans exposed to a single chemical agent at a time, and oftentimes, there may be multiple sources and routes of exposure to the same chemical, both of which can present challenges to the public health official responsible for making decisions on the relative magnitude of a particular risk associated with a specific source of exposure (e.g., a drinking water contaminant, or a pesticide residue on food). 'Exposure assessment' is a critical element of any risk assessment, and it is often the weak link in the overall risk assessment, usually because of lack of real-world measurements and/ or the use of default assumptions in the absence of real data. Default assumptions are by design 'risk averse,' tending to overestimate, rather than underestimate, actual exposures. For example, the US EPA and many other regulatory agencies assume that the typical adult consumes two liters of drinking water per day. This value is widely used in risk assessment of contaminants found in public water supplies. Yet numerous studies have demonstrated that typical consumption of tap water from the home is considerably less than this. Drewnowski et al. (2013) found that typical adult consumption of tap water was 0.65 liters, with a median range among different age groups and racial/ethnic groups between 0.38 L (Mexican-Americans) and 0.70 L (non-Hispanic Whites). The National Health and Nutrition Examination Survey (NHANES) from 2005 to 2008 found a similar value, 0.64 L per day, for average US adult (age 20+) tap water consumption (Sebastian et al. 2011). However, the risk-averse nature of many default assumptions is perhaps warranted, given that multiple different exposures to the same substance may occur via different routes, and/or concomitant exposures to similar substances may act in concert with the chemical of concern, but go unreported.

Indeed, the concept that we are constantly exposed to a plethora of potentially toxic substances, albeit generally at very low doses, has been brought to light in recent years through the concept of the 'exposome,' made possible by increasing sophistication of analytical instrumentation and the computational science of bioinformatics. The concept of the exposome was first introduced by Christopher Wild, at that time the director of the IARC in 2005 in considering potential links of multiple environmental exposures to cancer risk (Wild 2012). His original definition of the exposome, "[a]ll Exposures, from conception onward, including those from lifestyle, diet and the environment," has since undergone extensive refinement and expansion: "The cumulative measure of environmental influences and associated biological responses throughout the lifespan including exposure from the environment, diet, behavior and endogenous processes" (G. W. Miller 2020; Miller and Jones 2014). Although important in concept, actually measuring everything that a human is exposed to is perhaps an insurmountable challenge. However, a 'sister' approach, which is similar in concept, is measuring the 'metabolome' in biological samples. The metabolome is defined as "the study of the chemical metabolites that result from cellular processes"

(Miller 2020). However, the same analytical instrumentation (usually high-resolution mass spectrometry, HRMS) analyzing the same biological source (e.g., serum samples) is now capable of identifying not only metabolites of cellular processes but also potentially thousands of exogenous chemicals, and their metabolites, stemming from environmental exposures (including diet). The universe of these chemicals represents the fraction of total exposures (the true 'exposome') that are biologically available – i.e., absorbed into the bloodstream at some point in time. Of course, identifying specific chemicals that are responsible for the peaks and associated mass values seen in HRMS analysis of a blood sample is a monumental task and requires both an extensive database of known chemicals and their metabolites and bioinformatic approaches to make unambiguous associations between peaks and mass values to a specific chemical. But, if done successfully, an 'exposomics analysis' has the potential to quantitatively identify human exposures to hundreds, if not thousands of different environmental pollutants of potential interest in risk assessment. However, using such quantitative exposure data of hundreds to thousands of specific chemicals in a human risk assessment remains an enormous challenge. Nevertheless, quantitative measures of specific chemical metabolites in blood remain one of the most scientifically robust measures of human exposure, and such 'biomarkers of exposure' represent perhaps the most robust means of exposure assessment for quantitative risk assessment. Whether exposome data can be integrated in a biologically relevant manner into risk assessments in environmental health remains uncertain, but there are several approaches for conducting risk assessments for multiple chemical exposures, especially for chemicals that act via the same MOA.

E. Risk Assessment for Exposures to Multiple Chemicals

The traditional risk assessment paradigm is largely built around individual chemicals, with both the exposure assessment and toxicity evaluation focused on a single agent. But, as mentioned previously, in contrast to toxicological testing in experimental animals, humans are seldom exposed to only a single chemical at a time. One advantage of the AOP approach described earlier is that it is amenable to combining chemicals that act via a common MOA. For example, chemicals such as chlorinated dioxins, dibenzofurans, and certain PCBs exert most, if not all, of their toxicity via activating the AhR. The concept of 'toxic equivalence factors' (TEFs) was developed in the late 1990s, based on the relative ability of individual dioxin, dibenzofuran, or PCB congeners (a 'congener' is a specific chemical structure) to interact with and activate the AhR, with one congener, 2,3,7,8-tetrachlorodibenzofuran (TCDD) set to a value of 1. The potency for individual congeners, relative to that of TCDD, can vary by more than five orders of magnitude. Thus, by using a sum of the product of a specific TEF value and the concentration of that congener (TEF x (Congener)), one can estimate the overall 'Toxic Equivalence Quotient' (TEQ), in units of TCDD. This approach is widely used by US EPA, WHO, and most other regulatory agencies worldwide for assessment of complex mixtures of dioxins, dibenzofurans, and dioxin-like PCBs. Because it assumes a common 'key molecular event' (activation of the AhR) it is also amenable to an AOP approach to risk assessment of the mixture, as discussed previously.

Exposures to multiple chemicals continue to be a challenge for risk assessments used for regulatory purposes. Indeed, several regulations specifically call for consideration of 'cumulative risk assessment (CRA)' for multiple chemical exposures. For example, the US Food Quality Protection Act states that the US EPA shall base risk upon "available information concerning the cumulative effects on infants and children of (pesticide) residues and other substances that have a common mechanism of toxicity." And the US Superfund Regulation, under the Preliminary Remediation Goals for Non-carcinogens and the European Union Regulation (EC) No. 1107/2009 call for cumulative noncancer risks to be assessed (Moretto et al. 2017). The Health and Environmental Sciences Institute (HESI), has sponsored a series of reports over the past decade that explicitly deal with the challenges of CRA for multiple chemical exposures. Their process is illustrated in Figure 2.9.

HESI provides an online tool, called 'Risk21,' that provides graphical representation of exposures and responses on a 'risk continuum,' once exposure and toxicity data are entered. For a full description of Risk21 and the application of the tool for CRA, the reader is referred to Embry et al. (2014) Solomon et al. (2016), and Moretto et al. (2017).

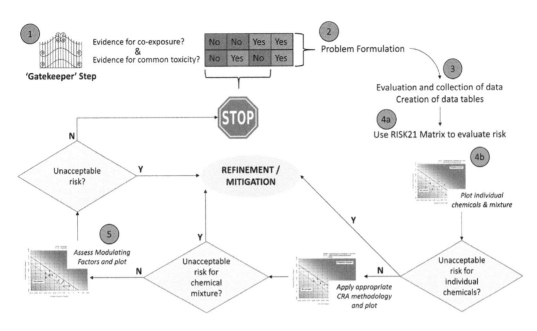

Figure 2.9   General conceptual framework of the HESI Risk21 approach to CRA.

RISK MANAGEMENT–RISK COMMUNICATION APPROACHES (SEE CHAPTER 17)

Exhibit 2.6 shows the key components for risk management and risk reduction through a variety of communication strategies. Finding appropriate technical language for effective two-way communication is an important responsibility (NRC 1989). We overuse powers of 10 (orders of magnitude) in our oral communication and documents, especially on the benefits of risk reduction. Many people seem to think that reducing estimated risks from 10^{-3} to 10^{-4} (from 1 in 1,000 to 1 in 10,000) is the same benefit as a further reduction to 10^{-5} (1 in 100,000). Figure 2.10 shows on a linear scale for the y-axis that the first risk-reduction step removes 90% of the risk, leaving only 10%; thus, the next step can remove only 9% of the original risk, usually at a far higher cost (Management 1997b).

Words matter. For example, safety officials and public health practitioners have campaigned for many years to expunge the word *accidents*, which implies "acts of God" and unpreventable events; instead, words like *incidents*, *injuries*, and *crashes* should be used (see BMJ 2001).

Exhibit 2.7 lists a broad range of approaches for reducing risks judged to be too high for protection of the public.

Engagement. The first, emphasized by the Risk Commission, is proactive engagement of stakeholders to learn the issues that matter in the community, to jointly formulate questions to be addressed in the risk assessment, and to build a basis for acceptable remedies. Such discussions, initiated as early as possible in the process (Figure 2.3), can help identify practical risk-reduction approaches that might be rejected by distant experts who do not compare the risks with the overall public health context in the community or are unaware of the modifications in behavior and

EXHIBIT 2.6   ESSENTIAL COMPONENTS FOR RISK REDUCTION

- Awareness of potential problems and context
- Engagement of the interested or affected publics
- Development of scientific knowledge
- Design of feasible alternative actions
- Affirmation of societal values
- Mobilization of political will

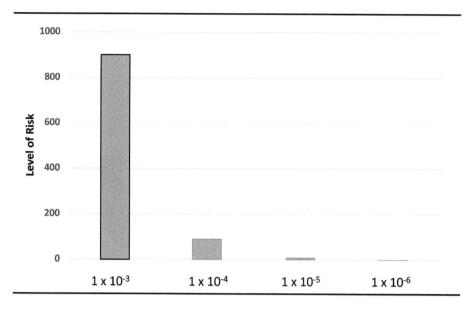

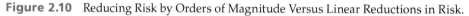

Figure 2.10 Reducing Risk by Orders of Magnitude Versus Linear Reductions in Risk.

Source: **Management (1997b).**

EXHIBIT 2.7   VARIOUS RISK MANAGEMENT AND RISK COMMUNICATION APPROACHES

- Engagement of stakeholders: Learning the issues and questions, finding what might be "acceptable"
- Risk-based (chemicals): *de minimis*, maximal contaminant levels (foods, water), bright lines, comparisons of similar risks
- Precautionary principle: Hippocrates' "Do No Harm," as low as reasonably achievable (ALARA), substantial equivalence (recombinant DNA)
- Best available technology (Clean Air Act)
- Benefit-cost analysis

---

therefore exposure that the affected community would consider quite acceptable. Such situations are well-documented in volume 1 of the Risk Commission reports.

Risk-based risk management approaches. These include determination by various methods (see (Faustman 2019)) of risks that policymakers may then declare to be *de minimis* levels of exposure and risk; bright lines for measurable levels of contaminants determined to be acceptable, as for food and water contaminants; and comparative analyses of similar risks from agents used for similar purposes, like pesticides or pharmaceuticals.

Intuitive approaches. Some alternatives do not require estimation of risk levels and uncertainty bounds. These include the following:

- The traditional engineering approach of ALARA with judgments about feasibility and cost

- The use of "best available technology," as mandated by Congress in the Clean Air Act Amendments of 1990, to be followed up later by risk-based determinations of whether additional reductions in emissions were warranted to be adequately protective of public health

The broad theme of *the precautionary principle* is a popular phrase in Europe and is compatible with traditional public health interventions in this country and with the dictum of Hippocrates to "do no harm." This last point highlights the importance of risk-risk trade-offs since many interventions themselves introduce new risks while reducing, hopefully, the targeted existing risks (Graham and Wiener 1995)

Risk perception. Careful social science studies of risk perception (Fischoff 1995; Kasperson et al. 2003, 1988; Slovic 1987, 1993; Slovic et al. 2004) have shown that people have somewhat predictable reactions to different kinds of risks. In general, exposures that are invisible or undetectable with the senses are feared more, dreaded consequences are magnified, and unfamiliar or new risks are more troublesome than such familiar, though much higher, risks as cigarette smoking, drinking alcoholic beverages, driving too fast, or engaging in hazardous recreational activities. Sometimes, public perceptions of risk and of acceptability of remedies change dramatically, as with seatbelts and infant car seats. Big changes in behavior generally require reinforcing and persistent actions and incentives, as occur in states with multimodality interventions to reduce cigarette smoking.

Information overload. Finally, there is a sense among many of the public that we inundate people with news about public health threats, some of which are quite unlikely, undercutting any sense of prioritization. A risk-based approach can help in this regard.

I know no safe depository of the ultimate powers of society but the people themselves; if we think them not enlightened enough to exercise their control with a wholesome discretion, the remedy is not to take it away from them, but to inform their discretion.

—Thomas Jefferson

THOUGHT QUESTIONS

1. Why do people who smoke or engage in very hazardous recreational sports seek extreme protection against low-level chemical risks?
2. Would health protection aimed at people at average risk be acceptable in light of presumed or known variation in susceptibility across the population?
3. How can we better evaluate risks from multiple simultaneous exposures?
4. How can public health practitioners and the media better communicate the nature and levels of risk?
5. What can be done to overcome the environmental injustice of the location of hazardous facilities in poor neighborhoods or failure to clean up areas near poorer populations in our society?

NOTE

1. https://www.epa.gov/tsca-inventory/how-access-tsca-inventory

REFERENCES

Albert, R. E. 1994. Carcinogen Risk Assessment in the U.S. Environmental Protection Agency. *Crit Rev Toxicol* 24: 75–85. 10.3109/10408449409017920.

Anderson, E. L. 1983. Quantitative Approaches in Use to Assess Cancer Risk. *Risk Anal* 3: 277–295. 10.1111/j.1539-6924.1983.tb01396.x.

Ankley, G. T., R. S. Bennett, R. J. Erickson, D. J. Hoff, M. W. Hornung, R. D. Johnson, and et al. 2010. Adverse Outcome Pathways: A Conceptual Framework to Support Ecotoxicology Research and Risk Assessment. *Environ Toxicol Chem* 29: 730–741.

Ankley, G. T., and S. W. Edwards. 2018. The Adverse Outcome Pathway: A Multifaceted Framework Supporting 21st Century Toxicology. *Curr Opin Toxicol* 9: 1–7. https://doi.org/10.1016/j.cotox.2018.03.004. https://www.ncbi.nlm.nih.gov/pubmed/29682628 file://vtx-s-fs1/data1/Library/Misc%20Papers/PCBs/Ankley%2018.pdf.

Bazelon, D. 1974. The Perils of Wizardry. *Amer J Psaich* 131 (12): 1535–7228. https://doi.org/Published Online: April 24, 2020 https://doi.org/10.1176/ajp.1974.131.12.1317.

BMJ. 2001. Editorial: BMJ Bans 'Accidents.' *Brit Med J* 322: 1320–1321.

Breslow, N. E., and N. E. Day. 1980. *The Analysis of Case-Control Studies.* Lyon, France: IARC.

Breslow, N. E., and N. E. Day. 1987. *The Design and Analysis of Cohort Studies.* Lyon, France: IARC.

Calkins, D. R., R. L. Dixon, C. R. Gerber, D. Zarin, and G. S. Omenn. 1980. Identification, Characterization and Control of Potential Human Carcinogens: A Framework for Federal Decision Making. *J NatCancer Inst* 64: 169–175. https://doi.org/10.1093/jnci/64.1.169.

Carusi, A, M. R. Davies, G. De Grandis, B. I. Escher, G. Hodges, K. M. Y. Leung, M. Whelan, C. Willett, and G. T. Ankley. 2018a. Harvesting the Promise of AOPs: An Assessment and Recommendations. *Sci Total Environ* 628–629: 1542–1555. https://doi.org/10.1016/j.scitotenv.2018.02.015.

Carusi, A., M. R. Davies, G. De Grandis, B. I. Escher, G. Hodges, K. M. Y. Leung, M. Whelan, C. Willett, and G. T. Ankley. 2018b. Harvesting the Promise of AOPs: An Assessment and Recommendations. *Sci Total Environ* 628–629: 1542–1556. https://doi.org/10.1016/j.scitotenv.2018.02.015. FILE:\\VTX-S-FS1\DATA1\Library\Misc%20Papers\PCBs\Carusi%2018.pdf.

Collins, F. S.. 2004. The Case for a U.S. Prospective Cohort Study of Genes an Environment. *Nature (London)* 429: 475–477. https://doi.org/10.1038/nature02628.

Drewnowski, A., C. D. Rehm, and F. Constant. 2013. Beverage Consumption Among Adults in The United States: Cross-Sectional Study Using Data from NHANES 2005–2010. *BMC Public Health* 13: 1068. https://doi.org/ http://www.biomedcentral.com/1471-2458/13/1068.

Embry, M. R., A. N. Bachman, D. R. Bell, A. R. Boobis, S. M. Cohen, M. Dellarco, I. C. Dewhurst, N. G. Doerrer, R. N. Hines, A. Moretto, and et al. 2014. Risk Assessment in the 21st Century: Roadmap and Matrix. *CRC Crit Rev Toxicol* 44: 6–16. https://www.tandfonline.com/loi/itxc20.

EPA. 2005a. *Supplemental Guidance for Assessing Susceptibility from Early-Life Exposure to Carcinogens. EPA/630/R-03/003F.* Available online at: https://www.epa.gov/risk/supplemental-guidance-assessing-susceptibility-early-life-exposure-carcinogens.

EPA. 2005b. *Guidance on Selecting Age Groups for Monitoring and Assessing Childhood Exposures to Environmental Contaminants.* (Washington, DC: Environmental Protection Agency).

EPA, NRDC v. 1987. Natural Resources Defense Council, Inc., Petitioner, v. U.S. Environmental Protection Agency and Lee M. Thomas, administrator, U.S. Environmental Protection Agency, Respondents, Vinyl Institute, Intervenor, 824 F.2d 1146 (D.C. Cir. 1987). https://law.justia.com/cases/federal/appellate-courts/F2/824/1146/122046/.

Estimation Programs Interface Suite™ for Microsoft® Windows. n.d. v 4.11. EPA, online.

Faustman, E. M. 2019. Risk Assessment. In C. D. Klassen (Ed.), *Toxicology: The Science of Poisons* (pp. 1010–1240). New York: McGraw-Hill.

Fischoff, B. 1995. Risk Perception and Communication Unplugged: Twenty Years of Process. *Risk Anal* 15 (2): 137–145. https://doi.org/0.1111/j.1539-6924.1995.tb00308.x.

Graham, J. D., and J. B. Wiener. 1995. *Risk vs. Risk: Tradeoffs in Protecting Health and the Environment.* Cambridge, MA: Harvard University Press.

IPEN. 2019. *2019/Stockholm Convention COP-9 White Paper: The Global PFAS Problem: Fluorene-Free Alternatives as Solutions.* Geneva, CH: IPEN.

Kasperson, J. X., R. E. Kasperson, N. Pidgeon, and P. Slovic. 2003. The Social Amplification of Risk: Assessing Fifteen Years of Research and Theory. In N. Pidgeon, R. Kasperson and P. Slovic (Eds.), *The Social Amplification of Risk*. London, UK: University Press Cambridge.

Kasperson, R. E., O. Renn, P. Slovic, E. S. Brown, J. Emel, R. Goble, J. X. Kasperson, and S. J. Ratick. 1988. The Social Amplification of Risk: A Conceptional Framework. *Risk Anal* 8 (2): 177–187.

Kleinstreuer, N. C., K. Sullivan, D. Allen, S. Edwards, D. L. Mendrick, M. Embry, J. Matheson, J. C. Rowlands, S. Munn, E. Maull, and W. Casey. 2016. Adverse Outcome Pathways: From Research to Regulation, Scientific Workshop Report. *Regul Toxicol Pharmacol* 76: 39–50. https://doi.org/10.1016/j.yrtph.2016.01.007.

Lave, L. B., F. Ennever, S. Rosenkranz, and G. S. Omenn. 1988. Information Value of the Rodent Bioassay. *Nature (London)* 336: 631–633.

Lave, L. B., and G. S. Omenn. 1986. Cost-Effectiveness of Short-Term Tests for Carcinogenicity. *Nature (London)* 324: 29–34.

Management, Presidential/Congressional Commission on Risk Assessment and Risk. 1997a. *A Framework for Environmental Health Risk Management*. US Government Printing Office. http://www.riskworld.com/Nreports/NR5ME001.HTM.

Management, Presidential/Congressional Commission on Risk Assessment and Risk. 1997b. *Risk Assessment and Risk Management in Regulatory Decision Making*. US Government Printing Office. http://www.riskworld.com/Nreports/NR5ME001.HTM.

Miller, G. W. 2020. *The Exposome: A New Paradigm for the Environment and Health*, 2nd ed. San Diego, CA: Elsevier/Academic Press.

Miller, G. W., and D. P. Jones. 2014. The Nature of Nurture: Refining the Definition of the Exposome. *Toxxicol Sci* 137: 1–2.

Moretto, A., A. Bachman, A. Boobis, K. R. Solomon, T. P. Pastoor, M. F. Wilks, and M. Embry. 2017. A Framework for Cumulative Risk Assessment in the 21st Century. *Crit Rev Toxicol* 47: 85–97. https://doi.org/10.1080/10 408444.2016.1211618.

Myatt, D. J., E. Ahlberg, Y. Akahori, D Allen, A. Amberg, L. T. Anger, A. Aptula, S. Auerbach, and et al. 2018. In Silico Toxicology Protocols. *Regul Toxicol Pharmacol* 96: 1–17. https://doi.org/10.1016/j.yrtph.2018.04.014.

NRC. 1983. *Risk Assessment in the Federal Government: Managing the Process*. Washington, DC: National Academies Press.

NRC. 1984. *Toxicity Testing: Strategies to Determine Needs and Priorities*. Washington, DC: National Academies Press.

NRC. 1989. *Improving Risk Communication*. Washington, DC: National Academies Press.

NRC. 1994. *Science and Judgment in Risk Assessment*. Washington, DC: National Academy Press.

NRC. 2009. *Science And Decisions: Advancing Risk Assessment*. Washington, DC: National Academies Press.

NRC. 2017a. *Global Health and the Future Role of the United States*. Nat. Acad. Sci. Press.

NRC. 2017b. *Using 21st Century Science to Improve Risk-Related Evaluations*. Washington, DC: National Academies Press.

Omenn, G. S.. 1996. Putting Environmental Risks in a Public Health Context. *Public Health Rep* 111 (6): 514–516. https://pubmed.ncbi.nlm.nih.gov/8955697.

Omenn, G. S. 2002. The Crucial Role of Public Health Sciences in the Postgenomic Era. *Genet Med* 4 (6): 21S–26S.

Omenn, G. S. 2003. On the Significance of 'The Red Book' in the Evolution of Risk Assessment and Risk Management. *Hum Ecol Risk Assess* 9: 1155–1167. https://doi.org/10.1080/10807030390240355.

Omenn, G. S., and E. M. Faustman. 2002. Risk Assessment and Risk Management. In R. Detels, J. McEwen, R. Beaglehole, and H. Tanaka (Eds.), *Oxford Textbook of Public Health* (Vol. 2. 4th ed.). Oxford, UK: Oxford University Press.

Omenn, G. S., S. Stuebbe, and L. Lave. 1995. Predictions of Rodent Carcinogenicity Testing Results: Interpretation in Light of the Lave-Omenn Value-of-Information Model. *Mol Carcinog* 14: 37–45. https://doi.org/10.1002/mc.2940140108.

Patlewicz, G., L. E. Lizarraga, D. Rua, D. G. Allen, A. B. Daniel, S. C. Fitzpatrick, N. Garcia-Reyero, J. Gordon, P. Hakkinen, A. S. Howard, A. Karmaus, J. Matheson, M. Mumtaz, A. N. Richarz, P. Ruiz, L. Scarano, T. Yamada, and N. Kleinstreuer. 2019. Exploring Current Read-Across Applications and Needs Among Selected U.S. Federal Agencies. *Regul Toxicol Pharmacol*. 106: 197–209.

Patterson, I. A., M. P. Whelan, and A. P. Worth. 2021. The Role of Validation in Establishing the Scientific Credibility of Predictive Toxicology Approaches Intended for Regulatory Application. *Comput Toxicol* 17. https://doi.org/10.1016/j.comtox.2020.100144.

Pawar, G., J. C. Madden, S. J. Enoch, A. Paini, and M. T. D. Cronin. 2020. A Review of In Silico Tools as Alternatives to Animal Testing: Principles, Resources and Applications. *Alt to Lab Animals* 48 (4): 146–172. https://doi.org/10.1177/0261192920965977.

Ruckelshaus, W. D. 1985. Risk Science, and Democracy. *Iss Sci Technol* 1 (3): 19–38 https://www.jstor.org/stable/43308875.

Sebastian, R. S., C. Cecilia Wilkinson Enns, and J. D. Goldman. 2011. *Drinking Water Intake in the U.S.: What We Eat In America, NHANES 2005–2008 Dietary Data Brief, Vol. 7*. Atlanta, GA: CDC.

Slovic, P. 1987. Perception of Risk. *Science (Washington)* 236: 280–285.

Slovic, P. 1993. Perceived Risk, Trust, and Democracy. *Risk Anal* 13: 675–682.

Slovic, P., M. Finucane, E. Peters, and D. G. MacGregor. 2004. Risk as Analysis and Risk as Feelings: Some Thoughts About Affect, Reason, Risk, and Rationality. *Risk Anal* 24 (2): 1–12.

Solomon, K. R., M. Wilks, A. Bachman, Boobis A. R., A. Moretto, T. P. Pastoor, R. Phillips, and M. R. Embry. 2016. Problem Formulation for Risk Assessment of Combined Exposures to Chemicals and Other Stressors. *Crit Rev Toxicol* 46: 835–844.

Tan, Y. M., M. Chan, A. Chukwudebe, J. Domoradzki, J. Fisher, C. E. Hack, P. Hinderliter, K. Hirasawa, J. Leonard, A. Lumen, A. Paini, H. Qian, P. Ruiz, J. Wambaugh, F. Zhang, and M. Embry. 2020. PBPK Model Reporting Template for Chemical Risk Assessment Applications. *Regul Toxicol Pharmacol* 115:104691. https://doi.org/10.1016/j.yrtph.2020.104691.

Tennant, R. W., J. W. Spaulding, S. Stasiewicz, and J. Ashby. 1990. Prediction of the Outcome of Rodent Carcinogenicity Bioassays Currently Being Conducted on 44 Chemicals by the National Toxicology Program. *Mutagenesis* 5 (1): 3–14. 10.1093/mutage/5.1.3.

Wild, C. P. 2012. The Exposome from Concept to Utility. *Int J Epidemiol* 24: 24–32.

Zhang, Q., J. Li, A. Middleton, S. Bhattacharya, and R. B. Conolly. 2018. Bridging the Data Gap From In Vitro Toxicity Testing to Chemical Safety Assessment Through Computational Modeling. *Front Public Health* 11 (6): 261. https://doi.org/10.3389/fpubh.2018.00261.

3 Risk Assessment and Regulatory Decision-Making in Environmental Health

Felicia Wu
Michigan State University, East Lansing, MI, USA

Joseph V. Rodricks
Ramboll US Consulting, Arlington, VA, USA

CONTENTS

Introduction 39
Food Constituents and Contaminants 40
Food Safety History: Origins of Federal Food Laws..41
A Brief Summary of Food Safety Risk Assessment..42
The Modern Food Supply...42
Food Additives: The Example of Non-nutritive Sweeteners..............................43
GRAS Substances 44
Veterinary Drug Residues..45
Substances Formed by Processing..45
Crop Protection Chemicals 45
Food Contaminants of Industrial Origin – The Organics 45
Heavy Metals – Food Contaminants of Industrial and Natural Origin............46
Food Allergies and Intolerances 48
Mycotoxins..48
Microbial Pathogens 49
Genetically Modified Organisms, Agricultural Biotechnology, and Food Safety 49
Future Directions..50
References..52

LEARNING OBJECTIVES

Students who complete this chapter will be able to

1. To identify important food contaminants and food additives in the United States and global food supply,
2. To understand the basic concepts of human health risk assessment applied to food contaminants, and
3. To learn the history of food safety regulations in the United States.

INTRODUCTION

Environmental health includes the safety and the quality of food. In the context of risk, food can become unsafe if it contains (1) *contaminants,* such as chemicals or microbes, that cause harm to human health; (2) *additives* that can compromise human health; or (3) *an unhealthful proportion of nutrients* – either undernutrition or overnutrition of macro- or micronutrients – leading to suboptimal health outcomes. A different category of food integrity is *food fraud*: mislabeling food (e.g., substituting one type of meat source for another) or tampering with expiration dates. As this is unrelated to environmental risks, food fraud discussions are not included in this chapter. The reader is referred to Spink et al. (2017) for a review of food fraud issues pertinent today.

This chapter addresses food safety risk analysis in the context of the first two of these categories: contaminants and additives to food. The health risks associated with suboptimal diets are a very important topic, but out of the scope of environmental risk assessment. The reader is referred to the US Department of Health and Human Services dietary guidelines page for further information

DOI: 10.1201/9780429291722-3

on healthful diets and risks to health through suboptimal diets: https://health.gov/our-work/food-nutrition.

Food contaminants are substances that, while not intentionally added to food, may come to be present in food at levels that can cause harmful human effects. There are many types of food contaminants, including viruses, bacteria, protozoan parasites, chemicals, and toxins. Industrial chemicals of many types that have become widespread environmental pollutants may find their way into foods, by a variety of mechanisms. While strictly speaking they are not contaminants, many foods naturally contain or produce substances that can be harmful if present at excessive levels. These include cassava cyanide and solanine, the chemical that turns potato skins green (Rodricks et al. 2020). Many other contaminants are inadvertently introduced into food, such as microbial pathogens that may occur on food as a result of washing or irrigating with polluted water. The different types of food contaminants are described in greater detail in the following section.

Food additives are substances that are added to food to enhance its technical characteristics in certain ways. For example, food preservatives are added to food to allow it to stay free of pathogenic microbes for longer or to stabilize flavor and extend shelf life. Food colors and flavors are added to enhance the sensory qualities of the food. Unlike food contaminants, food additives are deliberately introduced to the food supply, but like food contaminants, these additives must also be evaluated for safety along the same risk assessment guidelines: establishing what harmful health effects, if any, might take place from excessive exposure to these additives, and safe levels of these chemicals to add to food that would not increase the risk of human disease over a lifetime. Food additives and contaminants are subject to regulations of several types, all of which have arisen from the requirements of many laws relating to food safety.

FOOD CONSTITUENTS AND CONTAMINANTS

The immense, and probably uncountable, numbers of <u>natural constituents</u> of foods and beverages represent the major share of dietary chemicals. In addition to the chemicals that make up our macro- and micronutrients (proteins, carbohydrates, vitamins, minerals), there are thousands of chemicals that impart flavor, color, or natural defenses for plants. For example, coffee contains more than 600 distinct compounds (Smith 1991). Naturally occurring chemicals from the hundreds of herbs and spices used in food preparation number in the thousands.

Food processing can increase the numbers and types of chemicals in food. For example, fermentation alters the chemical content (as well as the taste and texture and safety) of food. Extruding, soaking, baking, boiling, and smoking foods may also change the chemical composition of foods. Additionally, food preservation and adding substances to color, sweeten, emulsify, flavor, and alter taste perception results in altered composition of foods. Aside from food processing-related chemicals, food can contain exogenous chemicals such as pesticide residues, feed additives or drugs from animal-source foods, and chemicals from packages that make contact with and migrate into food.

Environmental contaminants that make their way into food can jeopardize human health if present at excessive levels. These include toxins produced by bacteria or fungi growing on food, naturally occurring toxins that plants or animals produce in order to reduce the risk of predation, and heavy metals or antibiotics that may migrate to crop plants through soil or water used for food production. Industrial chemicals that have entered the environment can also become contaminants of food. Microbial pathogens such as *Salmonella* and *E. coli* – which cause the greatest global burden of disease from food (Havelaar et al. 2015) – can enter food through a variety of pathways along the food supply chain; starting with contamination in crop fields or livestock production, all the way through storage, transportation, processing, and even spoilage or cross-contamination in stores or households. Categories of the constituents and contaminants of food are summarized in Table 3.1 (Rodricks et al. 2020). Each of these classes, except for nutrients and alcoholic beverages, is discussed in this chapter.

Virtually all the aforementioned substances can, under certain conditions, pose risks to human health. The science of food safety is devoted to understanding those risks and their sources and to identifying ways to control them. Food safety science guides the actions of regulatory agencies, such as the US Food and Drug Administration (FDA) and the European Food Safety Authority (EFSA), in their missions to ensure adequate controls on risk are in place. Before we discuss these topics in detail, we offer a brief history of food safety in the United States.

Table 3.1: **Classes of Food Constituents and Contaminants**

Class	Description
Nutrients	Macronutrients (protein, carbohydrates, fats) and micronutrients (vitamins and minerals) that promote various aspects of human health.
Intentionally introduced substances	Food additives such as colors, flavorings, or preservatives; Generally Recognized as Safe (GRAS) substances;[a] pesticides; and veterinary drugs. These must be evaluated for safety for human health in the quantities added to food.
Chemicals produced during processing, preparation	Reaction products from food heating, or extrusion; chemically very diverse.
Contaminants	Substances not intended to be present that can harm human health, including industrial and natural chemicals and microbial pathogens.
Alcoholic beverages	Ethanol plus many fermentation products.

[a] GRAS: Generally Recognized as Safe. Refers to the regulatory status of certain food ingredients in the United States. See further in the following section.

FOOD SAFETY HISTORY: ORIGINS OF FEDERAL FOOD LAWS

As covered in greater detail in Wu and Rodricks (2020), the history of food safety regulation in the United States had a dramatic beginning over 100 years ago. Even before the Pure Food and Drug Act and the Meat Inspection Act were created in 1906, food workers and the general public were concerned about harmful food working conditions and unlabeled additives in foods. Then in 1906, Upton Sinclair's novel *The Jungle* was published, which highlighted the horrors of US meat operations: both in terms of worker unsafety and meat contamination. *The Jungle* helped catalyze the 1906 Pure Food and Drug Act, which prohibited trade of adulterated food and drugs, and required accurate labels on both. This act was enforced by the US Department of Agriculture's (USDA) Bureau of Chemistry, which became the FDA in 1930.

For the first time, the 1906 law required consideration of human health risks associated with chemicals that might be intentionally or unintentionally introduced into food through the revolutions in chemistry and chemical manufacturing of the late 19th century. Additionally, under this law, the government could take action against a substance it considered harmful only if it could demonstrate harm: the burden of proof of harm rested upon the government.

To take the process of foodborne chemical risk assessment further, in 1949, FDA published a report *Procedures for the Appraisal of the Toxicity of Chemicals in Food* (Lehman et al. 1955). This report introduced the notion of an acceptable (or allowable) daily intake (ADI) for chemicals introduced into food (such as flavors, preservatives, and colors), calculated using "safety factors" applied to toxicity findings in animal studies. These animal studies consisted of experiments in which laboratory animals received different doses of a food chemical, with the goal of determining the highest dose that caused no harmful effects in the animals (the No-Observed Adverse Effect Level, or NOAEL), and then dividing this dose by safety factors to arrive at a safe concentration for humans in the foodstuff.

Notably, this approach to determining a safe level of food additives (or contaminants) in human food relies on a concept stated by the 16th-century "Father of Toxicology" Paracelsus, who stated that anything can become toxic at a sufficiently high dose, but can be harmless at low doses. Thus arose the *threshold* hypothesis, adopted by those who began the systematic study of toxicity in the 20th century, and also the FDA approach to establishing safe intakes (ADIs) for food chemicals. A threshold is a dose of a chemical, below which it is assumed that there is no human health risk but above which, there may be some risk. This threshold is determined by dividing the NOAEL by safety factors as described in the previous paragraph. In somewhat modified form, but with one important exception to be described, this approach is still used by food safety regulators around the world (Wu and Rodricks 2020).

A challenge to this notion of a threshold arose in the 1950s with respect to any chemical that could cause cancer in humans. Congressman James Delaney of New York, who directed the House Select Committee to Investigate the Use of Chemicals in Food Products, held food safety hearings that focused on chemicals and passed amendments that altered food safety laws. Importantly, the "Delaney Clause" stated that FDA would not approve for use in food any chemical found to cause cancer in humans or animals (Food, Drug, and Cosmetic Act Section 409©). In other words, the previously described notion of a safe threshold was (and is) not used in the context of any chemical that might cause cancer.

Additionally, the amendments placed the burden of showing the safety of a foodborne chemical on the company seeking to introduce it into food. This applies to indirectly introduced chemicals as well: chemicals migrating from food contact materials, pesticide residues, and veterinary drugs used in livestock that become human food. The safety standard in the law is "reasonable certainty of no harm." The FDA considers intakes of a chemical at or less than its ADI to satisfy this standard. Food contaminants, on the other hand, described as "unavoidable" (meaning not present because of an intentional act of adulteration), are treated differently: the burden of demonstrating an unacceptable risk requiring regulation rests upon the government. Considerations of technical limitations associated with attempts to mitigate such risks can be considered in decisions to limit exposures.

A BRIEF SUMMARY OF FOOD SAFETY RISK ASSESSMENT

The approaches to risk assessment described throughout this book are also applied to food constituents and contaminants. In most cases, animal studies are used to study the adverse effects of chemicals, although in some cases, observational studies on human populations are available.

1. The safe level of intake for a food chemical is referred to as the ADI, expressed as weight of chemical per unit of body weight. The ADI is expected to be without significant health risk over a lifetime of exposure.

2. Risk assessment is used to derive the ADI for a specific substance. All of the hazardous properties of a substance (its toxicities) are reviewed and tabulated, and that occurring at the lowest dose (the most sensitive indicator of toxicity) is used as the critical effect for ADI development.

3. Generally, a NOAEL is identified in the study in which the critical effect is identified. The NOAEL is divided by one or more Uncertainty Factors (UFs) to account for expected variabilities in responses within the human population and between humans and animals. Other uncertainties in the data may result in the use of other UFs.

4. The ADI is generally a very small fraction of the NOAEL (it is far below any observable toxic dose).

5. If cancer is the toxicity of concern, laws such as the Delaney Clause, applicable to intentionally introduced food substances, will generally override any scientific considerations, and the additive will not be allowed at any level of addition. This clause is found only in US food law, but other countries often follow the same policy. In many cases, non-genotoxic carcinogens are treated as threshold agents, although substantial evidence to support a threshold will be required.

6. Carcinogens not subject to the Delaney Clause may sometimes be allowed if its risks are found to be tolerably small, generally in the range of 10^{-5} to 10^{-6} lifetime probabilities of cancer or less.

7. Carcinogenic contaminants are often not readily eliminated or readily controllable, and risk management models that include a determination of the maximum technically achievable risk reduction are used to guide regulatory decisions.

THE MODERN FOOD SUPPLY

The food we buy in grocery stores today is vastly different from what was available a century ago, and certainly in the centuries prior to the last. In very broad terms, in the United States, food production has increased enormously (all of meat, grains, and produce), food additives and contaminants are regulated by FDA, packaging has helped to preserve the freshness and shelf lives of various foods, refrigeration and freezing have reduced the risk of microbial pathogen contamination and food spoilage more generally, and there are novel concerns regarding agricultural chemical and veterinary medicine residues in food. Many of these topics will be dealt with in greater detail in this chapter.

From a broader perspective, food supply chains themselves have changed dramatically since a century ago and earlier. The number of "actors" in the food supply chain between the producers and the consumers has increased. There are relatively few Americans today who are completely self-sufficient in food production. Now, most food is mass-produced at the level of farms, which frequently specialize in just one or a few types of crops or animals (corn, apples, beef cattle, chickens, etc.). Oftentimes, when just one crop is produced year after year on a farm, the system is referred to as a "monoculture." These farmers then bring their crops or animals to various different processors, whether grain elevators or handlers or slaughterhouses, which will process the foodstuffs and may send these processed foods to other sites for further processing (e.g., a grain elevator will send grain to millers, companies manufacturing grain-based snacks or staples, flour producers). After substantial food processing, which often includes a packaging component, the foods are then distributed to grocery stores, convenience stores, restaurants, cafeterias and dining halls, and other venues for food distribution across the country. Finally, consumers can purchase the food.

Most of the food purchased by Americans undergoes at least five separate steps in the food supply chain: the producers, the handlers, the processors, the grocery stores or other distributors, and then the consumers. In some settings, such as farmers' markets or other localized markets, there may be just two or three steps: the producers and the consumers (with a possible processor in between).

Oftentimes, in the popular media, processed food is generalized as having undesirable qualities; for example, some foods might be bleached or stripped of fiber, or have sugar and salt added in large quantities. However, food processing can often improve food safety. Drying and cold and/or dry storage can reduce the risk of microbial pathogens and food spoilage. Processes such as extrusion, used to make corn grits or flakes out of milled corn, can reduce mycotoxin concentrations, while nixtamalization – soaking corn in a calcium carbonate solution for masa production – can also reduce mycotoxins and increase the bioavailability of niacin (Khlangwiset and Wu 2010).

Importantly, the Food Safety Modernization Act (FSMA), signed into law by President Barack Obama in 2011, sets regulations across the food supply chain to test for and reduce the risk of contaminants (FDA 2017). FSMA improves US food safety along several metrics: prevention of contamination, inspection and compliance of food supply chain actors, responses to contaminants and violations, and additional information requested on imported goods. The next several sections give greater detail on some of the items covered by FSMA and other food safety laws to protect US consumers.

FOOD ADDITIVES: THE EXAMPLE OF NON-NUTRITIVE SWEETENERS

No substance can be intentionally introduced into food unless it has been shown to have a technical function in the food and unless the estimated daily intake (EDI) resulting from its use is less than its ADI. In the United States, the FDA makes food additive approvals after the agency has received and reviewed a food additive petition (FAP) from the additive's sponsor. The FAP will contain all information necessary to verify an ADI and an EDI, and additional information pertaining to the purity of the additive, the methods of manufacture necessary to achieve required purity, and the analytical methods to be used to verify its presence in food at approved levels.

A number of substances have been approved for use in food as non-nutritive sweeteners (NNS). They impart sweetness but have no nutritional value and do not contribute calories, but sweetness is considered an allowable technical effect. The first of these to come into wide use was saccharin, a synthetic chemical discovered at the Johns Hopkins University in 1879 and found to be several hundred times sweeter than sucrose (table sugar). Saccharin was in wide use until the 1970s, when studies in laboratory rats demonstrated that the compound could, at extremely high doses, induce bladder cancers. The uses of saccharin virtually disappeared until the year 2000, when scientists from an arm of the National Institutes of Health (NIH) completed evaluations of a large number of human, animal, and mechanistic studies and found that the bladder cancer findings were almost certainly restricted to rats and to the extraordinarily high doses used in that study.

Saccharin uses are permitted, but a number of new substances, considered by regulatory authorities to have adequate safety characteristics, and having taste profiles superior to that of saccharin, have come into use. Among these are aspartame, acesulfame potassium, sucralose, and neotame. Each has its own commercial name.

These NNS were approved in the United States on the basis of information submitted by manufacturers in FAPs. Approvals rested on findings that the toxicology data were sufficient to establish ADIs, and the EDIs from all uses were less than the ADIs. The ADIs for some of these NNS are listed in Table 3.2. The EFSA has also established ADIs for these substances, also shown in Table 3.2.

The Joint Expert Committee on Food Additives (JECFA) of the World Health Organization and the Food and Agriculture Organization has evaluated all of these NNS (as well as hundreds of other food additives). JECFA has found these uses of NNS to be safe, and their evaluations are

Table 3.2: Comparison of ADIs for the United States and Europe

Non-Nutritive Sweetener	ADI (USFDA)*	ADI (EFSA)
Aspartame	50	40
Sucralose	5	5
Acesulfame-K	15	9

*mg/kg of body weight/day

used by the Codex Alimentarius Commission to support standards that are generally accepted by the 188 member states of the Commission.

There is some level of scientific controversy associated with all of these (and other) NNS. Much of the controversy relates to evidence that these substances may disrupt metabolic processes and thereby interfere with blood sugar and appetite control. Recently, some experiments have suggested that interactions of these additives with the gut microbiome may be a pathway to these effects. These matters remain under investigation in many research centers, but no regulatory body has considered the evidence to be sufficient to raise safety concerns.

There are more than 100 substances regulated as food additives, but many hundreds of others are regulated as GRAS substances (next section). The food additives have been the subjects of FAPs, submitted since 1958, following congressional approval of the various amendments to US food law discussed earlier. Some of the approved food additives are actually food contact materials and other so-called indirect food additives, substances indirectly becoming components of food because they are used in materials contacting foods and have the capacity to migrate from the contact materials into foods. Such indirect additives are required to meet the same safety standards as those required for direct food additives.

One final note concerning food additives pertains to those used to color foods (color additives). This class of additive is required to meet the same safety standards as required for other food additives, submitted to the FDA in a Color Additive Petition.

An additional requirement – certification of purity on a batch-by-batch basis by the FDA – is a necessary condition of approval for all synthetic colors. Color additives illustrate one additional feature of carcinogen risk management. Color additives that have been adequately tested and show no evidence of carcinogenicity are, if otherwise safe, allowed to be used in foods. But some such colors have been found to contain, presumably as residues from synthesis, trace amounts of known carcinogens. FD&C Green No.6 (FD&C indicates certification by the FDA), a well-tested and noncarcinogenic color, has been found to contain trace amounts of p-toluidine, a known animal carcinogen. The FDA has found the lifetime risk from p-toluidine to be less than 10^{-6} and has concluded that this risk is so small as to not warrant banning the use of the color additive. This use of risk assessment for decisions regarding trace contaminants of food ingredients is applied in a number of situations, not only to decisions about migrants from food contact materials.

GRAS SUBSTANCES

Under US federal law, some additives may meet the criteria for what are called GRAS substances. Substances having a documented history of safe use in food prior to the enactment of the new food additive amendments in 1958 were defined as GRAS. The lawmakers decided that there was no need to subject such substances to the animal testing requirements for new food additives. Moreover, the laws allowed experts in food safety (the authors of this chapter, for example), and not only the experts at the FDA, to judge whether a substance could be considered GRAS. The GRAS system remains in effect in the US, and most additives are allowed because they are considered to be GRAS. Even substances that have not had a long history of safe use can be considered GRAS if they are shown to be safe (as judged by any qualified scientist) after new testing. New evidence that a GRAS substance may no longer be safe is sufficient to end its use.

GRAS substances include a very wide range of the substances found in foods, including spices, natural flavoring agents, and substances such as caffeine, caramel, acetic acid, methyl cellulose, guar gum, lecithin, and hundreds more. It should be noted that a number of consumer advocacy groups contend that FDA's GRAS program has insufficient oversight of the safety of GRAS substances and have mounted substantial efforts with the goal of modifying the GRAS program. Note also that the GRAS system exists in no country except the United States.

VETERINARY DRUG RESIDUES

Use of drugs in animals that are sources of human food (meat, milk, eggs, fish, honey) may result in residues of those drugs or their metabolites in food. These drugs are, in a sense, another class of indirect food additives. Approvals for their uses, granted by the USFDA, require demonstrations of safety of the same types required for other additives. It is recognized that these veterinary drugs may be increasingly important to keeping livestock and poultry species healthy for the future of animal-source foods in global diets (NRC 2015), yet the presence of these drug residues in human food must be carefully controlled.

In many cases, the levels of drug residues present in edible products will exceed ADIs, and studies must be undertaken to learn how long it takes for residues to deplete to safe levels. Such studies will be used to establish times after drug administration (withdrawal times) when animal products can be safely consumed.

Among the more important uses of veterinary drugs in food-producing animals are those involving hormone implants used to enhance animal growth. The most significant such issue involved the use of the synthetic estrogen, diethylstilbestrol (DES), which was banned by the FDA in 1980 after 30 years of use. Use of other hormones is allowed, but with very strict limits; few concerns with those uses have been raised in recent times since it has been learned that the use of growth-promoting implants appears to have an extremely small effect on background levels of natural hormones.

SUBSTANCES FORMED BY PROCESSING

The use of heat in the processing and preparation of foods, as well as smoking and other processes, results in numerous chemical changes. A number of important carcinogens, such as polycyclic aromatic hydrocarbons (PAHs), which form when any type of organic matter is burned; N-nitrosamines; and the animal carcinogen acrylamide are some of the food constituents in this category. There are many studies of their risks, and efforts to find ways to reduce their occurrence. In some ways, such substances may be considered natural constituents of food, because the food preparation processes that produce them have been in use for millennia. Although these substances are not, strictly speaking, "contaminants" of food, they present difficult risk management challenges similar to those presented by contaminants (next section). No ideal risk management approach has yet been identified to deal with such substances (http://www.food.gov.uk).

CROP PROTECTION CHEMICALS

Use of pesticides in food production, regulated in the US by the Environmental Protection Agency (EPA), is allowed if food residues are determined to be safe. (Other safety issues, such as those relating to workers involved in pesticide application, and a variety of environmental risk issues, also need to be considered in pesticide approvals.)

Many pesticides, such as DDT and other chlorinated organics, were prohibited from use in the 1970s and 1980s because of safety concerns, in large part related to their chemical stability and long environmental persistence and bioaccumulation. Residues of some of those pesticides can still be found in fatty tissues and blood of humans and other animals. Early findings of the persistence and bioaccumulation of these pesticides drove concerns about a number of environmental pollutants that have been found to be important food contaminants (see next section).

FOOD CONTAMINANTS OF INDUSTRIAL ORIGIN – THE ORGANICS

A number of important products of the chemical industry, produced to serve a wide variety of industrial functions, have, for a variety of reasons, come to be widespread environmental contaminants, including contaminants of elements of the food supply. Perhaps the first of these to gain prominence were members of the class of polychlorinated biphenyls (PCBs). The class that includes dozens of PCB isomers was used as very effective dielectric fluids for capacitors and transformers, and by the 1960s were in very wide use. Early thinking about these uses suggested that the PCBs would be well contained and not capable of escaping to the environment. But this thinking turned out to be overly optimistic, and by the 1970s, PCB contamination of the environment – water systems and the fish contained in them – was clearly quite widespread. These chemicals shared many of the physical characteristics of the chlorinated pesticides (stability, persistence, bioaccumulation) and a variety of toxicities, and many actions have been taken by regulatory agencies around the world to limit consumption of PCB-contaminated fish. In parallel with concerns about PCBs arose concerns about similarly persistent and toxic polychlorinated dioxins, which arose as by-products of certain industrial processes, including those used to produce the herbicide that came to be known as Agent Orange, widely used in Vietnam during the war.

At present, another class of polyhalogenated compounds, known as polyfluoroalkyl substances (PFAS), is at the center of attention. The carbon-fluorine bond is stronger than the carbon-chlorine bond, so PFAS compounds are more persistent than chlorinated hydrocarbons. Many PFAS compounds degrade very slowly in the environment and are probably the most persistent organic contaminants of the environment (excluding heavy metals, which do not degrade at all).

In addition to a variety of industrial uses, including use in firefighting foams, PFAS compounds have been widely used in nonstick, stain-resistant, waterproof, and oil-resistant consumer products because of the hydrophobic and lipophobic properties of the PFAS molecules. These uses have included uses in food contact paper and paperboard (e.g., popcorn bags and pizza boxes) (Schaider et al. 2017). Because of the long residence times in the human body of the longer-chain PFAS, resistance to degradation in the environment, extensive worldwide dispersion, and concern for possible toxicity, major US manufacturers in cooperation with the US EPA have phased out production of the longer-chain PFAS, and EPA has taken action under the Toxic Substances Control Act (TSCA) to restrict manufacture or importation of these substances (EPA 2017). Shorter-chain PFAS, which show lower toxicity and shorter residence times in the body but share resistance to chemical degradation like their longer-chain analogs, have replaced the longer-chain forms in many industrial and consumer product uses.

Because of these concerns, some manufacturers have also withdrawn use of some of these materials for food contact purposes, and FDA has withdrawn approval for some indirect food additive uses in paper and paperboard (81 FR 83672), but food contact uses continue to appear in food packaging and in food (Schaider et al. 2017). Whether coming from food packaging materials or other sources, exposure to PFAS via the diet has been well documented in various countries (Domingo and Nadal 2017).

Health effects associated with some members of this class of compounds include effects on fetal/infant development, the immune system, the liver, and cancer. Detailed information of the toxicology of PFAS has been reviewed by DeWitt (2015), and the toxicology of two of the best-studied PFAS, perfluorooctanoic acid (PFOA) and perfluorooctane sulfonate (PFOS), have been reviewed by US EPA (2016a, 2016b). Most of the health effects information has thus far had its source in animal studies. Epidemiology studies have been difficult to conduct, and results have not been definitive.

HEAVY METALS – FOOD CONTAMINANTS OF INDUSTRIAL AND NATURAL ORIGIN

Various heavy metals and metalloids that can cause harm to human health occur naturally in food, particularly in certain geographic regions worldwide and in certain foodstuffs. Among these are arsenic, cadmium, lead, and mercury. These are the four main heavy metals of concern in the US and global food supplies, and have recently come to the public's attention because they were found at high levels in infant food pulled off grocery shelves in 2021 (Pilet 2021). Each of these will be described briefly, including the foods that are likely to contain these metals.

Arsenic is a naturally occurring metalloid that is found in both organic and inorganic forms. While isolated industrial sources provide significant exposures, the vast majority of individuals are chronically exposed to arsenic by ingestion of contaminated food or drinking water. Though the majority of human arsenic exposure is through drinking water, naturally occurring levels of arsenic in vegetables, grains, meats, and fish, as well as through food processed with water containing arsenic (e.g., cooking rice) presents a significant exposure affecting many millions of individuals worldwide (Oberoi et al. 2014). It is unlikely that there are individuals who are not exposed to some level of arsenic in food. However, the extent of human exposure to toxic forms of arsenicals in foods is difficult to estimate and highly variable due to the natural distribution of arsenic in soils and water. It is important to note that organic arsenicals found in seafood and food products from seaweed are inert and nontoxic.

Inorganic arsenic exposure causes multiple adverse health effects – both cancerous and non-cancerous effects – in humans. The International Agency for Research on Cancer (IARC) has concluded that arsenic in drinking water causes skin, bladder, and lung cancer, and that there is limited evidence of its causing kidney, liver, and prostate cancer (Straif et al. 2009). Oberoi et al. (2014) estimated that foodborne arsenic can account for over 100,000 lung, skin, and bladder cases per year. IARC has classified arsenic as a Group 1 carcinogen. Hypertension, myocardial infarction and ischemic disease, hyperkeratosis, peripheral vascular disease, and respiratory disease (Parvez et al. 2010) are the most common noncancer diseases (Chen et al. 2011; Parvez et al. 2010).

Multiple different foods can contain trace amounts of arsenic. These include rice, cereal grains, vegetables, pulses, meats, and seafood (primarily nontoxic organic arsenic in seafood). Crops and vegetables are more likely to have high arsenic levels if planted in soil that has high naturally occurring arsenic concentrations, or if arsenical pesticides were used on the land in the past. In the United States, this includes Maine, New Hampshire, Minnesota, Nevada (sites.dartmouth.edu/arsenicandyou/locations-with-higher-risk-of-arsenic-exposure/), and Louisiana (a site of arsenical pesticides applied to cotton in the 1800s; now growing rice). Worldwide, populations in South Asia, especially Bangladesh, have suffered high rates of arsenic-induced disease as a result of naturally high arsenic levels in the water. If food crops are irrigated with or cooked in this water, arsenic can migrate into the food.

Cadmium is both naturally occurring in soils, particularly from volcanic ash and an industrial by-product, from zinc oxide extractions and in products such as nickel-cadmium batteries and glazing for ceramics, glass, plastics, and metals (Rodricks et al. 2020). Foods that have higher levels of cadmium contamination include rice, cereal grains, seafood, meat, and leafy green vegetables. The amount of cadmium absorbed from food is relatively low compared with inhalation of cadmium (in mine tailings, smelting, and coal combustion). Although cadmium exposure has been linked to reduced kidney function as measured by reduced glomerular filtration rates, it was found in a recent study to cause at most only 0.2% of the global burden of chronic kidney disease (Zang et al. 2019). Cadmium toxicity is not considered to be high, and foodborne exposures are relatively lower than inhalation exposures.

Lead is well-known to cause neurotoxic effects in humans, including cognitive impairment as measured by decrements in IQ and other cognitive test scores (Carrington et al. 2019). Humans can be exposed to lead through inhalation or through ingestion of contaminated food or water. The waterborne route of lead exposure is more well-known in recent history: since 2014, lead contamination in drinking water in Flint, Michigan, has been linked to multiple adverse health effects, including skin rashes (Hana-Attisha et al. 2016).

In food, however, lead exposure has decreased substantially since the 1970s, as lead was phased out of soldering in cans. In this decade and the next, lead was also phased out of gasoline, as human studies found increasing evidence of lead's harmful neurocognitive effects (Needleman 1981). Indeed, a recent JECFA (2010) report determined that there was no safe dose of lead in food that would not cause harmful effects in humans. In the United States, however, a recent market basket survey conducted by FDA (2016), the Total Diet Study, found that less than 12% of foods collected in grocery stores across the nation were found to have detectable lead (Rodricks et al. 2020).

Mercury, or specifically *methylmercury*, found in foods, is similar to lead in its neurotoxicological effects that can lead to cognitive deficits (Bellinger et al. 2019). Methylmercury, which is the organic form of the metal mercury, is frequently found in seafood as a result of land-based pollution going into bodies of water. Because the risk seems to be highest for fetuses and young children, a recent systematic review has recommended that policies be taken to reduce maternal and child exposures to methylmercury in seafood (Sheehan et al. 2014). However, a conundrum is that seafood is frequently an important source of omega-3 fatty acids in the diet, which themselves promote neurocognitive health, so the risk of methylmercury must be weighed against the benefits to children of omega-3 fatty acid intake. This is why FDA, among other institutions, provides guidance documents emphasizing this benefit-risk trade-off and suggests fish that have lower methylmercury levels, particularly for pregnant women (www.fda.gov/food/consumers/advice-about-eating-fish). Generally, methylmercury levels are higher in fish "higher in the food chain" – those that are larger and consume smaller fish, thus bioaccumulating mercury.

The FDA has identified food safety as an area in which innovations in regulatory science are critical, particularly to address some of the heavy metal issues as described in this section (FDA 2010). Notably, regulation of foodborne chemicals and toxins does not adequately account for the risks to American consumers. On February 4, 2021, a US congressional investigation reported that dangerous levels of arsenic, cadmium, lead, and mercury were present in baby foods produced by seven leading manufacturers of both organic and conventional products. Moreover, the investigation found that no maximum levels have been established by FDA for these toxic metals in baby foods (US House of Representatives 2021). More policy work is needed to ensure US consumer safety in this area.

FOOD ALLERGIES AND INTOLERANCES

Many people are allergic (or hypersensitive) to certain food and food ingredients. In most cases, the reaction is immediate and reversible, but delayed-onset allergies also occur. These reactions involve the immune system, and a prior exposure to the allergenic agent is required to precipitate an event. Immunoglobins are typically involved, and reactions can be cutaneous (hives, dermatitis, rash), gastrointestinal (nausea, vomiting, diarrhea), or respiratory (asthma, wheezing, rhinitis) (Doull, 1081). Anaphylactic shock and death can also occur. Many foods have been reported to be allergenic, although the majority of cases involve peanuts and tree nuts, milk, fish, and shellfish. It appears that most allergic agents in food are large molecular weight glycoproteins, although closely related foods with similar proteins do not all cause allergies. The reaction is highly individualized and is not similar to the toxic responses described earlier. In recent years, there has been much public discussion about wheat gluten allergies, but there are many others. There is no available risk model to establish safe intake levels for individuals who are hypersensitive, and reactions are avoidable only by avoiding foods that are sources of the allergen.

Some types of genetic predisposition may lead to certain forms of food intolerance in individuals; these may resemble allergic reactions, but they are not immune mediated. In many cases, individuals lack certain enzymes necessary for the normal metabolism of food ingredients. Lactose intolerance, for example, results from the lack of the enzyme lactase, and this lack leads to excessive lactose accumulation in the bowel. Microbial fermentation of lactose in the bowel has an osmotic effect, leading to malabsorption and diarrhea. Lactose intolerance affects only a few percent of the population in Northern Europe but reaches 90% in Southern Italy and nearly 100% in Southeast Asia. Many people of African descent also have this intolerance. Other intolerances include those to fava bean (favism), chocolate (migraine), and red wine (similar to allergic reactions). "Asian flush syndrome" is seen in many Asians after alcohol consumption. No risk model is available to develop safe intake levels for people who experience these idiosyncratic reactions.

There are other categories of unusual reactions to certain foods, including anaphylaxis related to histamine content. Food-drug interactions of different kinds are not uncommon, and drug labeling is needed to warn people about them (such as warnings against grapefruit consumption for many drugs). Allergic and idiosyncratic reactions to certain foods and food constituents are unfortunately not manageable except by the individuals who are susceptible to them. Public health and regulatory authorities can only educate and provide warnings.

MYCOTOXINS

Mycotoxins are toxins produced by fungi, or molds, that colonize food, either in the field or in food storage conditions. Since the Middle Ages, mycotoxin poisoning in humans has been documented, although the cause was unknown at the time. Medieval European populations suffered frequent bouts of "St. Anthony's Fire" – a disease associated with hallucinations and eventual necrotizing of the fingers and toes and other extremities – which is now known to be caused by ergot alkaloids produced by the fungus *Claviceps purpurea* in rye (CAST 2003).

Aflatoxins, the first groups of mycotoxins to be identified in 1960, were discovered in moldy peanut meal in the United Kingdom, which led to the deaths of over 100,000 turkey poults (Kensler et al. 2011). Since that time, dozens of mycotoxins have been identified and characterized for toxicity and foodstuffs at risk of contamination. Of these, aflatoxins, fumonisins, deoxynivalenol (DON, vomitoxin), zearalenone, and ochratoxin A (OTA) are considered the most agriculturally important. In brief, Table 3.3 lists these major mycotoxin groups, the fungi that produce them, the crops in which they are found, and the known or postulated human health effects (Miller 1995; Kensler et al. 2011; Bulder et al. 2012; Wu et al. 2014a).

Food safety regulations on mycotoxins have had significant economic and trade impacts, although it is unclear whether there have been significant public health impacts. Several studies (Bui-Klimke et al. 2014; Wu 2008; Wu and Guclu 2012) found that aflatoxin regulations in pistachios, almonds, and maize have largely caused nations to shift trading partners, with stricter nations importing more from selected nations and nations with relaxed or no regulations against aflatoxin importing more highly contaminated foods. Likewise, OTA regulations may result in heavy economic losses to grain producing nations with not much health benefit (Wu et al. 2014b). Chen et al. (2019, 2021) found that even with currently existing DON regulations, many nations have DON exposures exceeding JECFA tolerable daily intakes, and even with a relatively new United Nations (UN) Codex Alimentarius Commission guidelines for DON in cereal grains, there may not be much motivation for UN member states to adopt these guidelines.

Table 3.3: **Major Mycotoxin Groups, the Fungi That Produce Them, the Crops in which They Are Found**

Mycotoxin Group	Fungi That Produce the Mycotoxin(s)	Foods Containing the Mycotoxin	Human Health Effects
Aflatoxins	*Aspergillus flavus, A. parasiticus*	Maize, peanuts, tree nuts, oilseeds	Liver cancer, immune system dysfunction, child growth impairment, acute aflatoxicosis
Fumonisins	*Fusarium verticillioides, F. proliferatum*	Maize	Postulated: neural tube defects in babies, esophageal cancer
Deoxynivalenol	*F. graminearum, F. culmorum*	Maize, wheat, barley, oats	Gastrointestinal illness, immune system dysfunction
Zearalenone	*F. graminearum, F. culmorum*	Maize, wheat, barley, oats	Estrogenic effects
Ochratoxin A	*Penicillium verrucosum, A. ochraceus*	Maize, wheat, barley, oats, coffee, tree nuts, chocolate, pork, grapes	Postulated: kidney disease

MICROBIAL PATHOGENS

Potential microbial pathogens in food include diverse bacteria, viruses, and protozoan parasites that can cause gastrointestinal illness and other adverse health effects in humans. About 1 in 10 people around the world each year become ill from food poisoning; mostly from microbial pathogens in food, which in immunocompetent persons may mean several days of gastrointestinal illness followed by complete recovery. However, in immunocompromised individuals, which can include the elderly and very young children, foodborne pathogens can increase the risk of death. In fact, food contamination is estimated to cause 420,000 deaths annually worldwide, one-third of which are in young children (under age 5 years). Diarrheal diseases are the largest cause of foodborne disease (can lead to death through dehydration and/or nutrient/weight loss). These diseases are caused primarily by the bacteria nontyphoidal *Salmonella enterica, S. typhi, E. coli*, and *Campylobacter*, as well as the virus norovirus, in food. Among parasites and chemicals/toxins, *Taenia solium* (pork tapeworm) and aflatoxin (mycotoxin produced by *Aspergillus* fungi in maize and nuts) caused the greatest disease burdens for their respective categories (Havelaar et al. 2015; WHO 2015).

In the United States, the Centers for Disease Control and Prevention (CDC) recently estimated that 31 foodborne pathogens cause about 9.4 million cases of food poisoning each year (Scallan et al. 2011). Interestingly, in the United States, as well as around the world, nontyphoidal *Salmonella enterica* is the bacterium causing the greatest number of foodborne disease cases: estimated at slightly over one million per year in the United States. The bacteria *Clostridium perfringens* and *Campylobacter* spp. follow. However, norovirus causes the greatest number of foodborne disease cases in the United States among all pathogens: about 5.5 million cases around the United States annually.

Although quantitative chemical risk assessment methods were systematized in *The Red Book* of the National Academies in 1983 (NRC 1983) and shared earlier in this chapter, quantitative *microbial* risk assessment (QMRA) is more complex for many reasons (Wu and Rodricks 2020). It is far more difficult to arrive at set "doses" of pathogens encountered in food if they are alive and growing in count: a very different situation from chemicals. The rate at which they multiply, if at all, in a food depends on multiple conditions, such as the food substrate itself, temperature, humidity, nutrients, and various other factors. Additionally, exposure models must account for pathogen growth and/or deactivation in different media. For a comprehensive primer on QMRA for food and water, the reader is referred to the USDA/EPA Interagency Microbiological Risk Assessment Guideline Workgroup (USDA/EPA 2012).

GENETICALLY MODIFIED ORGANISMS, AGRICULTURAL BIOTECHNOLOGY, AND FOOD SAFETY

Genetically modified organisms (GMOs) have received much media attention, largely negative, since their first planting in the United States and in other parts of the world in 1996. GMOs can be defined as organisms (usually crop plants) in which transgenes – genes from different species – are inserted into the genome of the host, such that the host is able to produce novel proteins for specific purposes. The major GMOs planted in the United States today include herbicide tolerant crops such as glyphosate-resistant soybean and corn and Bt crops that produce their own insecticides such as corn and cotton. Additionally, transgenic (GM) papaya is planted in Hawaii to prevent ringspot virus disease.

Three agencies oversee the safety evaluations of GMOs and other products of agricultural biotechnology in the United States. The 1986 Coordinated Framework for Regulation of Biotechnology, amended in 2017, held that existing federal statutes were sufficient to oversee biotechnology regulation, and designated the following responsibilities: the USDA to oversee agricultural and ecological risks, the US EPA to assess risks to human health and the environment of GMOs that produce pesticides, and the FDA to assess food safety risks. In 1992, FDA granted GMOs the status of GRAS, which meant that these foods were not required to undergo additional analyses with the FDA unless there was a claim of a nutritional or health benefit (57 *Federal Register* 22991). However, FDA has a voluntary consultation program for biotech foods that assesses the potential for toxicity or allergenicity and determines whether the biotech food has a significantly different nutritional profile from the conventionally produced food (Wu and Rodricks 2020). The EPA along with FDA assesses potential food safety/human health risks only of GMOs that produce pesticides in terms of toxicity, carcinogenicity, allergenicity, mutagenicity, teratogenicity, and oncogenicity, and evaluates environmental risks such as gene flow, impact to nontarget organisms, and evolution of insect resistance (US EPA 2001).

To date, no food safety concerns have arisen with any of the GMOs planted around the world. Interestingly, there may in fact be certain food safety benefits. For example, Bt corn, one of the most common transgenic crops worldwide, produces proteins that control certain insect pests. Because Bt corn suffers less insect pest damage than non-Bt isolines, farmers who plant it have experience increases in yields (Morel et al. 2002; Fernandez-Cornejo et al. 2014). Additionally, Perry et al. (2016) estimated that Bt corn planting in lieu of non-Bt corn has decreased insecticide use by over 10%, which means lower chemical exposures for farmworkers and lower pesticide residues in food for consumers. Importantly, because less insect pest damage means lower fungal infection risk, Bt corn has also been found to have lower mycotoxin levels than non-Bt isolines. Multiple field studies in the United States show lower fumonisin levels in Bt corn (Munkvold et al. 1999; Wu 2007; Weaver et al. 2017). In an analysis of aflatoxin-related insurance claims filed by corn growers, it was found that Bt corn planting correlates to lower aflatoxin risk, even when controlling for climatic factors and other grower practices (Yu et al. 2020).

In the case of glyphosate-tolerant crops, the total economic, environmental, and human health risks may be lower than if alternative herbicides were used (Ye et al. 2021). Relatively newer agricultural biotechnology methods applied to crops such as RNA interference (RNAi) and CRISPR (gene editing technologies) would further eliminate concerns of allergenicity – as no new protein is produced – and may hold promise for improvements in food safety and nutrition.

Of important recent news, the government of the Philippines approved, on July 21, 2021, the cultivation of the transgenic crop Golden Rice (https://www.philrice.gov.ph/filipinos-soon-to-plant-and-eat-golden-rice). Golden Rice has been under development for two decades: first modified with daffodil genes, and then corn genes in the modern varieties, to produce beta-carotene: the precursor to vitamin A. Golden Rice is meant to be cultivated in regions of the world where vitamin A deficiency currently causes blindness, increased risk of infectious diseases, and diarrheal deaths in children (Stevens et al. 2015). Although Golden Rice has been approved for human consumption by governments in many nations, the Philippines is the first nation to approve its cultivation in the field.

FUTURE DIRECTIONS

Although this chapter covers multiple chemicals (and to a lesser extent, microbes) that could be present in food, there are likely to be hundreds if not thousands of chemicals in food that have not yet been identified. Therefore, their health effects are as of yet unknown. At the same time, there are many aspects of human health and disease that remain unknown, such as the causes of some diseases, and the determinants of overall good health and recovery from disease. It is possible – and exciting to consider – that future generations of food scientists will discover these constituents of food that play an important role in human health and will have a range of new technologies and methods by which to elucidate food safety's challenges.

Generally, data from toxicology studies in mammalian species are limited to the oral route of exposure and indicate that glyphosate has limited toxicity at physiologically relevant exposure

BOX 3.1   RISK OF PESTICIDES IN THE ENVIRONMENT

Wattasit Siriwong

Pesticides are extensively used on agricultural land, in private gardens, along railways, highways, and in other public areas. The use of pesticides for crop protection is expected to increase based on a growing world population and the need for more food supplies. Over the last two centuries, chemicals have come to dominate human efforts at pest control and dramatically changed in 1939 after Paul Muller, a Swiss chemist, found a synthetic compound synthesized "Dichlorodiphenyltrichloroethane or DDT." It was an effective insecticide while boasting low mammalian toxicity and widely used during World War II and used in many parts of the world for vector control, particularly for malaria and other mosquito-borne diseases. While DDT and other chlorinated pesticides increase agricultural production, bioaccumulation and biomagnification through the food chain eventually became a risk to mammals and induce certain negative adverse health effects in humans such as neurobehavior, developmental, endocrine, and reproductive effects. These adverse effects were documented in Rachel Carson's book *Silent Spring*. Carson, a naturalist who loved to hear the songs of birds in the spring used the title because she envisioned a spring in which there would be no bird songs due to the loss of songbirds that followed DDT-induced thinning of eggshells. Carson argued that humankind was fatally tampering with nature by its reckless misuse of chemical pesticides, particularly the ubiquitous new wonder chemical DDT. Chlorinated hydrocarbons and organic phosphorus insecticides silently altered the cellular processes of plants, animals, and possibly humans. Carson suggested that the long-term effects of these contaminants in soil, water, vegetation, birds, and wildlife were detrimental to the continuation of human life in which they should not be called 'insecticides' but 'biocides.' Research at Lake Apopka, Florida, following contamination of the lake by the organochlorine pesticides, dibromochloropropane, and ethylene dibromide, has shown marked changes in the alligator population, including decreased testosterone levels, smaller genitalia, and altered gender ratios in newborns, findings attributed to the effects of pesticides. Recent work has shown similar endocrine and reproductive effects in other animals, the observations of demasculinization of atrazine-exposed frogs suggest that triazine compounds may have endocrine-disrupting effects. Many contemporary studies on persistent pesticides in Southeast Asia showed there is a potential risk to the health of wildlife. Although all of the chlorinated pesticides have been banned for many years as in Thailand, there are detectable levels of persistent organic pollutants (POPs, see Table 1.1) compounds in water, groundwater, sediment, soil, and aquatic species such as plankton, fishes, snail, bird, and turtle eggs.

Organophosphate pesticides (OPs) are hazardous compounds in the environment. Acute toxicity of OPs includes inhibition of acetylcholinesterase, resulting in neurotoxicity. Several studies show noncancer risks could be induced by OP exposures. At the same time, exposure to OPs could also lead to some adverse effects on human reproduction, including spontaneous abortions and preterm, delayed neuro-development during childhood, and male reproductive disorders. In the fetus, rapid growth and development occur during early development. Developing organs are sensitive to toxic substances. The developing brain is susceptible to neurotoxicants. Increasing evidence suggests that prenatal pesticide exposure may have a permanent effect on children's behavior and intelligence.

Today, traditional agriculture has changed to modern intensive agriculture to ensure food security for the world population. In the year 2020, global pesticide use was estimated to increase up to 3.5 million tons. Approximately, two million tons of pesticides are used annually worldwide. The three largest users of pesticides in agriculture are China, the United States, and Argentina. Although pesticides are beneficial for crop production, extensive use of pesticides still poses serious consequences directly or indirectly polluted in air, water, soil and overall ecosystem as followed health hazard for human being. Accordingly, the ideal pesticide is needed both safe and effective in the matter of human and environmental health and effective at controlling the target species, quick acting, and degraded rapidly to harmless in the environment.

BOX 3.2 ROUNDUP

Suren Bandara

Glyphosate [N-(phosphonomethyl)glycine: CAS 1071-83-6] is a broad-spectrum nonselective herbicide first registered for use by the US EPA in 1974 (ATSDR 2019). Glyphosate and glyphosate-containing products (GCPs; e.g., Roundup®), when applied directly to plant foliage, disrupt the shikimic acid pathway (an enzyme pathway limited to the plant kingdom) through the inhibition of the enzyme 5-enolpyruvylshikimate-3-phosphate synthase, resulting in subsequent plant growth inhibition and death (Eck 2013). Taking advantage of this highly specific mode of action and advances in recombinant DNA technology, glyphosate-tolerant genetically engineered crops, including soybean, corn, cotton, and canola, were first introduced in the United States in 1996. Owing to their effectiveness as a weed killer and crop protectant, glyphosate and GCPs are now commonly used in agriculture and in households for weed control (IARC 2019). In fact, in the United States, glyphosate is ranked as the second most used pesticide/herbicide for the home and garden setting (IARC 2019).

While agricultural workers, their families, and individuals living near farmland are at higher risk for glyphosate exposure, glyphosate has become so ubiquitous in the environment that the herbicide is routinely detected in various biological samples, even in the general population, and in all major food categories, but at varying frequency and quantity (Gillezeau et al. 2019). Due to its popularity and extensive use, concerns regarding human and environmental health from glyphosate or GCPs have been raised.

What is our current understanding of glyphosate human health risk?

Although several human health concerns with glyphosate exposure have been raised (e.g., respiratory, circulatory, and cerebrovascular disease and reproductive health), the most notable is cancer. Specifically, epidemiological studies on glyphosate in agricultural workers, their family members, and commercial applicators have reported increased incidences of cancers, including hematopoietic cancers such as non-Hodgkin's lymphoma and lymphocytic lymphoma in these populations. However, major confounders, including exposure characterization, and the lack of an observed biological gradient (i.e., exposure-response relationship) in most studies limit the evidence for an association between glyphosate or GCP exposure and adverse health effects (including cancers) among occupationally exposed workers and their family members.

concentrations. In fact, when toxicity is noted, these occur at doses or formulations fed to animals that are orders of magnitude higher than human exposure to glyphosate from the diet. Additionally, it is important to highlight that there are limited data for toxicity following the dermal route of exposure which is arguably the most relevant exposure route for workers and home gardeners. Currently, there is limited reliable mechanism of action data to support carcinogenesis from exposure to glyphosate or GCPs.

Based on available data, the safety of glyphosate has been evaluated and re-evaluated using accepted methods, principles, and procedures in toxicology by many regulatory agencies both within the United States and internationally. Among these agencies, the US EPA in its most recent evaluation classified glyphosate as a Group D (i.e., not classifiable as to human carcinogenicity) chemical based on both the epidemiological and nonclinical evidence, and noted that there are "no risks to the public health from the current registered uses of glyphosate" (US EPA 2019). Conversely, the IARC in its own evaluation of the human data reported that there is "limited evidence" in humans for the carcinogenicity of glyphosate – and noted that a positive association was found for non-Hodgkin lymphoma but "sufficient evidence" for carcinogenicity in nonclinical study data, concluding that glyphosate is "probably carcinogenic to humans (Group 2A)" (IARC 2019: p. 78). The debates regarding the accuracy of each agency's conclusions and the future use of glyphosate or GCPs are ongoing.

REFERENCES

Bellinger, D. C., B. Devleesschauwer, K. O'Leary, and H. J. Gibb. 2019. Global Burden of Intellectual Disability Resulting from Prenatal Exposure to Methylmercury. *Environ Res* 170: 416–421.

Bui-Klimke, T. R., H. Guclu, T. W. Kensler, J-M. Yuan, and F. Wu. 2014. Aflatoxin Regulations and Global Pistachio Trade: Insights from a Social Network Analysis. *PLoS ONE* 9(3): e92149.

Bulder, A. S., D. Arcella, M. Bolger, C. Carrington, K. Kpodo, S. Resnik, R. T. Riley, G. Wolterink, and F. Wu. 2012. Fumonisins (Addendum). In *Safety Evaluation of Certain Food Additives and Contaminants*, Vol. 65: 325–794. Geneva, Switzerland: World Health Organization.

Carrington, C., B. Devleesschauwer, H. J. Gibb, and P. M. Bolger. 2019. Global Burden of Intellectual Disability Resulting from Dietary Exposure to Lead, 2015. *Environ Res* 172: 420–429.

CAST (Council for Agricultural Science & Technology). 2003. Mycotoxins: Risks in Plant, Animal, and Human Systems. Task Force Report R139, Ames, IA.

Chen, C., K. Frank, T. Wang, and F. Wu. 2021. Global Wheat Trade and Codex Alimentarius Guidelines for Deoxynivalenol: A Mycotoxin Common in Wheat. *Glob Food Sec* 29: 100538.

Chen, C., N. Saha Turna, and F. Wu. 2019. Risk Assessment of Dietary Deoxynivalenol Exposure in Wheat Products Worldwide: Are New Codex DON Guidelines Adequately Protective? *Trends Food Sci Technol* 89: 11–25.

Chen, Y., J. H. Graziano, F. Parvez, M. Liu, V. Slavkovich, T. Kalra, M. Argos, T. Islam, A. Ahmed, M. Rakibuz-Zaman, R. Hasan, G. Sarwar, D. Levy, A. van Geen, and H. Ahsan. 2011. Arsenic Exposure from Drinking Water and Mortality from Cardiovascular Disease in Bangladesh: Prospective Cohort Study. *BMJ* 342: d2431.

DeWitt, J. C. 2015. *Toxicological Effects of Perfluoroalkyl and Polyfluoroalkyl Substances*. Switzerland: Humana Press (Springer International Publishing).

Domingo, J. L., and M. Nadal. 2017. Per-and Polyfluoroalkyl Substances (PFASs) in Food and Human Dietary Intake: A Review of the Recent Scientific Literature. *J Agric Food Chem* 65(3): 533–543.

FDA. 2016. *2016 FDA Food Safety Survey*. Center for Food Safety and Applied Nutrition.

FDA. 2017. *Full Text of the Food Safety Modernization Act (FSMA)*. https://www.fda.gov/food/food-safety-modernization-act-fsma/full-text-food-safety-modernization-act-fsma.

FDA (Food and Drug Administration). 2010. *Advancing Regulatory Science for Public Health*. Department of Health and Human Services. https://www.fda.gov/media/79184/download.

Fernandez-Cornejo, J., S. Wechsler, M. Livingston, and L. Mitchell. 2014. Genetically Engineered Crops in the United States. USDA Economic Research Service, Economic Research Report #162.

Hanna-Attisha, M., J. LaChance, R. C. Sadler, and A. C. Schnepp. 2016. Elevated Blood Lead Levels in Children Associated with the Flint Drinking Water Crisis: A Spatial Analysis of Risk and Public Health Response. *Am J Public Health* 106: 283–290.

Havelaar, A. H., M. D. Kirk, P. R. Torgerson, H. J. Gibb, T. Hald, R. J. Lake et al.. 2015. On Behalf of the World Health Organization Foodborne Disease Burden Epidemiology Reference Group. World Health Organization Global Estimates and Regional Comparisons of the Burden of Foodborne Disease. *PLoS Med.* 10.1371/journal.pmed.1001923.

Joint FAO/WHO Expert Committee on Food Additives (JECFA). 2010. Scientific Opinion on Lead in Food. Retrieved from https://www.efsa.europa.eu/en/efsajournal/pub/1570.

Lehman, A. J., et al. 1955. Procedures for the Appraisal of the Toxicity of Chemicals in Foods, Drugs, and Cosmetics. *Food Drug Cosmet Law J* 10, 679–748.

Kensler, T. W., B. D. Roebuck, G. N. Wogan, and J. D. Groopman. 2011. Aflatoxin: A 50-Year Odyssey of Mechanistic and Translational Toxicology. *Toxicol Sci* 120(Suppl. 1): S28–S48.

Khlangwiset, P., and F. Wu. 2010. Costs and Efficacy of Public Health Interventions to Reduce Aflatoxin–Induced Human Disease. *Food Addit Contam* 27: 998–1014.

Miller, J. D. 1995. Fungi and Mycotoxins in Grain: Implications for Stored Product Research. *J Stored Prod Res* 31:1–6.

Morel, B, R. S. Farrow, and F. Wu, E. A. Casman. 2002. Pesticide Resistance, the Precautionary Principle, and the Regulation of Bt Corn: Real Option and Rational Option Approaches to Decisionmaking. In R. Laxminarayan (Ed.), *Battling Resistance to Antibiotics and Pesticides* (204–233). Washington, DC: Resources for the Future. 10.4324/9781936331550

Munkvold, G. P., R. L. Hellmich, and L. G. Rice. 1999. Comparison of Fumonisin Concentrations in Kernels of Transgenic Bt Maize Hybrids and Nontransgenic Hybrids. *Plant Dis* 83: 130–138.

National Research Council (NRC). 1983. *Risk Assessment in the Federal Government: Managing the Process*. Washington, DC: The National Academies Press.

Needleman, H. L., ed. 1981. *Low Level Lead Exposure: Clinical Implications of Current Research*. New York: Raven Press.

NRC. 2015. *Critical Role of Animal Science Research in Food Security and Sustainability*. Washington, DC: The National Academies Press. ISBN: 978-0-309-31644-6.

Oberoi, S, A. A. Barchowsky, and F. Wu 2014. The Global Burden of Disease for Skin, Lung and Bladder Cancer Caused by Arsenic in Food. *Cancer Epidemiol Biomark Prev* 23: 1187–1194.

Parvez, F., Y. Chen, P. W. Brandt-Rauf, V. Slavkovich, T. Islam, A. Ahmed, M. Argos, R. Hassan, M. Yunus, S. E. Haque, O. Balac, J. H. Graziano, and H. Ahsan. 2010. A Prospective Study of Respiratory Symptoms Associated with Chronic Arsenic Exposure in Bangladesh: Findings from the Health Effects of Arsenic Longitudinal Study (HEALS). *Thorax* 65(6): 528–533.

Perry, E. D., F. Ciliberto, D. A. Hennessy and G. Moschini. 2016. Genetically Engineered Crops and Pesticide Use in US Maize and Soybeans. *Sci Adv* 2: e1600850.

Pilet, J. 2021. Lawsuits Piling Up Against Baby Food Firms Over Potential Damage to Infant Brain Development. *Food Safety News*, 23 June 2021.

Rodricks, J. V., D. Turnbull, F. Chowdhury, and F. Wu. 2020. Food Constituents and Contaminants. In M. Lippmann, and G. D. Leikauf (Eds.), *Environmental Toxicants: Human Exposures and Their Health Effects* (4th ed., 147–203). Hoboken, NJ: John Wiley & Sons.

Scallan, E, R. M. Hoekstra, F. J. Angulo, R. V. Tauxe, M-A. Widdowson, S. L. Roy, J. L. Jones, and P. M. Griffin 2011). Foodborne Illness Acquired in the United States – Major Pathogens. *Emerg Infect Dis* 17: 7–15.

Schaider, L. A., S. A. Balan, A. Blum, D. Q. Andrews, M. J. Strynar, M. E. Dickinson, D. M. Lunderberg, J. R. Lang, and G. F. Peaslee. 2017. Fluorinated Compounds in US Fast Food Packaging. *Env Sci Tech Lett* 4(3):105–111.

Sheehan, M. C., T. A. Burke, A. Navas-Acien, P. Breysse, J. McGready, and M. A. Fox. 2014. Global Methylmercury Exposure from Seafood Consumption and Risk of Developmental Neurotoxicity: A Systematic Review. *WHO Bull* 92: 254–69F.

Smith, R. L. 1991. Does One Man's Meat Become Another Man's Poison? *Trans Med Soc Lond* 11 6–17.

Spink, J., D. Ortega, C. Chen, and F. Wu. 2017. Food Fraud Prevention Shifts the Food Risk Focus to Vulnerability. *Trends Food Sci Technol* 62: 215–220.

Straif, K et al. 2009. A Review of Human Carcinogens – Part C: Metals, Arsenic, Dusts, and Fibers. *Lancet Oncol* 10: 453–454.

US House of Representatives. 2021. *Baby Foods Are Tainted with Dangerous Levels of Arsenic, Lead, Cadmium, and Mercury*. Subcommittee on Economic and Consumer Policy, U.S. House of Representatives, Washington, DC. https://oversight.house.gov/sites/democrats.oversight.house.gov/files/2021-02-04%20ECP%20 Baby%20Food%20Staff%20Report.pdf.

USDA/EPA (U.S. Department of Agriculture/Food Safety and Inspection Service and U.S. Environmental Protection Agency). 2012. *Microbial Risk Assessment Guideline: Pathogenic Organisms with Focus on Food and Water*. FSIS Publication No. USDA/FSIS/2012-001; EPA Publication No. EPA/100/J12/001.

US EPA. 2001. *Biopesticides Registration Action Document – Bacillus Thuringiensis Plant-Incorporated Protectants (2001)*. Washington, DC: Environmental Protection Agency.

US EPA. 2016a. *Health Effects Support Document for Perfluorooctanoic Acid (PFOA)*. EPA 822-R-16-003.

US EPA. 2016b. *Health Effects Support Document for Perfluorooctane Sulfonate (PFOS)*. EPA 822-R-16-002.

Weaver, M. A., H. K. Abbas, M. J. Brewer, L. S. Pruter, and N. S. Little. 2017. Integration of Biological Control and Transgenic Insect Protection for Mitigation of Mycotoxins in Corn. *Crop Prot* 98: 108–115.

World Health Organization (WHO). 2015. *WHO Estimates of the Global Burden of Foodborne Diseases: Foodborne Diseases Burden Epidemiology Reference Group 2007–2015*. Geneva, Switzerland: World Health Organization.

Wu, F. 2007. Bt Corn and Mycotoxin Reduction. *CAB Rev: Perspect Agric Vet Sci Nutr Nat Resour* 2(060): 8 pp.

Wu, F. 2008. A Tale of Two Commodities: How EU Mycotoxin Regulations Have Affected Food Industries. *World Mycotoxin J* 1: 71–8.

Wu, F., T. R. Bui-Klimke, and K. N. Shields. 2014b. Potential Economic and Health Impacts of Ochratoxin A Standards. *World Mycotoxin J* 7: 387–398.

Wu, F., J. D. Groopman, and J. J. Pestka. 2014a. Public Health Impacts of Foodborne Mycotoxins. *Annu Rev Food Sci Technol* 5: 351–372.

Wu, F., and H. Guclu. 2012. Aflatoxin Regulations in a Network of Global Maize Trade. *PLoS ONE* 7(9): e45141. 10.1371/journal.pone.0045151.

Wu, F., and J. V. Rodricks. 2020. Forty Years of Food Safety Risk Assessment: A History and Analysis. *Risk Anal* 40: 2218–2230.

Ye, Z, F. Wu, and D. A. Hennessy 2021. Environmental and Economic Concerns Surrounding Restrictions on Glyphosate Use in Corn. *Proc Natl Acad Sci* 118: e2017470118. 10.1073/pnas.2017470118.

Yu, J, D. A. Hennessy, and F. Wu. 2020. The Impact of Bt Corn on Aflatoxin-Related Insurance Claims in the United States. *Sci Rep* 10: 10046.

Zang, Y., B. Devleesschauwer, P. M. Bolger, E. Goodman, and H. J. Gibb 2019. Global Burden of Late-Stage Chronic Kidney Disease Resulting from Dietary Exposure to Cadmium, 2015. *Environ Res* 169: 72–78.

4 Exposure Assessment

The Ways We Measure Exposure and Its Application to Risk Assessment

Donghai Liang
Emory University Rollins School of Public Health, Atlanta, GA, USA

CONTENTS

Introduction 57
Basic Concepts and Key Components of Exposure Assessment..58
    Exposure 58
    Exposure Assessment 58
    Dose..60
Role of Exposure Assessment in Risk Assessment..63
Overview of the Exposure Assessment Process 64
    Step 1. Planning, Scoping, and Problem Formulation 65
    Step 2. Exposure Setting Characterization...65
    Step 3. Exposure Pathway Identification 66
    Step 4. Exposure Quantification...66
    Step 5. Uncertainty Assessment and Exposure Assessment Summary......................66
Approaches in Assessing and Quantifying the Exposure...67
    Direct Measurements Point-of-Contact Method..67
    Indirect Estimation – Scenario Evaluation...67
    Exposure Reconstruction – Biomonitoring and Reverse Dosimetry 68
Apply Exposure Assessment to Estimate Risk 68
References..71

LEARNING OBJECTIVES

Students who complete this chapter will be able to

1. Understand the basic concepts of exposure assessment,
2. Learn about the key components of exposure assessment,
3. Learn about the role of exposure assessment in risk assessment,
4. Understand the process and major steps involved in exposure assessment,
5. Become familiar with different methodologies and approaches applied to estimate exposure and dose, and
6. Learn about how to use exposure assessment in risk assessment.

INTRODUCTION

There are four major steps involved in risk assessment: hazard identification, dose-response assessment, exposure assessment, and risk characterization (US EP 2019). In risk assessment, to evaluate the nature and probability of adverse health effects in humans who may be exposed to chemicals in contaminated environmental media, we need to conduct exposure assessment to estimate the magnitude of actual and/or potential human exposures, the frequency and duration of these exposures, and the pathways by which humans are potentially exposed (US EPA 1989).

The use of exposure assessment in the fields of epidemiology, industrial hygiene, and health physics dates back at least to the early 20th century (US EPA 1992). Since the early 1970s, exposure assessment has become increasingly important with greater public awareness of environmental problems, and it has been widely applied in epidemiologic studies, occupational health settings, as part of routine surveillance, and in risk assessment, which is the primary application discussed herein. As an essential part of risk assessment for environmental health, exposure assessments are generally used to characterize and estimate environmental exposures to the general population

DOI: 10.1201/9780429291722-4

and occupational exposures in the workplace, such as emissions from industrial processes, contaminated soil, food, or water, as well as consumer products containing hazardous chemicals.

This chapter describes the concepts and key components of exposure assessment and its role in risk assessment. We will also cover various types of major methodologies and techniques applied to measure exposure and assess risk for environmental health.

BASIC CONCEPTS AND KEY COMPONENTS OF EXPOSURE ASSESSMENT

Exposure

Exposure is the contact of an agent with an external boundary of a receptor (exposure surface) for a specific duration (WHO 2004; Zartarian et al. 2005). Here, an agent can be a chemical, physical, or biological entity that contacts a receptor, and the receptor refers to any biological entity, such as an individual subject, human population, or life stage within a human population, that receives an exposure or dose. The exposure surface is the external boundary of a receptor where an agent is present and comes into contact with the receptor. For humans, the external exposure surfaces include the surface of the skin, the exterior of an eyeball, and conceptual surface over the nose and open mouth. There are also internal exposure surfaces, such as respiratory tract, gastrointestinal tract, and urinary tract lining. For exposure to occur, a receptor must be in contact with an agent in both space and time. In other words, if there exists an environmental contaminant but there is no human or other receptor in the same microenvironment concurrently, there will not be exposure.

Exposure Assessment

Exposure assessment is the process of estimating or measuring the magnitude, frequency, and duration of exposure to an agent and the size and characteristics of the population exposed (US EPA 2019). Generally, exposure assessment provides estimates of the exposure to the agent(s) of concern to the receptor and describes the receptor of concern. Exposure assessment principally characterizes the following key components and characteristics of exposures (NRC 1990, 2012; Sobus et al. 2010; US EPA 1992, 2009, 2019; WHO 2004, 2012; Zartarian et al. 2005; 2007):

- Magnitude of exposure – the total amount of substance (i.e., agent(s)) the receptor is exposed to (i.e., how much of the substance the receptor is in contact with). If we use a time-dependent profile of the exposure concentration to characterize the exposure over a period of time, the area under the curve of such profile (i.e., exposure concentration times time) is the magnitude of the exposure.

- Frequency of exposure – the number of exposure events in an exposure duration (i.e., how often the receptor is in contact with the substance).

- Duration of exposure – the length of time of contact with an agent (i.e., how long the receptor is in contact with the substance).

- Exposure period – the time of continuous contact between the agent and receptor.

- Exposure concentration – the concentration of an agent (e.g., chemical or contaminant) in its transport or carrier medium at the point of contact.

- Route of exposure – the way a chemical or pollutant enters an organism after contact. Agent(s) may have different toxicities depending on the routes of exposure. For humans, there are three most common routes of exposure to environmental contaminants, including inhalation, ingestion, and dermal absorption. Specifically, the following:

  Exposure by inhalation occurs when an individual breathes a chemical, which may directly affect the respiratory tract or enter the bloodstream through respiratory tract tissues, potentially affecting other systems of the body.

  Exposure by ingestion occurs when an individual drinks, eats, or inadvertently ingests a chemical into the gastrointestinal tract, where the chemical may directly target the tissues in the gastrointestinal tract or reach other systems of the body after being absorbed through the gut to enter the bloodstream.

  Exposure by dermal absorption occurs when a chemical contacts, acts on, or is absorbed through the skin to enter the bloodstream.

- Points of entry – the location where the receptor contacts the agent. For humans, these include the nose and mouth for inhalation, the mouth for ingestion, and the skin for dermal absorption.

- Source of exposure – the origin of an agent (i.e., where the chemical or substance comes from). The source significantly influences where and when stressors eventually will be found in the exposure assessment.

- Stressor – any physical, chemical, or biological entity that triggers an adverse response.

- Exposure medium – the material surrounding or containing an agent, such as air (ambient or indoor), water (groundwater or surface water, drinking or recreational), soil or sediments, biota (animals, plants, microorganisms), food, and consumer products.

- Exposure pathway – the physical course a chemical or pollutant takes from the source to the organism exposed (i.e., how the receptor comes into contact with a hazardous substance). A complete exposure pathway is one in which the stressor can be traced or expected to travel from the source to a receptor that can be affected by that stressor (US EPA OSWER 1997). The source, medium, exposure, route of exposure, and receptor are the five fundamental elements of a complete exposure pathway, and without any of them, exposure will not occur.

- Fate and transport – the process describing how contaminants move through and are transformed and degraded in the environment.

- Half-life – the amount of time necessary for a given amount of chemical or substance released into the environment to decrease to half of its initial value.

- Exposure factors – the factors related to human behavior and characteristics that help determine a receptor's exposure to an agent (i.e., the size and characteristics of the population exposed).

For most environmental contaminants, the magnitude, frequency, duration, timing (e.g., acute exposure, chronic exposure, and lifetime exposure), and route of exposure are all critical characteristics in determining the adverse effects of environmental exposures (US EPA 2019). To characterize these influential factors in exposure assessment, we will need to examine the stressor, the source of the contaminant, its transport and fate, its persistence in the environment, and the behaviors and activities of the receptor that lead to contact with the contaminant.

Specifically, to characterize the exposure pathway, we need to assess the fate and transport of the agent(s) by examining how it moves through and transforms in the environment and how it will come into contact with the receptor. Agents that can evaporate into air (i.e., volatilize) or dissolve in water can migrate considerable distances from where they are released. Humans, plants, wildlife, and domestic animals are more likely to be exposed to a chemical if it does not easily degrade or is dispersed widely in the environment. For example, if the target agent is the nitrogen oxides produced and emitted from a stack, we will need to consider both the surrounding ambient environment and the neighborhood community, especially in the direction of the prevailing winds when characterizing the exposure pathway. If the agents are the heavy metals emitted in the soil, we will need to consider the surrounding land and biota, where they may enter the human body through inhalation of dust, direct ingestion, or dermal contact of contaminated soil and consumption of vegetables and animals grown in contaminated fields. With biotransformation and metabolism, the chemical characteristic and toxicity of these heavy metal pollutants may change, so when humans consume the food grown in the contaminated soil, these environmental contaminants may be more or less toxic than when they were originally discharged into the soil. Many fat-soluble chemicals and heavy metals have a high potential for bioaccumulation, where these chemicals accumulate in living organisms so that their concentrations in tissues continue to increase. For example, very low concentrations of heavy metals in water can result in markedly higher concentrations in the tissue of fish at higher levels of the aquatic food chain, as well as in people or wildlife eating those fish.

In addition, one will need to consider the agent's potential for degradation in the environment. Some chemicals can be broken down rapidly into less toxic forms by sunlight, destroyed through reactions with other environmental substances, or metabolized by naturally occurring bacteria, while others may remain in the same form for a long time. We use persistence to indicate how resistant a chemical or substance is to degradation in the environment. Persistence can be described as the half-life of a chemical or substance in the specific environmental media such as air, water, soil, or sediment. Physical and chemical properties of a chemical or substance are essential determinants of their persistence and are important factors to consider when characterizing their fate and transport in the environment as well as in tissues (via absorption, distribution, metabolism, and excretion). For example, volatility is an influential factor of a chemical's half-life, where many volatile agents, including phosgene, chlorine, and hydrogen cyanide, are nonpersistent chemicals whose half-lives range from seconds to several hours, whereas less volatile agents like sulfur mustard and organosulfur are more persistent in the environment with their half-lives lasting for several days. Compared to nonpersistent chemicals, persistent chemicals generally possess greater threats to the environment and public health, especially for those high persistent chemicals with degradation half-life exceeding six months (Cousins et al. 2019). This is because for most short-lived chemicals, it is possible to rapidly cease environmental contamination by restricting or banning its use, which effectively minimizes the additional adverse effects caused by that chemical. In contrast, for those highly persistent chemicals, it is extremely challenging to cease environmental contamination within a reasonable time frame by simply restricting or banning their use. Moreover, since highly persistent chemicals are difficult to degrade and can bioaccumulate in the environment, environmental contamination by highly persistent chemicals and the corresponding effects related to this contamination will continue for years to decades. In particular, persistent organic pollutants, including polychlorinated biphenyl, chlorofluorocarbon, and per- and polyfluoroalkyl substance, are distributed widely around the globe and reach much higher concentrations than short-lived chemicals emitted at the same rate. Over the past several decades, these highly persistent chemicals have caused serious impacts on the environment and human health (Jepson and Law 2016) and extra caution must be taken in risk assessment and regulation of these chemicals.

Besides assessing the key characteristics of exposure, exposure assessment often generates estimates of exposure for both current and future scenarios to monitor status and trends in exposure over time. These assessments emphasize whether and how the exposure changes over time and what level the exposure is at a particular time. Specifically, current exposure estimates are useful for determining whether a threat exists based on existing exposure conditions at the study location, while future exposure estimates provide insights for decision-makers to gain a better understanding of potential future exposures and threats and include a qualitative estimate of the likelihood of such exposures occurring (US EPA 1989). The assessment of current and future exposure is critical for evaluation of the potential for emerging health risks and impact of risk mitigation actions. Additionally, exposure assessment provides key information on the individuals or populations exposed, the sources, routes, and pathways of exposure, which is critical to determine the most effective ways to reduce exposure and the corresponding risk. Prospective exposure assessments can also provide information on the overall impact of mitigation strategies, including both regulatory and nonregulatory actions (US EPA 2019).

The numerical output of an exposure assessment may be an estimate of either exposure or dose, depending on the purpose and objective of the exposure assessment (US EPA 1992). If being conducted as part of a risk assessment, the exposure assessment would be closely connected with the dose-response assessment, and therefore an estimate of dose is usually generated as its output. If the exposure assessment is done in other disciplines (e.g., as part of epidemiological studies), risk may be characterized without generating the estimates of dose by using empirically derived exposure-response relationships. Given the close connections and subtle differences between exposure and dose, we will introduce the concepts and characteristics of dose to gain a better understanding of the key components of exposure assessment.

Dose

By definition, dose is the amount of an agent that enters a receptor after crossing an external exposure surface (US EPA 2019), whereas exposure is the contact of an agent with an external boundary of a receptor for a specific duration. In other words, exposure mainly describes the potential of agent(s) to come into contact with the receptor at the external boundary, while dose reflects the actual amount of agent(s) available to cause affects within the receptor after crossing the outer boundary of an organism. To characterize dose, we will need to consider the following key factors (Sobus et al. 2010; US EPA 1992, 2009, 2019; WHO 2004, 2012; Zartarian et al. 2005, 2007):

■ Absorption barrier – the exposure surface that can slow down the penetration process of an agent into a receptor. Examples of absorption barriers for humans include the skin and other outer and inner exposed surfaces and tissues such as the eyes, lung surface, and intestinal tract.

- Intake – the process by which an agent crosses an outer exposure surface without passing an absorption barrier. Examples of an intake process for humans include breathing air into the lung and ingestion into the gut.

- Uptake – the process by which an agent crosses an outer exposure surface by passing an absorption barrier and results in an internal dose. Examples of an uptake process for humans include absorptions of chemicals or substances through the skin (i.e., dermal absorption) or other outer and inner exposed surfaces and tissues such as the eyes, respiratory tract lining, and gastrointestinal tract wall.

- Bioavailability – the extent to which an agent can be absorbed by a receptor and be available for metabolism or interaction with biologically significant receptors factor. Bioavailability is typically a function of chemical properties, the physical state of the material to which an organism is exposed, and the ability of the individual organism to physiologically take up the chemical.

- Applied dose or external dose – the amount of agent at an absorption barrier (i.e., skin, eye, respiratory tract, or gastrointestinal tract) that are available for absorption. Generally, the external dose of an agent is not necessarily equivalent to the internal dose, which is affected by how the agent is absorbed into the bloodstream. Given that many absorption barriers are internal to humans and thus not feasible to make a direct measurement, the potential dose is often measured to approximate the applied dose.

- Potential dose – the amount of agent that enters a receptor after crossing an exposure surface that is not an absorption barrier (i.e., the amount of the chemical ingested, inhaled, or in material applied to the skin).

- Absorbed dose or internal – the amount of agent that enters a receptor by crossing an exposure surface acting as an absorption barrier (i.e., the amount of a chemical that has been absorbed and is available for interaction with biologically significant receptors). Once absorbed, the agent can undergo metabolism, storage, excretion, or transport within the receptor.

- Delivered dose – the amount of agent transported to the location where the adverse effect occurs. Generally, the delivered dose constitutes only a small part of the total internal dose.

- Biologically effective dose – the amount of agent that reaches the target internal organ, tissue, or toxicity pathway where the adverse effect occurs. Similar to a delivered dose, a biologically effective dose may be only a small part of the total internal dose, but it is the most crucial part that contributes to adverse health effects.

Figure 4.1 illustrates these key components of exposure and dose in the three major routes of exposure in humans – namely, the dermal absorption route in the skin, the respiratory route (i.e., inhalation) in the respiratory tract, and the oral route (i.e., ingestion) in the gastrointestinal tract:

For the dermal route, exposure occurs when a chemical comes into contact with skin. Here, the amount of chemical applied to skin, regardless of being absorbed or not, is the potential dose, whereas the amount of chemical on the skin that can be absorbed by the body is the applied dose. The amount of chemical absorbed into the body from skin and available for interaction with organs and tissues is the internal dose or absorbed dose. Finally, the amount of the metabolized chemical that induces biological effects at the target organ and eventually results in health effects is the biologically effective dose. In the dermal route, uptake is the amount of chemical absorbed through the skin (i.e., internal dose).

In the respiratory route, exposure occurs when a chemical comes into contact with the external surface of the respiratory tract (i.e., the outer part of the mouth or the nose). The amount of chemical inhaled here after crossing the external surface of the mouth or nose is the potential dose, though not all would be absorbed. And the amount of the chemical at the absorption barrier of the respiratory tract that can be absorbed is the applied dose. The amount of chemical that crosses the absorption barrier (e.g., the exchange boundary in the lung) and has been absorbed into the systemic circulation (i.e., blood) is the internal dose or absorbed dose. Finally, the amount of the metabolized chemical that interacts with the internal target tissue or organ and eventually results in health effects is the biologically effective dose. Here, intake is the chemical crossing the outer part of the mouth or nose, and uptake is the chemical absorbed through the respiratory tract.

In the oral route, exposure occurs when a chemical comes into contact with the external surface of the gastrointestinal tract (i.e., the outer part of the mouth). And the amount of the chemical getting in the mouth and ingested is the potential dose, though not all would be

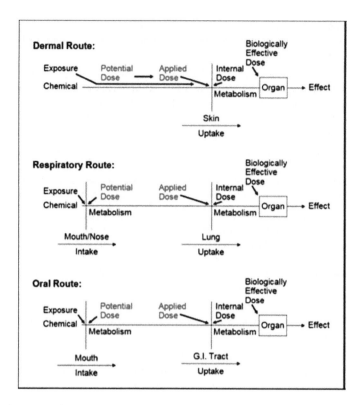

Figure 4.1 Schematic of exposure and dose terms by routes of exposure. (Adapted from US EPA 2019).

absorbed. The amount of the chemical that makes it into the gastrointestinal tract and is available for absorption is the applied dose. The amount of chemical that crosses the absorption barrier and has been absorbed into the blood is the internal dose or absorbed dose. Finally, the amount of the metabolized chemical that interacts with the internal target tissue or organ and eventually results in health effects is the biologically effective dose. Here, intake is the chemical crossing the outer part of the mouth, and uptake is the chemical absorbed through the gastrointestinal tract.

To estimate the dose for humans exposure to chemicals or substances, we will use this generic equation (US EPA 1992, 2004; ATSDR 2005):

$$\text{Dose} = (C \times IR \times AF \times EF)/BW$$

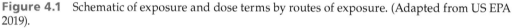

Where, C = contaminant concentration, IR = intake rate of contaminated medium, AF = bioavailability factor, EF = exposure factor, and BW = body weight. Here, for the inhalation route, the contaminant concentration is usually a measured or modeled value of air contaminant in the gas phase or particulate phase, or both; for the ingestion route, this can be either a measured or modeled concentration of contaminant in soil, water, food, or biota; for the dermal route, the C term is the absorbed dose, which is determined by the rate at which the contaminant is absorbed, and this will be a function of contaminant properties. For the IR term, it can be the inhalation rate (i.e., the volume of air inhaled over a specified time frame), the ingestion rate (i.e., the amount of contaminant that an individual ingests during a specific period of time), the permeability coefficient (for dermal contact with liquid), or the surface of the skin that is exposed (for dermal contact with solids). For inhalation and ingestion, the unit of intake rate is usually expressed in units of mass or volume per unit time, such as g/day or L/day. For dermal absorption, the unit of permeability coefficient is in cm/hr, and the unit of skin surface is in cm^2. For humans, the bioavailability factors reflect the total amount of a substance ingested, inhaled, or contacted that actually enters the bloodstream and is available to possibly harm a person. Bioavailability can vary by exposure pathway, chemical and medium, life stage of the individual, and other biological factors. When there is no data or information available to indicate otherwise, the bioavailability factor is usually assumed to be one for screening purposes, indicating that all the chemicals and substances to which a person is exposed are assumed to be absorbed. Exposure factor is usually estimated by averaging the dose over the period of exposure, where it can be calculated by multiplying the exposure frequency by the exposure duration and dividing by the time period during which the dose is to be averaged. For example, if an individual was exposed to polluted air three times a week during a three-year period, the exposure factor would be ([3 days/week × 52 weeks/year] × 3 years)/(3 years × 365 days/year) = 0.43. If the contaminant is persistent and ubiquitous, the exposure factor may equal to 1 in many instances, which indicates a daily exposure to the contaminant. Body weight is calculated by averaging the body weight of the individual during the entire exposure time period and when the individual data are not available, the default values for adults, children (age 1–6), and infants (6 to 1 months) are 70 kg, 16 kg, and 10 kg, respectively. Note that this is a generic equation and the way how dose is calculated varies by different types of exposure (e.g., nonradiant substances vs. radiation), the source of the exposure, the exposure medium and routes, and exposure factors (i.e., the characteristics of the study population). More details on how to calculate dose in various exposure scenarios can be found in US EPA Exposure Scenarios Assessment Tool (US EPA 2004) or in the Agency for Toxic Substances and Disease Registry Public Health Assessment Guidance Manual (ATSDR 2005).

ROLE OF EXPOSURE ASSESSMENT IN RISK ASSESSMENT

A source-to-outcome framework, as illustrated in Figure 4.2, helps visualize the processes and information important for exposure science (US EPA 2019). In risk assessment, the primary purpose of exposure assessment is to generate and provide estimates of the exposure or dose, or both, as well as their interpretations, to estimate risk. Specifically, risk assessors often combine exposure and dose information with data on exposure-response or dose-response relationships (usually from animal models) to describe and characterize risk. To illustrate the role of exposure assessment in risk assessment for environmental health, we use a source-to-outcome framework (US EPA 2019) to show the relationships of exposure and dose to risk and visualize how exposure assessment contributes to evaluating the nature and probability of adverse health effects in humans who may be exposed to chemicals in contaminated environmental media. As shown in Figure 4.2, exposure is clearly the critical linkage between the stressor and the receptor, where it

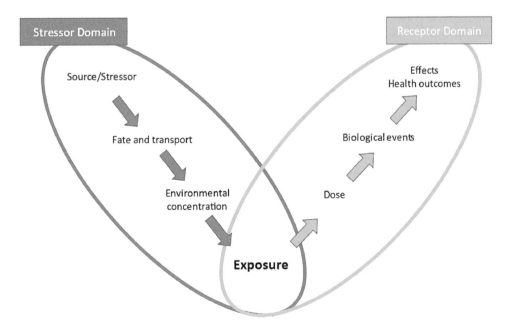

Figure 4.2 Exposure and dose in the source-to-outcome framework. (Adapted from US EPA 2019).

serves as the key component linking a hazard in the environment and the potential health effect in the exposed populations. Therefore, exposure is a critical element of risk, and without exposure, there is no risk. Moreover, both hazard and exposure are necessary for there to be a risk. Without hazard (i.e., source of harmful agents), there is no risk even with the presence of exposure. Similarly, if the exposure can be contained or prevented, then there may not be a risk even though there exists a hazardous agent in the environment. Hence, a hazardous chemical release does not necessarily result in a high-risk scenario if we can prevent the occurrence of exposure (i.e., contact between the stressor and receptor).

We will use traffic-related air pollution and respiratory diseases as examples to go over the key components in this source-to-outcome framework:

1. Source and Stressor. The combustion of fossil fuels in the vehicle releases numerous primary traffic-related air pollutants, including carbon monoxide, nitrogen oxides, hydrocarbons, and sulfur dioxide, from the tailpipe into the ambient environment.

2. Fate and Transport. Once released into the environment, these primary traffic-related air pollutants interact with other chemicals in the air and form secondary pollutants, including ozone (in the presence of sunlight) and particulate matters. These traffic-related air pollutants, along with their transformation products, move through the environment and can be found in various types of environmental mediums.

3. Environmental Concentration. The concentration levels of these traffic-related air pollutants in the ambient air (primary environmental medium) are key factors in determining the magnitude of the exposure.

4. Exposure. Exposure occurs when traffic-related air pollutants come into contact with individuals when they breathe in contaminated air.

5. Dose. Exposure becomes a dose when the traffic-related air pollutant moves across the respiratory tract and is absorbed into the body.

6. Biological Events. Once absorbed, the exogenous contaminant of traffic-related air pollutants disperses throughout the body in its native form, metabolized form, or both.

7. Effects and Health Outcomes. Finally, the biologically effective dose resulting from exposure to traffic-related air pollutants initiates the toxicity pathway and biological perturbations, which trigger the adverse effects at the target internal tissue, organ, or developing embryo or fetus.

Depending on the objective of the risk assessment, the role of exposure assessment may vary. In addition to estimating exposure or dose, exposure assessment can also (1) provide scientific evidence for specific chemical source regulations, such as point emission sources and pesticides, through establishing the connection of the source of exposure and the potentially exposed population; (2) evaluate both current and future exposure scenarios and monitor trends in exposure over time; (3) provide information on the overall impact of mitigation and remediation strategies, including both regulatory and nonregulatory actions; (4) provide critical information on the individuals or population exposed, the sources, routes, and pathways of exposure, to determine the most effective ways to reduce exposure and the corresponding risk; and (5) provide important data to understand and quantify health outcomes associated with environmental contaminants as they occur in various populations throughout the life span. To fulfill these important roles, the exposure assessors analyze and evaluate the exposure and dose information using different approaches, which we will introduce in the following sections.

OVERVIEW OF THE EXPOSURE ASSESSMENT PROCESS

The overarching goal of exposure assessment in risk assessment is to provide estimates of the magnitude, frequency, duration, and distribution of exposures in the exposed population. In any risk assessment, the information and data generated from the exposure assessment must be clearly linked to the hazard identification and exposure- or dose-response relationship to conduct an accurate risk characterization. Generally, the purpose of each risk assessment exposure, aspects of the hazard identification and dose-response relationships, and the health endpoints can vary widely, which will have an impact on how the exposure information needs to be collected and analyzed for the risk assessment. As such, we cannot strictly organize exposure assessment into a set format or protocol. Nevertheless, there are several major processes commonly involved in exposure assessment.

Step 1. Planning, Scoping, and Problem Formulation

According to the Environmental Protection Agency (EPA) guidelines for exposure assessment (US EPA 1992, 2019), planning, scoping, and problem formulation are essential and integral parts of exposure assessment, which promote efficient time and resource management. This step is usually the first step applied in exposure scenario evaluation, an indirect estimation approach commonly applied in exposure assessment (more details on this in the next section). Briefly, this process starts by initiating dialogue on the nature of the concern to establish objectives and goals. The next step is to assemble an exposure assessment team and identify stakeholders. Then, the exposure assessment team needs to develop a conceptual model, followed by a search and review of available information, approaches, options, data gaps, and needs for conducting the exposure assessment. Finally, the assessors will develop an exposure assessment plan and a communication plan. In this initial step of exposure assessment, the planning process identifies the underlying question on which the assessment is focused and the constraints under which the assessment is conducted (i.e., time frame, resources, data gaps, and needs). The scoping process defines the elements that will be included in the exposure assessment with a search and review of available information and approaches for conducting the exposure assessment. The problem formulation process develops preliminary hypotheses about how exposure occurs and why adverse effects might occur or have occurred and generates an analysis plan that lays out the approach for conducting the assessment.

Step 2. Exposure Setting Characterization

In this step, the exposure assessors mainly characterize the exposure setting by assessing the general characteristics of the physical environment and the characteristics of the population potentially exposed (US EPA 1989). To understand the physical environment where the potential exposure may occur, we will need to collect study site-specific information on the following physical characteristics:

- Climate and meteorological factors, including temperature, humidity, wind speed and direction, and precipitation
- Geologic setting, such as the physical location and characterization of the underlying rock strata
- Vegetation coverage, whether the area is unvegetated, grassy, or forested
- Soil type, whether the soil is acid, basic, sandy, or organic
- Groundwater properties, including depth, direction, and type of flow
- Surface water properties, including location, type, flow rates, and salinity

Meanwhile, to identify those who may come into contact with the chemical released into the environment, we will need to

- determine the distance and direction of the potentially exposed population from the study site;
- determine the current land use (i.e., if the study site is residential, commercial, industrial, or recreational);
- characterize the activities and activity patterns of the potentially exposed population by determining the length and percent of time spent in the contaminated site, microenvironment (i.e., if the activities occur indoors, outdoors, or both), seasonal pattern (i.e., if the activities occur more frequently in a particular season), site restriction (i.e., whether the study site is restricted for use or it is accessible to the local population), neighboring environment (i.e., if the study site is adjacent or in close distance to major commercial or recreational areas);
- determine if the land use of the study site will change in the future (i.e., if any activities associated with the current land use are likely to be different under an alternate future land use); and
- identify a subpopulation of potential concern by determining if any subpopulations at the study site are at greater risk or will be susceptible to increased risk in the future from the environmental exposures due to greater vulnerability and increased sensitivity (i.e., children, elderly, and those with preexisting conditions), behavior patterns that may result in high exposure, and previous or current exposures from other sources (i.e., occupational exposure).

Step 3. Exposure Pathway Identification

Identifying and characterizing the exposure pathway is an important step in exposure assessment, which will provide critical information on how individuals or populations come into contact with hazardous environmental contaminants. In the previous section, we learn that the exposure pathway describes the physical course a chemical or pollutant takes from the source to the organism exposed, and that the source, medium, exposure, route of exposure, and receptor are the fundamental elements of a complete exposure pathway. Therefore, to conduct a comprehensive exposure pathway identification, we will need to do the following:

- Identify the source of the contaminants based on monitoring data and information collected on the source location to analyze potential release mechanisms and map the source areas.

- Characterize the affected environment media (i.e., air, soil, water, biota, food, and consumer products) for which past, current, or potential future exposures exist using available information and monitoring data.

- Evaluate the fate and transport of the contaminant in the environment to connect the sources with the affected environmental media and to predict future exposures. The key questions to be answered in this step include what contaminants occur in the sources at the study site, how they were released, how they move through the environment and at what environmental media they occur, where and at what media they may occur in the future. To characterize the fate and transport, the assessors need to collect information on physical and chemical and environmental fate properties of the contaminants and also consider the site-specific characteristics that may influence fate and transport (e.g., local geologic, topographic, and climatic conditions).

- Determine the exposure points by investigating whether and where the potentially exposed individuals and populations can contact the contaminated environmental media. The site-specific information collected at Step 2 on population locations and activity patterns will also help identify the exposure point routes of exposure.

- Identify the routes of exposure (i.e., by inhalation, ingestion, or dermal absorption) using the information on the contaminated environmental media and the anticipated activities identified at the exposure points.

- Determine the complete exposure pathway that exists for the study site by integrating and summarizing information on all components of the exposure pathway, including source, potentially exposed populations, fate and transport, exposure media, exposure points, and exposure routes.

Step 4. Exposure Quantification

This is the critical step in exposure assessment where we quantify the magnitude, frequency, and duration of exposure for the populations and exposure pathways selected for quantitative evaluation in the previous steps. The assessors usually conduct the exposure quantification in two phases. In phase one, the assessors will estimate the concentrations of the contaminants over the exposure period using monitoring data or chemical transport and environmental fate models, or both. For prospective risk assessment, the assessor often uses a modeling approach to estimate future contaminant concentration in the environmental media that are currently contaminated or may become contaminated in the future (US EPA 1989). In phase two, the assessors will quantify the chemical-specific exposures for each exposure pathway identified in Step 3. The values of the intake will be calculated by normalizing the exposure estimates by body weight and the exposure averaging time. In the next section, we will go over different ways and approaches the assessors applied to quantify the exposure and intake for each exposure pathway.

Step 5. Uncertainty Assessment and Exposure Assessment Summary

Before the conclusion of the exposure assessment, the assessors shall evaluate and summarize the sources of uncertainty and the corresponding effect on the exposure estimates. Uncertainty assessment is critical for developing a robust and reliable exposure assessment that provides accurate information for risk assessors and decision-makers. We will discuss the sources and types of uncertainty in the exposure assessment in the last section of this chapter. Finally, after uncertainty evaluation, the assessors will conclude the exposure assessment by summarizing and reporting the pathway-specific intakes for current and future exposures to individual substances.

APPROACHES IN ASSESSING AND QUANTIFYING THE EXPOSURE

Many methods and approaches have been developed, validated, and applied in exposure assessment to estimate the pathway-specific intakes for current and future exposures to environmental contaminants. In general, there is no single method that will always capture all the needed exposure information across different scenarios. As such, a method that is best for assessing exposure to a given chemical at a particular exposure condition may not be the most appropriate method for assessing exposure to that same chemical at a different exposure condition. Depending on the design, complexity, population selection, estimation approach, and stressor evaluation, the exposure assessors may choose an exclusive approach, or combine multiple methods to estimate and quantify exposure. Each approach has its own unique characteristics, strengths, and limitations, and using them in combination will considerably strengthen the credibility of an exposure or risk assessment. Here, we will briefly describe the approaches commonly applied in exposure assessment and quantification, along with the strengths and weaknesses of each method.

Direct Measurements Point-of-Contact Method

Direct measurement, also called the point-of-contact method, is one of the three major types of quantitative approaches for estimating exposure. When using direct measurements, the assessors measure the exposure concentrations at the point of contact (i.e., the outer boundary of the body) during the occurrence of exposure over an identified period (i.e., a record of the length of time of contact at each concentration). Personal exposure monitoring techniques are established direct measurements commonly performed to evaluate an individual's direct exposures during a specific time period. Examples of personal monitoring include setting up a monitoring device at a breathing zone to collect samples to assess exposure to air pollutants (Sarnat et al. 2018), obtaining skin patch samples from individuals to characterize dermal exposures (Fenske et al. 1987), and collecting duplicate plates for food or other diet samples to measure an individual's exposure through dietary intake (Stockley 1985). In general, personal exposure monitoring provides reliable direct assessment of individual exposure to environmental contaminants with relatively high precision and accuracy. It can be also used to validate or verify results of assessments conducted using indirect estimation, such as scenario or population-based evaluations. Nevertheless, there are several limitations in applying personal exposure monitoring. For example, given that personal continuous-sampling devices need to be sensitive, selective, lightweight, easy to wear, and self-powered, the cost of these devices is often too high and thus cost-prohibitive for application in large-scale cohort studies. Since these direct measurements only characterize individual exposures, the estimates may not be representative of the entire study population. Many personal sampling measurements can be deployed in the field for a short period of time, and thus may require extrapolation from short-term sampling to long-term exposure. In addition, the measurements are usually not source-specific and thus limited in evaluating mixtures of environmental contaminants.

Indirect Estimation – Scenario Evaluation

Indirect estimation is the exposure assessment approach that does not actually involve personal direct measurements, but instead uses modeling, microenvironmental measurements, and questionnaires to assess exposure or dose (NRC 1990). Scenario evaluation is an indirect estimation approach commonly applied in exposure assessment to estimate exposure or dose by establishing exposure profiles. According to the EPA guidelines (US EPA 1992), an exposure scenario is "a combination of facts, assumptions and inferences that define a discrete situation in which exposures occur," and the scenario evaluation is "an approach to quantifying exposure by measurement or estimation of both the amount of a substance contacted, and the frequency or duration of contact, and subsequently linking these together to estimate exposure or dose." Different from the direct measurements, the assessors usually characterize the contaminant concentrations and time of contact separately when evaluating exposure scenarios. In this process, the assessors first characterize and estimate the chemical concentration by collecting data and information on the sources and releases of a stressor of interest, fate and transport mechanisms, and concentrations of contaminants at the point of exposure. Here, the contaminant concentrations are typically assessed indirectly by measuring, modeling, or using existing data on concentrations in the bulk media, rather than at the point of contact. Modeling approaches will be particularly helpful in determining the contaminant concentrations when some analytical data are available, but resources for additional sampling are limited. Then the assessors will evaluate the time of contact by examining the characteristics of the exposed individuals or population, and exposure factors (e.g., contact duration and frequency, activities during occurrence of exposure, contact rate). In this step, the assessors usually obtain information on the exposed population and the corresponding human behavior and physical characteristics by use of demographic data, survey statistics, behavior observation, activity diaries, and activity models, and if no relevant information is available, assumptions about behavior and activity pattern will be employed. Finally, the assessors will combine the chemical concentration, time of contact, and information on the exposed persons according to the applicable conceptual model structure to generate estimates of exposure and dose. In general, the indirect scenario evaluation approach is cost-effective and usually the least expensive exposure assessment approach. It is also particularly useful in prospective exposure and risk assessment to evaluate the impact and consequences of proposed regulatory actions and mitigation and remediation strategies. Given that scenario evaluation can be conducted with little or no data, the validity and soundness of the assessment will be greatly influenced by modeling choice and uncertainty of the underlying assumptions. To overcome the limitation, the assessors may consider combining both direct and indirect approaches to estimate the exposure, where the direct measurement (i.e., point-of-contact approaches) can be used to validate the results of scenario evaluation assessments.

Exposure Reconstruction – Biomonitoring and Reverse Dosimetry

Exposure reconstruction is one of the three major types of exposure assessment approach, where exposure can also be estimated from dose, which in turn can be reconstructed through internal biological indicators after the exposure has taken place. This reconstructive analysis is sometimes called reverse dosimetry (US EPA 2012). Different from direct measurement and indirect estimation, exposure reconstruction uses internal biological measurements rather than external measurements to estimate exposure or dose. Here, the information used in the exposure reconstruction is collected following the exposure and "downstream" of the point of exposure, while direct measurements and indirect estimation use information collected prior to exposure and "upstream" of the point of exposure (US EPA 2012). When reconstructing the exposure or dose, the assessors need to conduct biomonitoring after the occurrence of exposure and intake and uptake, and then use these measurements to back-calculate dose using pharmacokinetic models. Specifically, biomonitoring is the process where we assess human exposure to chemicals by collecting human tissues, body fluids, or specimens, such as skin, hair, blood, urine, to determine contaminant or biomarker concentrations. Combining with the information collected from the interviews and questionnaires on the use and timing of the chemical exposure in relation to the collection of the biospecimens, we can relate the biomonitoring data to the source of the exposure, which is critical for understanding internal dose and total exposure of an individual. Finally, the assessors will use the pharmacokinetic models and combine data about physiological and metabolic processes with biomarker concentrations or other biomonitoring data to mathematically estimate exposure or dose. If working with an established biomarker, the exposure reconstruction via biomonitoring can provide an accurate measurement of the internal exposure to the environmental contaminants with high precision. Another strength of reconstructing exposure using biomonitoring data is that both aggregate and cumulative exposure can be quantified. This approach also has several limitations. Generally, exposure reconstruction does not work for every chemical due to interferences or the reactive nature of the chemical. It may also not be possible to use biomonitoring to identify specific sources or routes of exposure (i.e., inhalation, ingestion, or dermal absorption). In addition, there is a very limited number of established biomarkers for use in environmental health, and biomonitoring has not been methodologically established to assess exposure to very many chemicals. The emerging omics technologies (Niedzwiecki et al. 2019), including high-resolution metabolomics (Liang et al. 2018), may help identify sensitive biomarkers to environmental contaminants through global detection and high throughput profiling of molecules and biological responses. In Chapter 5, we will learn about how biological monitoring is used to assess exposure to environmental chemicals throughout the life stages.

APPLY EXPOSURE ASSESSMENT TO ESTIMATE RISK

In general, direct measurement, indirect estimation, and exposure reconstruction can be viewed as different ways of estimating the same exposure or dose. Sometimes more than one approach is used to estimate exposure. Specifically, depending on the purpose of the risk assessment, the exposure assessor may analyze and evaluate the exposure and dose information in several different ways to emphasize certain areas in addition to quantifying the exposure and dose (US EPA 1992):

- If the purpose of the risk assessment is to set standards for environmental media, then the exposure assessment will emphasize the concentration levels in the medium that pose a particular risk level. In this case, the exposure assessment focuses more on connecting the concentration levels in the medium with the exposure and dose levels of those exposed, while it places less emphasis on the ultimate source of the chemical. Given the major goal of the assessment is to examine the relationship between the environmental media and the exposure levels of those exposed, conducting both media measurements and personal exposure monitoring in the exposure assessment will be very useful. In addition, modeling may provide support or complement these assessments.

- If the purpose of the risk assessment is to support environmental regulation on specific chemical sources (i.e., point emission sources, consumer products, or pesticides), then the exposure assessment will emphasize the relationship between the source and the exposed or potentially exposed population. In this scenario, source and fate models and exposure scenarios are often applied in the exposure assessment to trace chemicals from the source to the point of exposure. Specifically, the exposure assessors characterize and examine each individual component of an exposure scenario where they put emphasis on the factors that contribute the most to exposure. They may also use the exposure assessment to select possible actions to reduce risk (e.g., compare and select control or cleanup options). In most cases, the assessors employ the scenario evaluation to determine the relative risk reduction of each alternative by comparing the estimates of the residual risk associated with each of the alternatives under consideration to the baseline risk. Additionally, the assessors may employ the sample approach to make screening decisions about whether to further investigate a particular chemical. In these types of exposure assessments, personal or biological monitoring techniques are useful approaches for verification purposes.

- If the purpose of the risk assessment is to decide whether a waste site or chemical spill incident needs remediation, then the exposure assessment will focus on estimating the risk to an individual or small group and comparing it to an acceptable risk level, the result of which will decide what cleanup actions are appropriate to reach an acceptable risk. Since the source of chemical contamination may remain unknown in this case, the risk assessors need to evaluate both current and potential risks, as the exposure pathways and scenarios may change even if there is no risk identified in the current condition. As such, the exposure assessors primarily use modeling and scenario development techniques and focus on linking sources with the exposed individuals. If the chemical under investigation is not bioavailable even if the intake occurs, the assessors can use the established biological monitoring approach to determine if the exposure would actually result in a dose. Personal exposure monitoring may also be helpful, as it provides reliable estimates of the exposure or dose at the present time; however, it is limited in providing a good indication of future exposure scenarios.

- If the purpose of the risk assessment is to screen and set priorities, then the exposure assessment will focus on comparative risk levels, where risk estimates will be categorized into semi-quantitative categories (i.e., low, medium, high). Given the quick-sorting nature of the assessment where no decision will be made regarding direct cleanup or regulatory action, the cost-effective modeling and scenario developing approaches are the primary techniques applied in this case to set general priorities for future investigation of worst risk first.

- If the purpose of the risk assessment is to predict risk for prospective agents (i.e., chemicals yet to be manufactured), then the exposure assessment will emphasize examining the link between source and exposure individuals. Given that the agents may not even exist in the environment, the assessors mainly use modeling and scenario development to estimate the potential exposure and dose in this case.

In sum, each exposure assessment approach has its own unique characteristics, strengths, and weaknesses, and the approach selected for the assessment will determine which data are needed. Generally, there are multiple options available when selecting the approach for exposure assessment. If resources permit, applying more than one approach in exposure assessment can improve the validity of the exposure estimates. For example, the assessors can use point-of-contact

BOX 4.1   STRESS

Nancy Fiedler

Environmental stress includes a broad range of conditions occurring acutely, intermittently, or chronically that produce symptoms of stress. Exposure to noise, excessive heat, poor housing, toxic emissions, and natural disasters are only a few of the many environmental conditions associated with the stress response. Although references to stress often encompass external events and symptoms, it is important to clarify that stress is the symptomatic outcome of exposure to stressors that is influenced by the individual's interpretation of those stressors and the ability to cope. Hans Selye first identified the stress response as the alarm phase induced by the Hypothalamic Pituitary Adrenal axis that is relatively consistent across a variety of challenging situations or stressors. Over time, if the individual is unable to adapt to the stressor, stress can be manifested as psychological, physical, and behavioral symptoms. A person who is stressed may experience a combination of feelings of anxiety, physical symptoms such as gastrointestinal upset, and an inability to fulfill tasks at work or home. The individual's evaluation of an external event plays an important role in whether the individual adapts successfully or develops a maladaptive response that results in physical or psychological disability such as post-traumatic stress disorder. For example, the same event such as a financial loss may be regarded by one individual as a minor setback to be overcome while another individual may experience disabling symptoms of stress. Although some environmental stressors such as natural disasters or accidental chemical exposures may be considered universally stressful, even these stressors are interpreted differently by individuals depending on their coping resources and resilience. Characteristics of the environmental stressor and the exposed individual will increase or decrease the risk of developing stress symptoms and ultimately mental health disorders. For example, when individuals suffer serious physical injury, significant financial loss, or disruption in community and social networks as a result of natural disasters such as hurricanes or floods, the likelihood of stress symptoms and mental health disorders is increased. Technological disasters such as oil spills may have uncertain effects that result in persistent financial and health concerns. If the individual's cognitive appraisal of an environmental stressor is perceived as "human made" or exacerbated by failure to maintain infrastructure, the risk of stress-related symptoms is increased. Moreover, poor communication by government officials, reduced trust because systems to protect people have failed, and refusal to take responsibility for the disaster increases stress among individuals and communities and contributes to adverse health effects (e.g., the Flint, Michigan, water crisis). Individual characteristics such as exposure to previous traumatic events, lower education and income, and female sex also increase the risk of a stress disorder in response to acute environmental stressors. The increased vulnerability of these subgroups is due, in part, to fewer physical and psychological resources. For example, compared to men, a higher percentage of women stressed by Hurricane Katrina were unemployed. Thus, environmental stressors can induce an acute, predictable stress response and a more chronic stress disorder depending on the complex interaction of the individual, the characteristics of the environmental stressor, and the available social/psychological resources.

BOX 4.2   AIR POLLUTION EXPOSURE ASSESSMENT

Junfeng Zhang

Air pollution exposure is assessed for regulatory, research, and personal protection purposes. Depending on the purposes, the most appropriate and relevant methods can be selected to assess exposure. For example, air pollutants ubiquitously present in the atmosphere are regulated, under the US Clean Air Act, as criteria air pollutants (CAPs). National Ambient Air Quality Standards (NAAQS) are set for each of the six CAPs (particulate matter, nitrogen dioxide, ozone, sulfur dioxide, carbon monoxide, and lead). The regulation requires measurements of ambient concentrations at monitoring sites designed to represent population exposure. The primary purpose is to monitor whether pollutant concentrations at a specified monitoring site are in compliance with NAAQS. In contrast, 187 air pollutants classified as hazardous air pollutants (HAPs) are regulated at their sources of emission. HAP exposure is assessed for individuals or populations specifically affected by a particular source. The primary purpose of assessing HAP exposure is to estimate the health risk attributable to the emission source in the affected people.

Fixed-site monitoring is based on the premise that ambient concentrations serve as a reasonable proxy for population exposure. For the same premise, many air pollution epidemiologic studies have used these fixed-site concentrations to represent exposure usually at the population (or ecological) level. This approach has the clear advantage of using readily available data but may not capture spatial variability across the area that a single fixed site is designed to represent. This limitation has motivated the rapid advancement in various spatiotemporal models that can provide air pollution exposure assessment with high spatial and temporal resolutions. Many of these models have been published and utilized in more recent epidemiologic studies and risk assessments.

At the personal exposure level, however, air pollution exposure is determined not only by spatiotemporal variation in ambient (outdoor) pollutant concentration but also by indoor environments encountered and certain personal activities (e.g., active or passive tobacco smoking). To take into consideration of variability in pollutant concentration across different microenvironments (e.g., outside, inside homes, inside schools/offices, and in transit), time-averaged exposure can be assessed by measuring or estimating concentrations in microenvironments in conjunction with time-activity data associated with the microenvironments. Personal exposure can also be assessed via participants wearing so-called personal monitors or personal samplers, both small in size and light in weight. Personal samplers usually collect air pollutants on a sampling medium, and subsequent lab analysis is required to determine the pollutant concentration. In contrast, personal monitors often refer to a device that can provide real-time readings of pollutant concentration. Due to its convenience and real-time reading advantages, there has been a considerable amount of effort made in recent years to develop small, lightweight, and low-cost sensors to monitor common air pollutants (e.g., $PM_{2.5}$, O_3, and NO_2). These devices have a wide range of applications such as identifying air pollution "hot spots" within an area or community, identifying high-polluting microenvironments or activities, and identifying peak pollution periods. The data can provide personal-level exposure estimates for epidemiological studies and to guide risk-reduction measures (e.g., avoiding high-polluting places and times).

Despite the various advantages of low-cost sensors, their accuracy and precision are often a concern for research and regulatory purposes. Measurement methods for regulatory purposes must strictly follow the government (e.g., US EPA) designated methods including quality assurance/quality control (QA/QC) procedures. The designated methods use substantially more expensive and less portable technologies. For this reason, from a practical standpoint, low-cost sensors can be deployed to many locations to provide supplementary data to fixed-site monitoring data. For research purposes, adequate and proper calibrations are required. Commonly, sensors should be field calibrated by comparing the concentrations reported from the sensors to those reported from a designated monitor co-located with the sensors.

measurements to verify and validate the assessments made by scenario evaluation. As such, within an exposure assessment, the choices are not mutually exclusive, and an assessor may choose several approaches to estimate exposure and dose to evaluate the nature and probability of adverse health effects in humans who may be exposed to chemicals in contaminated environmental media.

REFERENCES

Agency for Toxic Substances and Disease Registry. 2005. *Appendix G: Calculating Exposure Doses*. Public Health Assessment Guidance Manual.

Cousins, I. T., C. A. Ng, Z. Wang, and M. Scheringer. 2019. Why Is High Persistence Alone a Major Cause of Concern? *Environ Sci Process Impacts* 21(5): 781–792.

Fenske, R. A., S. W. Horstman, and R. K. Bentley. 1987. Assessment of Dermal Exposure to Chlorophenols in Timber Mills. *Appl Ind Hyg* 2: 143–147.

Jepson, P. D., and R. J. Law. 2016. Persistent Pollutants, Persistent Threats. *Science* 352(6292): 1388–1389.

Liang, D., J. L. Moutinho, R. Golan, T. Yu, C. N. Ladva, M. Niedzwiecki, D. I. Walker, S. E. Sarnat, H. H. Chang, R. Greenwald, D. P. Jones, A. G. Russell, and J. A. Sarnat. 2018. Use of High-Resolution Metabolomics for the Identification of Metabolic Signals Associated with Traffic-Related Air Pollution. *Environ Int* 120: 145–154.

National Research Council. 1990. *Human Exposure Assessment for Airborne Pollutants: Advances and Applications. Committee on Advances in Assessing Human Exposure to Airborne Pollutants, Committee on Geosciences, Environment, and Resources, NRC.* Washington, DC: National Academy Press.

National Research Council. 2012. *Exposure Science in the 21st Century: A Vision and a Strategy.* Washington, DC: National Research Council.

Niedzwiecki, M. M., D. I. Walker, R. Vermeulen, M. Chadeau-Hyam, D. P. Jones and G. W. Miller. 2019. The Exposome: Molecules to Populations. *Annu Rev Pharmacol Toxicol* 59: 107–127.

Sarnat, J. A., A. G. Russell, D. Liang, J. L. Moutinho, R. Golan, R. J. Weber, D. Gao, S. E. Sarnat, H. H. Chang, R. Greenwald, and T. Yu, 2018. *Developing Multipollutant Exposure Indicators of Traffic Pollution: The Dorm Room Inhalation to Vehicle Emissions (DRIVE) Study.* Research Reports: Health Effects Institute, 2018.

Sobus, J., M. K. Morgan, J. D. Pleil, and D. B. Barr. 2010. Chapter 45. Biomonitoring Uses and Considerations for Assessing Human Exposures to Pesticides. In R. Krieger (Ed.), *Hayes' Handbook of Pesticide Toxicology* (3rd ed., Vol. 1, 1021–1036). Waltham, MA: Academic Press.

Stockley, L. 1985. Changes in Habitual Food Intake During Weighed Inventory Surveys and Duplication Diet Collections. *A Short Review Ecol Food Nutr* 17: 263–269.

US Environmental Protection Agency. 1989. *Risk-Assessment Guidance for Superfund. Vol. 1. Human Health Evaluation Manual. Part A. Interim Report (Final)* (No. PB-90-155581/XAB; EPA-540/1-89/002). Environmental Protection Agency. Washington, DC: Office of Solid Waste and Emergency Response.

US Environmental Protection Agency. 1997. Ecological risk assessment guidance for superfund: Process for designing and conducting ecological risk assessments – Interim final [EPA Report]. (EPA/540/R-97/006). Washington, DC: Office of Solid Waste and Emergency Response.

US Environmental Protection Agency. 1992. *Guidelines for Exposure Assessment.* https://www.epa.gov/sites/default/files/2014-11/documents/guidelines_exp_assessment.pdf.

US Environmental Protection Agency. 2004. *Example Exposure Scenarios.* https://ofmpub.epa.gov/eims/eimscomm.getfile?p_download_id=435481.

US Environmental Protection Agency. 2009. *A Conceptual Framework for U.S. EPA's National Exposure Research Laboratory.* (EPA/600/R-09/003). Washington, DC: National Exposure Research Laboratory, Office of Research and Development, U.S. EPA. https://cfpub.epa.gov/si/si_public_record_report.cfm?Lab=NERL&dirEntryId=203003.

US Environmental Protection Agency. 2019. *Guidelines for Human Exposure Assessment.* https://www.epa.gov/sites/default/files/2020-01/documents/guidelines_for_human_exposure_assessment_final2019.pdf

WHO. 2004. *IPCS Risk Assessment Terminology. Part 1, IPCS/OECD Key Generic Terms Used in Chemical Hazard/Risk Assessment; Part 2, IPCS Glossary of Key Exposure Assessment Terminology.* Geneva, Switzerland: IPCS Harmonization Project, WHO. http://www.who.int/ipcs/methods/harmonization/areas/ipcsterminologyparts1and2.pdf?ua=1.

WHO. 2012. *Harmonization Project Strategic Plan: Harmonization of Approaches to the Assessment of Risk from Exposure to Chemicals.* Geneva, Switzerland: IPCS Harmonization Project, WHO. http://www.who.int/ipcs/methods/harmonization/en/.

Zartarian, V. G., T. Bahadori, and T. McKone. 2005. Adoption of an Official ISEA Glossary. *J Expo Anal Environ Epidemiol* 15: 1–5.

Zartarian, V. G., W. R. Ott, and N. Duan. 2007. Chapter 2. Basic Concepts and Definitions of Exposure and Dose. In W. R. Ott, AC Steinemann, and L. A. Wallace (Eds.), *Exposure Analysis* (pp. 33–63). Boca Raton, FL: CRC Press. http://www.crcnetbase.com/doi/book/10.1201/9781420012637.

5 Biological Monitoring of Exposure to Environmental Chemicals throughout the Life Stages

Requirements and Issues to Consider for Birth Cohort Studies

Parinya Panuwet, P. Barry Ryan, and Dana Boyd Barr
Emory University, Atlanta, GA, USA

Warangkana Naksen
Chiang Mai University, Chiang Mai, Thailand

CONTENTS

Introduction 74
Exposure Assessment Methods and Their Uses..74
    Questionnaires and Ecologic Measures 76
    Direct Environmental Measurements..77
    Biological Monitoring or Biomonitoring..78
    Exposure Modeling...79
Biomonitoring and the Toxicokinetic Process of Environmental Chemicals........80
    The General Behavior of Chemicals in the Body..81
    Behavior of Specific Chemical Classes in the Body.......................................81
Assessing Exposure Throughout the Life Cycle..83
Biological Matrices for Exposure Assessment 84
    Blood or Blood Products (i.e., Plasma or Serum)...84
    Urine..84
    Breast Milk and Adipose Tissue..85
    Alternative Matrices 85
Exposure Measurement Considerations..86
    Biomolecular Adducts 86
    Sampling Time Frame..86
    Collecting Samples from Infants and Children...87
    Temporal Variability in Urine and Blood Samples..87
Chemical Analysis Methods..87
    Organic Chemicals 87
    Heavy Metals and Metalloids...88
Measurement Method Specificity and Sensitivity Requirements 88
Quality Assurance and Control 89
Conclusion 90
Thought Questions 90
Literature Cited 90
References...91

LEARNING OBJECTIVES

Students who complete this chapter will be able to

1. Understand the behavior of different classes of chemicals in the body after exposure has occurred,
2. Recognize the utility of biomonitoring in assessing exposure to environmental toxicants,
3. Recognize that different methodologies and techniques may affect the quality and ultimately the utility of selected biomonitoring measurements,
4. Learn the appropriate matrices to use for biomonitoring of exposure to selected classes of environmental chemicals, and
5. Learn about the temporal variability and uncertainties involved with biomonitoring of exposure to chemicals that have short environmental and biological lifetimes.

DOI: 10.1201/9780429291722-5

INTRODUCTION

Exposure assessment is an important component of risk assessment. When examining a population for adverse health impacts that result, in part, from environmental insults, it is essential to try to link those impacts with exposures to chemical, biological, and physical agents that occur in our daily environment. We consider not only the known toxicity and the concentration of a given chemical to which an individual or a population is exposed but also the frequency, duration, pathways, and routes of these exposures. In addition, the developmental life stage of the person(s) exposed is of fundamental importance (EPA 2001). For example, many researchers believe that some health endpoints that manifest themselves at various stages of development are a result of exposures that occurred soon after conception. The critical or most susceptible time period for environmental exposures and their related neurodevelopmental outcomes is thought to be in utero through childhood (Rauh and Margolis 2016). For reproductive health outcomes, some windows of susceptibility to toxicants include prenatal, childhood, puberty, and adulthood exposures depending on each endpoint (Buser et al. 2018). For instance, a research study suggests pre-pubertal exposures to high levels of 2,3,7,8-tetrachlorodibenzo-p-dioxin can later alter the male-to-female sex ratio of their children (Mocarelli et al. 2000). Nonetheless, identifying susceptible periods for developmental issues is quite challenging in the field of children's environmental health research (Braun and Gray 2017).

Various means exist for assessing children's exposures to environmental agents (Needham and Sexton 2000; Needham et al. 2005a, 2005b). Exposure is defined as contact between an agent and a target; contact takes place at an exposure surface over an exposure period (Zartarian et al. 1997). For many longitudinal birth cohort studies, the agents of concern are selected environmental chemical, biological, and physical agents; the targets are children; the exposure surfaces are the external surfaces of the children through which exposure can occur (i.e., skin, mouth, and nasal passage); and the exposure period is the child's lifetime or a defined portion of that lifetime (Needham et al. 2005b; Zartarian et al. 1997).

The continuum (Needham et al. 2005b) often used to describe the human exposure assessment pathway starts with the agent at its origin or its source, which, for example, can be a chemical manufacturing plant, automobile exhaust, or a chemical waste site. The agent can undergo various fate (such as transformation to another chemical) and transport (such as long-range air transport or movement from soil into groundwater) steps in the environment. This may lead to multiple intermediate sources in the pathway for a given agent; eventually, humans may have contact with the environmental media that contain the agent or its environmental transformation products, which is defined as exposure. This exposure may pass through membranes and enter into the body's circulatory system by three primary routes – ingestion, inhalation, and dermal absorption. Depending on the membrane absorption coefficients and other bioavailability factors, the agent (or its metabolite) can be absorbed into the bloodstream. This absorbed dose of the agent or metabolite (or its reaction product [adduct]) is also known as the internal dose. This internal dose can be either directly eliminated (usually a minor route); distributed within the body to other organs, including the target organ(s); metabolized and eliminated (usually in urine); metabolized and distributed within the body to other organs including the target organ; or some combination of these (Klaassen 2013; Needham and Sexton 2000).

A portion of the dose at the target organ may be biologically effective (biologically effective dose) (Needham et al. 2005b; Ozkaynak et al. 2005). The process of estimating or measuring the magnitude, frequency, and duration of exposure to an agent, along with the number and characteristics of the population exposed, is called an exposure assessment (EPA 2019; Needham et al. 2005b) and includes assessing the dose within the body as well as the actual contact with the agent. Exposure assessment can be a complex and costly process. The complexity only increases when physiologic changes occur during pregnancy and fetal development or when in a child at a young age (Barr et al. 2005, 2007; Needham et al. 2005b). Figure 5.1 presents the exposure-effect continuum during pregnancy.

EXPOSURE ASSESSMENT METHODS AND THEIR USES

A major goal in environmental epidemiology is to determine the association or lack of an association between exposure to environmental chemicals and morbidity and/or mortality, which provides a useful piece of information for risk assessment (Neutra 1983). In health studies, we prefer analytical chemistry data to define the biologically effective dose in a target organ that was sampled at the appropriate time to relate with the outcome of interest (Barr et al. 1999). However,

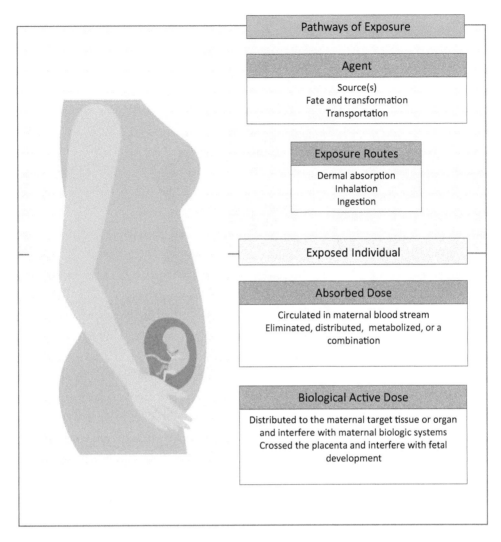

Figure 5.1   Maternal-fetal exposure diagram.

measurement of the biologically effective dose is seldom possible because we may not know the target organ, or if we do, the sampling of that organ is generally a quite invasive process (Barr et al. 1999). Therefore, the exposure status of an individual in health studies is classified based on his/her internal dose of that agent, its concentration in personal air samples, and/or the concentration of the agent in relevant environmental samples (Needham et al. 2005b; Ozkaynak et al. 2005). In addition, data from each of these measurements are coupled with questionnaire information to derive each person's exposure index. This index places each individual into an exposure category, such as distribution tertiles, and each category is examined for an association with a health outcome; the data are most powerful when a statistically significant trend between the assessed exposure and outcome is observed. Hence, to link exposure and disease status accurately, we must classify both the exposure and disease status. Other goals of health studies are to utilize exposure assessment information to diagnose disease, to treat disease, to prevent further disease, and to evaluate the effectiveness of each of these goals.

Exposures to the general population of the United States may be very difficult to assess accurately because we are generally exposed to low levels of environmental chemicals, and the exposure scenario may be episodic (occurring only occasionally) (Barr et al. 1999). The exposures may occur through various routes and pathways, including occupational, dietary, and nondietary ingestion. For assessing exposures to environmental agents, there is no single method that

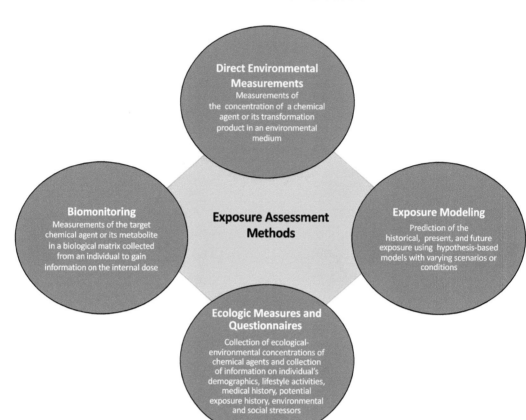

Figure 5.2 Exposure assessment methods.

will capture all the needed exposure information all the time (Barr et al. 1999; Needham 2005; Ozkaynak et al. 2005). This is true for children and adults but becomes even more relevant when attempting to assess exposures during the in utero and early childhood life stages. Therefore, a method that is "best" for assessing exposure to a given chemical at one life stage may not be the "best" method for assessing exposure to that same chemical at a different life stage (Needham et al. 2005b).

There are four main methods (questionnaires and ecologic data collection, direct/personal environmental monitoring, modeling, and biomonitoring; Figure 5.2) that are used to assess human exposures to chemical and biological agents (Needham et al. 2005b; Zartarian and Schultz 2010). All these methods seek to gain information on the concentrations of the agent(s) to which the person(s) may have been exposed and the duration and frequency of that exposure. From this information, exposure indices are constructed that are used to estimate or categorize an individual's exposure and ultimately the dose within a population. Other data that should be factored into the assessment, especially when the population studied includes fetuses as well as children and adults, is the timing of the exposure during critical susceptible periods of development.

Questionnaires and Ecologic Measures

Questionnaires seek information on an individual's demographics, lifestyle activities, medical history, potential exposure history, and environmental and social stressors that are essential in any study of human exposure to chemical agents. Questionnaires can be self-administered or administered by a trained interviewer. Both require a high level of expertise in developing the questionnaire and, for the latter, in administering the questionnaire. The questionnaire must acquire the necessary information in a clear unbiased manner yet not be too lengthy so as to present an undue burden (which leads to boredom and to inaccurate information) to the study participant. With respect to exposure, questionnaires seek to acquire information for developing exposure indices for the studied population. These indices consist of two types of information: the concentrations of the chemical to which individuals in the study population have contact (exposure), and the frequency/duration of that exposure. In general, questionnaires provide more accurate data on the frequency/duration aspect of the index as compared to the concentration component (Needham et al. 2005b).

In addition to the exposure situation itself, questionnaires can provide much needed information on factors that affect the chemical's toxicokinetics within an individual (absorption, distribution, metabolism [biotransformation], and elimination) and toxicodynamics. The individual toxicokinetics and toxicodynamics can dramatically influence the exposure-effect outcome (Fernandez et al. 2011). These factors include demographic factors (such as age, sex, and race/ethnicity), environmental (such as the built environment) and behavioral stressors, nutritional status, and other exposures, including medications and food supplements. Thus, questionnaires have the advantage of yielding information that cannot be gleaned readily by other methods, yet they suffer from the disadvantage of information bias, especially recall bias, which can lead to inaccurate exposure and outcome classifications. Information bias occurs when the accurate measurements of key variables are lacking, resulting from poor interviewing techniques or differing levels of recall by participants (Kesmodel 2018). Recall bias is caused by the tendency of an individual to remember more recent events or out-of-the-ordinary events better than everyday events, leading to systematic errors in obtaining relevant data for exposure classification. Also, questionnaires often provide no actual concentration data for the chemical/biological agent in the environment and in humans.

Information from other indirect methods, such as geographic information systems (GIS) and videotaping, is also limited by not providing actual concentration data for the agent in environmental and human specimens. However, videotaping has the advantages of tracing a given individual throughout his/her activities in daily life and observing potential contacts with the agent of concern and the frequency/duration of these contacts. Videotaping is particularly useful for recording the potential for transferring an agent from the outer surfaces of the body into, for example, the mouth; i.e., for recording such actions as hand-to-mouth activity (Ferguson et al. 2021, 2006). GIS uses computerized maps to integrate potential exposure data (e.g., from estimated pollution data) into a spatial form so that the data can be analyzed geographically. GIS data are often used when more direct monitoring data are not available, but we caution that measurements in environmental or biological samples should be performed to validate the exposure assessment derived from GIS.

Ecologic data are also widely used for exposure assessment (Needham et al. 2005b). These data reflect ambient exposures, often offering continuous monitoring, that may be assigned to a larger group depending upon their residence or work location. For example, larger cities may routinely monitor ozone or other criteria pollutants in specified regions, and those data can be used to assign exposure to specific subpopulations in the city, especially when you incorporate characteristics that may modify exposure such as land use, greenness, or climatic variables. These measurements are not as refined as other exposure assessment methods and are highly susceptible to exposure misclassification.

Direct Environmental Measurements

It is the measurement of a chemical agent or its transformation product in an environmental medium that provides information that can be used to track the chemical from its source throughout the environment – air, water, food, soil, dust, etc. Consequently, environmental measurements are especially useful in risk management, where one is concerned about interrupting the pathway of exposure and preventing further human exposure. In addition, direct measurements have been used widely as a metric for risk assessment. For example, reference concentrations/doses and cancer unit risks are expressed as an environmental concentration that can then be compared to an exposure estimate to determine whether an adverse health risk is likely. Environmental data are of most use when there is a single predominant environmental matrix, such as air, involved in the exposure scenario. If the exposure scenario is multimedia, then the number of potential measurements (and hence costs) increases dramatically, and the data are more difficult to model for the purpose of predicting human exposures and particularly for predicting internal doses (Ciffroy et al. 2016; Fantke et al. 2018; Shin et al. 2017).

In the exposure-effect continuum, environmental monitoring gives us information about the concentration of the chemical(s) to which humans are potentially exposed and potential pathways and routes of exposure, while questionnaire information provides data on the duration and frequency of exposure and the timing of the exposures. Thus, this combination of environmental monitoring and questionnaire information provides needed information on the potential dose. However, for health studies, we are most concerned with the biologically effective dose at the target organ of the exposed individual; therefore, models must then be developed to estimate the amount of the chemical to which the population is exposed and furthermore the amount that is absorbed into the body and becomes the internal dose and ultimately the biologically effective dose (Chou and Lin 2019; MacIntosh et al. 1999, 2000, 2001; Needham and Sexton 2000; Needham et al. 2005b; Ozkaynak et al. 2005; Pang et al. 2002; Ryan et al. 2000; Zartarian et al. 2000). These models, if possible, should be calibrated and validated before being used.

Air pollutants may be measured in the air itself or by personal exposure monitors (Ott 1990). Depending on several factors, including the chemicals to be monitored, active or passive sampling may be used. Active sampling involves drawing the air into the collection unit with a sampling pump, while passive sampling relies upon diffusion. In both sampling processes, the collection unit should be located within the "breathing zone" (i.e., 30 cm of the nose and mouth). Personal air monitoring is an important component in estimating exposure concentrations in certain exposure scenarios, but again, the uptake data for the chemical and pharmacokinetic data must be modeled for the exposed individual. Disadvantages of personal air monitoring and environmental air monitoring include the lack of accounting for differences in breathing rates and data on volumes of air inhaled among people or within a person, for example, during physical exercise.

A concern in human exposure assessment is the burden on the study population. The use of environmental monitoring plus questionnaire information may present no more burdens on the study population than the questionnaire itself. However, this is usually not the case. For example, if indoor air is monitored, equipment must be installed in the home; if food is monitored, then duplicate diets may be taken; and if personal air monitors are used, they must be installed on the individual. Assessing personal exposures in community health studies often relies upon partial information on measured concentrations of chemicals in various microenvironments of concern. Consequently, the use of limited outdoor or indoor monitoring information can lead to exposure misclassification biases, which in turn, may result in loss of statistical power or increase the potential for obtaining a null result when an association between exposure and disease exists (Ozkaynak and Spengler 1985; Ozkaynak et al. 1996). To minimize errors in estimating personal exposures, researchers identify key sources, media, routes, and pathways of concern for each environmental pollutant, and then determine an optimum sampling and analysis plan that will assure collection of environmental and/or questionnaire information for each of the significant media and route of exposure. In practice, of course, both the budgetary and technical constraints often limit the extent of an environmental monitoring program. The actual cost of environmental monitoring is dependent on the chemical compound, the number of matrices to be monitored, which matrices are monitored, the frequency of monitoring, and the cost of administering the questionnaire.

One advantage of environmental monitoring that is often overlooked is that certain chemicals are more toxic when they enter the body by a certain route. For example, chemicals such as manganese and polycyclic aromatic hydrocarbons that are bound to particulate matter are potentially more toxic when inhaled than when ingested. Therefore, if only biomonitoring (vide infra) is used for assessing exposure to these chemicals, the degree of exposure from these two routes cannot be differentiated, and thus the assessment of toxicity resulting from these exposures may be in error.

Biological Monitoring or Biomonitoring

Biomonitoring provides information on the internal dose integrated across environmental pathways and routes of exposure; thus, an advantage of biomonitoring is that it directly considers the amount of the chemical that is absorbed into the body's systemic circulatory system (Angerer et al. 2007). For persistent chemicals (those that have "long" half-lives on the order of months or years in the environment and in humans), biomonitoring data provide information as to what chemical and how much actually enters people and accumulates. These persistent chemicals are generally measured in blood or its components, such as serum and plasma, in adipose tissue, or in human milk. Following exposure to persistent chemicals, differences in pharmacokinetics among various people will affect the internal dose levels to some degree but typically will not interfere with proper classification of exposures in epidemiological studies. Thus, biomonitoring is generally considered to be the "gold standard" for assessing human exposure to persistent chemicals, provided the sample collection is feasible. In the event biomonitoring is not feasible, an exposure index derived by other methods for persistent chemicals, such as environmental sampling combined with questionnaires, should be considered.

For chemicals that have short half-lives, biomonitoring data may become much more difficult to interpret. If the exposure is continuous (constantly occurring) or even continual (repeatedly occurring but not constantly), then the exposure (not the chemical) could be deemed "persistent," and biomonitoring plays a vital role in assessing human exposure (Needham et al. 2005a); however, if the exposure is predominantly from one environmental medium, then environmental monitoring and questionnaire data should also be considered for assessing an exposure. Whenever exposures are inconsistent or episodic, then biomonitoring, like other techniques such as environmental monitoring, loses much of its ability to track these exposures. In this scenario, the frequency of sampling and hence the comparison of data from these samplings are extremely critical issues.

The collection of the biological sample to be analyzed may involve procedures that are invasive, such as the drawing of blood, to those with little intrusion, such as collecting urine samples from adults. If one neglects the burden on the person and the amount of blood that can be collected, blood has inherent advantages for biomonitoring. Regardless of the route of exposure, the chemical must be absorbed into the bloodstream and circulated to the tissues prior to an effect (exceptions would include direct inhalation effects on the lung and blistering agents on skin). Blood is also a "regulated" matrix; therefore, there is a constant amount of blood so that measurements can be "normalized" to this amount. The other most commonly monitored biological matrix is urine, which serves as a "sink" for many chemicals, especially nonpersistent chemicals; persistent chemicals are often eliminated primarily through feces. These nonpersistent chemicals are generally found in urine not only as their original "parent" structure but, more frequently, as metabolites including biomolecular adducts and degradation products.

Measuring these metabolites to assess exposure, however, may be problematic because (1) multiple chemicals may form the same metabolite, (2) individual genetic polymorphisms may cause a difference in metabolism (Nakajima et al. 2002), and (3) the environmental transformation product (for example, for organophosphate insecticide) may be the same chemical as the metabolite, thereby complicating interpretation. Nonetheless, urinary measurements can play a vital role in assessing human exposure to many environmental chemicals. To gain specificity, these nonpersistent chemicals, such as chlorpyrifos (an organophosphate insecticide) and many volatile organic chemicals, have been measured as the parent compound in blood (Needham et al. 2005c; Whyatt et al. 2004). Another way to gain specificity and increase the time window for the exposure assessment for certain nonpersistent chemicals is to measure their reaction products or adducts, such as hemoglobin, albumin, or DNA adducts.

It should be noted that there are some chemicals or physical agents for which we have no or little means to assess their exposure via biomonitoring. These include particulate matter, asbestos, some of the air criteria pollutants (such as oxides of nitrogen), and allergens. Several emerging environmental chemicals have incomplete information on human metabolism, making it difficult to monitor their metabolite(s) in humans. Also, for some chemicals, the nonspecificity of the metabolite biomarker (depending on the chemical and the biological matrix used) may make it difficult to determine the actual chemical to which the population or person was exposed. Another important point, especially for inorganic chemicals, is that both environmental and biological monitoring, include the biologically active specie(s) of the chemical – e.g., methyl mercury – for assessing exposure to mercury following fish consumption (Needham et al. 2005c).

Exposure Modeling

Exposure modeling offers an alternative strategy in exposure assessment methods, especially in cases where exposure data are not readily available or do not exist (Sexton and Ryan 1988). A few examples may clarify. Consider a case in which data have been collected using stationary monitors in multiple microenvironments, but personal exposure data are not available. However, data are available using, for example, a time-activity diary that affords an assessment of the amount of time individuals spend in each one of those microenvironments. A model can be constructed that accounts for the fractional time spent in each of these microenvironments, coupled with the concentration of contaminant in these microenvironments to get an estimate of what the exposure experienced by the individual is. Of course, there are compromises made in such an approach. There is an assumption of temporal homogeneity in the concentrations in each microenvironment. The variability expected, but not measured, can result in errors in the estimation of exposure. Further, the quality of the time-activity diary, which may suffer from recall biases and time-resolution inaccuracies, increases the likelihood of errors. Still, this type of approach has been used in numerous investigations as a hybrid measurement-modeling approach to exposure estimation (Mirabelli et al. 2015; Sarnat et al. 2014).

An alternative use of modeling is evident in retrospective exposure assessment. While many occupational studies use the Job-Exposure Matrix approach (Ryan 2016) to occupational exposure retrospectively, this is not an appropriate strategy for community-based exposure as no such "Job-Exposure Matrix" exists for the population at large. Yet such retrospective exposure assessment is often necessary in epidemiological investigations that require long-term exposure estimates where none exist. A recent example occurred in the large-scale epidemiologic investigations of perfluorooctanoic acid (PFOA) exposure experienced by individuals impacted by remissions from a manufacturing facility in West Virginia on the banks of the Ohio River (Shin et al. 2011a, 2011b, 2014; Steenland et al. 2020). To understand the measured concentrations of PFOA in the large (>40,000 individuals) population exposed over their entire lifetime, a modeling effort offered the only solution. In this case, multiple physical models (Ryan 1997) of release, transport, deposition, and groundwater movement were combined with intake models to arrive at an estimate of exposure for each individual for their entire lifetime, notwithstanding the lack of historical measurements of PFOA either in the environmental or internally in such cases, modeling is the only recourse in estimating exposures.

An additional use of modeling systems in exposure assessment is to evaluate alternative scenarios to that which is present in an environmental system. Consider the question: How would exposure to the population living in a specific community change if a new manufacturing facility were introduced in the community and it was a source of a specific type of contamination? Such scenario testing is the purview of models exclusively. Siting criteria for new facilities often require an environmental impact statement, part of which is the estimation of changes in the local environment. Models provide the only mechanism to explore such impact.

Human exposure models range from quite simple estimates using just one or two microenvironments and simple "back-of-the-envelop" calculations (Ryan et al. 1989) to highly sophisticated stochastic approaches invoking statistical arguments and distribution characteristics of multiple parameters to effect a population-based estimate of exposure distributions in a population (Isaacs et al. 2014). While the famous aphorism, "All models are wrong. Some are useful," attributed to the statistician George E. P. Box, is certainly true, exposure scientists have made use of models in exposure estimation for at least 50 years and will continue to do so due to their utility. In Box's point of view: "Some are useful."

CASE STUDY 1

INMA – INfancia y Medio Ambiente (Environment and Childhood) Project is a research network study created to assess exposure to environmental pollutants via air, water, and diet during pregnancy and early life, and their effects on child growth and development. The study area is Sabadell, a city of nearly 200,000 inhabitants situated in the metropolitan area of Barcelona, Spain. Women who visited the public health center of Sabadell in the 12th week of pregnancy and fulfilled the inclusion criteria were eligible to participate in the study. The main exclusion criteria were being < 16 years of age, nonsingleton pregnancy, not planning to deliver at the Hospital of Sabadell, and having followed an assisted reproduction program. Women were interviewed in the 12th and 32nd weeks of pregnancy using structured questionnaires to collect data on sociodemographic characteristics, health status, use of drugs, occupational data, environmental exposures, time-activity patterns, and food frequency intake. In this study, a GIS-based exposure to traffic-related air pollutants was also applied to examine the influence of time-activity patterns during pregnancy and the association between air pollution exposure and birth weight (Aguilera et al. 2009; Ribas-Fitó et al. 2006). Source: INMA web page (https://www.proyectoinma.org/en/)

BIOMONITORING AND THE TOXICOKINETIC PROCESS OF ENVIRONMENTAL CHEMICALS

Following an individual's exposure to a given chemical, a proportion of the chemical may be absorbed into the bloodstream, distributed among the bodily tissues, metabolized, and/or excreted (Mirabelli et al. 2015; Ryan 1997, 2016; Sarnat et al. 2014; Sexton and Ryan 1988; Shin et al. 2012, 2011a, 2011b, 2017; Steenland et al. 2020). These four complex steps (i.e., absorption, distribution, metabolism, and excretion (ADME)) make up the toxicokinetic process of a chemical

(Lehman-McKeeman 2008). In order to assess human exposure to a given chemical, biological measurements of the chemical can be made after the absorption step or during each of the subsequent steps of ADME.

Biomonitoring of exposure involves the measurement of the concentration of a chemical in each biological matrix during or after ADME, and its concentration level depends on the amount of the chemical that has been absorbed into the body, the pharmacokinetics (ADME) of the chemical, and the exposure scenario including the time sequence of exposure and time since last exposure (Sexton et al. 1995). Biomonitoring data are independent of the pathway of exposure (Albertini et al. 2006; Pirkle et al. 1995). Ideally, in order to link the dose with adverse health outcomes, measurements of the biologically effective dose, the dose at the target site that causes an adverse health effect, are preferred (La Rocca et al. 2012; Pirkle et al. 1995; Sabbioni et al. 2007). However, often the target organ is not known, and even if known, it is frequently not available for sampling. In these situations, we measure the level of the chemical in another biological sample to gauge the internal dose.

The General Behavior of Chemicals in the Body

Absorption of a chemical into the body occurs when the chemical enters the bloodstream by passing through absorption membrane barriers following contact of the chemical with an outer boundary (i.e., skin, nostrils, mouth, or eyes). Without absorption, there can be no direct internal toxic effect even if the chemical is toxic, although effects are possible at the absorption barrier (e.g., skin irritation, eye lens irritation). Once the chemical has been absorbed into the bloodstream, it undergoes a distribution to the primary deposition sites. Distribution is crucial to toxicity because if the chemical is never distributed to the target site, the toxic effect cannot occur. However, because the concentration of the chemical in the storage depot (e.g., adipose tissue) is in equilibrium with the concentration in the blood, the chemical is slowly released from the storage depot as it is eliminated from the blood, and low concentrations may reach the target organ.

Metabolism takes place primarily in the liver. The overall purpose of metabolism is to make the chemical less toxic and more hydrophilic so it can be easily eliminated in urine. Phase 1 metabolism of the chemical typically involves inserting or substituting a functional group to make the chemical more water-soluble. Phase 2 metabolism usually binds the chemical to a glucuronide or sulfate group, which increases the water solubility and facilitates elimination of the chemical in the urine. However, metabolism does not always render a chemical less toxic. Metabolized chemicals may be more hydrophilic and can be excreted in urine or may be passed into the feces. If the chemical is not absorbed, it can go straight into the feces. Lipophilic compounds are eliminated primarily in the feces. Volatile organic compounds (VOCs) can be excreted in the expired air. Chemicals can also be deposited in certain secretory structures and be excreted as tears, saliva, sweat, or milk in lactating women.

In addition to the internal movement of chemicals in the body, a pregnant woman can distribute the chemicals via the bloodstream through the placenta and into the fetal blood supply. Biomonitoring matrices unique to the fetus include amniotic fluid and meconium. In addition, cord blood, the placenta, and the umbilical cord can be collected at birth for exposure assessment purposes.

Behavior of Specific Chemical Classes in the Body

Persistent organic chemicals. Persistent organic pollutants or chemicals (POPs) include several chemicals such as polychlorinated dibenzo-p-dioxins, polychlorinated biphenyls, polybrominated diphenyl ethers, poly- and per-fluorinated alkyl substances (PFAS), and organochlorine insecticides (ATSDR 2017; Needham et al. 2005a). Polycyclic aromatic hydrocarbons (PAHs) are also often included in this class because they persist in the environment; however, because PAHs behave more like nonpersistent chemicals in the body, we have chosen to exclude them from POPs (Needham et al. 2005a). Several PFAS have recently been classified as highly persistent in the environment and humans (Cousins et al. 2020). The primary route of exposure to POPs is ingestion. POPs are readily absorbed into the blood supply by passive diffusion. Their blood level initially decays relatively rapidly, representing the alpha decay period (Flesch-Janys et al. 1996) except for chemicals like PFAS that do not sequester appreciably in deposition matrices but rather bind to albumin and continue circulating. During the alpha decay, the POP is distributed into the fatty portions of tissues and, in lactating women, in breast milk. The concentration of the POP in the fatty portions of tissues is in equilibrium with the concentration in the lipid portion of blood. The fat content of blood serum is 0.5%–0.6%, milk is ~4% lipid, and adipose tissue may be as much as 95% lipid. Thus, while the equilibrium concentrations of the chemical in the blood and fatty tissues may differ over orders of magnitude, they may be very similar when matrices are adjusted for lipid content.

In pregnant women, the POP may also distribute in the fetal compartment; therefore, other matrices such as cord blood or serum may be used for POP measurements. However, the lipid content of cord blood is lower than that of an adult, so the sensitivity of the analytical measurement may play a key role in obtaining a valid measurement in cord blood. Recently, placenta and fetal meconium have been explored for their potential in assessing POP exposures in the fetus (Jeong et al. 2016a, 2018; Zhao et al. 2007). Maternal blood or adipose tissue taken before or during pregnancy and maternal blood, milk, or adipose tissue taken soon after parturition (if breastfeeding or can be taken later if not breastfeeding) are considered the best matrices for estimating fetal exposures to POPs.

Because metabolism and excretion of POPs are very slow, they have a long half-life in the body, usually along the order of years (Bartell et al. 2010; Gribble et al. 2015; Zhang et al. 2013). However, because the lipophilic POPs accumulate in the breast milk of lactating women and the milk is removed from the woman's body, the half-life of POPs in lactating women is about six months (LaKind et al. 2000).

Nonpersistent organic chemicals. Nonpersistent organic chemicals, such as current-use pesticides, phthalates, phenols, and VOCs (Needham et al. 2005b), can be much more challenging to measure. Their primary routes of exposure for the general population, depending on the scenario, are generally ingestion or inhalation. These chemicals are rapidly metabolized, and their metabolites are eliminated in urine (Figure 5.3). The deposition matrices are minor matrices for monitoring because only small amounts of the chemical are deposited in the body. The major matrices for assessing exposure are excreta. Blood has also been used as a matrix for biomonitoring. Nonpersistent chemicals tend to have very short half-lives in blood (Figure 5.3), and the concentrations are usually about three orders of magnitude lower than urinary metabolite levels (Barr et al. 1999). Thus, if blood is used as a matrix, the sensitivity of the analytical method and the matrix volume available for analysis may become important. Blood can also be a valuable matrix for measuring biomolecular adducts such as hemoglobin, albumin, or DNA adducts, such as DNA-PAH adducts.

Saliva has also been explored as a matrix for measuring selected nonpersistent chemicals, such as bisphenols and phthalates (Panuwet et al. 2020; Russo et al. 2019; Silva et al. 2005). However, the exiting data do not suggest that it is a better matrix than urine or serum, despite the ease of sample collection. Because the concentrations present in saliva are often quite low, a very sensitive analytical technique is required. Further research on additional chemicals and the relationship between blood-saliva concentrations are required before saliva can routinely be used as a matrix for assessing exposure to nonpersistent chemicals.

To evaluate fetal exposures, maternal samples collected throughout pregnancy may be used. However, because these chemicals are, by definition, nonpersistent, urine or blood measurements

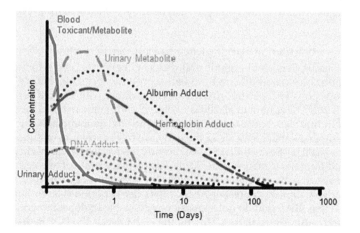

Figure 5.3 Theoretical postexposure fate of a nonpersistent chemical following a single-point exposure.

made at a single point in time during pregnancy will only address the exposures that may have occurred in the previous few days, unless the exposure is continuous (e.g., pervasive air levels of a chemical resulting from smokers in the home) or continual (e.g., eating the same foods daily with measurable levels of pesticides). To circumvent this problem, multiple biological samples can be taken every few days during pregnancy; however, this can be costly, logistically difficult to collect and store, and may present an undue burden on the participant. An alternative may be to collect multiple samples over particularly vulnerable stages of pregnancy if such stages can be appropriately identified. Another potential approach is to measure nonpersistent chemicals in fetal matrices such as cord blood or meconium.

Bioaccumulative metals and nonbioaccumulative metals. Bioaccumulative metals persist in the environment and bioaccumulate in humans. This group of chemicals includes some forms of mercury, lead, and cadmium (Needham et al. 2005a). For example, lead is readily absorbed, particularly in children, with distribution from the blood to its storage depots, i.e., bone and teeth (Aufderheide and Wittmers 1992). Both metabolism and excretion are slow, so monitoring lead levels is more straightforward. The best matrices to use would be blood, bone, and teeth. For general population exposures to mercury, methylmercury is the form of highest concern. Blood, hair, and nails are viable matrices for measuring methylmercury levels.

Nonbioaccumulative metals are readily absorbed into the body, and although some proportion may be distributed to various tissues, most will pass through the body rapidly. These metals are typically measured in urine to obtain information regarding the recent exposure dose (Horng et al. 1999). However, some of these nonbioaccumulative metals (such as arsenic) can also be measured in toenails (Rasheed et al. 2019; Signes-Pastor et al. 2021) to reflect long-term internal dose exposure.

Criteria pollutants and bioallergens. In general, biomonitoring has a limited role in the measurement of criteria pollutants (e.g., CO, NOX, ozone) and bioallergens (e.g., pollen, endotoxins) (Needham et al. 2005a). Exposure to carbon monoxide (CO) can be assessed by measuring the carboxyhemoglobin adduct (Luchini et al. 2009; Shenoi et al. 1998; Smith et al. 1998) or expired CO (Lapostolle et al. 2001; Paredi et al. 2002) in blood and breath, respectively. The adducts provide a longer-term dosimeter for the exposure than breath measurements because hemoglobin has a lifetime of about four months.

Bioallergen response can be measured by IgE in maternal, cord blood, or child blood (Carrer and Moscato 2004; Goodman and Leach 2004; Lee et al. 2004). Recently, responses to allergens can be quantified directly using urinary histamine and urinary n-methylhistamine levels (Raithel et al. 2015). Also, urinary leukotriene E4 has been proposed as a biomarker for allergen-specific IgE sensitization (Chiu et al. 2014). In addition, certain endotoxins or metabolites may be measured in blood or urine samples (Duquenne et al. 2013; Makarananda et al. 1998; Malír et al. 2004). Typically, the endotoxin measurements would reflect a more recent exposure, similar to nonpersistent chemical exposures.

ASSESSING EXPOSURE THROUGHOUT THE LIFE CYCLE

Biomonitoring measurements have been used for many years to assess exposures in adults (Angerer et al. 2007; Blount et al. 2000; Louro et al. 2019). Because the concern about children and adolescent health is growing, biomonitoring of children and adolescents has increased over the years (Adgate et al. 2001; Choi et al. 2017; Fenske et al. 2000; Gys et al. 2020; Schwedler et al. 2020). However, biomonitoring of fetuses and infants has been performed much less frequently due to difficulties in collecting biological samples. Various biological matrices have been used or considered for assessing environmental exposures throughout the life cycle. The mother or pregnant woman has generally been used as a surrogate to evaluate fetal exposures. The placenta plays a critical role in protecting the developing fetus from being exposed to toxic chemicals carried in maternal blood. However, recent evidence suggests that some toxic chemicals (such as phthalates, PFAS, phenols, and polychlorinated biphenyls) can cross the placental barriers and interfere with the developing fetus (Mitro et al. 2015; Rager et al. 2020). However, for many chemicals, their ability to transfer from the mother to the fetus via placenta and cord blood is not known and the relationship between maternal and fetal chemical levels has not been defined. Another potential option to evaluate fetal exposures is the use of meconium as a matrix of measurement since it begins accumulating in the bowels of the infant during the second trimester (Bearer 2003; Bearer et al. 2003; Jeong et al. 2016a; Ostrea et al. 1994). However, meconium use has many limitations. Meconium measurements are still in their infancy of development, and to date, no reliable way to relate these measurements to measurements in more commonly used matrices (e.g., urine and blood) exists. In addition, no information is gleaned from exposures that occurred in the first trimester. However, many have been shown to correlate well with reported maternal exposures to tobacco (Ostrea et al. 1994), drugs of abuse (Ostrea 1999), and alcohol consumption (Bearer et al. 2003), and this matrix shows promise for other chemical exposures of concern (Jeong et al. 2016a; Whyatt and Barr 2001; Zhao et al. 2007).

The period from birth through one year old is also very important (Needham and Sexton 2000; Needham et al. 2005b, 2005c). During this time, the infants may be breastfeeding, so they may be exposed to chemicals via breast milk. In addition, their microenvironments are often close to the floor and substantially different from an older child or adult. At this age, probably only urinary chemical measurements or breast milk measurements can be made. Although collection of infant urine samples via disposable diapers is a common practice for obtaining infant urine for assessing exposures to environmental agents, there are several analytic issues relating to the extraction of target chemicals or metabolites from the diapers, which results in poor extraction recoveries and the exposures being underestimated (Hu et al. 2004; Liu et al. 2012; Lucarini et al. 2021; Saito et al. 2014).

Once children start school, another environment with potential chemical contamination is included in the exposure scenario; however, biological sample collections become easier. At this stage in life, some blood can be collected, but it is often limited to a small amount. Urine and saliva samples can also be readily collected. As children approach adolescence and adulthood, more biological samples and/or a greater quantity of a matrix can be collected.

BIOLOGICAL MATRICES FOR EXPOSURE ASSESSMENT

The two primary matrices used to assess human exposure to chemicals are urine and blood (serum, plasma, blood cells, etc.) (Angerer et al. 2007; Barr et al. 1999; Choi et al. 2017; Needham and Sexton 2000).

Blood or Blood Products (i.e., Plasma or Serum)

Many persistent and nonpersistent chemicals can be measured in blood (Angerer 1988; Angerer and Hörsch 1992; Angerer et al. 2007; Barr et al. 2002; Leng et al. 1997). Although the amount of blood is nearly the same in all adults, the chemical composition of blood, such as lipid content, varies between individuals and within an individual, especially postprandial (Phillips et al. 1989). Blood concentrations of lipophilic chemicals are routinely normalized using blood lipid concentrations to allow a direct comparison of their concentrations within and among individuals, irrespective of the time of day the blood was collected. However, other chemicals that can be measured in the blood may not vary based on the blood lipid content. For example, fluorinated chemicals in blood are not dependent upon the lipid content; instead, they bind to blood albumin (Jones et al. 2003). Therefore, these measurements should not be adjusted based on the blood lipid content; however, other adjustments, such as for albumin content, may be required, if deemed appropriate.

Measuring a chemical in blood is inherently advantageous (Angerer et al. 2007; Barr et al. 1999). Because we know how much blood is in the body, we can calculate the body burden more accurately than if we measure the chemical or its metabolite in urine. However, blood collection is invasive, which may severely limit the ability to collect it from infants and small children. Blood volume changes during pregnancy may complicate interpretation of blood measurements as well. In addition, nonpersistent chemicals are usually found in very low concentrations in blood (Barr et al. 1999, 2002). Also, if testing is not performed soon after sample collection, long-term storage of blood may be problematic, depending upon what form of blood you are storing.

Urine

One of the major advantages of using urine in biomonitoring is the ease of its collection for spot urine samples (Barr et al. 1999; Needham et al. 2005c); however, the collection of 24-hour urine voids can be very cumbersome and result in nonadherence (Barr et al. 1999). Therefore, spot urine samples, whether first morning voids or "convenience" or "spot" samplings, are most generally used for biomonitoring purposes. The major disadvantages of spot urine samples include the variability of the volume of urine and the concentrations of endogenous and exogenous chemicals from void to void (Barr et al. 1999; Fromme et al. 2007). To overcome this issue, compositing a few urine samples collected at different time points together could reduce the temporal variability of the target chemicals or metabolites and potentially reflect the long-term exposure, depending on the collection time interval of the samples (Kim et al. 2021).

The issue of how best to adjust the urinary concentrations of environmental chemicals in a manner analogous to the adjustment of the concentrations of lipophilic chemicals in blood is a subject of continued research. Adjustment using urinary creatinine concentrations (i.e., dividing the analyte concentration by the creatinine concentration (in g creatinine/L urine)) is the most routinely used method for correcting for dilution. Analyte results are then reported as the weight of analyte per gram of creatinine (e.g., mg of analyte/g creatinine). This may work well when comparing analyte levels in a single individual because the intraindividual variation in creatinine excretion is relatively low; however, for diverse populations, the interindividual variation is extremely high (Barr et al. 2005). Further, creatinine excretion in growing children or in pregnant women does not display the same characteristics as adults, calling creatinine correction into question for these populations.

Breast Milk and Adipose Tissue

Many of the same chemicals measured in blood have been found in breast milk (LaKind et al. 2001; Lehmann et al. 2018; Mannetje et al. 2012) and adipose tissue (Lee et al. 2017; Patterson et al. 1986). Breast milk measurements are unique in that they provide data not only on ingestion exposures for the infant but also are indicators of maternal exposures. Breast milk and adipose tissue are lipid-rich matrices, more so than blood, so similar lipid adjustments are required for reporting concentrations of lipophilic analytes. Analytica methodologies for lipophilic compounds in breastmilk are cumbersome (Chen et al. 2014). In general, these lipophilic analytes partition among the lipid stores in blood, breast milk, and adipose tissue on nearly a 1:1:1 basis (Patterson et al. 1986). More laboratory work needs to be done on the partitioning of less bioaccumulative analytes in these matrices.

Alternative Matrices

Chemicals have been successfully measured in alternative matrices such as saliva (Lu et al. 1998; Panuwet et al. 2020), meconium (Bearer et al. 1999, 2003; Jeong et al. 2016b; Ostrea 1999; Ostrea et al. 1994; Whyatt and Barr 2001; Zhao et al. 2007), amniotic fluid (Barr et al. 2007; Bradman et al. 2003; Foster et al. 2002; Jiménez-Díaz et al. 2015), and exhaled breath (Amorim and de 2007; Geer Wallace et al. 2019; Pellizzari et al. 1992). Because many of these matrices are not commonly analyzed, the resulting chemical concentration data are more difficult to relate to measurements made in the more commonly used matrices such as urine, blood or breast milk; and consequently, may be more difficult to relate to exposure. However, because many of these matrices are available and could provide potentially useful information, they should not be discounted. Instead, preliminary studies evaluating the partitioning of chemicals in the various matrices should be conducted that will allow for comparison of data among matrices.

CASE STUDY 2

The Study of Asian Women and their Offspring's Development and Environmental Exposures (SAWASDEE) Cohort was established to investigate the impact of prenatal exposure to pesticides on neurodevelopment during infancy and early childhood in two farming districts of Chiang Mai province, Thailand. Recruitment began in July 2017 and was completed in June 2019. A total of 1298 women were screened, and of those, 394 women were enrolled. The mean gestational age at enrollment was 9.9 weeks (STD = 2.6). Multiple biospecimens were collected from the pregnant women participants and their children. During pregnancy, maternal urine samples were collected six times and composited to represent each trimester. Maternal urine samples were collected to measure urinary metabolites of organophosphate and pyrethroid insecticides. Maternal blood samples were collected three times in each trimester to primarily measure selected persistent organic chemicals and heavy metals. Maternal hair samples were also collected at the same time as blood samples. At delivery, an umbilical cord blood sample was collected to measure heavy metals and selected persistent organic chemicals. Placenta tissue was sampled and collected for transcriptomics. Meconium was collected from each neonate during the first week after birth. Breast milk samples were also collected three times during the breastfeeding period. Child urine samples were collected shortly after birth and during the follow-up visits when neurological testing was conducted to assess the child's neurodevelopment. Standardized questionnaires were administered during pregnancy and post-partum periods to collect demographic and general exposure characteristic data. All children will be followed until 3 years of age and undergo a series of neurodevelopmental tests to observe the effects of pesticide and other environmental chemical exposures on their developmental neurological trajectories (Baumert et al. 2021, In press).

CASE STUDY 3

MARBLES (Markers of Autism Risk in Babies – Learning Early Signs) is a longitudinal study for pregnant women who have a biological child with autism spectrum disorder (ASD). The MARBLES study, which began in 2006, aimed to investigate possible prenatal and postpartum biological and environmental exposures and risk factors that may contribute to the development of autism. Participants are primarily recruited from families receiving services for children with ASD through the California Department of Developmental Services.

Information about each participant's genetics and environment is collected through a number of sources, including blood, urine, hair, saliva, and breast milk (if the mother is breastfeeding), as well as through home dust samples, in order to obtain a comprehensive picture of the environment surrounding each pregnancy. Maternal biological samples were analyzed for selected chemicals (e.g. phthalates, phenols, PFAS). Demographic and exposure characteristic information is also obtained through interviews conducted with the mother using standardized questionnaires, and by accessing medical records in order to uncover more information about any behavioral aspects or trends that may contribute to the development of autism (Oh et al. 2021; Shin et al. 2018). Source: MARBLES Home (http://marbles.ucdavis.edu)

EXPOSURE MEASUREMENT CONSIDERATIONS

Biomolecular Adducts

Persistent and nonpersistent chemicals can also react with biomolecules such as DNA, hemoglobin, or fatty acids to form biomolecular adducts (Angerer et al. 1998, 2007; Hwa Yun et al. 2020; Schettgen et al. 2002). By measuring these adducts, we can increase the amount of time after exposure that we can measure a nonpersistent chemical because the amount of time the adduct remains in the body is largely dependent upon the lifetime of the biomolecule itself (Needham and Sexton 2000) (Figure 5.3). For example, the average life span of a red blood cell is about 120 days. If a chemical formed an adduct with hemoglobin on the day a red blood cell was created, the adduct should remain in the body for about four months, allowing a much longer time after exposure to collect the sample. Other adducts are formed with DNA, albumin, and other prominent proteins. Because adducts are not formed from every chemical molecule to which one is exposed, adduct measurements must be very sensitive, and usually, a large amount of matrix is required. In addition, the measurements are usually cumbersome and time-consuming, so the analytical throughput is very low, and the cost is very high (Hwa Yun et al. 2020; Sabbioni and Turesky 2017).

When measuring persistent chemicals, we do not gain much advantage by measuring them as adducts. Blood is still the matrix of choice because the concentration is higher in blood, and we have a wide window of opportunity (Barr and Needham 2002). To form an adduct, the chemical must have an electrophilic site for the nucleophile on the biomolecule (usually sulfur or nitrogen) to attack which forms a covalent bond, and hence, the adduct is formed.

Sampling Time Frame

For persistent organic chemicals, the time frame for sampling is reasonably straightforward. In general, a blood sample can be taken any time, up to several years, after exposure has occurred, and the exposure can still be accurately identified; however, no information about when the exposure occurred will be gained. For example, if a PCB concentration of 1,000 ng/g lipid was measured in a blood sample, it is impossible to know if a recent exposure to this amount of PCB occurred or whether a larger exposure occurred many years ago, and though a portion of the PCB has been eliminated from the body over time, this amount is still circulating in the bloodstream. By coupling questionnaire data with these biological measurements, it is possible to gain some information on the timing of the exposure (e.g., breastfeeding, subsistence food consumption).

The sampling time frame for nonpersistent chemicals is not straightforward. Because these chemicals have short biological half-lives, the samples, whether blood or urine, must be collected soon after the exposure in order to appropriately assess the exposure. For instance, the half-life of the herbicide glyphosate in humans is about 5–10 hours; therefore, samples must be collected sooner than 24 hours postexposure to assess the magnitude of exposure accurately (Connolly et al. 2019). If the primary exposure medium is the air and the exposure is continuous, a first morning void urine sample is probably the best biological sample for measuring the exposure. However, if the exposure is from a source related to personal grooming (e.g., VOCs from showers or phthalates from personal care products), a first morning void urine sample or an early morning blood sample (prior to showering) would likely miss the exposure from the following day. Rather, a late morning or early afternoon sample would more accurately characterize the daily exposure to these chemicals. Similarly, samples designed to evaluate dietary exposures, such as pesticides, should be collected several hours after mealtimes so that these exposures can be identified.

In general, sample collection for nonpersistent chemical measurements should reflect the residence time of the chemical in each individual matrix. The half-lives of nonpersistent chemicals in blood are typically much less than in urine samples, thus blood samples may need to be collected within minutes or hours after the exposure, whereas urine samples may be collected several hours, or in some instances days, after the exposure. Saliva samples will typically mimic blood, whereas meconium samples may provide a longer window for capturing the exposure. Measurements of biomolecular adducts need to consider the lifetime of the biomolecule, rather than the lifetime of the chemical, in the particular matrix; however, more adducts will likely be present immediately after exposure than several weeks after exposure.

Collecting Samples from Infants and Children

Difficulty is often encountered when collecting urine samples from infants and children who are not toilet trained. The traditional approach is similar to that in a clinical setting, using an infant urine collection bag. This technique is rather straightforward; however, it is usually bothersome to the child and often requires that the child be given liquids to encourage urination within a given time frame. Encouraging urination with drinks will usually dilute the urine and make the analytical measurement more difficult. Other approaches for urine collection, primarily from cloth diapers or cotton inserts, have also been investigated (Calafat et al. 2004; Hu et al. 2000). Another approach of ongoing investigation is the collection of the target analytes directly from the coagulated gel matrix of disposable diapers (Hu et al. 2004; Liu et al. 2012; Lucarini et al. 2021; Saito et al. 2014). If proven viable for isolating a broad array of target analytes, this method of collection would be most attractive, as it is the least burdensome on the participant and the most logistically practical.

Temporal Variability in Urine and Blood Samples

The variability of nonpersistent target analyte levels in samples collected from an individual over time, is of concern, whether the sample is biological or environmental. Temporal variability can include the variation of a given chemical in multiple samples collected on a single day or can include variation among days, months, or seasons (Fromme et al. 2007). For chronic exposures to nonpersistent chemicals, the exposure is repeated, thus the amount in each sample would likely represent the average exposure. However, for episodic exposures, the variability is often greater.

CHEMICAL ANALYSIS METHODS

Organic Chemicals

Most methods for measuring organic chemicals in biological matrices use a sample preparation step to isolate the target chemical(s) from the matrix, an analytical technique with a detection system, data processing, and quality assurance processes (Needham et al. 2005a). The sample preparation steps are usually the most common source of analytic error, whether systematic or random (Barr et al. 1999, 2006). If the chemical is inherently incompatible with the analytic system that follows, a chemical derivatization or reduction procedure may also be required. The addition of steps into the sample preparation procedure usually increases the overall imprecision of the method.

For the analyses of environmental organic chemicals or their metabolites in biological matrices, either gas chromatography (GC) or high-performance liquid chromatography (HPLC) coupled with mass spectrometry is commonly used. Depending on the chemical classes or their concentrations, the analyses can be done using either GC or HPLC coupled with electron capture, flame photometric, nitrogen phosphorus, fluorescence, and UV absorbance detection. Of the detection/analysis systems, mass spectrometers provide the most specificity, whereas UV absorbance

87

detection usually provides the least (Barr et al. 1999). Most mass spectrometry-based methods have limits of detection (LODs) that are typically adequate to detect levels in the general population. The analytical imprecision usually ranges from 10% to 20%.

Other analytic techniques that are often employed to measure organic chemicals in biological matrices are immunoassays and bioassays (Biagini et al. 1995; Brady et al. 1989; Hongsibsong et al. 2012; Huo et al. 2018; Vasylieva et al. 2015). For these techniques, a sample preparation step to isolate the chemical from the matrix may or may not be used. Many are commercially available for selected chemicals. However, their development for a new chemical is a lengthy process that typically requires the generation and isolation of monoclonal antibodies, then the development of the assay itself. Usually, UV, fluorescence, or radioactivity detection is used for the assays. They may be very specific for a given chemical or they may have a great deal of cross-reactivity that may limit their utility. Their LODs can vary widely; however, many have adequate sensitivity for measuring levels in the general population.

Heavy Metals and Metalloids

The sample preparation process for heavy metals and metalloids (HMMs) is typically much simpler than for organic chemicals. In some instances, the sample matrix just needs to be diluted with water prior to analysis. However, special precautions must be taken to avoid contamination, both pre-analytically and in the analytic system. For example, prescreened collection materials should be used for sample collection, all analytic supplies should be appropriately free of the target chemicals, and special clean rooms may be required for analysis.

Inductively coupled plasma-mass spectrometry (ICP-MS) has become the method of choice for the analysis of HMMs in biological matrices (Wilschefski and Baxter 2019). Less often, atomic absorption spectrometry (AAS) is used. For the ICP-MS, a dynamic collision cell may also be used to eliminate potentially interfering salts from the system. When various forms of HMMs are speciated, such as for arsenic, chromium, or mercury, the ICP-MS will be preceded in line by some chromatographic unit such as HPLC. For lead screening, an efficient portable lead analyzer can be used for in-field measurements. However, the portable analyzer has limited application for other metals.

MEASUREMENT METHOD SPECIFICITY AND SENSITIVITY REQUIREMENTS

Specificity – how specific an analysis method is for a particular exposure – and sensitivity – the ability to measure the chemical at the desired level – are critical parameters for analysis methods and both must be considered when deciding which matrix to measure. The half-life of a chemical may affect the sensitivity requirement; however, because persistent chemicals have long half-lives, it is not nearly as important as it is for nonpersistent chemicals, which metabolize rapidly. For instance, in adult men, 2,3,7,8-tetrachlorodibenzo-p-dioxin has a half-life of about 7.6 years (Pirkle et al. 1989) or the half-lives of long-chained PFAS were reported to be in a range from 1.77 to 2.93 years (Xu et al. 2021). When measuring exposure to persistent chemicals by analyzing adipose tissue, it does not make much difference which portion of the body the sample is taken from; however, because blood is easy to collect and readily available, blood is an ideal medium in which to measure persistent chemicals. In lactating women, milk is also frequently used.

The postexposure fate of a nonpersistent chemical is dramatically different (Figure 5.3) (Needham and Sexton 2000). After each exposure, the concentration of the nonpersistent chemical in blood declines rapidly. The window of opportunity for measuring nonpersistent chemicals in blood is narrow and requires the use of a very sensitive technique. By measuring these chemicals in blood as the intact, or parent, chemical, we gain information on the exact chemical to which one was exposed. For example, if someone was exposed to chlorpyrifos, we can measure chlorpyrifos in the blood rather than its metabolite, which is formed from more than one parent chemical and is also the same chemical as environmentally degraded chlorpyrifos (Huen et al. 2012). In addition to blood, certain nonpersistent chemicals, such as cotinine, have been measured in saliva because cotinine is in equilibrium in blood and saliva (Raja et al. 2016).

In urine, we generally measure metabolites of the chemical, which may lack the desired specificity for analysis; however, measurements in urine allow a much wider window of opportunity in which to take the sample. Generally, we assess exposure to nonpersistent chemicals by measuring their metabolites in urine, even though this method may not have the specificity of the blood measurement.

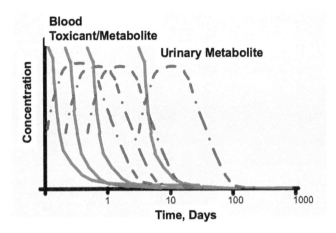

Blood Toxicant/Metabolite

Urinary Metabolite

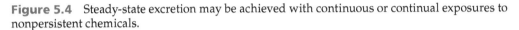

Concentration

Time, Days

Figure 5.4 Steady-state excretion may be achieved with continuous or continual exposures to nonpersistent chemicals.

When chronic exposure to a nonpersistent chemical occurs, the exposure is continually replenishing the chemical in the blood, and urinary elimination may reach a steady state (Figure 5.4). Therefore, urine becomes a better matrix for measurement because we integrate exposure over a longer period.

QUALITY ASSURANCE AND CONTROL

A vital component of all biomonitoring methodology is a sound quality assurance/control program (QA/QC). QA/QC programs typically require strict adherence to protocols and multiple testing procedures that easily allow the detection of systematic failures in the methodology. The general requirement for an analytical laboratory performing a method must be that it is able to demonstrate the method's accuracy, precision, specificity, linearity and range, limit of detection, and ruggedness/robustness.

For any mass spectrometric-based methods, a procedure for controlling and managing the matrix effects must be employed to ensure the accuracy of the data produced. Matrix effects are caused by co-eluting matrix components that alter the ionization of target analytes as well as the chromatographic response of target analytes, leading to reduced or increased sensitivity of the analysis. Matrix effects can lead to errors in analytical data, which results in exposure misclassification (Panuwet et al. 2016).

Once the analytical method is developed and validated and before the analysis of samples takes place, a QA/QC program must be established and enforced to easily allow the detection of systematic failures in the methodology and that ensures that these defined requirements are being maintained over time and among laboratories (Needham et al. 2002). The utilized testing procedures can include proficiency testing to ensure accuracy as measured against a known reference material, repeat measurements of known materials to confirm the validity of an analytical run and to measure analytical precision, "round robin" or interlaboratory studies to confirm reproducible measurement values among laboratories, regular verification of instrument calibration, daily assurance of minimal laboratory contamination by analyzing "blank" samples, and cross-validations to ensure that multiple analysts and instruments obtain similar analytical values.

QA/QC measures are applicable to not just the analytical method but to all aspects of the measurement process: from sampling design, sample collection (need to ensure no or a defined amount of contamination), transport and storage of samples, analytical method, and data reporting; therefore, all aspects of the measurement process must be subject to a stringent QA/QC protocol. Also, any new analytical method or any change in the measurement process must be documented and validated against the method being used. Figure 5.5 provides the considerations for maternal and fetal matrix selection, matrix storage condition, and analytical method selection for assessing exposures to environmental chemicals in a birth cohort study.

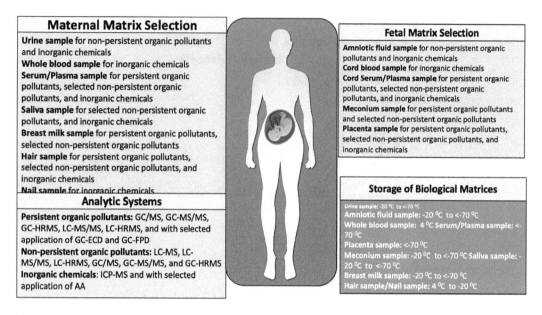

Maternal Matrix Selection

Urine sample for non-persistent organic pollutants and inorganic chemicals
Whole blood sample for inorganic chemicals
Serum/Plasma sample for persistent organic pollutants, selected non-persistent organic pollutants, and inorganic chemicals
Saliva sample for selected non-persistent organic pollutants, and inorganic chemicals
Breast milk sample for persistent organic pollutants, selected non-persistent organic pollutants
Hair sample for persistent organic pollutants, selected non-persistent organic pollutants, and inorganic chemicals
Nail sample for inorganic chemicals

Analytic Systems

Persistent organic pollutants: GC/MS, GC-MS/MS, GC-HRMS, LC-MS/MS, LC-HRMS, and with selected application of GC-ECD and GC-FPD
Non-persistent organic pollutants: LC-MS, LC-MS/MS, LC-HRMS, GC/MS, GC-MS/MS, and GC-HRMS
Inorganic chemicals: ICP-MS and with selected application of AA

Fetal Matrix Selection

Amniotic fluid sample for non-persistent organic pollutants and inorganic chemicals
Cord blood sample for inorganic chemicals
Cord Serum/Plasma sample for persistent organic pollutants, selected non-persistent organic pollutants, and inorganic chemicals
Meconium sample for persistent organic pollutants and selected non-persistent organic pollutants
Placenta sample for persistent organic pollutants, selected non-persistent organic pollutants, and inorganic chemicals

Storage of Biological Matrices

Urine sample: -20 °C to <-70 °C
Amniotic fluid sample: -20 °C to <-70 °C
Whole blood sample: 4 °C Serum/Plasma sample: <-70 °C
Placenta sample: <-70 °C
Meconium sample: -20 °C to <-70 °C Saliva sample: -20 °C to <-70 °C
Breast milk sample: -20 °C to <-70 °C
Hair sample/Nail sample: 4 °C to -20 °C

Figure 5.5 Maternal-fetal biological matrix selection and considerations for exposure assessment of environmental agents in a birth cohort study.

CONCLUSION

In general, persistent organic chemicals are more readily measured in blood-based matrices or other lipid-rich matrices. Maternal measurements serve as good surrogates for fetal exposures, and even early childhood exposures if levels are not reduced by breastfeeding. Assessments of exposure to nonpersistent chemicals are the most challenging, but they can be measured in multiple matrix types. Urine is the most commonly used matrix for measurement of these chemicals, but interpretation of the information obtained is often complicated by co-exposures, urine dilution, specificity issues, and the temporality of the measurement. To date, no ideal way exists to interpret many of these measurements without the use of additional measures, for example, repeat measurements or environmental measurements. Measurements of HMMs have been performed in many matrices over the years and are, in general, well-understood. Biomonitoring will likely have limited utility in the assessment of exposure to criteria pollutants and bioallergens.

THOUGHT QUESTIONS

1. What is biomonitoring and how does it differ from direct and personal environmental measurements?
2. What is the most used biological matrix for measuring nonpersistent chemicals?
3. Why are blood samples a common matrix for measuring persistent chemicals?
4. How many samples should be collected during pregnancy or other important time periods to overcome the temporal variability of nonpersistent chemicals in urine samples?
5. What are the methods of choice for measuring metals in blood samples?
6. What are the appropriate biological matrices for assessing prenatal exposure to environmental chemicals?

LITERATURE CITED

McConnell, E. E., G. W. Lucier, R. C. Rumbaugh, P. W. Albro, D. J. Harvan, J. R. Hass, and M. W. Harris. 1984. Dioxin in Soil: Bioavailability After Ingestion by Rats and Guinea Pigs. *Science* 223 (4): 1077–1079. 10.1126/science.6695194.

Umbreit, T. H., E. J. Hesse, and M. A. Gallo. 1986. Bioavailability of Dioxin in Soil from a 2,4,5-T Manufacturing Site. *Science* 232: 497–499. https://doi.org/DOI10.1126/science.396149.

REFERENCES

Adgate J. L., D. B. Barr, C. A. Clayton, L. E. Eberly, N. C. Freeman, P. J. Lioy, et al. 2001. Measurement of Children's Exposure to Pesticides: Analysis of Urinary Metabolite Levels in a Probability-Based Sample. *Environ Health Perspect* 109: 583–590.

Aguilera, I, M. Guxens, R. Garcia-Esteban, T. Corbella, M. J. Nieuwenhuijsen, C. M. Foradada, et al. 2009. Association Between GIS-Based Exposure to Urban Air Pollution During Pregnancy and Birth Weight in the INMA Sabadell Cohort. *Environ Health Perspect* 117: 1322–1327.

Albertini, R, M. Bird, N. Doerrer, L. Needham, S. Robison, L. Sheldon. et al. 2006. The Use of Biomonitoring Data in Exposure and Human Health Risk Assessments. *Environ Health Perspect* 114: 1755–1762.

Amorim, L. C., Z. D. Cardeal. 2007. Breath Air Analysis and Its Use as a Biomarker in Biological Monitoring of Occupational and Environmental Exposure to Chemical Agents. *J Chromatogr B Anal Technol Biomed Life Sci* 853: 1–9.

Angerer, J. 1988. *Determination of Toluene in Blood by Head-Space Gas Chromatography*. IARC Scientific Publication: 287–291.

Angerer, J, U. Ewers, and M. Wilhelm. 2007. Human Biomonitoring: State of the Art. *Int J Hyg Environ Health* 210: 201–228.

Angerer J, T. Goen, and A. Kramer, H. U. Kafferlein. 1998. N-Methylcarbamoyl Adducts at the N-Terminal Valine of Globin in Workers Exposed to n, N-Dimethylformamide. *Arch Toxicol* 72: 309–313.

Angerer, J., and B. Hörsch. 1992. Determination of Aromatic Hydrocarbons and Their Metabolites in Human Blood and Urine. *J Chromatogr* 580: 229–255.

ATSDR. 2017. *Interaction Profile for Chlorinated Dibenzo-P-Dioxins, Polybrominated Diphenyl Ethers and phthalates.* https://www.atsdr.cdc.gov/interactionprofiles/ip-14/ip14-p.pdf.

Aufderheide, A. C., and L. E. Wittmers Jr. 1992. Selected Aspects of the Spatial Distribution of Lead in Bone. *Neurotoxicology* 13: 809–819.

Barr, D. B., J. R. Barr, W. J. Driskell, R. H. Hill Jr., D. L. Ashley, L. L. Needham, et al. 1999. Strategies for Biological Monitoring of Exposure for Contemporary-Use Pesticides. *Toxicol Ind Health* 15: 168–179.

Barr, D. B., J. R. Barr, V. L. Maggio, R. D. Whitehead, Jr., M. A. Sadowski, R. M. Whyatt, et al. 2002. A Multi-analyte Method for the Quantification of Contemporary Pesticides in Human Serum and Plasma Using High-Resolution Mass Spectrometry. *J Chromatogr B Anal Technol Biomed Life Sci* 778: 99–111.

Barr, D.B., A. Bishop, L.L. Needham. 2007. Concentrations of Xenobiotic Chemicals in the Maternal-Fetal Unit. *Reprod Toxicol* 23: 260–266.

Barr, D. B., D. Landsittel, M. Nishioka, K. Thomas, B. Curwin, J. Raymer, et al. 2006. A Survey of Laboratory and Statistical Issues Related to Farmworker Exposure Studies. *Environ Health Perspect* 114: 961–968.

Barr, D. B., and L. L. Needham. 2002. Analytical Methods for Biological Monitoring of Exposure to Pesticides: A Review. *J Chromatogr B Anal Technol Biomed Life Sci* 778: 5–29.

Barr, D. B., R. Y. Wang, and L. L. Needham. 2005. Biologic Monitoring of Exposure to Environmental Chemicals Throughout the Life Stages: Requirements and Issues for Consideration for the National Children's Study. *Environ Health Perspect* 113: 1083–1091.

Bartell, S. M., Calafat, A. M., C. Lyu, K. Kato, P. B. Ryan, and K. Steenland. 2010. Rate of Decline in Serum PFOA Concentrations After Granular Activated Carbon Filtration at Two Public Water Systems in Ohio and West Virginia. *Environ Health Perspect* 118: 222–228.

Baumert, B. O., N. Fiedler, T. Prapamontol, P. Suttiwan, W. Naksen, P. Panuwet, et al. 2021. *The Study of Asian Women and Their Offspring's Development and Environmental Exposures (SAWASDEE): A Northern Thailand Birth Cohort Study.* JRP (in press).

Bearer, C. F. 2003. Meconium as a Biological Marker of Prenatal Exposure. *Ambul Pediatr* 3: 40–43.

Bearer, C. F., J. L. Jacobson, S. W. Jacobson, D. Barr, J. Croxford, C. D. Molteno, et al. 2003. Validation of a New Biomarker of Fetal Exposure to Alcohol. *J Pediatr* 143: 463–469.

Bearer, C. F., S. Lee, A. E. Salvator, S. Minnes, A. Swick, T. Yamashita, et al. 1999. Ethyl Linoleate in Meconium: A Biomarker for Prenatal Ethanol Exposure. *Alcohol Clin Exp Res* 23: 487–493.

Biagini, R. E., W. Tolos, W. T. Sanderson, G. M. Henningsen, B. MacKenzie. 1995. Urinary Biomonitoring for Alachlor Exposure in Commercial Pesticide Applicators by Immunoassay. *Bull Environ Contam Toxicol* 54: 245–250.

Blount, B. C., M. J. Silva, S. P. Caudill, L. L. Needham, J. L. Pirkle, E. J. Sampson, et al. 2000. Levels of Seven Urinary Phthalate Metabolites in a Human Reference Population. *Environ Health Perspect* 108: 979–982.

Bradman, A, D. B. Barr, B. G. Claus Henn, T. Drumheller, C. Curry, and B. Eskenazi. 2003. Measurement of Pesticides and Other Toxicants in Amniotic Fluid as a Potential Biomarker of Prenatal Exposure: A Validation Study. *Environ Health Perspect* 111:1779–1782.

Brady, J. F. F. J., R. A. Wilson, R. O. Mumma. 1989. Enzyme Immunoassay for Aldicarb. In R. G. F. C. Wang, R. C. Honeycutt, and J. C. Reinert (Eds.), *Biological Monitoring for Pesticide Exposure: Measurement, Estimation and Risk Reduction* (pp. 262–284). American Chemical Society.

Braun, J. M., and K. Gray. 2017. Challenges to Studying the Health Effects of Early Life Environmental Chemical Exposures on Children's Health. *PLoS Biolol* 15: e2002800.

Buser, M. C., H. G. Abadin, J. L. Irwin, and H. R. Pohl. 2018. Windows of Sensitivity to Toxic Chemicals in the Development of Reproductive Effects: An Analysis of ATSDR's Toxicological Profile Database. *Int J Environ Health Res* 28: 553–578.

Calafat, A. M., L. L. Needham, M. J. Silva, and G. Lambert. 2004. Exposure to di-(2-Ethylhexyl) Phthalate Among Premature Neonates in a Neonatal Intensive Care Unit. *Pediatrics* 113: e429–434.

Carrer, P., and G. Moscato. 2004. Biological Pollution and Allergic Diseases. *G Ital Med Lav Ergon* 26: 370–374.

Chen, X., P. Panuwet, R. E. Hunter, A. M. Riederer, G. C. Bernoudy, D. B. Barr, et al. 2014. Method for the Quantification of Current Use and Persistent Pesticides in Cow Milk, Human Milk and Baby Formula Using Gas Chromatography Tandem Mass Spectrometry. *J Chromatogr B Anal Technol Biomed Life Sci* 970: 121–130.

Chiu, C. Y., M. H. Tsai, T.C. Yao, Y. L. Tu, M. C. Hua, K. W. Yeh, et al. 2014. Urinary LTE4 Levels as a Diagnostic Marker for IgE-Mediated Asthma in Preschool Children: A Birth Cohort Study. *PLoS ONE* 9: e115216.

Choi, J, L. E. Knudsen, S. Mizrak, and A. Joas. 2017. Identification of Exposure to Environmental Chemicals in Children and Older Adults Using Human Biomonitoring Data Sorted by Age: Results from a Literature Review. *Int J Hyg Environ Health* 220: 282–298.

Chou, W.-C., and Z. Lin. 2019. Bayesian Evaluation of a Physiologically Based Pharmacokinetic (PBPK) Model for Perfluorooctane Sulfonate (PFOS) to Characterize the Interspecies Uncertainty Between Mice, Rats, Monkeys, and Humans: Development and Performance Verification. *Environ Int* 129: 408–422.

Ciffroy, P., B. Alfonso, A. Altenpohl, Z. Banjac, J. Bierkens, C. Brochot, et al. 2016. Modelling the Exposure to Chemicals for Risk Assessment: A Comprehensive Library of Multimedia and PBPK Models for Integration, Prediction, Uncertainty and Sensitivity Analysis – the MERLIN-EXPO Tool. *Sci Total Environ* 568: 770–784.

Connolly, A, K. Jones, I. Basinas, K. S. Galea, L. Kenny, P. McGowan, et al. 2019. Exploring the Half-Life of Glyphosate in Human Urine Samples. *Int J Hyg Environ Health* 222: 205–210.

Cousins, I. T., J. C. DeWitt, J. Glüge, G. Goldenman, D. Herzke, R. Lohmann, et al. 2020. The High Persistence of Pfas Is Sufficient for Their Management as a Chemical Class. *Environ Sci Process Impacts* 22: 2307–2312.

Duquenne, P., G. Marchand, and C. Duchaine. 2013. Measurement of Endotoxins in Bioaerosols at Workplace: A Critical Review of Literature and a Standardization Issue. *Ann Occup Hygiene* 57: 137–172.

EPA. 2001. *Summary Report of the Technical Workshop on Issues Associated with Considering Developmental Changes in Behavior and Anatomy When Assessing Exposure to Children: U.S.* Washington, DC: EPA.

EPA. 2019. *Guidelines for Human Exposure Assessment.* https://www.epa.gov/sites/default/files/2020-01/documents/guidelines_for_human_exposure_assessment_final2019.pdf, 25 August 2021.

Fantke, P., L. Aylward, J. Bare, W. A. Chiu, R. Dodson, R. Dwyer, et al. 2018. Advancements in Life Cycle Human Exposure and Toxicity Characterization. *Environ Health Perspect* 126: 125001–125001.

Fenske, R. A., J. C. Kissel, C. Lu, D. A. Kalman, N. J. Simcox, E. H. Allen, et al. 2000. Biologically Based Pesticide Dose Estimates for Children in an Agricultural Community. *Environ Health Perspect* 108: 515–520.

Ferguson, A., A. Dwivedi, F. Adelabu, E. Ehindero, M. Lamssali, E. Obeng-Gyasi, et al. 2021. Quantified Activity Patterns for Young Children in Beach Environments Relevant for Exposure to Contaminants. *Int J Environ Res Public Health* 18(6): 3274

Ferguson, A. C., R. A. Canales, P. Beamer, W. Auyeung, M. Key, A. Munninghoff, et al. 2006. Video Methods in the Quantification of Children's Exposures. *J Expo Sci Environ Epidemiol* 16: 287–298.

Fernandez, E, R. Perez, A. Hernandez, P. Tejada, M. Arteta, and J. T. Ramos. 2011. Factors and Mechanisms for Pharmacokinetic Differences Between Pediatric Population and Adults. *Pharmaceutics* 3: 53–72.

Flesch-Janys, D, H. Becher, P. Gurn, D. Jung, J. Konietzko, A. Manz, et al. 1996. Elimination of Polychlorinated Dibenzo-p-Dioxins and Dibenzofurans in Occupationally Exposed Persons. *J Toxicol Environ Health* 47: 363–378.

Foster, W. G., S. Chan, L. Platt, and C. L. Hughes Jr. 2002. Detection of Phytoestrogens in Samples of Second Trimester Human Amniotic Fluid. *Toxicol Lett* 129: 199–205.

Fromme, H., G. Bolte, H. M. Koch, J. Angerer, S. Boehmer, H. Drexler, et al. 2007. Occurrence and Daily Variation of Phthalate Metabolites in the Urine of an Adult Population. *Int J Hyg Environ Health* 210: 21–33.

Geer Wallace, M. A., J. D. Pleil, K. D. Oliver, D. A. Whitaker, S. Mentese, K. W. Fent, et al. 2019. Non-Targeted GC/MS Analysis of Exhaled Breath Samples: Exploring Human Biomarkers of Exogenous Exposure and Endogenous Response from Professional Firefighting Activity. *J Toxicol Environ Health Part A* 82: 244–260.

Goodman, R. E., and J. N. Leach. 2004. Assessing the Allergenicity of Proteins Introduced into Genetically Modified Crops Using Specific Human IgE Assays. *J AOAC Int* 87: 1423–1432.

Gribble, M. O., S. M. Bartell, K. Kannan, Q. Wu, P. A. Fair, and D. L. Kamen. 2015. Longitudinal Measures of Perfluoroalkyl Substances (PFAS) in Serum of Gullah African Americans in South Carolina: 2003–2013. *Environ Res* 143: 82–88.

Gys, C., Y. Ait Bamai, A. Araki, M. Bastiaensen, N. Caballero-Casero, and R. Kishi, et al. 2020. Biomonitoring and Temporal Trends of Bisphenols Exposure in Japanese School Children. *Environ Res* 191: 110172.

Hongsibsong, S, J. Wipasa, M. Pattarawarapa, S. Chantara, W. Stuetz, and F. Nosten, et al. 2012. Development and Application of an Indirect Competitive Enzyme-Linked Immunosorbent Assay for the Detection of p, p'-DDE in Human Milk and Comparison of the Results Against GC-ECD. *J Agric Food Chem* 60: 16–22.

Horng, C. J., J. L. Tsai, and S. R. Lin. 1999. Determination of Urinary Arsenic, Mercury, and Selenium in Steel Production Workers. *Biol Trace Elem Res* 70: 29–40.

Hu, Y, J. Beach, J. Raymer, and M. Gardner. 2004. Disposable Diaper to Collect Urine Samples from Young Children for Pyrethroid Pesticide Studies. *J Exp Sci Environ Epidemiol* 14: 378–384.

Hu, Y. A., D. B. Barr, G. Akland, L. Melnyk, L. Needham, E. D. Pellizzari, et al. 2000. Collecting Urine Samples from Young Children Using Cotton Gauze for Pesticide Studies. *J Expo Anal Environ Epidemiol* 10: 703–709.

Huen, K., A. Bradman, K. Harley, P. Yousefi, D. Boyd Barr, B. Eskenazi, et al. 2012. Organophosphate Pesticide Levels in Blood and Urine of Women and Newborns Living in an Agricultural Community. *Environ Res* 117: 8–16.

Huo, J., Z. Li, D. Wan, D. Li, M. Qi, B. Barnych, et al. 2018. Development of a Highly Sensitive Direct Competitive Fluorescence Enzyme Immunoassay Based on a Nanobody-Alkaline Phosphatase Fusion Protein for Detection of 3-Phenoxybenzoic Acid in Urine. *J Agric Food Chem* 66: 11284–11290.

Hwa Yun, B., J. Guo, M. Bellamri, and R. J. Turesky. 2020. DNA Adducts: Formation, Biological Effects, and New Biospecimens for Mass Spectrometric Measurements in Humans. *Mass Spectrom Rev* 39: 55–82.

Isaacs, K. K., W. G. Glen, P. Egeghy, M.-R. Goldsmith, L. Smith, D. Vallero, et al. 2014. SHEDS-HT: An Integrated Probabilistic Exposure Model for Prioritizing Exposures to Chemicals with Near-Field and Dietary Sources. *Environ Sci Technol* 48: 12750–12759.

Jeong, Y, S. Lee, S. Kim, S. Choi, J. Park, H. J. Kim, et al. 2016a. Occurrence and Prenatal Exposure to Persistent Organic Pollutants Using Meconium in Korea: Feasibility of Meconium as a Non-Invasive Human Matrix. *Environ Res* 147: 8–15.

Jeong, Y., S. Lee, S. Kim, S. D. Choi, J. Park, H. J. Kim, et al. 2016b. Occurrence and Prenatal Exposure to Persistent Organic Pollutants Using Meconium in Korea: Feasibility of Meconium as a Non-Invasive Human Matrix. *Environ Res* 147: 8–15.

Jeong, Y., S. Lee, S. Kim, J. Park, H. J. Kim, G. Choi, et al. 2018. Placental Transfer of Persistent Organic Pollutants and Feasibility Using the Placenta as a Non-Invasive Biomonitoring Matrix. *Sci Total Environ* 612: 1498–1505.

Jiménez-Díaz, I., F. Vela-Soria, R. Rodríguez-Gómez, A. Zafra-Gómez, O. Ballesteros, and Navalón, A.. 2015. Analytical Methods for the Assessment of Endocrine Disrupting Chemical Exposure During Human Fetal and Lactation Stages: A Review. *Anal Chim Acta* 892: 27–48.

Jones, P. D., W. Hu, W. De Coen, J. L. Newsted, and J. P. Giesy. 2003. Binding of Perfluorinated Fatty Acids to Serum Proteins. *Environ Toxicol Chem* 22: 2639–2649.

Kesmodel, U. S. 2018. Information Bias in Epidemiological Studies with a Special Focus on Obstetrics and Gynecology. *Acta Obstet Gynecol Scand* 97: 417–423.

Kim, K., H. M. Shin, S. A. Busgang, D. B. Barr, P. Panuwet, R. J. Schmidt, et al. 2021. Temporal Trends of Phenol, Paraben, and Triclocarban Exposure in California Pregnant Women During 2007–2014. *Environ Sci Technol* 55: 11155–11165.

Klaassen, C. D. 2013. *Casarett and Doull's Toxicology: The Basic Science of Poisons.* McGraw Hill Education.

La Rocca, C., E. Alessi, B. Bergamasco, D. Caserta, F. Ciardo, E. Fanello, et al. 2012. Exposure and Effective Dose Biomarkers for Perfluorooctane Sulfonic Acid (PFOS) and Perfluorooctanoic Acid (PFOA) in Infertile Subjects: Preliminary Results of the PREVIENI Project. *Int J Hyg Environ Health* 215: 206–211.

LaKind, J. S., C. M. Berlin, and D. Q. Naiman. 2001. Infant Exposure to Chemicals in Breast Milk in the United States: What We Need to Learn from a Breast Milk Monitoring Program. *Environ Health Perspect* 109: 75–88.

LaKind, J. S., C. M. Berlin, C. N. Park, D. Q. Naiman, N. J. Gudka. 2000. Methodology for Characterizing Distributions of Incremental Body Burdens of 2, 3,7,8-TCDD and DDE from Breast Milk in North American Nursing Infants. *J Toxicol Environ Health Part A* 59: 605–639.

Lapostolle, F, P. J. Raynaud, P. Le Toumelin, A. Benaissa, J. M. Agostinucci, F. Adnet, et al. 2001. Measurement of Carbon Monoxide in Expired Breath in Prehospital Management of Carbon Monoxide Intoxication. *Ann Fr Anesth Reanim* 20: 10–15.

Lee, C. H., H. Y. Chuang, C. C. Shih, S. H. Jee, L. F. Wang, H. C. Chiu, et al. 2004. Correlation of Serum Total Ige, Eosinophil Granule Cationic Proteins, Sensitized Allergens and Family Aggregation in Atopic Dermatitis Patients with or Without Rhinitis. *J Dermatol* 31: 784–793.

Lee, D. H., D. R. Jacobs Jr., H. Y. Park, and D. O. Carpenter. 2017. A Role of Low Dose Chemical Mixtures in Adipose Tissue in Carcinogenesis. *Environ Int* 108: 170–175.

Lehmann, G. M., J. S. LaKind, M. H. Davis, E. P. Hines, S. A. Marchitti, C. Alcala, et al. 2018. Environmental Chemicals in Breast Milk and Formula: Exposure and Risk Assessment Implications. *Environ Health Perspect* 126: 96001.

Lehman-McKeeman, L. D. 2008. Absorption, Distribution and Excretion of Toxicants. In C. D. Klaassen (Ed.), *Casarett and Doull's Toxicology: The Basic Science of Poisons, Part 5.* McGraw-Hill Publishing.

Leng, G., K. H. Kühn, H. Idel. 1997. Biological Monitoring of Pyrethroids in Blood and Pyrethroid Metabolites in Urine: Applications and Limitations. *Sci Total Environ* 199: 173–181.

Liu, L., T. Xia, L. Guo, L. Cao, B. Zhao, and J. Zhang, et al. 2012. Expressing Urine from a Gel Disposable Diaper for Biomonitoring Using Phthalates as an Example. *J Expos Sci Environ Epidemiol* 22: 625–631.

Louro, H., M. Heinälä, J. Bessems, J. Buekers, T. Vermeire, M. Woutersen, et al. 2019. Human Biomonitoring in Health Risk Assessment in Europe: Current Practices and Recommendations for the Future. *Int J Hyg Environ Health* 222: 727–737.

Lu, C, L. C. Anderson, M. S. Morgan, and R. A. Fenske. 1998. Salivary Concentrations of Atrazine Reflect Free Atrazine Plasma Levels in Rats. *J Toxicol Environ Health Part A* 53: 283–292.

Lucarini, F., M. Blanchard, T. Krasniqi, N. Duda, G. Bailat Rosset, A. Ceschi, et al. 2021. Concentrations of Seven Phthalate Monoesters in Infants and Toddlers Quantified in Urine Extracted from Diapers. *Int J Environ Res Public Health* 18: 6806.

Luchini, P. D., J. F. Leyton, L. Strombech Mde, J. C. Ponce, M. Jesus, and V. Leyton. 2009. Validation of a Spectrophotometric Method for Quantification of Carboxyhemoglobin. *J Anal Toxicol* 33: 540–544.

Mac Intosh, D. L., L. L. Needham, K. A. Hammerstrom, P. B. Ryan. 1999. A Longitudinal Investigation of Selected Pesticide Metabolites in Urine. *J Expo Anal Environ Epidemiol* 9: 494–501.

MacIntosh, D. L., C. Kabiru, S. L. Echols, and P. B. Ryan. 2001. Dietary Exposure to Chlorpyrifos and Levels of 3, 5,6-Trichloro-2-Pyridinol in Urine. *J Expo Anal Environ Epidemiol* 11: 279–285.

MacIntosh, D. L., C. Kabiru, K. A. Scanlon, P. B. Ryan. 2000. Longitudinal Investigation of Exposure to Arsenic, Cadmium, Chromium and Lead Via Beverage Consumption. *J Expo Anal Environ Epidemiol* 10: 196–205.

Makarananda, K., U. Pengpan, M. Srisakulthong, K. Yoovathaworn, and K. Sriwatanakul. 1998. Monitoring of Aflatoxin Exposure by Biomarkers. *J Toxicol Sci* 23 Suppl 2: 155–159.

Malír, F., V. Ostrý, M. Cerná, J. Kacerovský, T. Roubal, J. Skarková, et al. 2004. Monitoring the Important Mycotoxin Biomarkers (Ochratoxin a, Aflatoxin m1) in the Czech Population. *Cas Lek Cesk* 143: 691–696.

Mannetje, A., J. Coakley, J. F. Mueller, F. Harden, L. M. Toms, J. Douwes. 2012. Partitioning of Persistent Organic Pollutants (POPs) Between Human Serum and Breast Milk: A Literature Review. *Chemosphere* 89: 911–918.

Mirabelli, M. C., R. Golan, R. Greenwald, A. U. Raysoni, F. Holguin, P. Kewada, et al. 2015. Modification of Traffic-Related Respiratory Response by Asthma Control in a Population of Car Commuters. *Epidemiology* 26: 546–555.

Mitro, S. D., T. Johnson, and A. R. Zota. 2015. Cumulative Chemical Exposures During Pregnancy and Early Development. *Current Environmental Health Reports* 2: 367–378.

Mocarelli, P., P. M. Gerthoux, E. Ferrari, D. G. Patterson Jr., S. M. Kieszak, P. Brambilla, et al. 2000. Paternal Concentrations of Dioxin and Sex Ratio of Offspring. *Lancet* 355: 1858–1863.

Nakajima, M., Y. Kuroiwa, and T. Yokoi. 2002. Interindividual Differences in Nicotine Metabolism and Genetic Polymorphisms of Human CYP2a6. *Drug Metab Rev* 34: 865–877.

Needham, L. L. 2005. Assessing Exposure to Organophosphorus Pesticides by Biomonitoring in Epidemiologic Studies of Birth Outcomes. *Environ Health Perspect* 113: 494–498.

Needham, L. L., D. B. Barr, and A. M. Calafat. 2005a. Characterizing Children's Exposures: Beyond NHANES. *Neuro Toxicol* 26: 547–553.

Needham, L. L., H. Ozkaynak, R. M. Whyatt, D. B. Barr, R. Y. Wang, L. Naeher, et al. 2005b. Exposure Assessment in the National Children's Study: Introduction. *Environ Health Perspect* 113: 1076–1082.

Needham, L. L., D. G. Patterson Jr., D. B. Barr, J. Grainger, and A. M. Calafat. 2005c. Uses of Speciation Techniques in Biomonitoring for Assessing Human Exposure to Organic Environmental Chemicals. *Anal Bioanal Chem* 381: 397–404.

Needham, L. L., J. J. Ryan, and P. Furst, Technical Workshop on Human Milk S, Research on Environmental Chemicals in the United States. 2002. Guidelines for Analysis of Human Milk for Environmental Chemicals. *J Toxicol Environ Health Part A* 65: 1893–1908.

Needham, L. L., and K. Sexton. 2000. Assessing Children's Exposure to Hazardous Environmental Chemicals: An Overview of Selected Research Challenges and Complexities. *J Expo Anal Environ Epidemiol* 10: 611–629.

Neutra, R. 1983. Roles for Epidemiology: The Impact of Environmental Chemicals. *Environ Health Perspect* 48: 99–104.

Oh, J., D. H. Bennett, A. M. Calafat, D. Tancredi, D. L. Roa, R. J. Schmidt, et al. 2021. Prenatal Exposure to Per- and Polyfluoroalkyl Substances in Association with Autism Spectrum Disorder in the Marbles Study. *Environ Int* 147: 106328.

Ostrea, E. M. 1999. Testing for Exposure to Illicit Drugs and Other Agents in the Neonate: A Review of Laboratory Methods and the Role of Meconium Analysis. *Curr Probl Pediatr* 29: 41–56.

Ostrea, E. M. Jr., D. K. Knapp, A. Romero, M. Montes, and A. R. Ostrea. 1994. Meconium Analysis to Assess Fetal Exposure to Nicotine by Active and Passive Maternal Smoking. *J Pediatr* 124: 471–476.

Ott, W. R. 1990. Total Human Exposure: Basic Concepts, EPA Field Studies, and Future Research Needs. *J Air Waste Manage Assoc* 40: 966–975.

Ozkaynak, H., J. D. Spengler. 1985. Analysis of Health Effects Resulting from Population Exposures to Acid Precipitation Precursors. *Environ Health Perspect* 63: 45–55.

Ozkaynak, H., R. M. Whyatt, L. L. Needham, G. Akland, and J. Quackenboss. 2005. Exposure Assessment Implications for the Design and Implementation of the National Children's Study. *Environ Health Perspect* 113: 1108–1115.

Ozkaynak, H., J. Xue, J. Spengler, L. Wallace, E. Pellizzari, P. Jenkins. 1996. Personal Exposure to Airborne Particles and Metals: RESULTS from the Particle Team Study in Riverside, California. *J Expo Anal Environ Epidemiol* 6: 57–78.

Pang, Y., D. L. MacIntosh, D. E. Camann, and P. B. Ryan. 2002. Analysis of Aggregate Exposure to Chlorpyrifos in the NHEXAS-Maryland Investigation. *Environ Health Perspect* 110: 235–240.

Panuwet, P., P. E. D'Souza, E. R. Phillips, P. B. Ryan, and D. B. Barr. 2020. Salivary Bioscience and Environmental Exposure Assessment. In D. A. Granger, and M. K. Taylor (Eds.), *Salivary Bioscience: Foundations of Interdisciplinary Saliva Research and Applications* (pp. 349–370). Cham: Springer International Publishing.

Panuwet, P., R. E. Hunter Jr., P. E. D'Souza, X. Chen, S. A. Radford, J. R. Cohen, et al. 2016. Biological Matrix Effects in Quantitative Tandem Mass Spectrometry-Based Analytical Methods: Advancing Biomonitoring. *Crit Rev Anal Chem* 46: 93–105.

Paredi, P., S. A. Kharitonov, and P. J. Barnes. 2002. Analysis of Expired Air for Oxidation Products. *Am J Respir Crit Care Med* 166: S31–37.

Patterson, D. G. Jr., R. E. Hoffman, L. L. Needham, D. W. Roberts, J. R. Bagby, and J. L. Pirkle, et al. 1986. 2,3,7,8-Tetrachlorodibenzo-p-Dioxin Levels in Adipose Tissue of Exposed and Control Persons in Missouri. An Interim Report. *J Am Med Assoc* 256: 2683–2686.

Pellizzari, E. D., L. A. Wallace, and S. M. Gordon. 1992. Elimination Kinetics of Volatile Organics in Humans Using Breath Measurements. *J Expo Anal Environ Epidemiol* 2: 341–355.

Phillips, D. L., J. L. Pirkle, V. W. Burse, J. T. Bernert Jr., L. O. Henderson, and L. L. Needham. 1989. Chlorinated Hydrocarbon Levels in Human Serum: Effects of Fasting and Feeding. *Arch Environ Contam Toxicol* 18: 495–500.

95

Pirkle, J. L., L. L. Needham, K. Sexton. 1995. Improving Exposure Assessment by Monitoring Human Tissues for Toxic Chemicals. *J Expo Anal Environ Epidemiol* 5: 405–424.

Pirkle, J. L., W. H. Wolfe, D. G. Patterson, L. L. Needham, J. E. Michalek, J. C. Miner, et al. 1989. Estimates of the Half-Life of 2,3,7,8-Tetrachlorodibenzo-p-Dioxin in Vietnam Veterans of Operation Ranch Hand. *J Toxicol Environ Health* 27: 165–171.

Rager, J. E., J. Bangma, C. Carberry, A. Chao, J. Grossman, K. Lu, et al. 2020. Review of the Environmental Prenatal Exposome and Its Relationship to Maternal and Fetal Health. *Reprod Toxicol* 98: 1–12.

Raithel, M., A. Hagel, H. Albrecht, Y. Zopf, A. Naegel, H. W. Baenkler, et al. 2015. Excretion of Urinary Histamine and N-Tele Methylhistamine in Patients with Gastrointestinal Food Allergy Compared to Non-Allergic Controls During an Unrestricted Diet and a Hypoallergenic Diet. *BMC Gastroenterol* 15: 41.

Raja, M., A. Garg, P. Yadav, K. Jha, and S. Handa. 2016. Diagnostic Methods for Detection of Cotinine Level in Tobacco Users: A Review. *J Clin Diagn Res* 10: Ze04–06.

Rasheed, H., P. Kay, R. Slack, and Y. Y. Gong. 2019. Assessment of Arsenic Species in Human Hair, Toenail and Urine and Their Association with Water and Staple Food. *J Expos Sci Environ Epidemiol* 29: 624–632.

Rauh, V. A., and A. E. Margolis. 2016. Research Review: Environmental Exposures, Neurodevelopment, and Child Mental Health – New Paradigms for the Study of Brain and Behavioral Effects. *J Child Psychol Psychiatry* 57: 775–793.

Ribas-Fitó, N., R. Ramón, F. Ballester, J. Grimalt, A. Marco, and N. Olea, et al. 2006. Child Health and the Environment: The INMA Spanish Study. *Paediatr Perinat Epidemiol* 20: 403–410.

Russo, G, F. Barbato, D. G. Mita, and L. Grumetto. 2019. Simultaneous Determination of Fifteen Multiclass Organic Pollutants in Human Saliva and Serum by Liquid Chromatography-Tandem Ultraviolet/ Fluorescence Detection: A Validated Method. *Biomed Chromatogr* 33: e 4427.

Ryan, P.B. 1997. Historical Perspective on the Use of Exposure Assessment in Human Risk Assessment. In M. C. Newman and C. Strojan (Eds.), *Risk Assessment: Logic and Measurement*. CRC Press. First Edition.

Ryan, P. B. 2016. Exposure Assessment, Industrial Hygiene and Environmental Management. In H. Frumkin (Ed.), *Environmental Health: From Local to Global*, 3rd ed. Lewis Publishers.

Ryan, P. B., C. P. Hemphill, I. H. Billick, N. L. Nagda, M. D. Koontz, and R. C. Fortmann. 1989. Estimation of Nitrogen Dioxide Concentrations in Homes Equipped with Unvented Gas Space Heaters. *Environ Int* 15: 551 556.

Ryan, P. B., N. Huet, and D. L. MacIntosh. 2000. Longitudinal Investigation of Exposure to Arsenic, Cadmium, and Lead in Drinking Water. *Environ Health Perspect* 108: 731–735.

Sabbioni, G., O. Sepai, H. Norppa, H. Yan, A. Hirvonen, Y. Zheng, et al. 2007. Comparison of Biomarkers in Workers Exposed to 2,4,6-Trinitrotoluene. Biomarkers: Biochemical Indicators of Exposure, *Res Susceptibility Chem* 12: 21–37.

Sabbioni, G., and R. J. Turesky. 2017. Biomonitoring Human Albumin Adducts: The Past, the Present, and the Future. *Chem Res Toxicol* 30: 332–366.

Saito, S., J. Ueyama, T. Kondo, I. Saito, E. Shibata, M. Gotoh, et al. 2014. A Non-Invasive Biomonitoring Method for Assessing Levels of Urinary Pyrethroid Metabolites in Diapered Children by Gas Chromatography–Mass Spectrometry. *J Expos Sci Environ Epidemiol* 24: 200–207.

Sarnat, J. A., R. Golan, R. Greenwald, A. U. Raysoni, P. Kewada, A. Winquist, et al. 2014. Exposure to Traffic Pollution, Acute Inflammation and Autonomic Response in a Panel of Car Commuters. *Environ Res* 133: 66–76.

Schettgen, T., H. C. Broding, J. Angerer, H. Drexler. 2002. Hemoglobin Adducts of Ethylene Oxide, Propylene Oxide, Acrylonitrile and Acrylamide-Biomarkers in Occupational and Environmental Medicine. *Toxicol Lett* 134: 65–70.

Schwedler, G., E. Rucic, R. Lange, A. Conrad, H. M. Koch, C. Pälmke, et al. 2020. Phthalate Metabolites in Urine of Children and Adolescents in Germany. Human Biomonitoring Results of the German Environmental Survey GerES V, 2014–2017. *Int J Hyg Environ Health* 225: 113444.

Sexton, K., M. A. Callahan, and E. F. Bryan. 1995. Estimating Exposure and Dose to Characterize Health Risks: The Role of Human Tissue Monitoring in Exposure Assessment. *Environ Health Perspect* 103 Suppl 3:13–29.

Sexton, K., and B. Ryan. 1988. Assessment of Human Exposure to Air Pollution: Methods, Measurement and Models. In A. Y. B. R. Watson, and D. Kennedy (Eds.), *Air Pollution, the Automobile, and Public Health*, (pp. 207–238). Washington, D.C.: National Academy Press.

Shenoi, R., G. Stewart, and N. Rosenberg. 1998. Screening for Carbon Monoxide in Children. *Pediatr Emerg Care* 14: 399–402.

Shin, H. M., T. E. McKone, and D. H. Bennett. 2017. Model Framework for Integrating Multiple Exposure Pathways to Chemicals in Household Cleaning Products. *Indoor Air* 27: 829–839.

Shin, H.-M., P. B. Ryan, V. M. Vieira, and S. M. Bartell. 2012. Modeling the Air–Soil Transport Pathway of Perfluorooctanoic Acid in the MID-OHIO VALLEY USING Linked Air Dispersion and Vadose Zone Models. *Atmos Environ* 51: 67–74.

Shin, H.-M., R. J. Schmidt, D. Tancredi, J. Barkoski, S. Ozonoff, D. H. Bennett, et al. 2018. Prenatal Exposure to Phthalates and Autism Spectrum Disorder in the Marbles Study. *Environ Health* 17: 85.

Shin, H. M., K. Steenland, P. B. Ryan, V. M. Vieira, and S. M. Bartell. 2014. Biomarker-Based Calibration of Retrospective Exposure Predictions of Perfluorooctanoic Acid. *Environ Sci Technol* 48: 5636–5642.

Shin, H. M., V. M. Vieira, P. B. Ryan, R Detwiler, B. Sanders, K. Steenland, et al. 2011a. Environmental Fate and Transport Modeling for Perfluorooctanoic Acid Emitted from the Washington Works Facility in West Virginia. *Environ Sci Technol* 45: 1435–1442.

Shin, H. M., V. M. Vieira, P. B. Ryan, K. Steenland, and S. M. Bartell. 2011b. Retrospective Exposure Estimation and Predicted Versus Observed Serum Perfluorooctanoic Acid Concentrations for Participants in the C8 Health Project. *Environ Health Perspect* 119: 1760–1765.

Signes-Pastor, A. J., E. Gutiérrez-González, M. García-Villarino, F. D. Rodríguez-Cabrera, J. J. López-Moreno, E. Varea-Jiménez, et al. 2021. Toenails as a Biomarker of Exposure to Arsenic: A Review. *Environ Res* 195: 110286.

Silva, M. J., J. A. Reidy, E. Samandar, Herbert, A. R., L. L. Needham, and A. M. Calafat. 2005. Detection of Phthalate Metabolites in Human Saliva. *Arch Toxicol* 79: 647–652.

Smith, C. J., T. D. Guy, M. F. Stiles, M. J. Morton, B. B. Collie, B. J. Ingebrethsen, et al. 1998. A Repeatable Method for Determination of Carboxyhemoglobin Levels in Smokers. *Hum Exp Toxicol* 17: 29–34.

Steenland, K., T. Fletcher, C. R. Stein, S. M. Bartell, L. Darrow, M. J. Lopez-Espinosa, et al. 2020. Review: Evolution of Evidence on PFOA and Health Following the Assessments of the C8 Science Panel. *Environ Int* 145: 106125.

Vasylieva, N., K. C. Ahn, B. Barnych, S. J. Gee, B. D. Hammock. 2015. Development of an Immunoassay for the Detection of the Phenylpyrazole Insecticide Fipronil. *Environ Sci Technol* 49: 10038–10047.

Whyatt, R. M., and D. B. Barr. 2001. Measurement of Organophosphate Metabolites in Postpartum Meconium as a Potential Biomarker of Prenatal Exposure: A Validation Study. *Environ Health Perspect* 109: 417–420.

Whyatt, R. M., V. Rauh, D. B. Barr, D. E. Camann, H. F. Andrews, R. Garfinkel, et al. 2004. Prenatal Insecticide Exposures and Birth Weight And Length Among an Urban Minority Cohort. *Environ Health Perspect* 112: 1125–1132.

Wilschefski, S. C., and M. R. Baxter. 2019. Inductively Coupled Plasma Mass Spectrometry: Introduction to Analytical Aspects. *Clin Biochem Rev* 40: 115–133.

Xu, Y., C. Nielsen, Y. Li, S. Hammarstrand, E. M. Andersson, H. Li, et al. 2021. Serum Perfluoroalkyl Substances in Residents Following Long-Term Drinking Water Contamination from Firefighting Foam in Ronneby, *Sweden Environ Int* 147: 106333.

Zartarian, V. G., W. R. Ott, and N. Duan. 1997. A Quantitative Definition of Exposure and Related Concepts. *J Expo Anal Environ Epidemiol* 7: 411–437.

Zartarian, V. G., H. Ozkaynak, J. M. Burke, M. J. Zufall, M. L. Rigas, and E. J. Furtaw Jr. 2000. A Modeling Framework for Estimating Children's Residential Exposure and Dose to Chlorpyrifos Via Dermal Residue Contact and Nondietary Ingestion. *Environ Health Perspect* 108: 505–514.

Zartarian, V. G., and B. D. Schultz. 2010. The EPA's Human Exposure Research Program for Assessing Cumulative Risk in Communities. *J Expos Sci Environ Epidemiol* 20: 351–358.

Zhang, Y., S. Beesoon, L. Zhu, and J. W. Martin. 2013. Biomonitoring of Perfluoroalkyl Acids in Human Urine and Estimates of Biological Half-Life. *Environ Sci Technol* 47: 10619–10627.

Zhao, G., Y. Xu, W. Li, G. Han, and B. Ling. 2007. Prenatal Exposures to Persistent Organic Pollutants as Measured in Cord Blood and Meconium from Three Localities of Zhejiang, China. *Sci Total Environ* 377: 179–191.

6 Role of Epidemiology in Environmental Health Research

Wil Lieberman-Cribbin and Emanuela Taioli
Icahn School of Medicine at Mount Sinai Hospital, New York, NY, United States

CONTENTS

Definition of Environmental Epidemiology..99
How Epidemiology Addresses Environmental Health Problems 99
Spatial Analysis in Environmental Epidemiology 100
Biomarkers in Environmental Epidemiology 101
Addressing Environmental Health Effects of Disasters 105
The Exposome 106
Conclusions..107
Appendix...107
References..109

DEFINITION OF ENVIRONMENTAL EPIDEMIOLOGY

Epidemiology is a broad scientific discipline that includes observational studies of the role that lifestyle factors, such as smoking, drugs, and drinking habits, play on individuals' health status; estimations of the risks associated with occupational exposures; and controlled clinical evaluations of different treatment methods.

Whatever the subject of epidemiologic evaluation, the basic theoretical and general principles are ruled by well-defined scientific methods that build on statistical and biological knowledge of the phenomenon under study, with the main goal to assess if observed rates of a given phenomenon differ significantly from those that would be expected under specified conditions (Miettinen 1985).

The application of epidemiology to the study of environmental exposures is key to validating the models used in predicting hazards and can characterize the actual and potential health effects of certain exposures. It is also a tool for studying risks associated with environmental exposures and defining a dose threshold for environmental, physical, and chemicals agents.

The commonly accepted definition of *environmental epidemiology* (NRC 1991) is the study of the effect on human health of physical, biological, social, and chemical factors in the external environment. By examining specific populations or communities exposed to different environmental factors, environmental epidemiology seeks to clarify the relationship between the various components of such an environment on human health. This broad definition incorporates two important concepts. One is understanding disparities in exposure that result through the intersection of the built environment and physical environment, and how this affects the health of some sections of the population. The other is the relevance of biomarkers in the understanding of the biological effects of exposure on human health. Often, exposures occur months or even years before health conditions become apparent, and linking exposure to disease becomes complex. Biomarkers can facilitate this link by measuring residues and indicators of past exposures or their transient or persistent biological effects on the body.

HOW EPIDEMIOLOGY ADDRESSES ENVIRONMENTAL HEALTH PROBLEMS

Although environmental epidemiology relies on classical epidemiologic methods to address the health effects of environmental hazards, there are additional specific approaches that environmental epidemiologists use when designing a study to address a specific question.

One common approach epidemiologists use is to identify a study population suspected to be exposed to unsafely or disproportionately high levels of the agent of interest. This is a generally common condition for occupationally exposed groups; therefore, occupational studies are often the first step when studying the association between an environmental exposure and health. The advantage of this approach is that any suspected biological effect or health outcome, if it exists, will be amplified and more likely present in these populations of either highly, or chronically exposed individuals. For example, early studies on the carcinogenicity of asbestos were conducted in insulators and pipe fitter workers highly exposed to the carcinogen for years (Nicholson et al., 1982). Another example is the study of cholangiocarcinoma in vinyl-chloride workers (Fralish and Downs, 2002). Although occupational studies are extremely useful and necessary, they have several limitations: the population under study, occupationally exposed workers, is not representative of the general population potentially exposed. In fact, those employed in these occupations are generally males, younger, and healthier than the general population and comparing this occupational group to the general population can introduce bias as a result of the "healthy worker effect." Another limitation is that the type and amount of exposure experienced in occupational settings are very different from what happens in the general population. Usually, occupational exposures last several hours a day, plausibly six to eight depending on the job shifts, and can continue daily for years, resulting in biological effects that could differ from what is observed in other exposure settings.

For these reasons, a study of subjects environmentally exposed to the toxic substance of interest is as important as occupational studies and usually follows that evidence, building on the results of occupational studies. One important addition of environmental exposure studies is the assessment of the biological effects of low doses of exposure to a certain agent. This in turn can help define the minimum safe dose allowed to be present in air, water, or soil without major predictable risks for the general population. This understanding is relevant to how the US Environmental Protection Agency (EPA) regulates contaminants in water and emission standards for air pollutants. An illustrative example of these concepts is studying benzene, a compound found in the air from emissions from burning coal and oil, gasoline service stations, and motor vehicle exhaust. Acute and chronic effects of exposure to benzene were first studied in occupational settings. Acute inhalation exposure to benzene may cause drowsiness, dizziness, headaches, as well as eye, skin, and respiratory tract irritation, and, at high levels, unconsciousness. Chronic inhalation exposure has caused various disorders in the blood, including reduced numbers of red blood cells and aplastic anemia, and increased incidence of leukemia. These results, combined with the results of laboratory experimental studies, brought the EPA to classify benzene as a known human carcinogen for all routes of exposure, with a maximum time-weighted average (TWA) exposure limit of one part of benzene vapor per million parts of air (1 ppm) for an 8-hour workday and the maximum short-term exposure limit (STEL) of 5 ppm for any 15-minute period. However, it was through several studies of environmentally exposed populations that new guidelines were established stating that no safe level of exposure can be recommended and that the unit risk of leukemia per 1 $\mu g/m^3$ air concentration is 6×10^{-6}, while the concentrations of airborne benzene associated with an excess lifetime risk of 1/10,000, 1/100,000, and 1/1,000,000 are 17, 1.7, and 0.17 $\mu g/m^3$, respectively (Harrison et al., 2010).

SPATIAL ANALYSIS IN ENVIRONMENTAL EPIDEMIOLOGY

Waldo Tobler popularized the idea of spatial autocorrelation with the phrase "everything is related to everything else, but near things are more related than distant things" (Tobler 1970). Taking spatial proximity into account is central in applying geographic tools to epidemiology and can be useful for identifying spatial clustering. Spatial clustering is defined as a "geographically bounded group of occurrences of sufficient size and concentration to be unlikely to have occurred by chance" (Knox 1989). In environmental health research, it is necessary to ask if an environmental exposure or disease outcome has a spatial component; that is, is the distribution related across space. One example is studying the release of toxic emissions. We can understand and visualize that the distribution of emitters is not uniform in space; they are often concentrated in specific areas, with distributions potentially proportional to population size, just as shopping stores can be more concentrated in malls. An environmental epidemiology approach can then ask what, if any, are the consequences of this grouping of emitters across space and/or time. We can imagine the impacts could be consequential to those living closer to the sources of pollution, and further lines of questioning could incorporate demographic, socioeconomic, and other population-level characteristics to understand how exposures influence people's health.

There are many further examples of the role of geography in environmental health research, such as studying the spatial clustering of cancer cases. In a 2016 paper by Liu et al., spatial clusters of patients with myelodysplastic syndromes (MDS) were identified, and the characteristics of patients in areas of high MDS incidence were compared to those residing in areas of low MDS incidence. This comparison helped elucidate that smokers and older patients with MDS were more likely to be in areas of high incidence. This epidemiologic analysis was performed in a software called 'SaTScan,' which is a free tool supported by the National Cancer Institute. However, there are many tools and statistical programs that can be applied to environmental health research that can analyze spatial and temporal trends in data, such as R Studio and QGIS. Cluster analysis can also be applied to study composite sociodemographic variables. For example, there are epidemiologic reports that flooding after Hurricane Sandy in New York was more common in areas of lower median household income. This type of analysis can contribute to the understanding of how socioeconomic factors may be associated with exposure type and concentration, and how this relates to disease outcomes (Figures 6.1 and 6.2).

BIOMARKERS IN ENVIRONMENTAL EPIDEMIOLOGY

The US Food and Drug Administration and the National Institutes of Health (NIH) Biomarker Working Group define a biomarker as "[a] defined characteristic that is measured as an indicator of normal biological processes, pathogenic processes or responses to an exposure or intervention." Although concise, these agencies also introduce many subclasses of biomarkers, including 'monitoring,' 'diagnostic,' 'pharmacodynamic/response,' 'predictive,' 'prognostic,' 'safety,' and 'susceptibility/risk.' Extensive literature has been written about the usefulness of biomarkers in improving measurement of the exposure, in the identification of subpopulations particularly susceptible to exposure, and in the assessment of the long-lasting biological effects of exposure, including the identification of biological links between exposure and carcinogenicity.

One prominent application of biomarkers is in assessing exposure to a suspected toxicant. To discuss this and other applications of biomarkers, we will use the example of the 9/11 terrorist attacks on the World Trade Center (WTC) in New York City (NYC) within a common framework (Figure 6.3).

In the 9/11 example, exposure from the terrorist attacks included a mixture of dust, smoke, chemicals, and carcinogens, among which were benzene, volatile organic compounds, asbestos, silica, cement dust, glass fibers, heavy metals, polycyclic aromatic hydrocarbons, polychlorinated

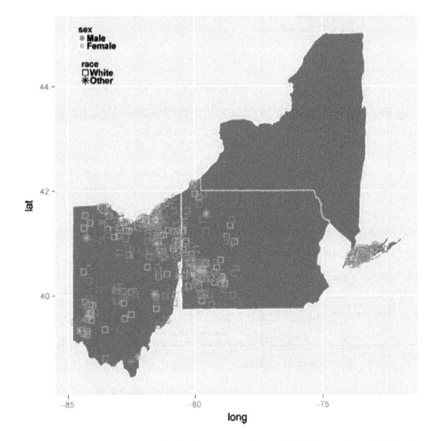

Figure 6.1   Locations of all the myelodysplastic syndrome (MDS) cases (*n* = 984) in the study area (Ohio, western Pennsylvania, and Long Island, New York) include in the spatial analysis. Lat, latitude; long, longitude. (Previously published in Liu B, Kerath SM, Sekeres MA, Fryzek JP, Sreekantaiah C, Mason CR, Kolitz J, Taioli E. Myelodysplastic syndromes spatial clusters in disease etiology and outcome. Leukemia & lymphoma. 2016 Feb 1, 57(2): 392–399.)

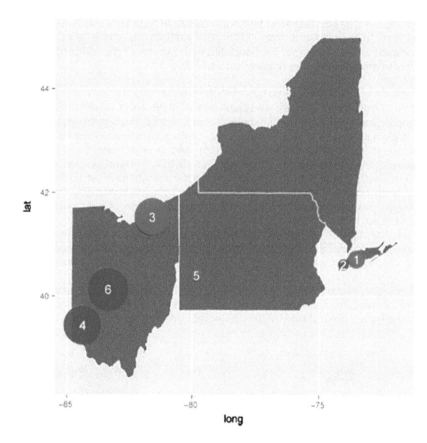

Figure 6.2   :pcatopm pf the ,pst ;ole;u c;ister (Cluster 1) and the five secondary clusters (Clusters 2–6) in high (in red color, Clusters 1, 3, and 5) and low (in blue color, Clusters 2, 4, and 6) myelodysplastic syndrome (MDS) incidence in the study area. (Previously published in Liu B, Kerath SM, Sekeres MA, Fryzek JP, Sreekantaiah C, Mason CR, Kolitz J, Taioli E. Myelodysplastic syndromes spatial clusters in disease etiology and outcome. Leukemia & lymphoma. 2016 Feb 1, 57(2): 392–399.)

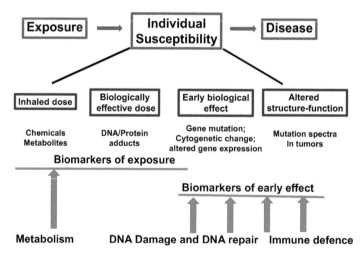

Figure 6.3   Continuum of biomarkers.   **Previously published in Tomasetti M, Santarelli L. Biomarkers for early detection of malignant mesothelioma: diagnostic and therapeutic application.** *Cancers.* **2010 Jun, 2(2): 523–548.**

biphenyls, and polychlorinated dibenzofurans and dioxins. This exposure mixture was complex and rapidly changing in concentration and composition. From an exposure assessment perspective, in retrospect, it would have been useful to collect urine and blood in the immediate period after the terrorist attacks to characterize the types and concentrations of exposures in biological samples. Utilizing biomarkers in this manner would have been useful in identifying subgroups of individuals who had hazardously high levels of exposure to particularly dangerous compounds, and therefore were at increased risk of a possible health-related outcome. This example illustrates how biomarkers could help identify affected populations and drive subsequent research. Biomarkers of biologically effective doses, in order to better understand the acute biological effects of the exposure, would have also been extremely precious in the population of WTC responders. For example, if we observed the presence of DNA adducts in a certain subgroup of the exposed population, we could expect further problems related to DNA replication in these subjects; these important hints could have been the focus of further research in the population. Unfortunately, this early information as well as biological samples from the exposed cohorts are missing.

While the WTC health program has documented exposure from first responders in questionnaires and interviews, new techniques based on DNA methylation have emerged to predict cancer risk and early biological effects associated with exposure (Kuan et al. 2019). Additional analyses of WTC-exposed women reported methylation differences between WTC-exposed and unexposed women (Arslan et al., 2020). Further, these analyses identify pathways that are enriched among the exposed participants, such as mitogen-activated protein kinase and Ras-associated protein-1 (Figure 6.4).

WTC research has also identified biological differences in tumors as a consequence of exposure. In a 2019 study by Gong et al. (2019), the expression of immunologic and inflammatory genes was compared across prostate cancer patients with a history of WTC exposure and prostate cancer cases without WTC exposure using the NanoString assay, a laboratory test that assesses gene expression of a panel of 800 inflammatory and immune-related genes. The results point at a different functional spectrum in WTC cancer cases, specifically upregulation of genes involved with immune and inflammatory responses. This could be a sign that WTC exposure is associated with more aggressive tumors, as suggested by the remarkable inflammatory pattern coupled with immune dysregulation observed in prostate cancer tissues from WTC responders in comparison to nonexposed WTC prostate cancers. The visualization of gene expression data is usually accomplished through a volcano plot, which can identify which genes are differentially expressed (upregulated or downregulated) between the two groups, WTC-exposed and non-WTC-exposed cancer cases (Figure 6.5).

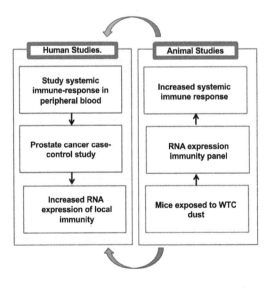

Figure 6.4   Example of studies using both human and animal samples.   **Previously published in Lieberman-Cribbin W, Tuminello S, Gillezeau C, van Gerwen M, Brody R, Donovan M, Taioli E. The development of a Biobank of cancer tissue samples from World Trade Center responders.** *Journal of Translational Medicine.* **2018 Dec, 16(1): 1–0.**

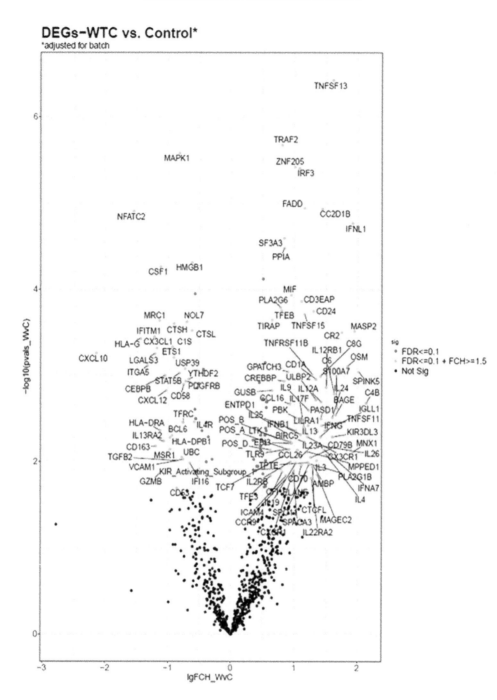

Figure 6.5

Taken together, WTC research represents a unique example of how biomarkers can be used to identify exposure and associations of exposure on disease biology (Figure 6.5).

In order to offset the limitations of human studies, and in the example of 9/11, the lack of early samples to better define WTC exposure and its early biological effects, resulted in data from animal models to be utilized. Generally, biomarkers can also be studied in animal models to inform environmental epidemiology studies. In the 9/11 example, mice and rodents exposed to WTC dust were studied for various cardiovascular and cancer-related endpoints. Rodents exposed to WTC dust have also exhibited changes in gene expression related to lung inflammation, oxidative stress,

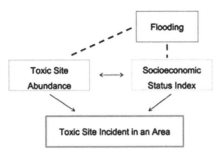

Figure 6.6 The interplay between toxic site abundance, socioeconomic status, flooding, and toxic incidents occurring in an area. (Previously published in Lieberman-Cribbin W, Liu B, Sheffield P, Schwartz R, Taioli E. Socioeconomic disparities in incidents at toxic sites during Hurricane Harvey. *Journal of Exposure Science & Environmental Epidemiology.* 2021 May, 31(3): 454–460.)

and cell cycle control (Cohen et al. 2015). The endpoints noted in this research have the translational research capacity to identify parallel early biological effects of exposure in WTC-exposed humans and identify subgroups at risk (Figure 6.4).

ADDRESSING ENVIRONMENTAL HEALTH EFFECTS OF DISASTERS

Among the numerous examples of epidemiological studies in environmental health research, an important and growing place is epidemiological studies centered around disaster events. There are several historical examples of natural as well as man-made disasters that resulted in populations exposed to chemical compounds or high-doses of radiation. These can be considered as moments to investigate the biological and health effects of certain exposures. For example, Hurricane Harvey in 2017 resulted in extensive flooding and power outages across greater Houston, Texas, which released toxic substances from chemical, waste, and petroleum facilities in this heavily industrialized area. Some of these toxic releases have been well-characterized, which include flooding of Superfund sites, releases of carcinogens such as benzene into the atmosphere, and releases of oil, sewage bacteria, and other chemicals into floodwaters. In this example, it is vital to characterize the type and magnitude of exposure, the spatial distribution of exposure, and if certain areas or populations were disproportionately exposed. In disaster-epidemiology, understanding the health effects of an exposure must also consider environmental justice concerns in exposure. For example, there is a legacy of environmental justice research following Hurricane Katrina, where Black and low-income residents of New Orleans, Louisiana, were disproportionately exposed to flooding and experienced extensive displacement from their homes.

The example of Hurricane Harvey exposure shows very clearly how an interplay exists between toxic site abundance, socioeconomic status, flooding, and toxic incidents occurring in an area (Figure 6.6).

Additionally, research following Hurricane Harvey found that racial and ethnic minority communities, as well as lower socioeconomic status communities, faced more extensive flooding. Additionally, areas of lower socioeconomic status were also more likely to have a toxic release incident. This indicated that disproportionate exposure occurred in more socioeconomically vulnerable communities and how it is essential to frame an environmental exposure event from an environmental justice and epidemiology perspective to construct the full story and consequences of an exposure. Using epidemiologic methods to answer environmental health questions in this manner is essential to inform public health interventions and prevent adverse consequences of exposure from happening again (Figure 6.7).

Another example of how epidemiology integrates with environmental health is in studying the impacts of COVID-19. The unique situation of lockdowns provided an opportunity to study the effect of decreased mobility on disease and pollution outcomes. Epidemiology can assess how much human activity has changed, and if there are patterns or specific types of mobility (bus, subway, car, plane) that have decreased as a consequence of COVID-19. From an environmental health perspective, we can also measure air pollutant concentrations over time and link these with health outcomes. In NYC, cell phone data used as a proxy for mobility has shown that mobility decreased during COVID-19 lockdown periods (Figure 6.7). It has also been shown that mobility has a sociodemographic component, as racial and ethnic minority populations, essential workers,

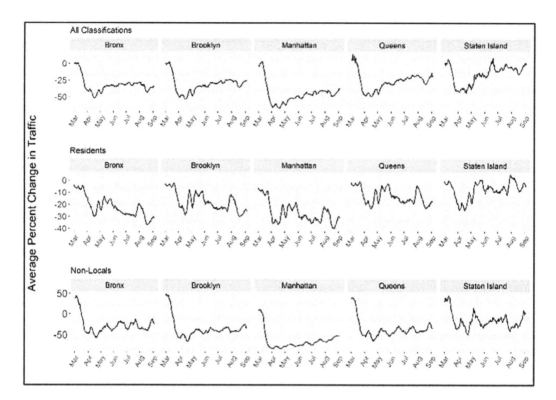

Figure 6.7

and those with lower household incomes had more mobility during the lockdown and also more disease burden from COVID-19 (Sy et al. 2021). While different segments of the population experienced different changes in mobility, lockdown periods did have an impact on air pollution. The phases of reopening in NYC serve as natural benchmarks where increasing proportions of the population become more mobile. Therefore, if we aim to reduce future air pollution in NYC, a mobility analysis can understand which segments of the population and which types of transportation have the greatest contributions. While the long-term effects of COVID-19 in NYC will continue to be studied, this situation represents a strong example of the intersection between epidemiology and environmental health.

THE EXPOSOME

As the field of environmental epidemiology moved forward, it became clear that the interplay between lifetime exposures and the individual's response to such exposures is more complex than previously thought and that it is important to incorporate the idea of the exposome into study design, analysis, and implications of research findings. The exposome was first introduced in 2005 by Wild to encompass the "life-course environmental exposures from the prenatal period onwards" (Wild 2005). One's cumulative exposures throughout the life span include exposures from the environment, diet, and lifestyle and are tied to an individual's genetics, physiology, and epigenetics (Center for Disease Control, 2022). Epidemiologists are interested in the exposome in relation to how past exposures contribute to disease occurrence, which inherently requires accurate measures of these exposures. While past approaches tried to achieve this through using biomarkers, more recently, the exposome model proposes to additional domains related to as 'social,' 'lifestyle,' ecosystems,' and 'physical-chemical' factors. To emphasize this approach, the National Institute for Environmental Health Sciences (NIEHS) currently funds the Health and Exposome Research Center: Understanding Lifetime Exposures (HERCULES) at Emory University, as well as the Children's Health Exposure Analysis Resource (CHEAR), and Human Health Exposure Analysis Resource (HHEAR). These approaches show the commitment to exposome-focused research, with emphasis on the development of new technology to study the exposome, as well as applications in children and individuals throughout the life course (Figures 6.8 and 6.9).

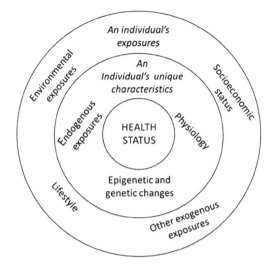

Figure 6.8 Concept of the exposome. An individual has many sources of exposure. How those exposures are modulated and impact health depends on the individual's unique characteristics. (Previously published in DeBord DG, Carreón T, Lentz TJ, Middendorf PJ, Hoover MD, Schulte PA. Use of the "exposome" in the practice of epidemiology: a primer on-omic technologies. *American Journal of Epidemiology*, 2016 Aug 15, 184(4): 302–314.)

CONCLUSIONS

Epidemiology in environmental health research is inherently interdisciplinary that encompasses classical epidemiology, molecular biology, social epidemiology, behavioral science, health disparities, environmental justice, and toxicology. The field has changed markedly over the years and is now moving toward a more complete view of the intersection between personal and social factors, biological markers, and lifetime exposure. Environmental epidemiologists have contributed greatly to the understanding of the acute and chronic health effects of occupational and environmental exposures, and have instructed and directed public health officials on how to mitigate and ameliorate the health status of the population (Figure 6.10).

The future goals of environmental epidemiology must consider to be interdisciplinary in order to navigate and understand complex exposures and how they influence health outcomes in order to work toward a more just and healthier world.

APPENDIX

The following is a list of sources of large datasets that can be useful for environmental epidemiology.

National Health and Nutrition Examination Survey (NHANES): NHANES is a nationally representative cross-sectional survey, designed to assess the health and nutritional status of the noninstitutionalized population in the United States. The NHANES program is administered by the National Center for Health Statistics (NCHS) and includes demographic and health interview questions, physical examinations, and laboratory tests (available at https://www.cdc.gov/nchs/nhanes/about_nhanes.htm).

Departments of Health Surveys: Local health departments may administer their own surveys to assess the health of their populations. For example, NYC administers the Community Health Survey (CHS) to provide estimates on chronic diseases and risk factors. Environmental topics include the presence of pests or mold in the home and the use of pesticides. Other examples of NYC data include Child Health Data, the Youth Risk Behavior Survey, and Child Lead Data. NYC also maintains a World Trade Center Health Registry with periodic surveys of responders and survivors of 9/11 (available from https://www1.nyc.gov/site/doh/data/data-sets/data-sets-and-tables.page).

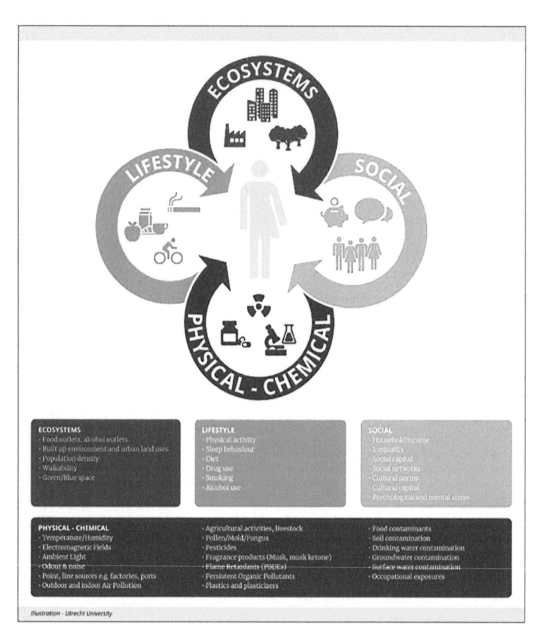

Figure 6.9 The exposome concept. (Previously published in Vermeulen R, Schymanski EL, Barabási AL, Miller GW. The exposome and health: where chemistry meets biology. *Science*, 2020 Jan 24, 367(6476): 392–396.)

Neighborhood Atlas and Area Deprivation Index (ADI): The Neighborhood Atlas is maintained by the University of Wisconsin and includes measures of neighborhood disadvantage, including health systems, not-for-profit organizations, and government agencies. The ADI ranks neighborhoods by socioeconomic disadvantage at either the state or national level (available at https://www.neighborhoodatlas.medicine.wisc.edu/).

PolicyMap: PolicyMap draws from hundreds of data sources to make geographic data widely accessible. It includes 50,000 indicators on demographics, incomes, housing, economics, education, health, and environment and disaster risk (available at https://www.policymap.com/).

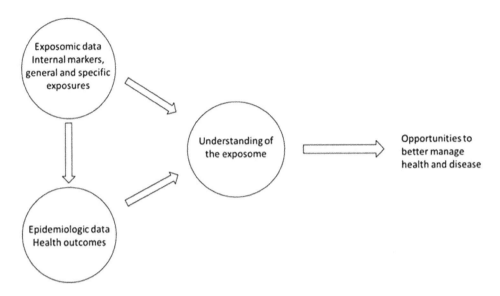

Figure 6.10 Exposome-informed epidemiologic research, (Previously published in: DeBord, D.G., Carreón, T., Lentz, T.J., Middendorf, P.J., Hoover, M.D. and Schulte, P.A., 2016. Use of the "exposome" in the practice of epidemiology: a primer on-omic technologies. *American Journal of Epidemiology, 184*(4): 302–314.)

US Census Data: The US Census Bureau conducts a series of ongoing surveys to assess vital information about the people of the United States. Examples of surveys include the American Community Survey (ACS) and the American Housing Survey (AHS). ACS provides information at the community level on topics, including demographics, education, employment, health, housing, and income, while the AHS provides detailed information on housing, including accessibility, housing quality (including exposure to pests, heating and water problems, structural issues, and mold), cost, neighborhood, and food insecurity (available from https://www.census.gov/data.html).

Air Quality: The EPA provides data from outdoor air quality monitors across the United States. Data can be used to estimate area-level ambient pollution levels and to derive area-level environmental health risks (available from https://www.epa.gov/outdoor-air-quality-data).

State and Local Departments of Health: Local health departments, as well as the Centers for Disease Control and Prevention (CDC) frequently report statistics on health conditions. For example, the CDC reports data on COVID-19 testing, cases, hospitalizations, deaths, and vaccines (available from https://covid.cdc.gov/covid-data-tracker/#datatracker-home). NYC reports similar statistics for geographic units within the city (available from https://www1.nyc.gov/site/doh/covid/covid-19-data.page). Statistics are often reported by area, sociodemographic factors, and geographic characteristics.

REFERENCES

Arslan, A.A., Tuminello, S., Yang, L., Zhang, Y., Durmus, N., Snuderl, M., Heguy, A., Zeleniuch-Jacquotte, A., Shao, Y., and Reibman, J., 2020. Genome-wide DNA methylation profiles in community members exposed to the World Trade Center disaster. *International Journal of Environmental Research and Public Health*, 17(15), 5493.

Center for Disease Control. Exposome and Exposomics. 2022. https://www.cdc.gov/niosh/topics/exposome/default.html

Cohen, Mitchell D., et al. 2015. Acute high-level exposure to WTC particles alters expression of genes associated with oxidative stress and immune function in the lung. *Journal of Immunotoxicology*, 12(2), 140–153.

Fralish, M.S., and Downs JW. 2022. Vinyl chloride toxicity. [Updated 2022 Jun 21]. In: StatPearls [Internet]. Treasure Island (FL): StatPearls Publishing; January. Available from: https://www.ncbi.nlm.nih.gov/books/NBK544334/

Gong, Y., Wang, L., Yu, H., Alpert, N., Cohen, M.D., Prophete, C., Horton, L., Sisco, M., Park, S.H., Lee, H.W., and Zelikoff, J. 2019. Prostate cancer in World Trade Center responders demonstrates evidence of an inflammatory cascade. *Molecular Cancer Research*, 17(8), 1605–1612.

Harrison, R., Delgado Saborit, J.M., Dor, F., et al. 2010. Benzene. In: *WHO Guidelines for Indoor Air Quality: Selected Pollutants*. Geneva: World Health Organization; 1. Available from: https://www.ncbi.nlm.nih.gov/books/NBK138708/

Knox, E. George. 1989. *Detection of clusters. Methodology of Enquiries into Disease Clustering*. London: Small Area Health Statistics Unit 17, 20.

Kuan, Pei-Fen, et al. 2019. Enhanced exposure assessment and genome-wide DNA methylation in World Trade Center disaster responders. *European Journal of Cancer Prevention: The Official Journal of the European Cancer Prevention Organisation (ECP)*, 28(3), 225.

Miettinen, O.S. 1985. *Theoretical Epidemiology: Principles of Occurrence Research in Medicine*. New York: John Wiley & Sons, p. 359.

NanoString PanCancer Immune Profiling Panel Analysis of archived WTC and non-WTC PCa samples. Differentially expressed genes (DEG) with FDR≤0.1 and Fold Change(FCH)≥1.5 (using non-WTC as the reference) represented in a volcano plot with batch-adjusted expression values. X axis: Fold changes in log2. Y axis: –p value in log 10 n.d.

NRC (National Research Council). 1991. *Environmental Epidemiology. Public Health and Hazardous Wastes*. Washington, DC: National Academy Press. 282 pp.

QGIS Development Team. 2022. *QGIS Geographic Information System*. Open Source Geospatial Foundation Project. Available from: http://qgis.osgeo.org.

RStudio Team. 2020. *RStudio: Integrated Development for R. RStudio*. Boston, MA: PBC. Available from: http://www.rstudio.com/

Sy, Karla Therese L. et al. 2021. Socioeconomic disparities in subway use and COVID-19 outcomes in New York City. *American Journal of Epidemiology*, 190(7), 1234–1242.

Tobler, Waldo R. 1970. A computer movie simulating urban growth in the Detroit region. *Economic Geography*, 46(sup1), 234–240.

Vermeulen, Roel, et al. 2020. The exposome and health: Where chemistry meets biology. *Science*, 367(6476), 392–396.

Wild, C.P., 2005. Complementing the genome with an "exposome": The outstanding challenge of environmental exposure measurement in molecular epidemiology. *Cancer Epidemiology Biomarkers & Prevention*, 14(8), 1847–1850.

7 Toxicological Basis for Risk Assessment

Mark G. Robson
Rutgers University, Piscataway, NJ, United States

William A. Toscano
University of Minnesota School of Public Health, Minneapolis, MN, United States

CONTENT

References and Further Reading...146

LEARNING OBJECTIVES

Students who complete this chapter will be able to

1. describe historical uses of toxins,
2. contrast a toxin from a toxicant,
3. discuss the exposomes and exposure to environmental agents,
4. discuss how the psychosocial affects toxicity in humans,
5. explain the difference between acute and chronic toxicity,
6. compare and contrast dose-response models,
7. identify Phase I and Phase II metabolic pathways,
8. describe the action of metabolism in the toxic response,
9. discuss gene-environment interactions,
10. describe systems toxicology,
11. identify how molecular biology informs toxic mechanisms, and
12. compare and contrast models used in toxicology studies.

Alle Ding sind Gift und nichts ohn "Gift; allein die Dosis macht, das ein Ding kein Gift Ist." or, All things are poison and nothing (is) without poison; the dose alone makes a thing not a poison – Paracelsus, 1493–1541.

Toxicology is the scientific underpinning for risk assessment. Philippus Aureolus Theophrastus Bombastus von Hohenheim (Paracelsius) was an innovator in medicine who has been called the "father of modern toxicology." He proposed the concept of dose response (Beaudoin et al. 2013) with his famous quote; he was the first to document that dose of a drug was related to either its therapeutic efficacy or its toxicity. His observation was similar to the advice given by our grandmothers who, like millions of other grandmothers cautioned us that "everything in moderation is best" (Figure 7.1).

These statements are most useful when evaluating a risk; anything, if taken to excess can cause harm. Data suggest one or two cups of coffee are protective against several health risks and that coffee naturally contains a variety of compounds that display antioxidant properties. These include chlorogenic acids and melanoidins, which act as antioxidants. Additionally, there is an association between caffeine consumption and an increase in alertness and performance. Caffeine may also increase insulin sensitivity and reduce the risk of developing type 2 diabetes in women and

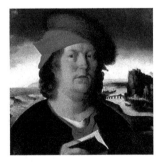

Figure 7.1 Philippus Aureolus Theophrastus Bombastus von Hohenheim (Paracelsius; 1493–1543), the "father of toxicology."

Source: **Alamy.com.**

DOI: 10.1201/9780429291722-7

men (Beaudoin et al. 2013), but excessive caffeine consumption may negatively affect sleep patterns (Lazarus et al. 2011). Moderate red wine consumption may reduce the risk of several cancers, but excessive wine consumption can lead to impairment, addiction, dementia, depression, and liver diseases. There is no chemical, natural or synthetic, that is not potentially toxic. The science of toxicology provides the means to generate data about chemicals and describe the associated risks of harm from exposure to those chemicals.

Risk assessment provides the context of the potential harm of a given chemical exposure under defined conditions. Toxicity is unique to a particular agent; minimizing the exposure will minimize the risk of harm. There are more than 100,000 chemicals in commerce, most of which were developed since 1945 (Stanton and Kruszewski 2016). Approximately 2800 compounds are high production volume chemicals, i.e., are manufactured in a volume of one million pounds annually (A. J. Williams et al. 2021). Toxicology historically is described as "the science of poisons" and has a colorful history of the use of poisons that range from hunting for food to removing undesirables, like Socrates, from society (Wexler and Hayes 2019). A contemporary description of toxicology is the study of the adverse actions of chemical, physical, or biological agents on living organisms and the ecosystem, including the prevention and mitigation of those adverse actions.

The observed adverse actions of a substance can be acute (immediate) or chronic (over time). The acute changes are easy to recognize; chronic actions are less obvious and often more complex. These actions can occur in a particular organ or cell type. The time from the initial exposure to the manifestation of the toxic response is called the latent period. An acute response may occur immediately and may last a few days. Chronic toxicity may last for months or even years. In the past five decades, the understanding of mechanisms by which toxic agents act in humans has progressed enormously because of advances in exposure science and molecular biology.

A toxicant may be either natural or synthetic. It is a common misbelief that only synthetic chemicals can be toxic; however, the first toxic agents used were all naturally occurring substances. A summary of the associated risks of natural and synthetic chemicals is given in Figure 7.2. Of particular note are the number of naturally occurring compounds in food that may be toxic.

Risk can be defined as the probability that harm will arise after exposure to a chemical or physical agent under a particular set of conditions. These events include injury, onset of a disease, or death. When the toxicological data about a particular chemical are known, a risk can be calculated. Risk assessment is the identification and quantification of risk resulting from exposure and toxicology studies that are used to set exposure limits. The integration of risk assessment and risk management enables policymakers to make decisions regarding the use of a particular chemical and the procedures and regulatory tools that can be used to reduce the risks either through administrative or regulatory policies (Figure 7.3).

While toxicology drives risk assessment, political, social, economic, and engineering factors drive risk management. Together risk assessment, exposure control, and risk monitoring can be applied to develop a workable risk management plan.

Hazard identification is based on the physicochemical properties of a chemical. Thus, hazard, or potential to do harm, is intrinsic to the substance. Toxicology data are often generated for a single chemical under a specific set of circumstances. However, humans are exposed to mixtures of chemicals under numerous conditions. Each of the chemicals in a mixed exposure may have its own adverse effect, or they may interact to yield additive, synergistic, or antagonistic toxicities.

Exposure assessment identifies the source; measures how much, how long, how often, and how many humans are exposed to a pollutant (Harper et al. 2015). Exposure in laboratory studies measures the action of a chemical as in a dose-response experiment. Dose response is an important concept in toxicology. The relationship between dose and response correlates exposure with health outcomes (Tsatsakis et al. 2018). In the broadest sense, the higher the dose the greater the response. A dose-response curve is based on observational data from studies in animals and *in vitro* experiments in laboratories.

The intensity of the response to a chemical at a single dose identifies resistant or sensitive individuals (see Figure 7.4). The affected individuals typically follow a normal distribution. The x-axis is the response and y-axis is the percent of individuals responding.

For the dose-response experiment, the logarithm of the administered dose, usually in mg/kg, is plotted on the x-axis and the response or number of individuals affected on the y-axis, this is typically expressed in percent (Figure 7.5). We can compare different chemicals by plotting them on a dose-response curve and observe the difference in the slope, the threshold, and the shape of the curve (see Figure 7.6).

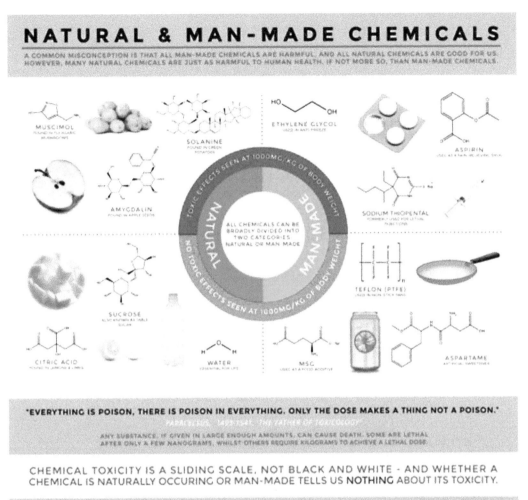

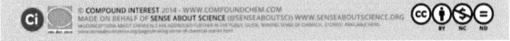

Figure 7.2   Natural and man-made chemicals.

Source: http://pbs.twimg.com/media/CTn6HlDWwAEB1Jc.png:large, Creative Commons license.

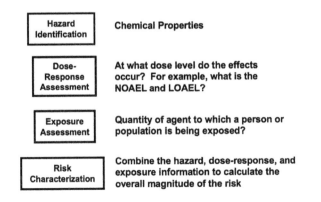

Figure 7.3   Steps in a typical risk assessment.

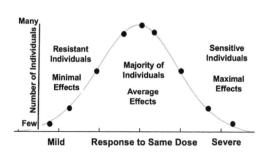

Figure 7.4 Range-finding for a complete dose-response study. The data obtained from this type of study yields the range in which the action of a chemical may be measured.

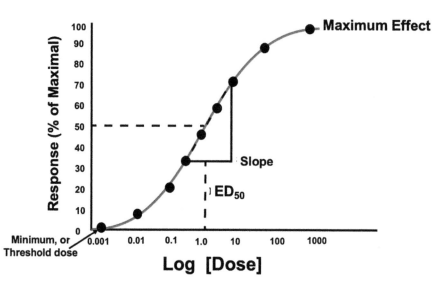

Figure 7.5 A typical dose-response curve where percent response is plotted vs. the logarithm of the concentration of a xenobiotic in mg/kg.

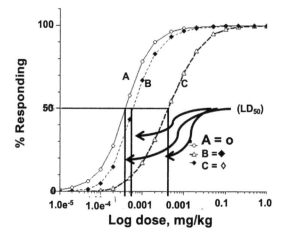

Figure 7.6 LD_{50} of three different compounds to compare relative toxicity of three analogous compounds in a Structure-Activity Relation (SAR). These experiments can be used to assess compounds of similar structure to determine their respective toxicity (Chung and Cerniglia 1992; Farhadi et al. 2018).

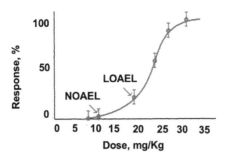

Figure 7.7 A dose-response curve showing doses where the NOAEL and LOAEL occur for a substance.

Table 7.1: **Summary of the Use of Safety Factors to Adjust for Uncertainties in Risk Assessments**

Safety Factor	Condition for Application
10	Valid chronic human exposure data available
100	No or inconclusive chronic human exposure data are available; long-term exposure data for several species of animals are available
1,000	No chronic or acute human exposure data available, scanty available animal exposure data

The slope of the curve yields the rate of response (positive or negative) and can be used to identify a threshold for the lowest observable effective dose (LOAEL) for a particular chemical or agent (see Figure 7.7). For comparison purposes, when lethality is the measured effect, the term "Lethal Dose 50," the dose at which 50% of the animals or cells die (LD_{50}) is used. This is a crude measure of toxicity, hardly used in clinical situations, but is an assessment tool to do a quick look at which chemical in a list of chemicals would be the most or least acutely toxic Figure 7.6.

To determine the range of doses to be used in the dose-response experiment (Figure 7.4) the doses at which all the animals die (the LD_{100}) is important as a maximum dose, or the cutoff dose to start an experiment of a protocol to see where the lethality is low, such as 10% the LD_{10} could be calculated. The LD_{50} is used as an estimate for the chronic toxicity of a compound; it is far from exact but provides an approximate level in most cases. The LD_{50} is associated with toxic or adverse effects; however, the pharmaceutical literature will also contain terms like ED_{50} for Effective Dose and TD_{50} for Therapeutic Dose to measure a particular effect. In environmental health risk assessment, the focus is on the harmful or toxic effects. Because these numbers are estimates rather than exact, and because individuals vary in response to a xenobiotic (a foreign substance of no nutritional value), safety factors are applied. Margins of Safety (MOS) are usually multiples of ten (Table 7.1). There is no biological basis for using these MOS values. Most of the techniques used to compensate for toxicity assessment uncertainties (such as the use of safety factors, conservative assumptions, and extrapolation models) are designed to err on the side of safety.

Thus, once a No Observed Adverse Effect Level (NOAEL) is identified, the highest acceptable level is 10, 100, or 1,000 times less, under defined conditions.

It is common when doing a risk assessment to apply several safety factors in establishing a safe level or standard. Much of the toxicity data that are derived for risk assessment come from animal studies using inbred strains. There is a difference between humans and rats or humans and mice; consequently, most agencies would apply a safety factor of ten for the difference between animals and humans. To account for variation in susceptibility within human populations, another safety factor of ten would be applied.

In the past decade, more concern about the specific risks to infants and small children has arisen because of outcomes from maternal exposure to diethylstilbesterol, known as DES, thalidomide, or other teratogens (Jamkhande, Chintawar, and Chandak 2014). It is often pointed out that children are not just little adults. The changes in physiology and metabolism that occur during the life-span account for many of the differences in response to toxic exposures during the life cycle, from womb to tomb (Arnoldussen and Kiliaan 2014). Given the risks that certain chemicals pose to developing organ systems, another safety factor of ten is applied. For example, if a safe drinking water standard for a compound is set at 1 ppm, but that compound could only be remediated to a level greater than the standard, what would the level be for the published standard for the compound at issue? If a safety factor of 10X is applied for species variation, then another 10x for human variation 10x, and then another 10X for child protection, a recommended standard of 1 ppb would be published, because 1 divided by $10 \times 10 \times 10 = 0.001$ ppm (or 1 ppb). Many people would argue that these levels are overly conservative and not realistic. Often, the regulation that follows the determination of a risk number will be modified based on additional scientific and practical data, and economic and political considerations.

There are two important doses that must be considered when looking at toxicological data and applying those doses to risk assessment. First is the "No Adverse Effect Level," *NOAEL*, which is the *highest dose at which there was not an observed toxic or adverse effect.* Equally important is the *"Lowest Observed Adverse Effect Level"* (LOAEL), which *is the lowest dose at which there was an observed toxic or adverse effect* (Figure 7.7.)

The abbreviations NOEL and LOEL were used in the older literature when although there was an effect, nothing was observed. However, more sensitive analytical methods and more sensitive measures of physiological changes are available to measure effects that could not have been observed previously. In present-day terms, NOAEL is used where the emphasis is on the "adverse" effect. If the effect is not one considered to be adverse, then the effect is of little consequence. For many years, exposure was the weak link in toxicology studies for risk assessment. Much of the data came from ambient area – or personal – monitoring of a toxicant, or retrospective "expert opinion" modeling (Dahm et al. 2015; Spengler and Soczek 1984; Tosteson and Ware 1990). New technology to measure exposures has been developed, which includes more sensitive analytical chemistry instruments, better biomarkers, new sensors, and remote detection to better understand the complex nature of how environmental exposure affects health (Lioy 2010; Weichenthal, Hatzopoulou, and Brauer 2019).

Exposure assessment or the process of estimating or measuring the magnitude, frequency, and duration of exposure to an agent, along with the number and characteristics of the population exposed (Moya et al. 2011) are brought together in the Exposome (Wild 2012).

Modern toxicology uses the exposome, which was proposed as a complement to the genome, as a measure of the entirety of human exposures from preconception to death (Wild 2005) that range from the external to the internal environment (see Canali 2020 for a review). The paradigm of exposome-genome interaction together with epigenetics (see Chapter 10) is a valuable tool to understand the risk of the onset of environmentally driven complex disease (Plusquin, Saenen, and Naweot 2019).

After exposure, a toxicant enters the body *via* the oral cavity, lungs, gastrointestinal tract, or the skin. Once inside the body, toxicants are distributed to the organs (see Chapter 4) and enter the cell by crossing a membrane. Xenobiotics need to cross cellular membranes (Figure 7.8) to elicit a biological response. Five processes are used: passive diffusion, filtration, facilitated diffusion, active transport, and phago- or pinocytosis (Hall and Hall 2021). The manner in which the toxicant crosses a membrane depends on the chemical makeup of the agent and the organ. Absorption occurring primarily by passive diffusion shows first-order kinetics and is generally rapid and efficient. Agents that are not soluble in the hydrophobic moiety of membranes enter the cell through a process called facilitated diffusion, whereby the toxicant binds to a carrier protein and is carried into the cell. Active transport is a process where the compound of interest requires energy to move against a gradient, i.e., from an area of low concentration to one of a higher concentration. Carrier proteins are also involved in active transport. Facilitated diffusion and active transport show saturation kinetics (Figure 7.9).

Lungs have a large surface area and are vascularized. Gases enter alveoli by passive diffusion. The barrier between air in lung and blood supply is as little as two cell membranes thick. Absorption occurs primarily by passive diffusion; generally rapid and efficient, particulate matter is taken up by phagocytosis (Hall and Hall 2021; Wang et al. 2019)

The gastrointestinal (GI) tract is an important site for xenobiotic absorption. The microenvironment changes throughout the length of the GI tract, with internal pH ranging from pH ~7 in

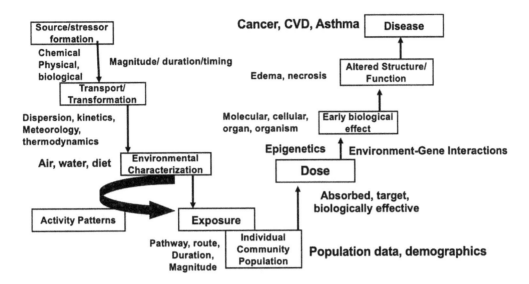

Figure 7.8 Source-exposure-dose-effects continuum.

Source: Moya et al. (2011).

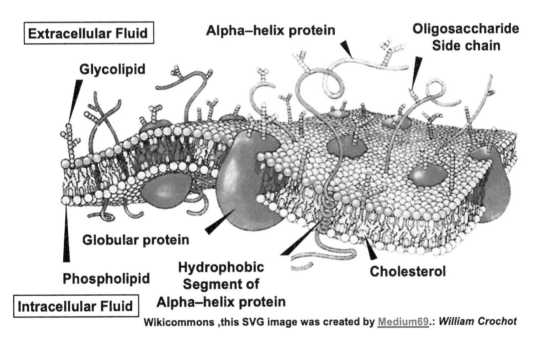

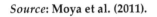

Figure 7.9 Structure of a cellular membrane. External and internal surfaces are negatively charged phospholipids, the interior of the membrane is hydrophobic, proteins, some of which span the membrane, float in the membrane matrix.

the mouth and ~2 in the stomach; the degree of vascularization differs over its large surface area (human small intestine: >200 m²). Lipid soluble, nonionized compounds can be absorbed anywhere in the GI tract. Ionizable compounds will only be absorbed if they are un-ionized at the pH of a particular site and are also lipid soluble. Weak acids can be absorbed by the small intestine (pH 6) because of large surface area, good blood flow, and ionization of the compound in blood at pH 7.4. Absorption mechanisms in the GI tract include the following: passive diffusion for weak acids/bases, nonionizable compounds; carrier-mediated transport for weak acids, peptides, sugars, strong acids and bases, permanently charged compounds; phagocytosis for large molecules and particles.

Xenobiotic exposures are either unintentional or predicted. An unintentional exposure is often hard to quantitate. Very often, regulators, emergency responders, and emergency department physicians have to estimate these exposures quickly without a lot of precision. Predicted exposures can be calculated with a high degree of certainty based on *in vitro* and *in vivo* studies, controlled environmental studies, and regular monitoring of environmental conditions such as for air toxics or water pollutants.

Laboratory and monitoring studies provide data for the setting of Tolerable Daily Intake (TDI), Acceptable Daily Intake (ADI), Threshold Limit Values (TLV), and Reference Doses (RfD). Then, based on what is known about an RfD or an ADI, an acceptable level of exposure can be computed and risk predicted.

Risk assessment determines acceptable exposure levels for humans or other living organisms; acceptable exposure is determined through the risk management process. These processes are essential to determine what are acceptable or unacceptable levels of exposure to a particular substance.

Animal studies are based on the principle that all vertebrate animals share a common physiology with humans. It is known, however, that even among rodent species, there are differences in physiology. Toxicity studies using rodents have been criticized as summarized in Table 7.2.

The dose of xenobiotics required to observe toxicity in rodent models often is much higher than that to which humans are exposed and thus has been criticized as not relevant to the human condition. Animals that respond to exposure levels similar to that of humans include zebrafish (*Danio rerio*), or Japanese rice fish, or Medaka fish (*Orryzias lapites*) (Hobbie et al. 2010; Laing et al. 2016; Wang et al. 2020).

To address the criticism that toxicity found in animals is not relevant to human risk assessment, the cultivation of human cells became useful for screening human toxicants at relevant doses. Human cell culture has proven to be a valuable tool in elucidating toxicogenomic mechanisms and yielding a better understanding of risk than traditional toxicological testing (Bourdon-Lacombe et al. 2015). This method can be used for rapid screening of toxicity but has met some criticism because of the inability to assess systemic actions in these models (D. Wang et al. 2020). Attempts to address organ toxicology studies and organ-organ interactions have led to the development of new cell culture techniques, such as 3D and tissue chips (organ on a chip, Figure 7.10) were developed. With advances in fluidics, it became possible to develop multiple organs on a chip, or the so-called Body Chip (Ma et al. 2021) (Figure 7.11).

Growth of a single organ on a chip was a big advance in technology but did not address organ-organ interactions. Capability to cultivate multiple organs on a single chip started to address the issue, and the number of organs that could be used is being expanded. The NCATS at NIH and partners in the Tissue Chip Consortium (https://ncats.nih.gov/tissuechip/partnerships) are developing the "Human Chip" and "Female Reproductive Systems Chip" (Low et al. 2021; Skardal et al. 2017; Picollet-D'hahan et al. 2017; Wang et al. 2020), which will dramatically advance studies of organ-organ interaction in risk assessment in humans (Figure 7.12).

Toxicology has evolved from the science of measuring death from acute poisoning to investigating complex disease onset brought on by exposure to one or more toxicants. Prior to the sequencing of the human genome, the coupling of environmental toxicology and epidemiology with genetic methods was a linear science that investigated single exposures and single genes. This reductionist approach is reminiscent of the ancient Indian parable of the blind men describing an

Table 7.2: Some Issues with Data Obtained from a Toxicological Risk Assessment Study

Hazard Identification	a. Use of animals
	b. Epidemiology studies with negative human data
Dose Response	Animal studies:
	a. High-low dose exposure extrapolation
	b. Animal-human extrapolation, linear vs. threshold
Exposure Evaluation	a. Ambient vs. biological monitoring
	b. Monitors vs. modeling

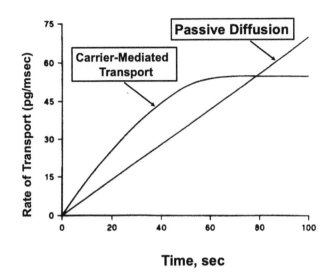

Figure 7.10 Kinetics of transport. Comparison of the kinetics of passive diffusion, first order, and facilitated diffusion, which show typical Michaelis–Menten saturation kinetics. For a video demonstration of transport through a membrane, see Tox Tutor "Absorption," https://www. toxmsdt.com/100-section-10-overview.html (viewed November 30, 2021).

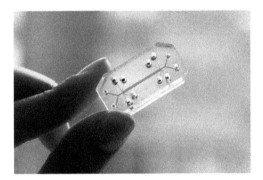

Figure 7.11 This lung-on-a-chip serves as an accurate model of human lungs to test for safety or toxicity.

Source: **National Center for Advancing Translational Sciences, NCATS; NIH.**

elephant, where conclusions were drawn depending on which part of the elephant each person touched (Baldwin 2019). The reductionist approach to understanding toxic mechanisms is being phased out because new technologies are being applied that allow a systems toxicology approach to study complex biological processes. Because of the large number of toxicology research approaches over the years, and much of the data being generated in different systems – *in vivo, in vitro, and large data sets generated from* "omics" approaches – the field of systems toxicology was developed (Strurla et al. 2014). Systems toxicology is an approach that utilizes data from different branches of toxicology and integrates them to provide a holistic understanding of the adverse effects of xenobiotics on biological systems (Heijne et al. 2014). Using systems toxicology to gain an in-depth understanding of biological networks is being applied to gain new insights into how toxicants perturb the tightly regulated signal networks to yield a deeper understanding of mechanisms of environmentally caused disease. Systems toxicology relies heavily on mathematical and computational models to link the data from various systems. The main driving force behind the development of systems toxicology approaches is that the whole risk assessment process is a time-consuming and expensive process, and often yields incomplete information (Krewski et al. 2009).

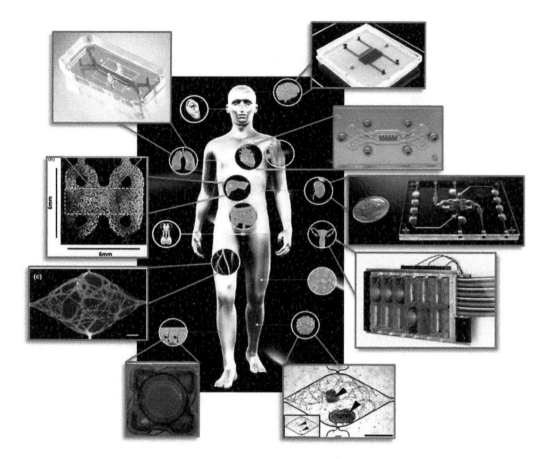

Figure 7.12 Human on a chip. New methods in organ culture and fluidics now allow for multiple, interacting organs to be grown on a single chip, to perform dose-response experiments to screen toxicants *in vitro*, minimizing the use of animals in human health risk assessment.

Source: **NCATS; NIH https://ufluidix.com/circle/wp-content/uploads/2019/10/organ-on-chip-systems.png (visited November 20, 2021).**

The benefit of systems toxicology is that it allows the determination of various points along the exposure-disease pathway to assess risk and to be used in risk management as places in the pathway to prevent disease (Akarapipad et al. 2021; Meng et al. 2013).

The sequencing of the human genome in 2000 (Venter et al. 2001) led to many promises of a deeper understanding of biology and disease mechanisms. The anticipated deep understanding of biology did not materialize immediately.

In an interview in the *New Yorker*, Craig Venter, a leading sequencer of the genome, recognized that the genome sequence itself didn't really inform biology, but it was the genome interacting with the environment, broadly defined, that resulted in a healthy or ill phenotype (Preston 2000). In other words, humans are more than a bag of DNA sequences. The need to develop new tools to investigate mechanisms of the toxicant-disease paradigm became apparent in the postgenomic era.

The exposome interacting with human genomes leads to chronic, noncommunicable diseases. These diseases are common and complex because multiple exposures and multiple genes are involved. These "ecogenomic" diseases occur through altering gene expression, commonly through epigenetic mechanisms (see Chapter 10). In an average year, approximately 56 million people die (Ritchie and Roser 2018). Historically, most diseases were thought to be caused by acute infections, exposure to specific chemicals, or physical injuries. Today, more people present with chronic illnesses that last for years and are rarely cured. The four most common preventable complex diseases are listed in Table 7.3. These common complex illnesses have been called "diseases

Table 7.3: **Preventable Common Complex Diseases**

Complex Condition	Tobacco Use	Unhealthy Diet	Misuse of Alcohol	Lack of Physical Activity
Cardiovascular	✓	✓	✓	✓
Diabetes	✓	✓	✓	✓
Cancer	✓	✓	✓	✓
Chronic Respiratory Disease	✓		✓	✓

Source: WHO

of civilization" (E. Ziegler 1968), based on studies of changes in cancer patterns among Japanese women and African Americans of West African descent after settling in a new country with different exposomes (R.M. Ziegler et al. 1993; Fregene and Newman 2005). Humans live in exposomes that are changing more rapidly than our genomes can adapt. Some of the exposomes in which people live are health promoting, while others are unhealthy exposomes (Canali 2020; Cui and Balshaw 2019; Giurgescu et al. 2019; Niedzwiecki et al. 2019; Nieuwenhuijsen et al. 2014)

The EXPOsOMICS project is a European Union–funded group that is developing novel approaches to assess exposure to high-priority environmental pollutants (see https://www.epa.gov/sites/production/files/2015-09/documents/priority-pollutant-list-epa.pdf viewed December 1, 2021) by characterizing the external and the internal components of the exposome during critical periods of life.

Modern toxicology uses the tools developed for molecular biology (summarized in Table 7.4.) to elucidate potential harmful effects of exposures. Genomics is a useful tool to identify and explain structure and gene-gene communication. Gene chips are used to measure gene expression from cells exposed to a toxicant. Transcriptomics focuses on the entire complement of mRNA. Proteomics studies the entire cellular complement of proteins, including posttranslational modification processes, which are associated with active enzymes (Madiera and Costa 2021). Metabolomics is the study of the entire cellular complement of metabolites and the enzymes that produce those metabolites. The control of metabolites, proteins, and nucleic acid macromolecules are interconnected as networks; thus, these postgenomic sciences anticipated systems biology, which considers the cellular –omes as a unit. Taken together, the EXPOsOMICS project is assessing environmental chemicals and their mixtures to find links to disease risk through an "exposome–wide association study (EWAS)," which promises to be a more effective tool than genome wide association studies (GWAS) to better understand exposure-disease links (Vineis et al. 2017) (Figure 7.13).

Humans can be exposed to approximately 100,000 xenobiotic compounds. A Toxin–Toxin-Target Database (T3DB – www.t3db.ca) (Wishart et al. 2015) was established as a resource to facilitate a detailed understanding of the properties of chemical toxicants. Together with the CTD, http://ctdbase.org/ (see Box 7.1), these informatics-based resources provide a more complete set of toxicology data to better inform risk assessment. The Toxic Substance Control Act (TSCA) inventory

Table 7.4: **Omics Tools Used in Toxicology and Risk Assessment**

Field of Study	Description
Genomics	Structure, function, evolution, and mapping of genomes
Transcriptomics	The study of the entire compliment of messenger RNAs
Proteomics	The study of the entire cellular component of proteins
Metabolomics	The study of the complete set of metabolites, including xenobiotic metabolites
Exposomics	The study of new approaches to measure these complex exposures that include individual and population exposure data in combination with biological modifications and health outcomes
Informatics	Study of computational systems for storing and integrating data generated from studies of genomics, transcriptomics, proteomics, and metabolomics
Systems Toxicology	Quantitative understanding, modeling, and prediction of the response of cells to toxicants and expand the model to model organ and body systems for accurate risk assessment

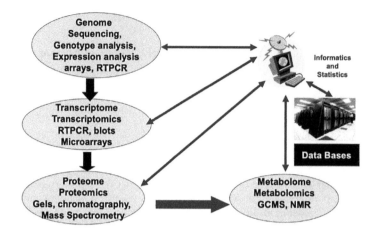

Figure 7.13 Molecular biological tools applied to toxicology. Sequencing of the human genome opened new avenues of computer data handling and has created new fields of informatics that combine biology and mathematical sciences to establish biomolecular networks.

BOX 7.1   THE COMPARATIVE TOXICOGENOMICS DATABASE (CTD)

Carolyn Mattingly

Most human diseases involve interactions between genetic and environmental factors. Although the environment is implicated in most chronic diseases, the etiology and mechanisms of action underlying these diseases remain unclear. It is estimated that more than 80,000 chemicals are currently used in commerce, challenging elucidation about chemical mechanisms of action and prioritization of environmental health research. Integration of diverse data with novel analysis approaches is required to understand environment-disease associations, mechanistic pathways of toxicity, regulation, and development of effective therapeutic interventions.

Launched in 2004, the CTD; http://ctdbase.org) is a publicly available toxicological resource that identifies connections between environmental exposures, molecular mechanisms, and consequent biological effects. CTD provides manually curated information from peer-reviewed literature that links chemicals, genes/proteins, phenotypes, anatomy, diseases, and population-based exposures. Data curation uses community-accepted ontologies and controlled vocabularies to (a) standardize information, allowing it to be computable; (b) ensure adherence to Findable, Accessible, Interoperable and Reusable principles; (c) enable integration across manually curated data and with key external data sets; and (d) allow discovery of novel data connections.

Curated data unique to CTD is presented in two ways. DIRECT information comprises descriptive statements, manually curated from the scientific literature, describing how chemicals affect the expression, activity, or modification of genes and proteins; induce phenotypes; and are associated with diseases as well as complex exposure study parameters and outcomes. Experimental data is provided from a range of model systems (in vitro, in vivo, and from over 600 species) to facilitate cross-species, comparative studies. INFERENCES are constructed via integration of curated and external datasets; they are computationally predicted relationships intended to identify connections that would otherwise appear disconnected in the literature. Information in CTD is accessible via user-friendly queries and a range of analytical tools that allow batch queries, complex data comparisons, molecular pathway construction, and analysis of user-defined data sets.

Identifying correlations between chemical exposures and adverse outcomes (e.g., air pollution-cardiovascular disease, pesticide-Parkinson's disease, endocrine disrupting chemicals-cancer, metals-diabetes) is a key first step to improving our understanding of environmental influences on health. Closing the knowledge gaps about the mechanisms *underlying* these correlations is a critical next step to developing more effective preventative, regulatory, and clinical interventions. By virtue of integrating population-based exposure with mechanism-based model systems studies, CTD provides new opportunities to discover pathways that connect exposures with outcomes and highlights factors that may explain interindividual susceptibility to exposures. The scope and integration of chemicals and molecular data in CTD have far-reaching applications, including predictive toxicity studies about chemical mixtures, identification of evolutionarily conserved environmental responses, tissue-specific toxicity, chemical classification by biological response, and elucidation of complex environmental pathways. All curated data, tools, and many examples of functionality have been documented extensively (http://ctdbase.org/about/publications/). Custom curation (e.g., chemicals) is available upon request (http://ctdbase.org/help/contact.go).

list compiled by the US Environmental Protection Agency (US EPA) contains 86,557 nonconfidential chemicals; of these, 41,864 are active. See https://www.epa.gov/tsca-inventory/how-access-tsca-inventory (accessed June 11, 2021). Approximately 2,000 new chemicals are introduced for use in consumer products each year. These include additives and dyes, personal care products, food, prescription drugs, household cleaners, and lawn care products. The effect of many of these chemicals on our health is unknown (Figure 7.14).

Humans can be exposed to many potentially toxic chemicals through daily activities (see Table 7.5). Occupational exposures occur during the manufacture, distribution, or disposal of those chemicals. When disposed of, the ingredients and products become pollutants in the air, water, or soil.

Safeguarding public health depends on identifying the actions of these chemicals and the levels of exposure that may become toxic to humans (Erickson 2017). Toxicology data show that the relationship between dose and effect is very different depending on the nature of the chemical, the frequency of the exposure, age, sex, and genetic makeup of the individual. There are cases where a lower dose exposure may have a more deleterious effect than a higher dose, or sometimes a low dose of a toxicant may have a beneficial health effect as demonstrated by the so-called inverted U (see Figure 7.15). This effect is called hormesis, first discovered in the late 1800s and applied to toxicology and medicine in 2000 (Calabrese and Baldwin 2001). It has been argued that hormesis will allow for a better understanding of mechanisms of environmental agents, the ability of humans to adapt to them, and more accurate risk assessments (Calabrese and Mattson 2017) (Table 7.6).

When considering the toxicity of a particular chemical, it must first be determined whether the xenobiotic is a systemic or an organ-specific toxicant. As the name implies, a systemic toxicant affects the entire organism. Organ toxicants affect a specific organ and do not cause damage to the entire individual. Benzene and lead are two examples of organ-specific toxicants.

Both the matrix containing a chemical (air, soil, water, food) and the route of uptake are important factors to consider when performing a risk assessment. There are multiple pathways of xenobiotic uptake. The three most common are, dermal (through the skin), inhalation (via breathing), and ingestion (taken by mouth). Whether the exposures are acute or chronic must also be part of the experimental design. All substances to which people are exposed are not absorbed equally. An individual's body mass (size) age, gender, and exposome in which they live also influence the toxicity of a compound and ultimately, the risk.

When a compound or process is evaluated, sensitive or vulnerable populations, children, the elderly, the immunocompromised, and individuals with comorbidities are of particular concern. Children are of special interest because they represent future generations. (discussed in more detail in Chapter 14). There is an obvious connection with the size of a child (the EPA standard is 10 kg), which is considerably less than that of an adult (the EPA standard is 70 kg), but the EPA is quick to point out that children are not just little adults (https://www.epa.gov/children/children-are-not-little-adults; last accessed June 20, 2021). The age and stage of physiological development are more important than body mass when determining childhood toxicity (Landrigan et al. 2004). Body surface area is especially important when the exposure pathway is *via* the dermal route.

Another issue particular to children is that they are growing and their organ systems are developing rapidly. The influence of a xenobiotic on a neonate is greater and often more lethal than a comparable dose for an adult. However, neonates may be less susceptible to a toxicant that must be metabolized to exert an effect, if the metabolic system is less developed in the child than in an adult (Bruckner 2000; Lau et al. 2000).

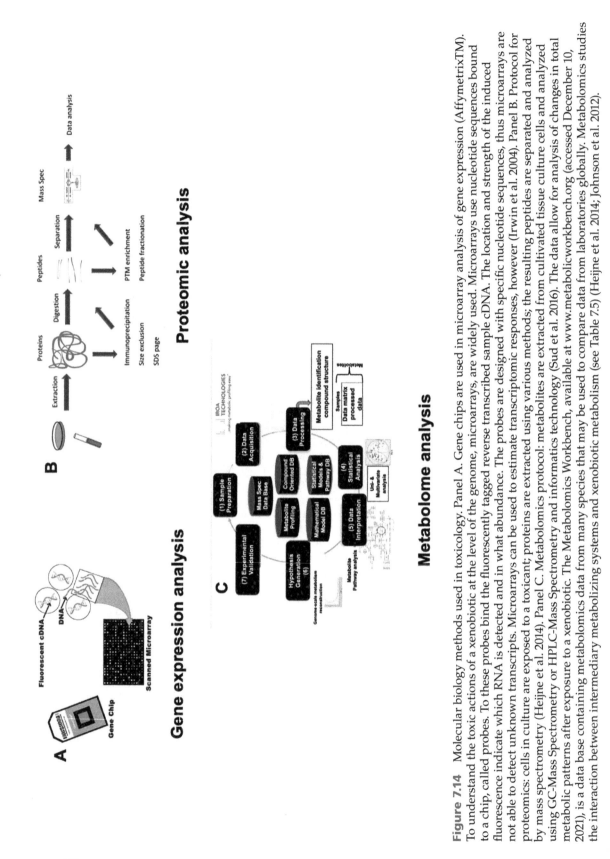

Figure 7.14 Molecular biology methods used in toxicology. Panel A. Gene chips are used in microarray analysis of gene expression (AffymetrixTM). To understand the toxic actions of a xenobiotic at the level of the genome, microarrays, are widely used. Microarrays use nucleotide sequences bound to a chip, called probes. To these probes bind the fluorescently tagged reverse transcribed sample cDNA. The location and strength of the induced fluorescence indicate which RNA is detected and in what abundance. The probes are designed with specific nucleotide sequences, thus microarrays are not able to detect unknown transcripts. Microarrays can be used to estimate transcriptomic responses, however (Irwin et al. 2004). Panel B. Protocol for proteomics: cells in culture are exposed to a toxicant; proteins are extracted using various methods; the resulting peptides are separated and analyzed by mass spectrometry (Heijne et al. 2014). Panel C. Metabolomics protocol: metabolites are extracted from cultivated tissue culture cells and analyzed using GC-Mass Spectrometry or HPLC-Mass Spectrometry and informatics technology (Sud et al. 2016). The data allow for analysis of changes in total metabolic patterns after exposure to a xenobiotic. The Metabolomics Workbench, available at www.metabolicworkbench.org (accessed December 10, 2021), is a data base containing metabolomics data from many species that may be used to compare data from laboratories globally. Metabolomics studies the interaction between intermediary metabolizing systems and xenobiotic metabolism (see Table 7.5) (Heijne et al. 2014; Johnson et al. 2012).

Table 7.5: Common Groups of Xenobiotics to which Humans Are Exposed

Group	Number
Pesticides	1,000
Active drugs	4,000
Drug additives	2,500
Food additives	5,500
Other chemicals	80,000

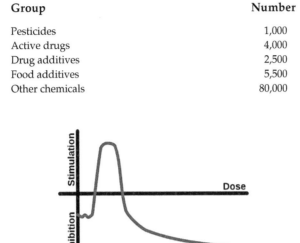

Figure 7.15 An example of the in verted U-shaped dose-response curve.

Contact with a xenobiotic can vary from a one-time acute exposure to a sustained chronic exposure. Duration of exposure must be considered in any discussion of toxicology as applied to risk assessment. Thus, Toxicity = Dose × Time (Rozman 2000), which is the basis for setting standards. Standard setting is discussed in more detail in Chapter 12. In a workplace, the norm for exposure is typically an eight-hour day, consequently, a safe or unsafe level is based on an exposure over the course of a typical work shift, with a unit for exposure of mg/kg/Day. For some workplaces with an 8-hour work shift, a safe dose or exposure would be established for a typical 40-hour week.

The US EPA released the first *Exposure Factors Handbook* in 1989. This was a landmark document that provided a summary of the available statistical data on various factors used in assessing human exposure. This handbook was written as a guide for exposure assessors inside the US EPA as well as outside in an effort to have a set of data on standard factors to calculate human exposure to toxic chemicals. As more data are collected and standardized for a wider range of compounds under a greater number of exposure scenarios, the *Exposure Factors Handbook* (Moya et al. 2011) becomes a more valuable tool. The US EPA last revised the *Exposure Factors Handbook* in 2011 (Moya et al. 2011), but individual chapter updates have been released since 2017. To access the updates to the handbook, go to: https://www.epa.gov/expobox/about-exposure-factors-handbook (accessed on June 20, 2021). There is also a "Child-Specific Exposure Scenarios Examples" document that is

Table 7.6: Toxic and Lethal Doses of Common Chemicals

Substance	Nontoxic (Beneficial) Dose	Toxic Dose	Lethal Dose
Alcohol	0.05%	0.1% (Ethanol blood level)	0.5%
Carbon Monoxide	<10%	20%–30% (Percent hemoglobin bound)	> 60%
Secobarbitol	0.1 mg/dL	0.7 mg/dL (Blood level)	>1 mg/dL
Aspirin	650 mg (2 tablets)	9.75 g (30 tablets; acute oral dose)	34 g (105 tablets)
Ibuprofen	400 mg (2 tablets)	1.4 g (7 tablets; acute oral dose)	12 g (60 tablets)

(Adapted from T. Gossel and J. Bricker, eds.)

a companion to the *Exposure Factors Handbook* on the US EPA website, this can be found at: https://cfpub.epa.gov/ncea/efp/recordisplay.cfm?deid=262211 (accessed on June 20, 2021).

It is not possible to measure the dose of a xenobiotic directly in an uncontrolled situation. For example, if the potential exposure to a pesticide taken up in food by an individual is to be calculated, the amount of that particular food can be measured; the concentration of pesticide in the food can be determined from the residue data cataloged by the US EPA, Food and Drug Administration (FDA) or similar agency. Dose is calculated from

$$\text{Dose}\,(\text{mg}/\text{kg}) = \text{Food}_g \times (\text{Xenobiotic}_{mg/g})/\text{Body Mass}_{kg}.$$

Where, Food is in grams; Xenobiotic concentration is in mg/gram of food, divided by Body Mass (kg).

Heavy metals, such as lead, and arsenic, are of particular concern in children's health. Lead toxicity has been known for more than 2,000 years (ATSDR 2020). Lead is an element obtained from mined ores. The modern sources of concern about lead contamination are from anthropogenic activities, such as smelters, deteriorating paint, gasoline, tires, children's playthings, sand, soil, and water (see Box 7.2) (H. W. Mielke and Gonzales 2008; H. W. Mielke et al. 2007; H.W.

BOX 7.2 HEAVY METALS, LEAD, AND MERCURY

A. Lead in Drinking Water

Robert Rottersman

Lead has been used for the conveyance of drinking water for millennia. In fact, the word "plumbing" derives its name from "plumbum," the Latin word for lead. This bluish metal is widespread in the earth's crust, easily extracted, durable, has a low melting point, and is malleable at room temperature, making it ideal for early drinking water infrastructure. Lead pipes were famously used to distribute and drain water from Roman cities. The use of lead for pipes, fittings, fixtures, and solder continued for centuries and has been described by the World Health Organization (WHO) as "almost universal in practice." In the United States, lead pipes were commonly used for service connections in many cities through at least the 1950s and were installed in some areas through 1986.

The science and understanding of the health effects of lead have evolved over time, but decisions about, and the practicality of, meaningful reduction of the use of lead in drinking water systems have taken decades to implement and were largely overshadowed by the phasing out of lead in gasoline and paint in the 1970s. A 1986 amendment to the Safe Drinking Water Act banned the use of lead pipes for drinking water infrastructure and limited the allowable use of lead in brass and solder to 8%, which was defined by the regulation as being "lead-free." In 2011, the Reduction of Lead in Drinking Water Act reduced the definition of lead-free to 0.25% and went into effect in 2014. "Lead-free" solder and brass components, containing up to 8% lead, were routinely used in commercial and residential pipes and fixtures for approximately 28 years. These rules have resulted in a hodgepodge of systems where neighboring buildings, even adjacent restrooms, could have different concentrations of lead in drinking water depending on when they were constructed or remodeled, regardless of whether or not the main service line contains lead.

The concentration of lead in water released at the tap is much more complicated than simply the presence, or perceived absence, of lead in the water conveyance system. Galvanic corrosion can occur when new copper pipes are joined with old lead pipes. This electrochemical reaction can increase the amount of lead released into drinking water at concentrations above what may have been released from lead pipes alone. This is just one of many ways metallurgy can influence lead concentrations. The water within the pipes also plays an important role in oxidizing disinfectants (chlorine or chloramines) reacting with pipes and fittings to form a more soluble form of lead. Drinking water engineers often use treatments to form films or scale on the inner surface of pipes to reduce the amount of lead that enters the water.

In 1991 the EPA issues the Land and Copper Rule (LCR). The LCR recognizes that lead can enter drinking water from plumbing materials, including pipes and fixtures located in the building of the water users. For this reason, the LCR established a "treatment technique regulation" for lead and copper as opposed to a maximum contaminant level (MCL) commonly used for other drinking water contaminants. The LCR requires water providers to control the corrosivity of the water and to periodically test for lead at the taps of representative end users. Additional action is required if lead concentrations exceed 15 parts per billion (ppb) in more than 10% of the samples.

There has been debate, and now appears to be consensus, that the LCR may not be sufficiently protective for higher-risk populations, and both the EPA and CDC have indicated that there is no known safe level of lead in a child's blood. Based on this, many state and local agencies have passed their own regulations. For example, in 2017, Illinois required every elementary school to test every fixture that may be used for drinking water. Levels above 2 ppb, the reporting limit for the analytical method, required follow-up action, and levels above 5 ppb required public notification of results. It is important for professionals performing lead risk assessments to understand current requirements under LCR, as well as any local regulations related to lead content in drinking water.

Because of its simplicity and ease of use, lead has been used to transport drinking water for millennia. After thousands of years, the legacy of lead is now an extraordinarily complex interaction of health risk assessment, chemistry, and public policy.

B. Reducing Childhood Lead Exposure

Michael Gochfeld and *Joanna Burger*

The reduction of lead in the environment is one of the great public health stories of the past 50 years. The toxicity of lead has been known since antiquity, yet lead poisoning, particularly among young children, persists as a public health problem. Lead and lead compounds have found many industrial and commercial uses, some related to the physical properties of the metal (bullets) and some to its toxic properties (lead in paint). The addition of tetraethyl lead to gasoline resulted in millions of vehicles around the world emitting lead, resulting in lead pollution in soil along highways and in the air, particularly in dense urban areas. During the same period, lead was widely advertised as a healthful additive to indoor paint. By the 1950s, lead exposure was widespread, and as the white paint deteriorated in older housing, children were exposed, both indoors and out. Although blood lead testing did not become routine until the 1970s, the average blood lead of city dwellers was about 15 micrograms/DL (= 0.72 μmol/L). In the 1970s a blood level > 60 mcg/dL was considered "elevated," and children with lead levels >100 mcg/dL would appear in urban emergency rooms with lead encephalopathy, which left a residual of physical and mental impairment in survivors.

A series of regulations and policies beginning with the removal of lead from automotive gasoline and banning of lead in indoor paints, coupled with universal testing of toddlers and the efforts to remove lead from the household environment, had a dramatic impact on blood lead levels through the 1980s and 1990s (see Figure 7.1). Hand in hand with the decline in blood lead was the lowering of the health criterion for an elevated level, from 60 to 40 to 25 to 10 and now to 5 mcg/dL. Even at these levels, large neurobehavioral studies detect a negative impact on cognitive development in toddlers. Hence there is a move to lower blood leads even further. Lead is one of the few widespread toxics for which the EPA has declined to set a Reference Dose, based on its determination that there is no threshold below which there is no "appreciable risk."

Today, the average blood lead among children is below 1 mcg/dL. A level > 5 mcg/dL is considered elevated, and efforts are devoted toward detecting and eliminating the sources of lead for toddlers with blood lead > 5 mcg/dL. Although the exposure and poisoning of children from ingesting lead paint dust or chips was well-known in the 1970s, it took the Flint water disaster to catapult lead to front page news. Flint became iconic of urban communities nationwide and worldwide, where in the 1800s, lead piping was used to conduct water from water mains to houses. As water sat in the pipes overnight, the first morning draw would often contain significant amounts of dissolved lead. Society learned that adding a phosphate buffer to the drinking water supply would inhibit the leaching of lead and render the water source "safe."

When Flint, a once thriving industrial city, suffered the loss of industry and jobs, and its economy flagged, the governor put the city under a manager. To cut costs, the manager switched the Flint water supply from Lake Michigan to the Flint River. As the river water was sometimes

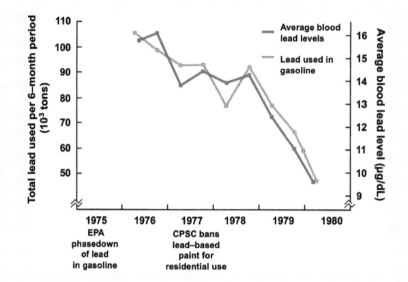

Figure Box 7.2-1

rusty or bad tasting, the community became outraged at having to drink polluted water, but it wasn't lead they were tasting. When an astute pediatrician, Dr. Mona Hanna-Attisha, reported that the number of children with blood leads > 5 mcg/dL had doubled since the water switch occurred, the community and the media made the logical connection that the lead was coming from the river water. This made national headlines. As the "Flint story" unfolded, it was discovered that when the switch to River water was made, the orthophosphate buffer used to prevent pipe corrosion was not added. The river water was leaching lead from the hundred-year-old service lines.

The Flint experience has multiple lessons to teach us and served as a wake-up call to communities nationwide to investigate old lead distribution pipes as a source of lead exposure. Many communities have discovered their own lead pipes and found blood lead levels even higher than those measured in children from Flint. The costly process of replacing these piping systems is underway in many cities. It is important and gratifying to see the widespread response, but it would be a mistake to assume that lead exposure is thereby a thing of the past. Experimenting with the EPA *Integrated Exposure Uptake Biokinetic, known as the IEUBK Model* of childhood lead exposure reveals that drinking water is a relatively minor source of elevated blood lead, compared, for example, to paint chips/dust. (The model is available free online at https://www.epa.gov/superfund/lead-superfund-sites-software-and-users-manuals.) Other sources continue to expose children and interfere with critical developmental processes. There are still children with blood leads > 25 mcg/dL who would benefit from identifying and eliminating the source(s) of their lead exposure. This may require diligent detective work to identify the household sources. But there is also a societal benefit in having fewer children with significant cognitive impairment. Society will theoretically benefit from the IQ points gained by lowering blood lead levels from 5 to below 5 mcg/dL, the subject of ongoing research.

Figure Box 7.2-1 shows the impact of regulations in reducing blood lead from mean values around 14 mcg/dL in the 1970s to below 2 mcg/dL by 2002.

Although strictly a correlation study, this graph shows blood lead levels closely tracking the quantity of lead added to gasoline in the United States (1975–1980).

C. Methylmercury Exposure from Fish Consumption: Balancing Risks and Benefits

Joanna Burger and Michael Gochfeld

Mercury is a pan-toxicant. All forms of mercury are toxic to all organisms that have been studied. Unlike many metals, but like lead and cadmium, mercury is not essential for any organism or physiologic process. The very toxic properties of mercury account for many of its uses as a biocide to inhibit mold, kill bacteria, and stabilize vaccines. Mercury occurs naturally in seawater, and ambient mercury levels range from 1–10 ng/L. About 80% of the global pool of mercury results from mining, processing, industrial uses, and disposal of elemental mercury and mercury compounds. About 20% is contributed to the atmosphere from natural processes, erosion, volcanism, and evasion from the ocean surface.

In the 1970s, Swedish ecologists discovered that elemental and inorganic mercury that entered lakes and sank to the bottom could be biomethylated by bacteria, particularly by anaerobic bacteria in the lake sediment. Microorganisms may take up the methylmercury, and as they are consumed by plankton, and then small fishes, medium-sized fishes, and larger predatory fishes, there is bioconcentration at each stage, resulting in a cumulative increase in the methylmercury content at each trophic level on the food chain. This phenomenon of bio-amplification explains why methylmercury can reach high levels in top-level predators (e.g., sharks, tuna, and swordfish). As an example, if the concentration in plankton is 1 part per billion, it might reach 10 ppb in small fish, 100 ppb in medium-sized fish, and 1 ppm in large fish. Even higher levels are encountered in large predatory fish, such as sharks and swordfish. Fish consumers, both wildlife and humans, can accumulate toxic doses of mercury by consuming large fish frequently. Even the common health-recommended diet of a can of tuna fish every day can result in mercury poisoning, depending on whether one chooses "white" (averaging 0.3 ppm) or "light" (averaging 0.1 ppm) of mercury.

Through 50 years of clinical practice, it has become apparent that the people most at risk of developing symptoms of mercury toxicity are those who eat fish very often, more than twice a week up to two meals daily. Patients evaluated for mercury poisoning at the Rutgers Environmental and Occupational Health Sciences Institute (EOHSI) Clinical Center present a variety of symptoms and report a strong preference for eating tuna and swordfish, large predatory species, high on the food chain, and high in mercury. The classic symptoms of methylmercury poisoning, beginning with paresthesias (pins and needles around the mouth) and eventually in the fingers and feet, feet, tremors, incoordination and unsteady gate, and constriction of visual fields, progressing to deafness, blindness, coma, and death.

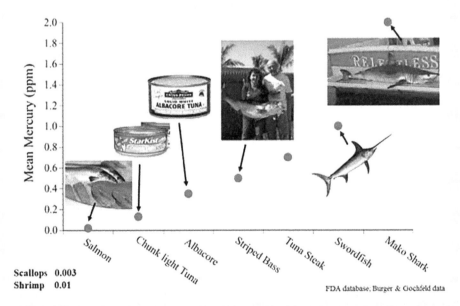

Figure Box 7.2-2 The average mercury concentration (wet weight) in selected fish species increases from very low levels in shrimp and scallops, to levels below 0.1 ppm in salmon and up to 1 ppm in swordfish, and over 2 ppm in sharks.

This progression is based on the well-studied epidemics of organic mercury ingestion of fungicide-treated grain in Iraq and Guatemala. This progression was also documented in the tragic laboratory-acquired organic mercury poisoning of Dartmouth professor Karen Wetterhahn over the six-month period of her decline and demise. Fortunately, our patients at EOHSI seek treatment before reaching such severity. They typically report the paresthesias, tremors, and incoordination, but also cognitive effects. The treatment is to stop eating fish, particularly high-mercury fish for several months. Mercury levels decline and symptoms typically improve, and fish can be cautiously reintroduced to the diet. Chelation is seldom indicated.

Fetal neurologic development can be seriously impaired by mercury that crosses the placenta from the mother. Hence the advice for pregnant women to avoid eating high-mercury fish. Severe fetal mercury poisoning can result in multiple abnormalities referred to as congenital Minamata disease. This is named after the Minamata Bay in southern Japan, where a major epidemic of methylmercury poisoning occurred in the 1950s among people who regularly at fish from Minamata Bay, contaminated by industrial effluent.

But it is not a simple story. Many studies have shown that eating fish often, up to once or twice a week, confers health benefits, particularly cardiovascular benefits. Concerns that the mercury risk message might discourage people from eating fish have led the FDA to downplay the mercury risk. The benefits are attributed to various nutrients including the polyunsaturated fatty acids in the fish oil, as well as other nutrients such as selenium. Selenium particularly reacts with mercury and may mitigate some of its toxicity. But too much selenium is toxic in its own right.

People who eat fish rarely (less than once a month) may experience health benefits from eating fish more frequently, up to twice a week. Eating more than two fish meals (12 ounces) a week does not appear to increase the benefit. People who eat fish frequently, more than twice a week, will benefit from choosing fish that are low in mercury content (< 0.1 mcg/g or 0.1 ppm). An occasional high-mercury meal can be enjoyed, providing that most of the fish and seafood consumed are low in mercury. The FDA website lists average mercury levels in fish and shellfish. This is a good source of information on which fish are low in mercury. Salmon provide a good trade-off between high fish oil content and low mercury concentration (they are low on the food chain).

The benefits of eating fish are complex. Clinical trials of fish oil capsules do not validate the benefits ascribed to this component. It may be that people who eat fish frequently, also follow other healthful life styles, including avoiding red meat and Twinkies.

Figure Box 7.2-2 shows the average mercury content of several types of seafood, emphasizing the low mercury content of shellfish and salmon and the high-mercury concentration in large predatory fish (source: https://www.fda.gov/food/metals-and-your-food/mercury-levels-commercial-fish-and-shellfish-1990-2012). The numbers are for total mercury. Methylmercury averages about 90% of the total mercury across many species of fish.

Mielke, Laidlaw, and Gonzales 2010). The data that are used to define the risk for a particular compound or mixture drives the toxicity testing, and those data inform the risk assessment. The data are often evaluated based on the health impact on an organism. The testing process attempts to understand the mode of action and evaluate the physiological impact of the chemical at the cellular level. The sex of an organism may influence the toxicity of a number of xenobiotics. There are, of course, physiological differences among the sexes of an animal. The differences influence the clearance and metabolism of a chemical through effects on pharmacokinetics, pharmacodynamics, and metabolome. Examples that are often cited are studies in animals, which have identified gender-related differences. Two classic examples are studies of pesticide action that show male rats were ten times more sensitive than females to liver damage from DDT (Sierra-Santoyo et al. 2005) and a study that showed female rats were twice as sensitive to parathion as male rats (Agarwal et al. 1982).

Aromatic and aliphatic hydrocarbons tend to accumulate in animals to levels that can be toxic. Thus, xenobiotic metabolism evolved as a mechanism to remove those xenobiotics from the body. Xenobiotic metabolism is divided into two phases, Phase I and Phase II (R.T. Williams 1975). Phase I metabolism involves adding a functional group to the xenobiotic, usually a hydrophobic

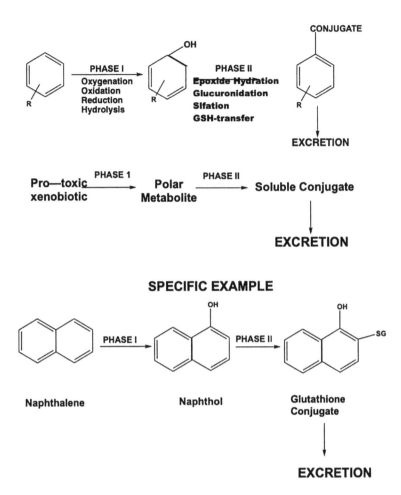

Figure 7.16 Summary of Phase I and Phase 2 xenobiotic-metabolizing enzyme systems. After exposure to a xenobiotic and distribution to organs, the xenobiotic is metabolized by Phase I enzymes to yield a more polar metabolite, which may be more toxic than the parent compound. The polar metabolite is further metabolized by Phase II enzymes, which results in a soluble metabolite, which may be excreted, but in some cases undergoes a second round of Phase I metabolism to yield another toxic species.

molecule, resulting in a polar metabolite. The enzymatic product may be more reactive, and possibly more toxic. The most studied group of Phase I enzymes are called Cytochromes P450 (CYPs), which activate and split oxygen (Omura and Sato 1962; Rendic and Guengrich 2021). One atom of the activated oxygen is inserted into the xenobiotic, while the other forms water. Xenobiotic-transforming enzymes, localized in the endoplasmic reticulum, require a great deal of metabolic energy and are closely linked with ATP-generating systems of the mitochondrion.

Products of Phase I metabolism provide sites for conjugation reactions, called Phase II. Phase II enzymes are conjugating enzymes and can directly interact with polar xenobiotics or with metabolites produced by Phase I enzymes. Phase II metabolism involves conjugation of a metabolite from intermediary metabolism onto an activated molecule from Phase I metabolism. These steps are summarized in Figure 7.16.

Alcohols, such as ethanol, methanol, isopropanol, and ethylene glycol are common poisoning hazards in humans. These agents are found in a number of products kept around the house, including antifreeze, windshield deicers, hand sanitizers, window cleaners, and rubbing alcohols. In 2019, 14,269 single exposures to isopropanol (from sources including rubbing alcohol, cleaning agents, and hand sanitizers) were reported to the US Poison Control Centers. Of these, 71 patients were classified as experiencing "major" morbidity, but no deaths were reported (Cederbaum 2012).

Table 7.7: Relative Toxicities of Alcohols and Aldehyde Metabolites. Typically, the Aldehyde Metabolite Is More Toxic than the Parent Compound

Parent Compound	LD_{50} (mg/kg)	Metabolite	LD_{50} (mg/kg)
Ethanol	10,470	Acetaldehyde	1,930
Methanol	5,630	Formaldehyde	646
Isopropanol	5,045	Acetone	5,800
Ethylene glycol	4,700	Glycol aldehyde	280
Propylene glycol	20,000	Lactaldehyde	None Found

The metabolism of alcohol is carried out by several enzyme systems, including alcohol dehydrogenases (ADH) (Suddendorf 1989), catalase (Hanby–Mason et al. 1997), and a monooxygenase, CYP2E1 (Chen et al. 2019). Alcohol metabolism is a good example of metabolism increasing the toxicity of a xenobiotic (see Table 7.7).

As shown in Figure 7.17, the aldehyde product of the alcohol metabolizing enzymes is metabolized by the corresponding aldehyde dehydrogenases (ALDH). Ethyl alcohol has a high metabolic rate for a xenobiotic, ~ 0.016% per hour in a nonalcoholic individual and higher in an alcoholic. Alcohol and aldehyde dehydrogenases are polymorphic. ADH2* 2 and ADH3* 1 alleles encode for the high–activity ADH isoform. ALDH1 and ALDH2, respectively, convert acetaldehyde to the nutrient, acetic acid, which enters the tricarboxylic acid cycle (TCA or Krebs cycle) as acetyl coenzyme A (AcCoA), connecting metabolism of this xenobiotic to the metabolome. The ALDH2*

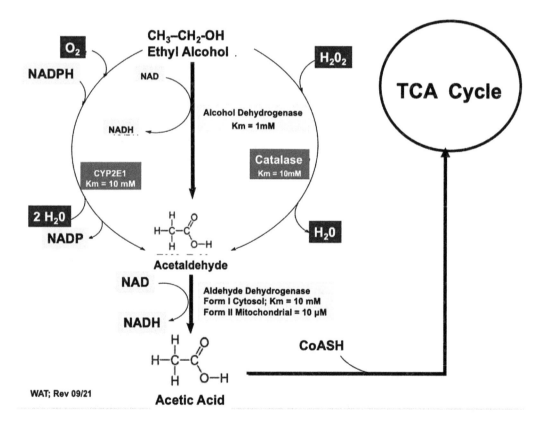

Figure 7.17 Metabolism of alcohols by Phase I metabolizing enzymes. The example shown is for ethyl alcohol (ethanol). Alcohol dehydrogenases catalyze the first step in metabolism of alcohols, leading to the formation of the corresponding aldehyde, which is usually more toxic than the parent compound (Til et al. 1988).

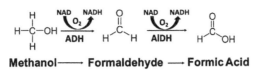

Methanol⟶ Formaldehyde ⟶ Formic Acid

Figure 7.18 Methanol is slowly metabolized by alcohol dehydrogenase to formaldehyde, which can cause severe acidosis; formaldehyde is further metabolized to formic acid, which is directly toxic to retinal cells and leads to blindness.

2 allele of the mitochondrial matrix encodes for a low-activity isoform that leads to acetaldehyde accumulation over time.

East Asians are more likely to have the ADH2* 2 and ALDH2* 2 alleles, which lead to more acetaldehyde accumulation and increased toxicity. These individuals are less likely to become alcoholics because of the adverse reactions they experience after consuming alcohol (Suddendorf 1989) and accumulation of toxic acetaldehyde (O'Brien, Siraki, and Shangari 2005).

Alcohols are probably the most common toxicants to which humans are exposed, having both beneficial and deleterious actions (Thakker 1998). Dose-response curves indicate a biphasic, inverted U shape. Some of the benefits of moderate ethanol intake include reducing risk of heart disease and stroke. Heavy alcohol consumption or binge drinking leads to alcohol use disorder (AUD), liver or pancreatic diseases, various cancers, and strokes (Thakker 1998). Characteristics of AUD include failure to fulfill responsibilities at home, school, or work. Approximately 1.4 million Americans suffer from AUD, overburdening the emergency departments (White et al. 2018), and 95,000 die per year in the United States because of alcohol (see: https://www.niaaa.nih.gov/publications/brochures-and-fact-sheets/alcohol-facts-and-statistics; last viewed June 18, 2021).

Methyl alcohol (methanol) is found in some fuels and as an adulterant in ethyl alcohol and rubbing alcohols, and in industrial solvents, ingestion of ~ 100 mL can be fatal (Liesivuori and Savolainen 1991). The first steps in the metabolism of methanol are shown in Figure 7.18.

In mid-2020, Médecins Sans Frontières reported ~7,000 cases and 1,607 deaths related to methanol poisoning globally (Arnold 2020), evidently caused by exposure to methanol in hand sanitizers (Hassanian-Moghaddam et al. 2020; Mousavi-Roknabadi et al. 2021). Demand for alcohol-based hand sanitizer in the community has increased since the onset of the COVID-19 pandemic in 2020 (Sandle 2020). Because of shortages, some unscrupulous vendors substituted methanol for ethanol in the product. Methanol must never be used in hand sanitizers because oral, pulmonary, or skin exposures can result in severe systemic toxicity and sometimes death (Beradi et al. 2020; Holzman et al. 2021). The FDA issues periodic advisory information on which hand sanitizers to avoid because of toxic chemicals added to the basic (FDA 2021) (Figure 7.19).

Negative health outcomes of pregnant women drinking alcohol have been recognized since antiquity. Aristotle noted that drunken women bore abnormal children, and Plato admonished that no alcohol should be taken at conception. In the early part of the 20th century, it was suggested that "giving pregnant women alcohol will tend to eliminate bad individuals, and inasmuch as from an economic viewpoint they may not do much good or amount to much, why not use this means to eradicate them?" (Stockard 1912a, 1912b). Public health has been working diligently to reduce drinking while pregnant, but the latest data suggest that alcohol consumption while pregnant has increased. Between 2011 and 2013, about 3.1% of pregnant women drank alcohol, but between 2015 and 2017, 10.2% drank alcohol, although extensive research has demonstrated that no level of alcohol intake while pregnant is safe (England et al. 2020). Fetal alcohol syndrome (FAS) and fetal alcohol spectrum disorder (FASD) are conditions resulting from *in utero* exposure to alcohol (Bailey and Sokol 2011; Denny, Coles, and Blitz 2017). The global prevalence of FASD is estimated to be ~ 8 in 1,000 in the general population, but the rate can be much higher in certain high-drinking populations. Global FASD prevalence is not a trivial issue: the rate is about eight times greater than Down's syndrome, which is 1 per 1,000. South Africa has the highest global rate of FASD. It has been postulated that high alcohol consumption takes place in rural areas where the workers were paid in alcohol (Lang et al. 2017).

That a disease could be caused by exposure *in utero* was not seriously considered until the late 20th century, when FAS was officially recognized as a disease in 1973 (Jones and Smith 1973) about

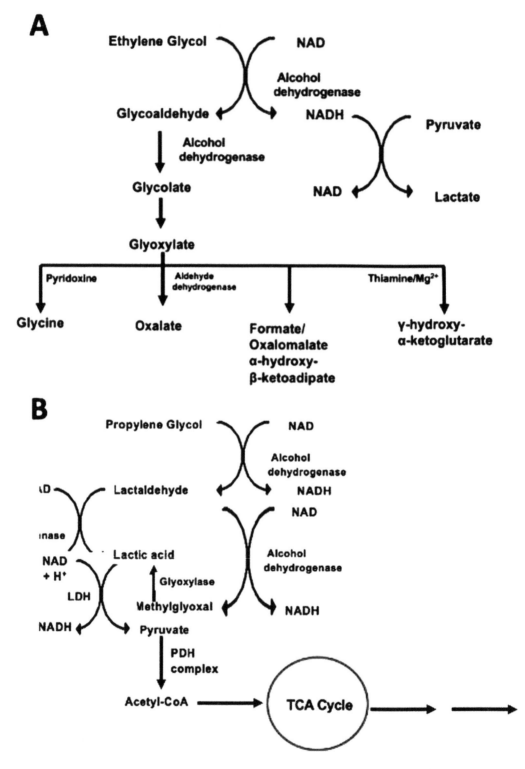

Figure 7.19 Metabolic pathways of the di alcohols, A. ethylene glycol and B. propyl alcohol. Ethylene glycol (LD_{50} = 4,700 mg/kg) is toxic because the accumulation of oxalic acid in the blood combines with Ca2+, which accumulates in the kidney and results in nephrotoxicity. Propylene glycol (LD_{50} = 20,000 mg/kg) is much less toxic because the metabolic products enter intermediary metabolism through acetyl CoA and the TCA (Holyoak, Fraser, and Gelperowicz 2011).

the same time that diethyl stilbesterol (DES) was recognized as a teratogen (Wilson 1973; also see Box 7.3). Characteristics of FASD include growth deficiency either before or after birth, distinctive abnormal facial characteristics, and central nervous system disorders, including cognitive deficits, developmental delays, behavioral impairments, and learning disabilities (Glass and Mattson 2017; May et al. 2009). Today, it is widely accepted that *in utero* exposure to xenobiotics or their metabolites has dramatic effects on birth outcomes (Barker 2004), which is a new branch of toxicology called developmental origins of health and disease, known as DOHaD (Gluckman, Hanson, and Mitchell 2010; Gluckman et al. 2009).

BOX 7.3   HEALTH EFFECTS OF ARSENIC

Paul Tchounwou

Arsenic, a naturally occurring element, is widely distributed throughout the environment and is found in various concentrations in the air, water and land. It is also produced industrially and used in many pesticide and defoliant formulations, in the manufacture of glass, ceramics, electrical semi and photoconductors, pigments, fireworks and some type of alloys, and in the preparation of arsenic-based drugs. Human exposure to arsenic can occur through ingestion of contaminated water, foods, and arsenic-based drugs, inhalation of arsenic-contaminated air, aerosols and suspended particles, and/or dermal contact with arsenic products.

Arsenic ranks among the top ten chemicals that have been identified by the WHO to be of global public health concern. It is now estimated that over 200 million people around the world are exposed to arsenic in drinking water at concentrations higher that the recommended guideline/standard of 10 µg/L. Outbreaks of arsenicosis and other adverse health effects associated with ground water contamination in Argentina, Bangladesh, Chili, China, Mexico, India, Thailand, Taiwan, and Uruguay are good examples of such concerns. From a public health point of view, arsenic and arsenic-containing compounds are divided into three groups that include the elemental, inorganic, and organic forms. The magnitude of toxic effects has been linked to the arsenic species as well as to its dose and length of exposure. In general, the inorganic species are more toxic than the organic forms, although arsine appears to be the most toxic.

There are many case reports of death in humans due to ingestion of high doses of arsenic. The clinical manifestations of poisoning depend on the type of arsenical involved and on the duration of exposure. Symptoms of acute intoxication usually occur within 30 minutes of ingestion, but may be delayed if arsenic is taken with food. In nearly all cases, the most immediate effects are severe nausea and vomiting, colicky abdominal pain, profuse diarrhea with rice stools, gastrointestinal hemorrhage and death may ensue from fluid loss and circulatory collapse. Drowsiness and confusion are often seen along the development of psychosis associated with paranoid delusions, hallucinations and delirium. Finally, seizures, coma and death, usually due to shock, may ensue. Cardiac manifestations include acute cardiomyopathy, subendocardial hemorrhages, and electro cardiographic changes. Hypertension and increased cardiovascular disease mortality have also been observed. The pathological lesions described in patients with rapidly fatal arsenic intoxication are fatty degeneration of the liver, hyperemia and hemorrhages of the gastrointestinal tract, renal tubular necrosis, and demyelination of peripheral nerves. There are also several epidemiological studies reporting an association between exposure to inorganic arsenic and increased risk of adverse developmental effects such as congenital malformations, low birth weight, and spontaneous abortion.

Chronic exposure to arsenic affects the gastrointestinal tract, circulatory system, skin, liver kidneys, nervous system and heart. *In utero* and early childhood exposure has been linked to negative impacts on cognitive development and increased deaths in young adults. There is clear evidence from epidemiological studies that exposure to inorganic arsenic increases the risk of cancer. Dermatologic effects including hyperpigmentation, hypopigmentation, keratosis and Bowen's disease, constitute the most common signs and symptoms and the most sensitive indicators of arsenicosis that have been observed in patients. When exposure occurs by the oral route, the main carcinogenic effect is increased risk of skin cancer. In addition to skin cancer, increased risk of other internal tumors (mainly of liver, kidney, lung, and bladder) have been reported with chronic arsenic exposure.

Several biochemical mechanisms of action including the induction of oxidative damage, activation of mitosis, and genotoxic damage, interference with the methyl transfer to DNA, decrease of DNA repair mechanisms; perturbation of signaling cascades, disruption of transcriptional and translational activities, histone perturbations, differential microRNA expression, cytotoxicity and regenerative hyperplasia resulting from inorganic arsenic interaction with protein sulfhydryls, and changes in genes and proteins expression, have been linked to arsenic carcinogenicity in humans.

Because of its high potential to cause adverse effects in exposed persons, a number of regulatory guidelines have been established for various inorganic and organic forms of arsenic by international, federal, and state agencies. The MCL has been fixed at 10 µg/L. The WHO TDI for inorganic arsenic is 2 µg/kg BW. The action level for arsenic in the air is 5 µg/m³. The permissible exposure limit-total weighted average (PEL – TWA) is 10 µg/m³ for inorganic arsenicals, and 500 µg/m³ for organic arsenicals. BAL or 2,3-Dimercaptopropanol) has been used to treat acute dermatitis, and the pulmonary symptoms associated with arsenic exposure. However, because of the side effects associated with BAL, other agents such as Dimercapto-propane sulfonate (DMPS) and meso-2,3-Dimercaptosuccinic acid (DMSA) are being tested for the chelation therapy of arsenic poisoning (note that these agents have not yet been FDA approved). Removal of arsenic by appropriate technologies is one of the most important control and management strategies. Several treatment methods including chemical precipitation (coagulation processes), ion exchange, reverse osmosis/electrodialysis, use of activated alumina or carbon, and oxidation, have been recommended for arsenic removal in water. The most important action in arsenicosis-endemic areas is to prevent further exposure by providing a safe water supply for drinking, food preparation and irrigation of food crops. Steps should also be taken to reduce occupational exposure, and to educate the communities on the nature and magnitude of the problem as well as to engage them in the development and implementation of prevention/control strategies.

Direct interactions between xenobiotic metabolism and intermediary metabolism that makes up the metabolome occur with both Phase I and Phase II xenobiotic metabolism. Polymorphisms in the aryl hydrocarbon receptor (AhR), a nuclear receptor involved in regulating CYP1A1 and CYP1B1 induction are involved in AhR-mediated immune suppression (Neavin et al. 2018) through interaction with the genome in such a way that results in toxic responses independent of xenobiotic metabolism.

Phase II metabolism involves the conjugation of a product of intermediary metabolism to a xenobiotic metabolite containing a polar group (see Figure 7.18).

The ability of a given exposure of a xenobiotic compound to cause disease varies among individuals (Figure 7.20). Cytochrome P450s have broad specificity and metabolize a wide range of xenobiotics. Other Phase I enzymes include flavin-dependent monooxygenases (FMO) (Cashman and Zhang 2006), hydrolases, and epoxide hydratases have a narrower range of xenobiotic metabolites. Flavin-monooxygenases are involved in pesticide metabolism, through desulfuration, and oxidation at N, S, and P groups, as shown in Figure 7.24, and the Phase II enzymes such as glutathione transferases (GSTs) and sulfotransferases (SULTs), and glucuronyl transferases. Hydrolytic reactions are unusual in that they are the only Phase I reactions that do not use energy and their major cofactor, water, is never limited. Metabolism can activate a xenobiotic to produce a more toxic compound, as in the case of benzo(α)pyrene metabolism to benzo(α)pyrene,7,8 epoxide (see Figure 7.21), but more frequently, metabolism decreases the toxicity of a compound through a Phase II detoxication reaction step.

Products of Phase I metabolism and other xenobiotics that contain functional groups: hydroxyl, epoxide, amino, carboxyl, or a halogen, undergo conjugation reactions with endogenous metabolites, which include sugars, amino acids, sulfate, methyl-, acetyl- groups, and glutathione (GSH). Conjugation products resulting from Phase II metabolism, with rare exceptions, are more polar, less toxic, and more readily excreted than their parent compounds. Conjugation reactions usually involve activation by some high-energy intermediate.

Phase II metabolism is classified into two general types: Phase $II_{Type\ I}$, in which an activated conjugating agent combines with the substrate to yield the conjugated product, and Phase $II_{Type\ II}$, in which the substrate is activated and then combines with an amino acid to yield a conjugated product (Omiecinski et al. 2011). Conjugation products, of Phase II metabolism typically are more water soluble, less toxic, and more readily excreted than the parent compound. Conjugation

A

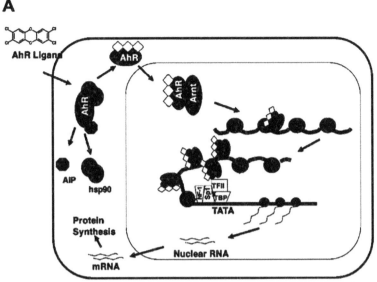

(Adapted from Whitlock, Ann. Rev. Pharmicol. Toxicol.

B

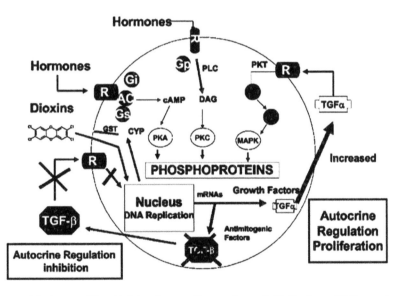

Figure 7.20 AhR Action. The AhR is a heterodimer of two β–Helix–loop–Helix nuclear proteins, Aryl hydrocarbon Receptor Nuclear transferase (ARNT) and AhR. On binding of a ligand such as TCDD or benzo(α)pyrene enters the nucleus this ligand-activated transcription factor. Activation of AhR mediates the expression of target genes (e.g., CYP1A1) by binding to dioxin response element (DRE) sequences in their promoter region (A). The AhR system also mediates action of physiological regulators (B) (Rothammer and Quintana 2019).

reactions usually involve activation by some high-energy intermediate that uses ATP. Substrates that undergo Phase II metabolism are products from Phase I metabolism or polar xenobiotics. Some examples are shown in Figure 7.22

Examples of Phase II$_{Type I}$ metabolism include formation of glycosides and sulfates and acetylation. Glucuronidation is one of the major pathways for elimination of many hydrophobic xenobiotics from the body. Glucuronidation, which is catalyzed by a superfamily of enzymes, called

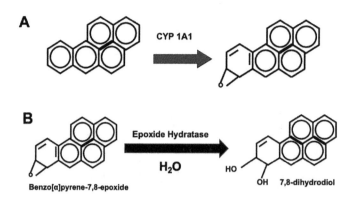

Figure 7.21 Metabolism of benzo(α)pyrene. Panel A. Activation of a pro carcinogen to a carcinogen through Phase I metabolism; Panel B. Deactivation of an aryl epoxide by epoxide hydrase.

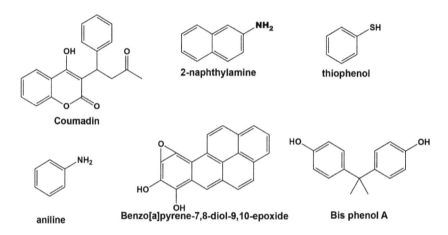

Figure 7.22 Some example substrates for Phase II xenobiotic metabolism. Substrates are either products of Phase I or xenobiotics containing a functional group, including hydroxyl, amines, mercaptyl, epoxide.

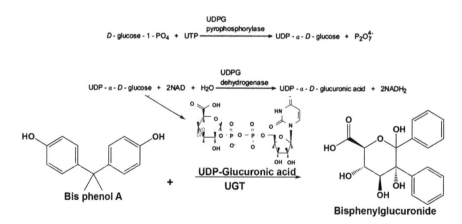

Figure 7.23 Phase II xenobiotic metabolism using glucuronidation. Glucose-1-phosphate reacts with uridine-5′triphosphate (UTP) catalyzed by UDPG pyrophatase to yield UDP-α-D-glucose, which is oxidized to UDP-glucuronic acid, which conjugates to the polar xenobiotic, and is then excreted through urine or feces from the body.

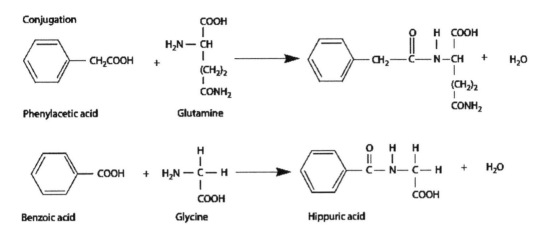

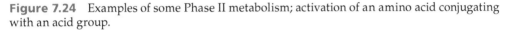

Figure 7.24 Examples of some Phase II metabolism; activation of an amino acid conjugating with an acid group.

UDP-glucuronosyltransferases (UGT), involves the reaction of one of many possible functional groups (R-OH, Ar-OH, R-NH$_2$, Ar-NH$_2$, R-COOH, Ar-COOH) with the sugar derivative, uridine 5′-diphosphoglucuronic acid (UDPGA).

Phase II$_{Type\ II}$ conjugation, in which the substrate is activated and then combines with an amino acid to yield a conjugated product of glycosides and sulfates (Figure 7.23).

The polar metabolites of Phase II metabolism are eliminated through urine or feces. Most xenobiotics are cleared through multiple enzymes and pathways. The relationship between chemical concentrations, enzyme affinity, copy number, and cofactor pools can determine which metabolic reaction dominates in a particular individual.

Phase I enzymes are typically membrane associated, but Phase II enzymes can exist as membrane-bound or soluble. Reaction schemes of selected Phase I and Phase II enzymes are shown in Figure 7.24).

Benzene is an organ-specific toxicant, targeting bone marrow. Chronic exposure to benzene results in deterioration of the hematopoietic system. According to the Agency for Toxic Substances and Disease Registry (ATSDR), benzene is rapidly absorbed through the lungs; approximately 50% of the benzene in air is absorbed. Over 90% of ingested benzene is absorbed through the gastrointestinal tract. Absorbed benzene is rapidly distributed throughout the body and tends to accumulate in fatty tissues. The liver serves an important function in benzene metabolism, which results in the production of several reactive metabolites https://www.atsdr.cdc.gov/toxguides//toxguide-3.pdf). At low exposure levels, benzene is rapidly metabolized and excreted predominantly as conjugated urinary metabolites. At higher exposure levels, metabolic pathways appear to become saturated, and a large portion of an absorbed dose of benzene is excreted as parent compound in exhaled air. The metabolism of benzene by Phase I and Phase II metabolism is summarized in Figure 7.25.

Glucuronidation is an important detoxication pathway involved in the metabolism of aniline, a very toxic substance (Kao, Faulkner, and Bridges 1978). Aniline toxicity occurs through methemoglobin formation in blood. Intoxication by aniline results in cyanosis or blue skin because the formation of methemoglobin interferes with the capacity of erythrocytes to bind oxygen. Aniline can be detoxified by Phase II metabolism with glucuronic acid to yield glucuronides, with activated sulfate (PAPS) to yield sulfate conjugates. The glucuronide and sulfate greatly increase water solubility. When aniline is acetylated using acetyl CoA, the solubility of the metabolite decreases (see Figure 7.26).

Xenobiotic metabolism can be modified by many factors, including the exposome and an individual's physiology. It has been suggested that many changes in toxicity are caused by the changes in metabolism of the toxicant, resulting from events that lead to overt toxicity by either activation or lead to detoxication (Dorne, Walton, and Renwick 2005).

Individuals may metabolize various xenobiotics differently because of gene polymorphisms (a gene for which 1% of the population has a variant allele). The gene may include single nucleotide polymorphisms (SNPs) or copy number variations, which may influence susceptibility to disease

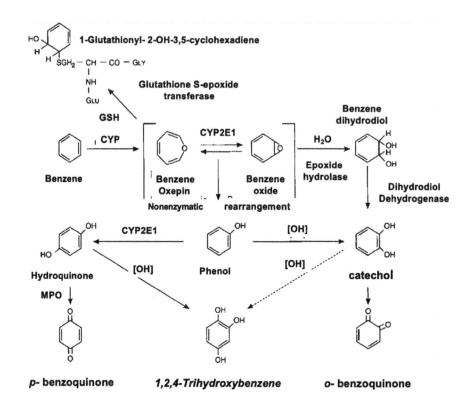

Figure 7.25 Summary of benzene metabolism. **Reproduced from *Environmental Health Perspectives* with permission (Snyder and Hedli 1996).**

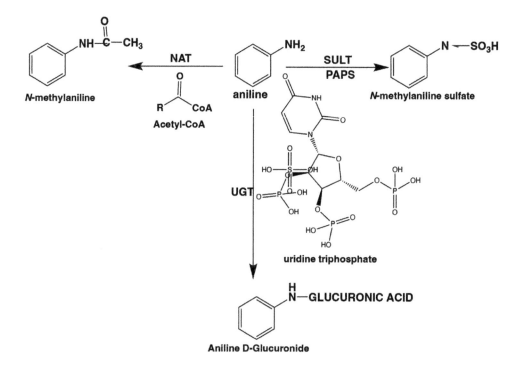

Figure 7.26 Conjugation of primary amines using aniline as an example. Conjugation of primary amines is carried out by UGT, SULT, or N-acetyl transferase (NAT) (Figure 7.27).

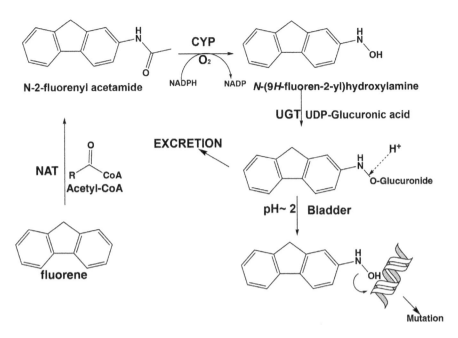

Figure 7.27 Metabolism of fluorene. Fluorene undergoes an N–acetylation reaction catalyzed by N-acetlytransferase, a Phase II reaction, to form N-2-fluorenylacetamide, which undergoes N–oxygenation catalyzed by cytochrome P450 to form N(9H-fluoren-2-yl)hydroxylamine, a carcinogen, which undergoes glucuronidation and is carried in urine to the bladder, where the glucuronide, which is acid labile, and the carcinogenic compound are regenerated (Miller and Miller 1981).

Table 7.8: Example SNPs in Various Populations

Trait	European Origin (%)	African Origin (%)	Asian Origin (%)
NAT2*4 (Fast)	20–25	36–41	50–60
NAT2*5B (Slow)	44	25–27	2–6
CYP 2D6 (Poor)	6–10	5	1
α-2 Adrenergic	37	49	59

Adapted from Rothstein, ed., *Pharmacogenomics*, Wiley (2020).

BOX 7.4   ENVIRONMENTAL JUSTICE

Angele White

The primary environment that human beings occupy is a community; a community includes the places where people live work and play. For this reason, the space occupied by humans – shared with other living things – exists within an environment that definitely has an overall impact on health. For instance, the pollution in the air we breathe, chemical/radiation exposure, unhygienic and/or unsanitary water, loud-decibel sounds in the atmosphere, and hazardous agricultural practices plausibly contribute to a toxic environment. In tandem with occupational risks – individually or collectively – environmental pollutants have been shown to detrimentally change the climate of the planet, thereby risking the distribution of land-to-water ratios that are necessary for the planet to be functional for all living creatures.

Justice relates to the equitable use, presence, or state of existence between different living entities. Furthermore, it is a moral, ethical perspective based on or guided by truth. To be "just" is to "do the right thing" based on the principles of fairness in the eyes of the law and in the consciousness of humanity.

Consequently, when a community becomes too polluted to carry out the basic functions of its environment, and when the cause of the pollution is not within the control of the people, but rather is outwardly imposed upon the community, human environmental justice is challenged and infringed upon.

As defined by the US Environmental Justice Order (E.O.) 12898, established in 1994, *environmental justice* focuses upon the environmental and human health effects of federal actions on minority and low-income populations with the goal of achieving environmental protection for *all* communities. The three directives of E.O. 12898 are to (1) identify and address the disproportionately high and adverse human health or environmental effects of their actions on minority and low-income populations to the greatest extent practicable and permitted by law, (2) develop a strategy for implementing environmental justice, and (3) promote non-discrimination in federal programs that affect human health and the environment, as well as provide minority and low-income communities access to public information and public participation.

The toxic and hazardous risks forced upon communities of color and those too economically disadvantaged to move away from environmental injustices are, in many cases, systemic and generational constructs supported by many of the "powers that be" – within the locality or from corporate interests abroad. Those propagating environmental injustices do so mainly for monetary profit and indirectly sustain racial inequities. The efforts of environmental justice – then and now – seek to correct the current paradigm of environmental racism and an inequitable mindset/philosophy held by those working in industry (and their stockholders/ financial beneficiaries), government, economic/business sector, and others who choose to continue disregarding the risks put upon residents living, working, playing in communities where the overall quality of life is desecrated by continual leaking, spraying, spilling, dropping, building, or injecting toxic and hazardous pollutants into communities. Some people think that because the environmental pollution is "**NIMBY**" or "Not In My Back Yard," the negative risks to human health and ecology are insignificant compared to the benefits to the general economy, while the negative environmental risks impact only people of color and/ or low-income people who may feel they have no influence on where polluting chemicals or processes are sited. Yet, having to exist in detrimental environments, they are subjugated to economic and educational impairments, and being swallowed into psychosocial degradation can have exaggerated negative health outcomes on those communities. For some, constantly being afraid of deadly natural, physical, and human environmental risks transforms the emotion of fright into a charge to battle for human and ecological survival. The desirable endgame: a just transition to protect human life and progeny, repair ecological surroundings, and restore balance in favor of life instead of environmental destruction. Protection, repair, and restoration are key reasons environmental justice is sought after, fought for, and must prevail.

Pollutants do not differentiate by class, status, race, socioeconomic status, religion, gender, or age; the pervasiveness of pollutants does not follow "NIMBY" rules. Therefore, it is important for all citizens to embrace environmental justice and equitable distribution of environmental risks because eventually, environmental risks will appear "**IMBY**." Investing in environmental justice is a risk unto itself: lots of time, health, money are often lost during long periods of protest and litigation. However, by doing the right thing for the well-being of people and the planet by decreasing deleterious environmental risks in minority and low-income communities, we purposefully choose another step toward "justice for ALL."

(i.e., gene-environment interaction). Polymorphisms in genes regulating enzymatic metabolism may result in higher or lower levels of active metabolites, which in turn can lead to increased interaction with DNA or other macromolecules (Cai et al. 2018; Cai and Xiang 2020). For example, polymorphisms in the CYP1A1 9 gene (**ile**[462]→**val**) have been associated with a moderate to high increase in the risk of lung cancer in the Japanese population (Venzlaff et al. 2005). A summary of some important polymorphisms in Phase I or Phase II metabolic enzymes in various populations is shown in Table 7.8.

That economic health is an important determinant of physical and mental health has been recognized by public health professionals since the 1800s. Human health effects of a chemical depend on many factors beyond dose. As mentioned earlier, the exposome takes into account cumulative environments and exposures and the resulting biological responses from preconception until death (Niedzwiecki et al. 2019). A growing body of literature on the impact of poverty and the importance of social determinants of health show significant health disparities of the disadvantaged in disease outcome. Awareness of the disparity in health outcomes has been amplified in recent years from popular press reports on COVID deaths (van Dorn, Cooney, and Sabin 2020).

Often, chronic conditions appear in a family where there is no immediate relative with that condition. These disorders often arise from exposures that occur *in utero* (Neophytou et al. 2019). The impact of poverty in the early years of life has a lifelong effect on the biology of an individual.

BOX 7.5   GEOGRAPHIC INFORMATION SYSTEMS (GIS)

Yannis Vassilopoulos

As far back as the time of Hippocrates (460–370 BCE), epidemiologists have observed that certain diseases seem to occur in some places and not in others. Hippocrates studied the effects that produced disease due to climate, water, clothing, and diet. The Hippocratic concept of health and disease stressed the relationship between humans and their environment.[1]

Fast forward to the 19th century with arguably the seminal role of GIS in public health in 1854 London, England. British physician John Snow mapped cholera outbreak locations. That "Cholera Map" led him to conclude that the epicenters of transmission were water pumps dispersed around the city and the clusters of high disease incidence evidently proximate (Map 7.5-1).

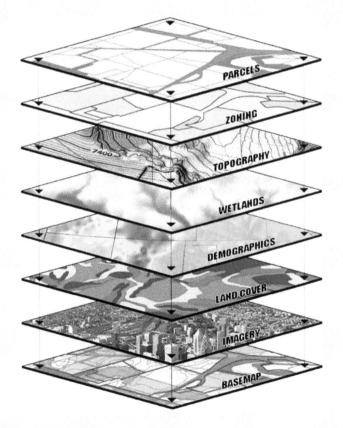

Figure Box 7.5-1   GIS data layers visualization.

Credit: **USGS (public domain), Ontario County, New York.**

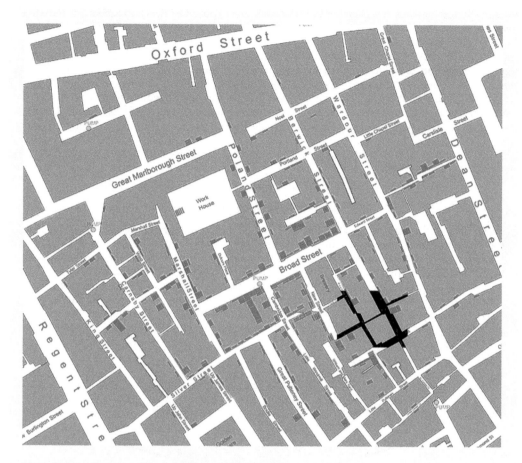

Map 7.5-1   Section of Dr. John Snow's Cholera Map.

Credit: **Wikimedia Commons, the free media repository.**

In its shorter computer-aided 60-year life span. GIS has evolved from a paper-driven implement to become a prized digital apparatus in support of public health and, more particularly, risk assessment endeavors. So, what are GIS? They are computer-based frameworks used to store, visualize, analyze, and interpret geographic (spatial) data (GIS in health). GIS can use any information that includes location. The location can be expressed in many ways, such as latitude and longitude, address, or ZIP code (Nat Geo Res Libr.) GIS data layer visualizations (Figure Box 7.5-1) can include roads, natural or man-made borders between counties, states, or countries, climate or environmental hazards, disease instances, healthcare resources, demographics, all of which can be overlaid on a map.

More specifically, GIS hardware and software implementations in public health include expertise from geographers, geospatial scientists, epidemiologists, statisticians, and other scientists. The involved parties work with raster and vector data to implement hazard surveillance, establish tracking frameworks, provide analytical methods to better visualize emerging patterns, and construct predictive assessments. *CDC uses GIS to study the spatial aspects of health and illness. For example: where are diseases found? How are diseases related to the environment? Where do people go to seek health care?* (GIS and Public Health at CDC).

In recent years, GIS evolved to offer powerful prediction and mitigation tool sets for risk assessment. Embedded layers of information can convey critical values like population density, threats, causes, and temporal events. Subsequently, GIS can create "threat maps" to assess risk to life or health from natural hazards (extreme weather, fires), man-made hazards (pollution, overpopulation, crime, resource contention), or diseases

Table Box 7.5-1: **GIS in Five-Step Risk Assessment**

Step 1. Identify hazards	Create data requirements and acquire corresponding raster and vector data for a hazard area to be mapped.
Step 2. Identify who may be harmed and how	Create GIS map layers that represent vulnerability based on location, density, hazard proximity, and temporal parameters.
Step 3. Assess risks and design control measures	Calculate risks based on quantifiable patterns, and construct a GIS user interface driven by databases (spatial and relational), human exposure models, and fate/transport models.
Step 4. Record and implement findings	Catalogue the long-term behavior of the hazard area, as well as the timing, cost, and feasibility of mitigation measures.
Step 5. Review the risk assessment and update	Analyze historical data (GIS maps of events and trends), assess probability and severity of future events, and revise risk assessment based on hazard analysis.

(origins, spread, containment). The ability to add or subtract data layers onto a GIS map offers risk assessors a unique perspective focused on a carefully selected geographic area with variable information fields and through different timeframes.

An example of how GIS complements the five-step process of risk assessment is shown in Table Box 7.5-1.

Currently, GIS is an indispensable tool set applied by numerous local, state, and federal government agencies, corporations, and academic institutions. There are several GIS platforms, but ArcGIS by ESRI is the golden standard offering multifarious customization capabilities with a remarkable track record.

REFERENCES

GIS in Health, Geospatial World. Retrieved from https://www.geospatialworld.net/article/gis-in-health/ (accessed on October 12, 2021)

Nat Geo Res Libr. Encyclopedic Entry. Retrieved from https://www.nationalgeographic.org/encyclopedia/geographic-information-system-gis/ (accessed on October 12, 2021)

GIS and Public Health at CDC. GIS and Public Health at CDC. Retrieved from https://www.cdc.gov/gis/index.htm (accessed on October 12, 2021)

If no intervention occurs within the first year, a 15-year difference in life span is observed between the child born into a family of low social economic status (SES) and an individual born into a family of higher SES (Hanson and Gluckman 2011; Marmot 2017; McCrory et al. 2019).

Using the exposome-genome approach as a study system yields significant new information on the link between exposure and disease. The traditional approach of studying the actions of a single chemical provides limited understanding of the environment-health link because humans are exposed to mixtures of chemicals. Although genomic analyses demonstrate a 99.9% congruence among humans, there are interindividual differences in responses to various exposures. These variations result from SNPs in the individual, the exposome in which the individual lives, microbiome differences (Das et al. 2016; Milani et al. 2017), and social stressors.

Our individual metabolomes and differences among individual microbiomes affect xenobiotic metabolism by inducing or repressing enzymes. The adverse outcome pathway framework (**see Chapter 9 for an in-depth discussion**) recognizes that many chemicals converge on similar metabolomic pathways (Nymark et al. 2018). Systems toxicology integrates classical toxicology and the quantitative analyses of large networks of molecular and functional changes that occur across levels of biological organization. Systems toxicology uses *in silico* methodology to devise molecular testing to better predict toxicant action yielding more accurate risk assessments (Strurla et al. 2014; Hartung et al. 2017), thus assessing risk by using systems toxicology approaches will be more informative than looking at single targets, and thus give more insight into environmental disease. The systems approaches are likely to advance meaningful risk assessments (Iskandar et al. 2013).

REFERENCES AND FURTHER READING

Agarwal, D. K., D. Misra, S. Agarwal, P. K. Seth, and J. D. Kohli. 1982. Influence of Sex Hormones on Parathion Toxicity in Rats: Antiacetylcholinesterase Activity of Parathion and Paraoxon in Plasma, Erythrocytes, and Brain. *J. Toxicol. Environ. Health* 9: 451–459.

Akarapipad, P., K. Kaarj, Y. Liang, and J.-Y. Yoon. 2021. Environmental Toxicology Assays Using Organ-on-Chip. *Annu. Rev. Anal. Chem.* 14: 155–183. https://doi.org/10.1146/annurev-anchem-091620-091335.

Arnold, C. 2020. Tainted Sanitisers and Bootleg Booze Are Poisoning People. Science. National Geographic Society. Accessed December 20. https://www.nationalgeographic.co.uk/science-and-technology/2020/08/tainted-sanitizers-and-bootleg-booze-are-poisoning-people.

Arnoldussen, I. A. C., and A. J. Kiliaan. 2014. Impact of DHA on Metabolic Diseases from Womb to Tomb. *Mar.* 12: 6190–6212. https://doi.org/10.3390/md12126190.

ATSDR, Toxicol.& Env. Med. August 2020 *Toxicological Profile on Lead.* Atlanta, GA: Center for Disease Control and Protection.

Bailey, B. A., and R. J. Sokol. 2011. Prenatal Alcohol Exposure and Miscarriage, Stillbirth, Preterm Delivery, and Sudden Infant Death Syndrome. *Alcohol Res. Health* 34: 86–91.

Baldwin, J. 2019. The Blind Men and the Elephant. *Short Story of the Day*, March 10, 2019. Accessed June 21, 2021.

Barker, D. J. P. 2004. Developmental Origins of Adult Health and Disease. *J. Epidemiol. Community Health* 58: 114–115.

Beaudoin, M.-S., B. Allen, G. Mazzetti, P. J. Sullivan, and T. E. Graham. 2013. Caffeine Ingestion Impairs Insulin Sensitivity in a Dose-Dependent Manner in Both Men and Women. *Appl. Physiol. Nutr. Metab* 38: 140–147. https://doi.org/dx.doi.org/10.1139/apnm-2012-0201

Beradi, A., D. R. Perinelli, H. A. Merchant, L. Bisharat, I. A. Basheti, G. Bonacucina, M. Cespi, and G. F. Palmieri. 2020. Hand Sanitisers Amid CoViD-19: A Critical Review of Alcohol-based Products on the Market and Formulation Approaches to Respond to Increasing Demand. *Int. J. Pharmacol.* 30 (584): 119431. https://doi.org/10.1016/j.ijpharm.2020.119431.

Bourdon-Lacombe, J. A., I. D. Moffat, M. Deveau, M. Husain, S. Auerbach, D. Krewski, R. S. Thomas, P. R. Bushel, A. Williams, and C. L. Yauk. 2015. Technical Guide for Applications of Gene EXPRESSION Profiling in Human Health Risk Assessment of Environmental Chemicals. *Regul. Toxicol. Pharmacol.* 72: 292–309. https://doi.org/10.1016/j.yrtph.2015.04.010.

Bruckner, J. V. 2000. Differences in Sensitivity of Children and Adults to Chemical toxicity: The NAS Report. *Reg. Toxicol. Pharmacol.* 31: 280–285.

Cai, J., R. G. Nichols, I. Koo, Z. A. Kalikow, L. Zhang, Y. Tian, J. Zhang, P. B. Smith, and A. D. Patterson. 2018. Multiplatform Physiologic and Metabolic Phenotyping Reveals Microbial Toxicity. *m Systems* 3: e00123–18. https://doi.org/10.1128/mSystems.00123-18.

Cai, W., and X Xiang. 2020. Introducion and Principles of Pharmacogenomics in Precision Medicine. In *Pharmacogenomics in Precision Medicine: From a Perspective of Ethnic Differences*, edited by W. Cai, Z. Liu, L. Miao and X. Xiang, 13–83. Singapore: Springer Nature.

Calabrese, E. J., and L.A. Baldwin. 2001. Hormesis: U-Shaped Dose Responses and Their Centrality in Toxicology. *Trends Pharmacol. Sci* 22: 285–289. https://doi.org/10.1016/S0165-6147(00)01719-3.

Calabrese, E. J., and M. P. Mattson. 2017. How Does Hormesis Impact Biology, Toxicology and Medicine. *npj Aging and Mech Dis* 3(13). https://doi.org/10.1038/s41514017-0013-z.

Canali, S. 2020. What Is New about the Exposome? Exploring Scientific Change in Contemporary Epidemiology. *Int. J. Environ. Res. and Public Health* 17 (8): 2879–2887. https://doi.org/10.3390/ijerph17082879.

Cashman, J. R., and J. Zhang. 2006. Human Flavin-containing Monooxygenases. *Annu. Rev. Pharmacol. Toxicol.* 46: 65–100.

Cederbaum, A. I. 2012. Alcohol Metabolism. *Clin. Liver Dis.* 16: 667–685. doi:https://doi.org/10.1016/j.cld.2012.08.002.

Chen, J., S. Jiang, J. Wang, J. Renukuntla, S. Sirimulla, and J. Chen. 2019. A Comprehensive Review of Cytochrome P450 2E1 for Xenobiotic Metabolism. *Drug Metab. Rev* 51 (2): 178–196. https://doi.org/10.1080/03602532.2019.1632889.

Chung, K.-T., and C. F. Cerniglia. 1992. Mutagenicity of Azo Dyes: Structure–Activity Relationships. *Mutation Res.* 277: 201–220.

Cui, Y., and D. Balshaw. 2019. From the Outside In: Integrating External Exposures into the Exposome Concept. In *Unraveling the Exposome: A Practical View*, edited by S. Dagnino and A. Macherone, 1135–1239. New York: Springer.

Dahm, M. M., S. Bertke, S. Allee, and R. D. Daniels. 2015. Creation of a Retrospective Job-exposure Matrix Using Surrogate Measures of Exposure for a Cohort of US Career Firefighters from San Francisco, Chicago and Philadelphia. *Occup. Environ. Med.* 72: 670–677. http://dx.doi.org/10.1136/oemed-2014-102790.

Das, A., M. Srinivasan, T. S. Gosh, and S. S. Mande. 2016. Xenobiotic Metabolism and Gut Microbiomes. *PLoS One* 11 (10). https://doi.org/10.1371/journal.pone.0163099.

Denny, L. A., S. Coles, and R. Blitz. 2017. Fetal Alcohol Syndrome and Fetal Alcohol Spectrum Disorders. *Amer. Fam. Physician* 15: 515–522.

Dorne, J. L. C. M., K. Walton, and A. G. Renwick. 2005. Human Variability in Xenobiotic Metabolism and Pathway–related Uncertainty Factors for Chemical Risk Assessment: A Review. *Food Chem. Toxicol.* 43: 201–216.

England, L., C. Bennett, C. H. Denny, M. A. Honein, S. M. Gilboa, S. Y. Kim, Jr. G. P. Guy, E. L. Tran, C. E. Rose, M. K. Bohm, and C. A. Boyle. 2020. *Alcohol Use and Co-Use of Other Substances Among Pregnant Females Aged 12–44 Years — United States, 2015–2018.* (Atlanta, GA: Centers for Disease Control & Prevention).

Erickson, B. E. 2017. How Many Chemicals Are in Use Today? *Chem. & Eng. News* 95 (9): 23–24.

Farhadi, F., B. Khameneh, M. Iranshahi, and M. Iranshahy. 2018. Antibacterial Activity of Favonoids and their Structure–Activity Relationship: An Update Review. *Phytotherapy Res.*: 1–28. https://doi.org/10.1002/ptr.6208.

FDA. 2021. FDA Updates on Hand Sanitizers Consumers Should Not Use. Food and Drug Administration. Accessed January 8. https://www.fda.gov/drugs/drug-safety-and-availability/fda-updates-hand-sanitizers-consumers-should-not-use (Accessed January 6, 2022).

Fregene, A., and L. A. Newman. 2005. Breast Cancer in Sub-Saharan Africa: How Does It Relate to Breast Cancer in African-American Women? *Cancer* 103: 1540–1550.

Giurgescu, C., A. L. Nowak, S. Gillespie, T. S. Nolan, C. M. Anderson, J. L. Ford, D. B. Hood, and K. B. Williams. 2019. Neighborhood Environment and DNA Methylation: Implications for Cardiovascular Disease Risk. *J. Urban Health* 96, no. 1: S23–S34. https://doi.org/10.1007/s11524-018-00341-1.

Glass, L., and S. N. Mattson. 2017. Fetal Alcohol Spectrum Disorders: A Case Study. *J. Pediatr. Neuropsychol.* 3 (2): 114–135. https://doi.org/10.1007/s40817-016-0027-7.

Gluckman, P. D., M. A. Hanson, T. Buklijas, and A. S. Beedle. 2009. Epigenetic Mechanisms that Underpin Metabolic and Cardiovascular Diseases. *Nat. Rev. Endocrinol.* 5: 401–408.

Gluckman, P. D., M. Hanson, and M. D. Mitchell. 2010. Developmental Origins of Health and Disease: Reducing the Burden of Chronic Disease in the Next Generation. *Genomic Med.* 2: 14.

Hall, J. E., and M. E. Hall. 2021. Transport of Substances through Cell Membranes. In *Guyton and Hall Textbook of Medical Physiology 14th Ed.*, edited by J. E. Hall and M. E. Hall, 51–58. New York, NY: Elsevier.

Hanby–Mason, R., J. J. Chen, S. Schenker, A. Perez, and G. I. Henderson. 1997. Catalase Mediates Acetaldehyde Formation from Ethanol in Fetal and Neonatal Rat Brain. *Alcoholism: Clin. Experim. Res.* 21 (6): 1063–1072. https://doi.org/10.1111/j.1530-0277.1997.tb04255.x.

Hanson, M., and P. D. Gluckman. 2011. Developmental Origins of Noncommunicable Disease: Population and Public Health Implications. *Am. J. Clin. Nutr.* 94: 1754S–1758S.

Harper, M., C. Wies, J. D. Pleil, B. C. Blount, A. Miller, M. D. Hoover, and S. Jahn. 2015. Commentary on the Contributions and Future Role of Occupational Exposure Science in a Vision and strategy for the Discipline of Exposure Science. *J. Exp. Sci Environ. Epidemiol.* 25: 381–387.

Hartung, T., R. E. FitzGerald, P. Jennings, G. R. Mirams, M. C. Peitsch, A. Rostami-Hodjegan, I. Shah, M. F. Wilks, and S. J. Sturla. 2017. Systems Toxicology: Real World Applications and Opportunities. *Chem. Res. Toxicol.* 30: 870–882.

Hassanian-Moghaddam, H., N. Zamani, A-A. Kolahi, R. McDonald, and K. E. Hovda. 2020. Double Trouble: Methanol Outbreak in the Wake of the COVID-19 Pandemic in Iran—A Cross-sectional Assessment. *Crit. Care.* 24 (1): 1–3. https://doi.org/10.1186/s13054-020-03140-w.

Heijne, W.H.M., A.S. Keinhuis, B. van Ommen, R. H. Stierum, and J. P. Groten. 2014. Systems Toxicology: Application of Toxicogenomics, Transcriptomics, Proteomics and Metabolomics in Toxicology. *Expert Rev. Proteomics* 2: 767–780.

Hobbie, K. R., A. DeAngelo, L. C. King, R. N. Wilnn, and M. A. Law. 2010. Toward a Molecular Equivalent Dose: Use of the Medaka Model in Comparative Risk Assessment. *Comp.Biochem. Physiol.* 149, no. CToxicol. Pharmacol.: 141–151.

Holzman, S. D., J. Larson, R. Kaur, G. Smelski, S. Dudley, and F. M. Shirazi. 2021. Death by Hand Sanitizer: Syndemic Methanol Poisoning in the Age of COVID-19. *Clin. Toxicol.* 59 (11): 1009–1014. https://doi.org/10.1080/15563650.2021.1895202.

Irwin, R. D., G. A. Boorman, M. L. Cunningham, A. N. Heinloth, D. E. Malarkey, and R. S. Paules. 2004. Application of Toxicogenomics to Toxicology: Basic Concepts in the Analysis of Microarray Data. *Toxicol. Pathol.* 32, no. Suppl. 1: 72–83.

Iskandar, A. R., F. Martin, M. Talikka, W. K. Schlage, R. Kostadinova, C. Mathis, J. Hoeng, and M. C. Peitsch. 2013. Systems Approaches Evaluating the Perturbation of Xenobiotic Metabolism in Response to Cigarette Smoke Exposure in Nasal and Bronchial Tissues. *BioMed. Res. Int.* 2013, Article ID 512086: 14. http://dx.doi.org/10.1155/2013/512086.

Johnson, C.H., A. D. Patterson, J. R. Idle, and F. J. Gonzalez. 2012. Xenobiotic Metabolomics: Major Impact on the Metabolome. *Annu. Rev. Pharmacol. Toxicol.* 52: 37–56.

Jamkhande, P. G., K. G. Chintawar, and P. G. Chandak. 2014. Teratogenicity: A Mechanism Based Short Review on Common Teratogenic. *Asian Pac. J. Trop. Dis.* 4: 421–432.

Jones, K. L., and D. W. Smith. 1973. Recognition of the Fetal Alcohol Syndrome in Early Infancy. *Lancet* 302: 999–1001

Kao, J., J. Faulkner, and J. W. Bridges. 1978. Metabolism of Aniline in Rats, Pigs and Sheep. *J. Pharmacol. Exp. Therapeut.* 6: 549–555.

Krewski, D., M. E. Anderson, E. Mantus, and L. Zeise. 2009. Toxicity Testing in the 21st Century: Implications for Human Health Risk Assessment. *Risk Anal.* 29 (4): 474–479. https://doi.org/10.1111/j.1539-6924.2008.01150.x.

Laing, L. V., J. Viana, E. L. Dempster, M. Trznadel, L. A. Trunkfield, T. M. U. Webster, R. van Aerle, G. C. Paull, R. J. Wilson, J. Mill, and E. M. Santos. 2016. Bisphenol A Causes Reproductive Toxicity, Decreases dnmt1 Transcription, and Reduces Global DNA Methylation in Breeding Zebrafish (*Danio rerio*). *Epigenetics* 101, no. 7: 526–538. https://doi.org/10.1080/15592294.2016.1182272.

Landrigan, P. J., C. A. Kimmel, A. Correa, and B. Eskenazi. 2004. Children's Health and the Environment: Public Health Issues and Challenges for Risk Assessment. *Environ. Health Perspect.* 112: 257–265. https://doi.org/:10.1289/ehp.6115; http://dx.doi.org/.

Lang, S., C. Probst, G. Gmel, J. Rehm, L. Burd, and S. Popova. 2017. Global Prevalence of Fetal Alcohol Spectrum Disorder Among Children and Youth: A Systematic Review and Meta-analysis. *JAMA Pediatr* 17: 948–956. https://doi.org/10.1001/jamapediatrics.2017.1919.

Lau, C., M. E. Anderson, D. J. Crawford-Brown, R. J. Kavlock, C. A. Kimmel, T. B. Knudson, K. Muneoka, J. M. Rogers, R. W. Setzer, G. Smith, and R. Tyl. 2000. Evaluation of Biologically Based Dose–Response Modeling for Developmental Toxicity: A Workshop Report. *Reg. Toxicol. Pharmacol.* 31: 190–199.

Lazarus, M., H.-Y. Shen, Y. Cherasse, W-M. Qu, Z-L. Huang, C. E. Bass, R. Winsky-Sommerer, K. Semba, B. B. Fredholm, D. Boison, O. Hayaishi, Y. Urade, and J.-F. Chen. 2011. Arousal Effect of Caffeine Depends on Adenosine A2A Receptors in the Shell of the Nucleus Accumbens. *J. Human Neurosci.* 31: 10067–10075

Liesivuori, J., and A. H. Savolainen. 1991. Methanol and Formic Acid Toxicity: Biochemical Mechanisms. *Basic Clin. Pharmacol. Toxicol..* 69 (3): 157–163. https://doi.org/10.1111/j.1600-0773.1991.tb01290.x.

Lioy, P. J. 2010. Exposure Science: A View of the Past and Milestones for the Future. *Environ. Health Persp.* 118: 1081–1090. doi:https://doi.org/10.1289/ehp.0901634 (Lioy).

Low, L. A., C. Mummery, B. R. Berridge, C. P. Austin, and D. A. Togle. 2021. Organs-on-chips: Into the Next Decade. *Nature Rev. Drug Discovery* 20: 345–361. https://doi.org/10.1038/s41573-020-0079-3.

Ma, C., Y. Peng, H. Li, and W. Chen. 2021. Organ-on-a-Chip: A New Paradigm for Drug Development. *Trends Pharmacol. Sci.* 42: 119–133. https://doi.org/10.1016/j.tips.2020.11.009.

Madiera, C., and P. M. Costa. 2021. Proteomics in Systems Toxicology. *Adv. Protein Che, Struct. Biol.* 127: 55–91. https://doi.org/10.1016/bs.apcsb.2021.03.001.

Marmot, M. 2017. Social Justice, Epidemiology and Health Inequalities. *Eur. J. Epidemiol.* 32 (7): 537–546. https://doi.org/10.1007/s10654-017-0286-3.

May, P. A., P. Gossage, W. O. Kalberg, L. K. Robinson, R. Brien, D. Buckley, M. Manning, and H. E. Hoyme. 2009. Prevalence and Epidemiologic Characteristics of FASD from Various Research Methods with an Emphasis on Recent in-school Studies. *Dev. Disabil. Res. Rev.* 15: 176–192.

McCrory, C., G. Fiorito, C. Ni Cheallaigh, S. Polidoro, P. Karisola, H. Alenius, R. Layte, T. Seeman, P. Vineis, and R. A. Kenny. 2019. How Does Socio-economic Position (SEP) Get Biologically Embedded? A Comparison of Allostatic Load and the Epigenetic Clock(s). *Psychoneuroendocrinology* 104: 64–73.

Meng, Q., M.-P. Mäkinen, H. Luk, and X. Yang. 2013. Systems Biology Approaches and Applications in Obesity, Diabetes, and Cardiovascular Diseases. *Curr. Cardiovasc. Risk Rep.* 7: 73–83.

Mielke, H. W., and C. Gonzales. 2008. Mercury (Hg) and Lead (Pb) in Interior and Exterior New Orleans House Paint Films. *Chemosphere* 72: 882–885. http://doi.org/10.1016/j.chemosphere.2008.03.061.

Mielke, H. W., C. R. Gonzales, E. Powell, M. Jartun, and P. W. Mielke Jr. 2007. Nonlinear Association between Soil Lead and Blood Lead of Children in Metropolitan New Orleans, Louisiana: 2000–2005. *Sci. Total Environ.* 388: 43–53. http://doi.org/10.1016/j.scitotenv.2007.08.012.

Mielke, H.W., M. A. Laidlaw, and C. Gonzales. 2010. Lead (Pb) Legacy From Vehicle Traffic in Eight California Urbanized Areas: Continuing Influence of Lead Dust on Children's Health. *Sci. Total Environ.* 408: 3965–3975. http://doi.org/10.1016/j.scitotenv.2010.05.017.

Milani, C., S. Duranti, F. Bottacini, E. Casey, F. Turroni, J. Mahoney, C. Belzer, S. Delgado-Palacio, S. A. Montes, L. Mancabell, G. A. Luigi, J. M. Rodriguez, L. Bode, W. deVos, M. Gueimonde, A. Margolles, D. vanSinderen, and M. Ventura. 2017. The First Microbial Colonizers of the Human Gut: Composition, Activities, and Health Implications of the Infant Gut Microbiota. *Microbiol. Mol. Biol. Rev.* 81 (4): e00036–17. https://doi.org/10.1128/MMBR.00036-17.

Miller, E. C., and J. A. Miller. 1981. Searches for Ultimate Chemical Carcinogens and Their Reactions with Cellular Macromolecules. *Cancer* 47: 2327–2345.

Mousavi-Roknabadi, Razieh Sadat, Melika Arzhangzadeh, Hosain Safaei-Firouzabadi, Reyhaneh Sadat Mousavi-Roknabadi, Mehrdad Sharifi, Nazanin Fathi, Najmeh Zarei Jelyani, and Mojtaba Mokdad. 2021. Methanol Poisoning During COVID-19 Pandemic: A Systematic Scoping Review. *Am. J. Emerg. Med.* 52: 69–84.

Moya, J., L. Phillips, L. Schuda, P. Wood, A. Diaz, R. Lee, R. Clickner, R. Jeffries, B. N. Adjei, P. Blood, K. Chapman, R. de Castro, and K. Mahaffey. 2011. *U.S. EPA Exposure Factors Handbook.* Edited by J. Moya, L. Phillips, L. Schuda, P. Wood, A. Diaz, R. Lee, R. Clickner, R. Jeffries, B. N. Adjei, P. Blood, K. Chapman, R. de Castro and K. Mahaffey. Washington, DC: US EPA.

Neavin, D. R., D. L. Liu, B. Ray, and R. M. Weinshilboum. 2018. The Role of the Aryl Hydrocarbon Receptor (AHR) in Immune and Inflammatory Diseases. *Int. J. Mol. Sci.* 19. https://doi.org/3851; https://doi.org/10.3390/ijms19123851.

Neophytou, A. M., S. S. Oh, D. Hu, S. Huntsman, C. Eng, J. R. Rodríguez-Santana, R. Kumar, J. R. Balmes, E. A. Eisen, and E. G. Burchard. 2019. *In utero* Tobacco Smoke Exposure, DNA Methylation, and Asthma in Latino Children. *Environ. Epidemiol.* 3 (3): e048. https://doi.org/10.1097/EE9.0000000000000048.

Niedzwiecki, M. M., D. L. Walker, R. Vermeulen, M. Chadeau-Hyam, D. P. Jones, and G. W. Miller. 2019. The Exposome: Molecules to Populations. *Annu. Rev. Pharmacol. Toxicol.* 59: 107–127.

Nieuwenhuijsen, M. J., D. Donaire-Gonzalez, M Foraster, D. Martinez, and A. Cisneros. 2014. Using Personal Sensors to Assess the Exposome and Acute Health Effects. *Int. J. Environ. Res. Public Health* 11: 7805–7819. https://doi.org/10.3390/ijerph110807805.

Nymark, P., L. Rieswijk, F. Ehrhart, N. Jeliazkova, G. Tsiliki, H. Sarimveis, C. T. Evelo, V. Hongisto, P. Kohonen, E. Willighagen, and R. C. Grafstrom. 2018. A Data Fusion Pipeline for Generating and Enriching Adverse Outcome Pathway Descriptions. *Toxicol. Sci.* 162: 264–275.

O'Brien, P. J., A. G. Siraki, and M. Shangari. 2005. Aldehyde Sources, Metabolism, Molecular Toxicity Mechanisms, and Possible Effects on Human Health. *Crit. Rev. Toxicol.* 35 (7): 609–662. https://doi.org/10.1080/10408440591002183.

Omiecinski, C., J. P. Vanden Heuvel, G. H. Perdue, and J. M. Peters. 2011. Xenobiotic Metabolism, Disposition, and Regulation by Receptors: From Biochemical Phenomenon to Predictors of Major Toxicities. *Toxicol. Sci.* 120 (S1): S49–S75. doi:https://doi.org/10.1093/toxsci/kfq338.

Omura, T., and R. Sato. 1962. The Carbon Monoxide–Binding Pigment of Liver Microsomes I. Evidence for its Hemoprotein Nature. *J. Biol. Chem.* 239: 2370–2386.

Picollet–D'hahan, N., M. Dolega, D. Frieda, D. K. Martin, and X. Gidrol. 2017. Deciphering Cell Intrinsic Properties: A Key Issue for Robust Organoid Production. *Trends Biotechnol.* 35: 1035–1048.

Plusquin, M., N. D. Saenen, and T. S. Naweot. 2019. Epigenetics and the Exposome. In *Unraveling the Exposome*, edited by S. Dagnino and A. Macherone, 562–665. New York: Springer.

Preston, R. 2000. The Genome Warrior. *The New Yorker* 76: 66–83.

Rendic, S. P., and F. P. Guengrich. 2021. Human Family 1-4 Cytochrome P450 Enzymes Involved in the Metabolic Activation of Xenobiotic and Physiological Chemicals: An Update. *Arch. Toxicol.* 95: 395–472.

Ritchie, H., and M. Roser. 2018. Causes of Death. *Our World in Data.* Accessed June 2021.

Rothammer, V., and F. J. Quintana. 2019. The Aryl Hydrocarbon Receptor: An Environmental Sensor Integrating Immune Responses in Health and Disease. *Nat. Rev. Immunol.* 19: 184–197. https://doi.org/10.1038/s41577-019-0125-8.

Rozman, K. K. 2000. The Role of Time in Toxicology or Haber's CXT Product. *Toxicology* 149: 35–42.

Sandle, T. 2020. Coronavirus Pandemic Shortages and the Rsks of Using Ineffective Hand Sanitisers in Cleanrooms. *Clean Air Contam. Rev.* 43 (3): 12–14.

Sierra-Santoyo, A., M. Hernandez, A. Albores, and M. E. Cebrian. 2005. DDT Increases Hepatic Testosterone Metabolism in Rats. *Arch. Toxicol.* 79: 7–12.

Skardal, A., S. V. Murphy, M. Devarasetty, I. Mead, H. W. Kang, Y. J. Seol, Y. Shrike Zhang, S. R. Shin, L. Zhao, J. Aleman, A. R. Hall, T. D. Shupe, A. Kleensang, M. R. Dokmeci, S. Jin Lee, J. D. Jackson, J. J. Yoo, T. Hartung, A. Khademhosseini, S. Soker, C. E. Bishop, and A. Atala. 2017. Multi-Tissue Interactions in an Integrated Three-Tissue Organ-On-A-Chip Platform. *Sci Rep* 7 (1): 8837. https://doi.org/10.1038/s41598-017-08879-x.

Snyder, R., and C. C. Hedli. 1996. An Overview of Benzene Metabolism. *Environ. Health. Perspect* 104, no. Suppl. 6: 1165–1171.

Spengler, J. D., and M. L. Soczek. 1984. Evidence for Improved Ambient Air Qualitv and the Need for Personal Exposure Research. *Environ. Sci. Technol.* 18: 268A–280A.

Stanton, K., and F. H. Kruszewski. 2016. Quantifying the Benefits of Using Read-Across and In Silico Techniques to Fulfill Hazard Data Requirements for Chemical Categories. *Reg. Toxicol. Pharmacol.* 81 (23): 250–259.

Stockard, C. M. 1912a. An Experimental Study of Racial Regeneration in Mammals Treated with Alcohol. *Arch. Int. Med.* 10: 381.

Stockard, C. M. 1912b. Is the Control of Embryonic Development a Practical Problem? *Proc. Am. Phil. Soc.* 51: 191–200.

Strurla, S. J., A. R. Boobis, R. E. FitzGerald, Hoeng, J., R. J. Kavlock, K. Schirmer, M. Whelan, M. F. Wilks, and M. C. Peitsch. 2014. Systems Toxicology: From Basic Research to Risk Assessment. *Chem. Res. Toxicol.* 27: 314–329.

Sud, M., E. Fahy, D. Cotter, K. Azam, I. Vadivelu, C. Burant, A. Edison, O. Fiehn, R. Higashi, K. S. Nair, S. Sumner, and S. Subramaniam. 2016. Metabolomics Workbench: An International Repository for Metabolomics Data and Metadata, Metabolite Standards, Protocols, Tutorials and Training, and Analysis Tools. *Nucleic Acids Res.* 44 (D463–D470): D463–D470. https://doi.org/10.1093/nar/gkv1042.

Suddendorf, R. F. 1989. Research on Alcohol Metabolism Among Asians and Its Implications for Understanding Causes of Alcoholism. *Publ. Health Repts.* 104: 615–620.

Thakker, K. D. 1998. An Overview of Health Risks and Benefits of Alcohol Consumptin. *Alcohol Clin. Exptl. Res.* 22, no. 7: 285S–298S. https://doi.org/10.1097/00000374-199807001-00003

Tosteson, T. D., and J. Ware. 1990. Designing a Logistic Regression Study Using Surrogate Measures for Exposure and Outcome. *Biometrika* 77: 11–21. https://doi.org/10.1093/biomet/77.1.11.

Tsatsakis, A. M., L. Vassilopoulou, L. Kovatsi, C. Tsitsimpikou, M. Karamanou, G. Leon, J. Lesivouri, A. W. Hayes, and D. A. Spandidos. 2018. The Dose Response Principle from Philosophy to Modern Toxicology: The Impact of Ancient Philosophy and Medicine in Modern Toxicology Science. *Toxicol. Reports* 5: 1107–1113.

van Dorn, A., R. E. Cooney, and M. L. Sabin. 2020. COVID-19 Exacerbating Inequalities in the US. *Lancet* 295: 1243–1244.

Venter, J.C., M. D. Adams, Eugene W. Myers, P. W. Li, R. J. Mural, G. G. Sutton, H. D. Smith, M. Yandel, C. A. Evans, and R. A. Holt. 2001. The Sequence of the Human Genome. *Science (Washington)* 291 (5507): 1304–1351.

Venzlaff, A. S., M. L. Cote, S. J. Land, S. K. Santer, D. R. Schwartz, and A. G. S. Schwartz. 2005. CYP1A1 and CYP1B1 Polymorphisms and Risk of Lung Cancer Among Never Smokers: A Population-Based Study. *Carcinogenesis* 26: 2207–2212.

Vineis, P., M. Chadeau-Hyam, H. Gmuender, J. Gulliver, Z. Herceg, J. Kleinjans, M. Kogevinas, S Kyrtopoulos, M. Nieuwenhuijsen, D. H. Phillips, N. Probst-Hensch, A. Scalbert, R. Vermeulen, C. P. Wild, and The EXPOsOMICS Consortium. 2017. The Exposome in Practice: Design of the EXPOsOMICS Project. *Int. J. Hyg. Environ. Health* 220: 142–151.

Wang, D., Y. Zhang, J. Li, R. A. Dahlgren, H. Huang, and H. Wang. 2020. Risk Assessment of Cardiotoxicology to Zebrafish (Danio rerio) by Environmental Exposure to Triclosan and its Derivatives. *Environ. Pollut.* 265 https://doi.org/10.1016/j.envpol.2020.114995.

Wang, G., X. Zhang, X. Liu, J. Zheng, R. Chen, and H. Kan. 2019. Ambient Fine Particulate Matter Induce Toxicity in Lung Epithelial-Endothelial Co-Culture Models. *Toxicol. Lett.* 301: 133–145. https://doi.org/10.1016/j.toxlet.2018.11.010.

Weichenthal, S., M. Hatzopoulou, and M. Brauer. 2019. A Picture Tells a Thousand…Exposures: Opportunities and Challenges of Deep Learning Image Analyses in Exposure Science and Environmental Epidemiology. *Environ. Int.* 122: 3–10.

Wexler, P., and A. N. Hayes. 2019. Journey of Toxicology: A Historical Glimpse. In *Cassarett & Doull's Toxicology: The Basic Science of Poisons, 9th Edition*, edited by C. D. Klassen, 3–23. New York: McGraw-Hill.

White, A. M., M. E. Slater, G. Ng, and R. B. Hingson. 2018. Trends in Alcohol-related Emergency Department Visits in the United States: Results from the Nationwide Emergency Department Sample, 2006 to 2014. *Alcoholism: Clin. Experim. Res.* 42: 352–359.

Wild, C. P. 2005. Complementing the Genome with an "Exposome": The Outstanding Challenge of Environmental Exposure Measurement in Molecular Epidemiology. *Cancer Epidemiol. Biomarkers Prev.* 14 (8): 1847–1850.

Wild, C. P. 2012. The Exposome from Concept to Utility. *Int. J. Epidemiol.* 24: 24–32.

Williams, A. J., J. C. Lambert, K. Thayer, and J.-L. C. M. Dorne. 2021. Sourcing data on Chemical Properties and Hazard Data from the US-EPA CompTox Chemicals Dashboard: A Practical Guide for Human Risk Assessment. *Environ. Intl.* 154. Accessed June 2021. https://doi.org/10.1016/j.envint.2021.106566.

Williams, R. T. 1975. Detoxication Mechanisms. In *Metabolism and Detoxication of Drugs, Toxic Substances and Other Organic Compounds, 3rd* ed., edited by R. T. Williams. New York: Wiley.

Wilson, J. G. 1973. Present Status of Drugs as Teratogens in Man. *Teratology* 7: 3–15.

Wishart, D., D. Arndt, A. Pon, T. Sajed, A. C. Guo, Y. Djoumbou, C. Knox, M. Wilson, Y. Liang, J. Grant, Y. Liu, S. A. Goldansaz, and S. M. Rappaport. 2015. T3DB: The Toxic Exposome Database. *Nucleic Acids Res.* 4: D–928–D934.

Ziegler, E. 1968. Zur Prophylexe der Zivilisationskrqnkheiten (Ziegler). *Praxis* 23: 1032–1035.

Ziegler, R. M., R. N. Hoover, M. C. Pike, A. Hildesheim, A. M. Y. Nomura, D. W. West, A. H. Wu-Williams, L. N. Kolonel, P. L. Pamela, L. Horn-Ross, J. F. Rosenthal, and M. B. Hyer. 1993. Migration Patterns and Breast Cancer Risk in Asian-American Women. *J. Nat. Cancer Inst.* 85: 1819–1827.

8 The Application of Physiologically Based Pharmacokinetic (PBPK) Modeling to Risk Assessment

Raymond S. H. Yang
Colorado State University, Fort Collins, CO, USA

Yasong Lu
Quantitative Clinical Pharmacology, Daiichi Sankyo, Inc., Basking Ridge, NJ USA

Zhoumeng Lin
University of Florida, Gainesville, FL, USA

CONTENTS

Introduction: The Need for PBPK Modeling in Risk Assessment 154
What Is PBPK?..154
    Differences between Classical Pharmacokinetic Models and PBPK Models 155
    Conceptual Model: Graphical Representation..155
    Mathematical Model: Mass Balance Differential Equations 156
    A Priori Prediction vs. Curve Fitting...156
    Biological Relevance 156
How Does a PBPK Model Work?..157
    PBPK Modeling 157
    Data Requirements for PBPK Modeling 157
    Data Sets Used for Model Building and Model Validation...158
    Available Software Comparison..158
    Explanation of an Example of Computer Code for a PBPK Model in Berkeley Madonna 160
    Numerical Integration 166
    Sensitivity and Uncertainty 166
        Sensitivity Analysis 166
        Uncertainty Analysis...167
PBPK Models for Chemical Interactions (Multiple Chemical Interactive PBPK Models)
    in Chemical Mixtures...167
An Example of Application of PBPK Modeling in Dichloromethane Risk Assessment and
    Its Recent Development in Bayesian Population Approach 169
The Potential Applications of AI to PBPK Modeling...170
Acknowledgments 172
References..172

LEARNING OBJECTIVES

Students who complete this chapter will be able to

1. Understand why physiologically based pharmacokinetic (PBPK) modeling is needed in risk assessment,
2. Learn what PBPK modeling is,
3. Understand how PBPK modeling is done, particularly in its application to risk assessment,
4. Learn how PBPK modeling of chemical mixtures may be carried out, particularly some new considerations, and
5. Follow some of the latest development in the application of PBPK modeling in risk assessment.

DOI: 10.1201/9780429291722-8

Physiologically based pharmacokinetic (PBPK) modeling is an area of science that can be traced back to the 1920s. In June 2005, the first book on PBPK (Reddy et al. 2005) was published, and its contents encompassed over 1,000 publications on PBPK modeling. Since then, two more PBPK modeling books appeared (Fisher et al. 2020; Peters 2012); the former is oriented toward pharmacology and the latter toward toxicology and risk assessment. Despite the fact that it is a mature science with about a hundred years of history, active development is still going on in this area, and this chapter will also provide a glimpse of some of these latest advances. It is important to emphasize that this chapter, though a learning tool, will only provide some of the fundamentals to stimulate your interests. This chapter alone will not make you a PBPK modeler. To be proficient, there is no alternative but to attend specific training workshops and, most importantly, to "get your hands dirty" by doing PBPK modeling. Through repeated practice, reading, and making all the mistakes everyone else made before you, you would then open the window to a very useful and powerful technology.

INTRODUCTION: THE NEED FOR PBPK MODELING IN RISK ASSESSMENT

In earlier days, risk assessment was done based on exposure dose or administered dose. This is neither accurate nor satisfying because an exposure or administered dose will go through absorption, distribution, metabolism, and excretion (ADME) in our body before a sufficient amount of the dose reaches the target organ to exert its toxicity. To be able to follow, on a time-course basis, the ADME processes of a given chemical in our body and, further, to follow an active component (say, from a technical formulation) or a reactive species (from metabolic transformation) require the understanding of pharmacokinetics of that chemical. PBPK modeling is a very useful tool for the integrated computer simulation of pharmacokinetics of a chemical or chemicals and its or their metabolites. Therefore, the need for PBPK modeling in risk assessment arises when we want to incorporate state-of-the-science technology to conduct a more accurate risk assessment. Additional arguments in favor of the incorporation of PBPK modeling into the risk assessment process include deliberations from the following perspectives:

A. Toxicological Interactions of Multiple Chemicals
B. Minimizing Animal Experiments
C. Food Quality Protection Act and the Subsequent Development of Cumulative Risk Assessment at the US Environmental Protection Agency (US EPA)
D. Internal Dose
E. Exposure Dose Reconstruction and Human Biomonitoring
F. In vitro to in vivo extrapolation (IVIVE)
G. Interspecies Extrapolation (e.g., from animals to humans)
H. Systems Biology

A great deal of discussion under many of these perspectives was provided in the earlier edition of this book (Robson and Toscano 2007); please refer to that edition for additional information. Detailed discussion on some of the other perspectives is beyond the scope of this chapter, and the readers are encouraged to study the literature on their own.

In addition to the aforementioned points, risk assessment is about a population, not an individual. Thus, Bayesian Population PBPK Modeling utilizing Markov Chain Monte Carlo (MCMC) simulations is an active area of advancement in PBPK modeling application to risk assessment. For a more thorough discussion on this, please see Yang et al. (2015).

WHAT IS PBPK?

The concept of PBPK had its embryonic development in the 1920s. PBPK modeling blossomed and flourished in the late 1960s and early 1970s in the chemotherapeutic area due mainly to the efforts of investigators with expertise in chemical engineering. In the mid-1980s, work on PBPK modeling of volatile solvents by Dr. Melvin E. Andersen and colleagues started yet another "revolution" in the toxicology and risk assessment fields. Today, PBPK modeling is frequently part of the safety evaluation and risk assessment in the regulatory arena. For more historical perspectives on PBPK modeling, please refer to Reddy et al. (2005) and Fisher et al. (2020).

Differences between Classical Pharmacokinetic Models and PBPK Models

"Classical pharmacokinetics" refers to those empirical noncompartmental or compartmental pharmacokinetic studies routinely practiced in the pharmaceutical industry (van de Waterbeemd and Gifford 2003). Classical pharmacokinetic modeling is based on observed data and is also termed a data-driven, "top-down" approach. As will be illustrated later, the compartments of a PBPK model have distinct anatomical and physiological significance. This is a major difference from empirical noncompartmental or compartmental pharmacokinetic modeling approaches. Another major difference is that PBPK modeling is *a priori* prediction of kinetic behaviors of the chemical(s) of interest based on a mathematical model formulated with the incorporation and integration of all known physicochemical, physiological, biochemical, pharmacological, toxicological, and other information of the chemical(s) and organism(s) of interest. Thus, it is also termed the "bottom-up" approach and is not curve fitting (see more details in the Section of *A Priori Prediction vs. Curve Fitting*). PBPK models can be used to describe concentration-time profiles in individual tissues/organs and in the plasma or blood. When the concentration in a certain target tissue, rather than in the plasma, is highly related to a compound's efficacy or toxicity, PBPK modeling will be a more useful tool than classical pharmacokinetic models for describing the pharmacokinetic/pharmacodynamic (PK/PD) relationship and thus make a better prediction of the time course of drug effects resulting from a certain dose regimen for the compound of interests. Furthermore, PBPK models in combination with absorption simulation and quantitative structure-activity relationship (QSAR) approaches could bring us closer to a full prediction of drug disposition for pharmaceutical new entities and help streamline the selection of lead drug candidates in the drug discovery process (van de Waterbeemd and Gifford 2003). Lastly, unlike empirical noncompartmental and compartmental pharmacokinetics, PBPK modeling is a powerful tool for extrapolation, be it for interspecies, inter-routes, inter-doses, inter-life stages, IVIVE, etc.

Conceptual Model: Graphical Representation

A PBPK model graphically and conceptually illustrated in Figure 8.1 reflects the incorporation of basic physiology and anatomy.

The compartments correspond to anatomic entities, such as the liver and fat, while the blood circulation conforms to basic physiology. In the specific model in Figure 8.1, a PBPK model for hexachlorobenzene (HCB) in the rat (Lu et al. 2006), the exposure routes of interest are either oral gavage or intravenous as indicated. Depending on the need, other routes of exposure can be added easily. The liver is modeled as an individual compartment, as it is the major target organ of toxicity as well as the principal organ of metabolism of HCB; whereas fat is included as an individual compartment because HCB, being lipophilic, can accumulate in fat, thus it is a kinetically important compartment. Some tissues are "lumped" together [e.g., richly (rapidly) or poorly (slowly) perfused tissues in Figure 8.1] when they are "kinetically" similar, for the specific chemical(s) studied. On the other hand, a given tissue can be split off as needed. In this case, HCB is known to bind with

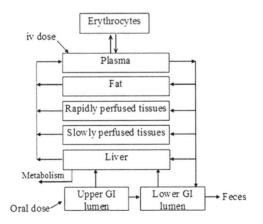

Figure 8.1 A graphic or conceptual PBPK model for HCB following iv or oral exposure. For an iv exposure, the uptake in the upper GI lumen was turned off, and the excretion of metabolites was tracked. For oral exposures, the reverse was true. (redrawn from Lu et al. (2006).)

erythrocytes, and the blood compartment is split into two subcompartments: the erythrocytes and plasma. Similarly, because of the complexity related to the absorption and exsorption (plasma-to-gastrointestinal (GI) lumen passive diffusion) processes of HCB, the GI lumen compartment is split into upper and lower portions. In conceptualizing the PBPK model, the Law of Parsimony should always be applied to keep the model as simple as possible. When the needs arise and experimental data are available, complexity can be incorporated.

Mathematical Model: Mass Balance Differential Equations

A mathematical model, regarding PBPK modeling, is generally represented by a set of computer code(s) in such a way that it can be executed by the modeling software to simulate the kinetic behavior of a chemical(s) in the body of an organism (e.g., rat, mouse, fish, human). A key element of such a mathematical model is a set of mass balance differential equations representing all of the interlinked compartments such as liver or fat. This set of mass balance differential equations is formulated to express a mathematical representation, or model, of the biological system. This model can then be used for computer simulation to predict the time-course behavior of any given chemical included in the model.

These mass balances are essentially molecular accounting statements that include the rates at which molecules enter and leave the compartment, as well as the rates of reactions that produce or consume the chemical. For instance, a general equation, for chemical j in any tissue or organ i, is

$$V_i \frac{dC_{ij}}{dt} = Q_i(CA_j - CV_{ij}) - \text{Metab}_{ij} - \text{Elim}_{ij} + \text{Absorp}_{ij} - \text{Pr} Binding_{ij}, \tag{8.1}$$

where V_i represents the volume of tissue group i, Q_i is the blood flow rate to tissue group i, CA_j is the concentration of chemical j in arterial blood, and C_{ij} and CV_{ij} are the concentrations of chemical j in tissue group i and in the effluent venous blood from tissue i, respectively. Please note that C_{ij} here refers to the "free" (i.e., not bound to macromolecules, e.g., proteins, that hinder redistribution of the chemical out of the tissue) chemical concentration; in toxicology literature, C_{ij} under similar conditions may mean total chemical concentration (free and bound) and the equation would be different from Equation 8.1. A typical example is the 2, 3, 7, 8-tetrachlorodibenzo[p]dioxin (TCDD) PBPK models (Leung et al. 1988; Mills and Andersen 1993). $Metab_{ij}$ is the rate of metabolism for chemical j in tissue group i; liver, being the principal organ for metabolism, would have significant metabolic rates, while, with some exceptions, $Metab_{ij}$ is usually equal to zero in other tissue groups. $Elim_{ij}$ represents the rate of elimination from tissue group i (e.g., biliary excretion from the liver); $Absorp_{ij}$ represents uptake of the chemical from dosing (e.g., oral dosing), and $PrBinding_{ij}$ represents protein binding of the chemical in the tissue. These terms are zero unless there is definitive knowledge that the particular organ/tissue of interest has such processes and, more importantly, that such processes will have significant impact on the pharmacokinetics of the chemical(s).

A Priori Prediction vs. Curve Fitting

Once a PBPK model is validated (see the section titled "Data Sets Used for Model Building and Model Validation"), it has the predictive capability in carrying out *a priori* computer simulations given a set of initial conditions such as animal species of interest, dosing route, dosing levels, and regimen. Certain validation experiments under precise simulation conditions can then be conducted to test the predictive capability of the PBPK model by comparing experimental results with the *a priori* computer simulation results. Therefore, PBPK modeling should not be considered curve-fitting exercises.

Biological Relevance

As the name "physiologically based" implies, another important consideration in PBPK modeling is that whenever an equation and its related parameter(s) are introduced into the model, they must have biological relevance. In many ways, the mass balance differential equations in PBPK modeling can be translated into simple English. For instance, the mass balance equation for the liver compartment in Figure 8.1 is

$$VL \times \frac{dCL}{dt} = QL \times (CA - CVL) - KMET \times CVL + KGILV1 \times AGIUp + KGILV2 \times AGILow. \tag{8.2}$$

It looks like a rather formidably long equation. However, the English translations for both sides of the equation are really quite easy to follow:

Left side: A small (infinitesimal) change in the amount of chemical (HCB in this case) with respect to a small (infinitesimal) change in time. We talk about "amount" (or mass) because when volume of the liver (VL in mL) multiplies the concentration in the liver (CL in mg/mL), it becomes amount (mg). Note the unit on the left side is finally amount/time or, more specifically, mg/hr.

Right side: Amount coming into the liver from general circulation (1st term) minus the amount metabolized (2nd term) plus amount absorbed from the upper GI lumen (3rd term), and plus amount absorbed from the lower GI lumen (4th term). The 1st term is derived from blood flow rate (QL in mL/hr) to and from the liver times the differential concentration between arterial blood (CA in mg/mL) and venous blood (CVL in mg/mL). In the 2nd term, KMET is the metabolic rate constant with a unit of mL/hr. In the 3rd and 4th terms, KGILV1 and KGILV2 are absorption rate constants from upper and lower GI lumen with a unit of 1/hr whereas AGIUp and AGILow are the amounts of HCB in the two GI lumen subcompartments. Note the unit for each term on the right side is also mg/hr.

The exercise simply illustrates that all the mass balance equations and their respective parameters in a PBPK model should be explainable by biologically relevant concepts and terminologies.

HOW DOES A PBPK MODEL WORK?

PBPK Modeling

The fundamentals of PBPK modeling are to identify the principal organs or tissues involved in the disposition of the chemical of interest and to correlate the chemical ADME within and among these organs and tissues in an integrated and biologically plausible manner. Individual pieces of how PBPK modeling works have been given in the section "What Is PBPK?" However, we will briefly summarize it in its entirety in this section.

After a conceptual model is developed (*e.g.*, Figure 8.1), time-dependent mass balance equations are written for a chemical(s) in each compartment. A set of such mass balance differential equations representing all of the interlinked compartments are formulated to express a mathematical representation, or model, of the biological system. This model can then be used for computer simulation to predict the time-course behavior of any given chemical, under specific dosing conditions, included in the model. Computer simulations may be made for any number of desired time-course endpoints such as the blood levels of the parent compound, liver level of a reactive metabolite, and similar information on different species, at lower or higher dose levels, and/or via a different route of exposure. The experimental pharmacokinetic data may then be compared with a PBPK model simulation. If the model simulation does not agree with the experimental measurements, the model might be deficient because critical scientific information might be missing or certain assumptions are incorrect. The investigator, with knowledge of the chemical and a general understanding of the physiology and biochemistry of the animal species, can design and conduct critical experiments for refining the model to reach consistency with experimentation. This refinement process may be repeated again and again when necessary; such an iterative process is critically important for the development of a PBPK model. In that sense, PBPK modeling is a very good hypothesis-testing tool in toxicology, and it may be utilized to conduct many different kinds of experiments on the computer (i.e., *in silico* toxicology). It should be noted that there is always the possibility that a good model may not be obtained at the time because of the limitation of our knowledge of the chemical. Validation of the PBPK model with data sets other than the working set (or training set) to develop the model is necessary. One should remember that a model is usually a simplification of reality; thus, "all models are wrong, some are useful," as stated by George Box. The more data sets against which a model is validated, the more robust is that model in its predictive capability. Once validated, the PBPK model is ready for extrapolation to other animal species, including humans.

Data Requirements for PBPK Modeling

What are the specific data needed for building PBPK models? Obviously, well-conducted *in vivo* pharmacokinetic data are important, and usually, the more data sets (e.g., different doses, routes, species) the better. In each study, time-course blood and tissue concentration data are important.

These time-course data should include at least the following tissues and organs: blood (or plasma if blood cell binding is not an issue), liver (organ of metabolism), kidney (representing rapidly perfused organs/tissues), muscle (representing slowly perfused organs/tissues), and target organ(s)/tissue(s). It should be noted that, in recent years, there have been proposals that in vitro and in silico data be used instead of in vivo data to minimize animal killings (OECD 2021).

Three sets of parameters are needed for PBPK model building: physiological parameters (e.g., ventilation rates, cardiac output, organs as % body weight), thermodynamic parameters (e.g., tissue partition coefficients, protein binding), and biochemical parameters (e.g., K_m and V_{max}). Most, if not all, of the physiological parameters for laboratory animals, food animals, and humans are available in the literature (Brown et al. 1997; Li et al. 2021; Lin et al. 2020; Wang et al. 2021); other parameters, chemical specific, are sometimes available in the literature as a result of chemical profiling from in vitro or in vivo studies. When information gaps exist, needed data can be obtained or estimated via experimentation, allometric extrapolation, usually based on a power function of the body weight (Lindstedt 1987), or quantitative structure-activity relationships.

Data Sets Used for Model Building and Model Validation

When building a PBPK model, certain experimental data sets are necessary for comparing with simulation results to see if the theoretical data (computer simulations) are super-imposable to the observed data (experimental results). During this phase of the work, we are trying to: (1) test our hypotheses of the pharmacokinetic fate of the chemical(s) of interest in the given biological system, (2) assess the appropriateness of the assumptions that we made for the PBPK model, and (3) find appropriate values for those parameters that can neither be derived experimentally nor estimated theoretically. The data sets used in this model-building phase should be considered a "Training Set" or "Working Set." Once a PBPK model is constructed, the next phase is model validation. This is where *a priori* simulations under a specific exposure scenario can be carried out, and the simulation results are then compared with available experimental data. Superimposition of the two suggests validity of model prediction under that set of conditions. The more data sets against which a model is validated, the more robust is that model in its predictive capability. Validation of the PBPK model with data sets other than the training set (or working set) used to develop the model is essential. It is prudent to indicate that the authors of this chapter like to stick to the simplest usage of the word "validation" (e.g., "an act, process, or instance of validating" defined by *Merriam-Webster* as searched online using Google, January 2021) without considering any legal implications. As such, a scientist's personal judgment or bias is inevitable in the process of validation.

Available Software Comparison

A PBPK model generally is a system of coupled ordinary differential equations, which is solved with the aid of computer tools. The available computer tools for PBPK modeling include programming languages, simulation software, and spreadsheets. An excellent list of these tools, along with their developers/vendors, salient features, and application examples, has been compiled in a report on PBPK modeling (US EPA 2005) and in a more recent peer-reviewed paper by Lin et al. (2017), as well as in the discussions and examples in the book by Fisher et al. (2020) and the PBPK guidance document from the Organisation for Economic Co-operation and Development (OECD 2021). Earlier, Rowland et al. (2004) presented a somewhat different list. Certain commonly known examples in these lists are Berkeley Madonna (University of California at Berkeley, California), R (R Core Team, Vienna, Austria), MATLAB (MathWorks, Natick, Massachusetts), SAAM II (University of Washington, Seattle, Washington), SCoP (Simulation Control Program, Simulation Resources Inc., Redlands, California), SimuSolv (Dow Chemical Company, Midland, Michigan), and the ACSL (Advanced Continuous Simulation Language) series of software (e.g., ACSL, ACSL Tox, and acslX (AEgis Technologies Group, Huntsville, Alabama), as well as the recently available Magnolia software). These pieces of software for PBPK modeling vary in flexibility and user-friendliness. Regardless of the variation in flexibility, PBPK software should at least have proper algorithms for integration, optimization, and sensitivity analysis. Given the diversity in the software in use, concerns have been expressed about standardizing the software for PBPK modeling (Rowland et al. 2004). In the toxicology community, Berkeley Madonna, acslX, and R were the most commonly used software according to a survey in 2017 (Paini et al. 2017), but acslX was discontinued in 2015, and its usage has been decreasing. Programming in R for PBPK modeling is gaining popularity; however, because of the rapid advancement and frequent changes and updates in the R community, unless you are proficient in R programming and a faithful user in the R community, it is difficult for the rest of us to keep up.

Two PBPK simulation programs used in our laboratories, Berkeley Madonna and acslX, are briefly introduced here. Both programs are general-purpose differential equation solvers with high flexibility. The modeling process in each program follows the procedure of representing models graphically or in equations, compiling model equations into machine code, and reporting results. Berkeley Madonna is more affordable, easier to learn, more user-friendly, and requires less programming knowledge.

The critical components of a model in both Berkeley Madonna and acslX are the equations and statements that represent the parameter settings, model structure, integration method, and other related conditions. In Berkeley Madonna, the equations are not required to follow a particular order or structure. The equations will be automatically sorted into proper order for execution. For readability and ease to debug, however, coding in the following order is recommended: integration method and related conditions, parameters, parameter scaling, exposure conditions, and mass balance for each compartment. In the following sections, we first provide a general explanation of the blocks for a model written with ACSL. We then provide a detailed explanation of a PBPK model written with Berkeley Madonna. This seemingly preferential treatment of Berkeley Madonna is due to the fact that Berkeley Madonna is more affordable for students and easier to use. We believe that there is a higher likelihood that the readers of this book will be interested in starting their PBPK modeling experience with Berkeley Madonna.

In acslX, the model equations, saved in a CSL (Continuous Simulation Language) file, are organized to a specific structure with several blocks (AEgis Technologies Group, Huntsville, Alabama):

```
PROGRAM

    INITIAL
    Statements executed before the run begins.
    State variables do not contain the initial conditions yet.
    END

    DYNAMIC
        DERIVATIVE
        Statements to be integrated continuously.
        END

        DISCRETE
        Statements executed at discrete points in time.
        END
        Statements executed each communication interval.
    END

    TERMINAL
    Statements executed after the run terminates.
    END

END
```

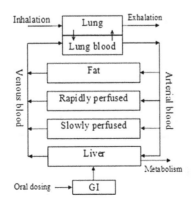

Figure 8.2   PBPK model structure for 1,1,1-trichloroethane in the rat. (From Lu et al. (2008).

Equations should be placed in the appropriate blocks; misplacement of equations may prevent the code from running or produce wrong results. In the DERIVATIVE block, however, the equations can be grouped in whatever way the modeler likes. Readers can refer to Thomas et al. (1996a), Easterling et al. (2000), and Fisher et al. (2020) for the codes in ACSL and Magnolia that are structurally very similar to those in acslX.

After a model code is executed, both Berkeley Madonna and acslX are amenable to *in silico* experimentation, including, but not limited to, tabulating and plotting simulation results, examining the effects of a parameter on model outputs, visual optimization, statistical optimization, sensitivity, and Monte Carlo analysis. In this regard, Berkeley Madonna offers a user-friendly interface such that those manipulations can be achieved by selection of the self-explanatory options from the tool menu. AcslX, however, requires some acquaintance with the specific command language which is a challenge to a new user. Also, while Berkeley Madonna is an ideal tool to learn and perform common PBPK analyses, one caveat is that its functionality is somewhat limited when it comes to more advanced analyses, such as MCMC simulation, global sensitivity analysis, and conversion of the PBPK model from computer code to a web-based PBPK interface, which will require more flexible tools, such as R (Li et al. 2019).

Explanation of an Example of Computer Code for a PBPK Model in Berkeley Madonna

A PBPK model code written in Berkeley Madonna is explained in detail in this section. The code simulates the exposure and pharmacokinetics in the rat of 1,1,1-trichloroethane, a volatile organic chemical, which is lipophilic and metabolized in the liver; detailed information can be found in Reitz et al. (1988) and in the original code in SimuSolv, kindly provided by Dr. Reitz. It should be noted that the transformation of the model code to Berkeley Madonna format was part of a contract from the EPA conducted in our laboratory at Colorado State University as described in Lu et al. (2008). Prior to explaining the code, we need to sequentially define the foundations on which the code is based: (1) exposure conditions, (2) PBPK model structure, and (3) necessary assumptions/simplifications and mass balance differential equations for all compartments.

Exposure conditions: Two exposure pathways, not taking place simultaneously, are involved in this case. At time 0, a rat is orally administered 1,1,1-trichloroethane water solution at the dose of 14.2 mg/kg body weight, or it starts inhaling 1,1,1-trichloroethane vapor at 150 ppm continuously for 6 hours. The time-course concentrations of 1,1,1-trichloroethane in the exhaled air and venous blood, respectively, are determined.

PBPK model structure: The model structure (Figure 8.2) is determined according to the exposure conditions and the pharmacokinetic characteristics of 1,1,1-trichloroethane.

As 1,1,1-trichloroethane is lipophilic and metabolized in the liver, the fat and liver are included in the model structure. The other organs and tissues have no individually distinct impacts on the pharmacokinetics and thus are lumped into rapidly and slowly perfused compartments. The lung/lung blood and GI compartments accommodate the inhalation and oral dosing exposures, respectively.

We assume that each of the compartments is homogeneous, that the chemical uptake in each tissue compartment is perfusion limited (i.e., the diffusion of the chemical into the tissue is rapid, and the rate-limiting step is the blood perfusion rate), and that 100% of the oral dose in the GI compartment is absorbed. The amount of change of 1,1,1-trichloroethane in an infinite small time interval (dt) in the fat (F) compartment can be expressed as

$$\frac{dAF}{dt} = QF \times (CA - CVF) = QF \times \left(CA - \frac{CF}{PF} \right), \tag{8.3}$$

where AF is the amount in fat, QF is the blood flow rate into fat, CA is the arterial blood concentration, and CVF is the concentration in the effluent blood from the fat, which is related to the fat concentration (CF) divided by a factor of fat partition coefficient (PF). Equation 8.3 can be applied to the rapidly (R) and slowly (S) perfused compartments by replacing the "F" with "R" and "S", respectively.

The differential equation for the liver is a little more complicated than Equation 8.3 because the absorption from the GI compartment and the metabolism should be considered therein:

$$\frac{dAL}{dt} = QL \times (CA - CVL) + \frac{dAB}{dt} - \frac{dAM}{dt}, \tag{8.4}$$

where dAB/dt represents the rate of absorption from the GI compartment into the liver via blood (B), and dAM/dt represents the rate of metabolism (M) which results in a negative change in the chemical amount in the liver.

The differential equation for the GI lumen is

$$\frac{dAGI}{dt} = -\frac{dAB}{dt} = -KAB \times AGI, \tag{8.5}$$

where AGI stands for the amount in the GI compartment, and KAB is the rate constant of absorption from the GI to the liver. The minus sign indicates that the amount left in the GI compartment decreases with time because of absorption.

The venous blood concentration, CV, can be expressed using an algebraic equation:

$$CV = (QF \times CVF + QL \times CVL + QR \times CVR + QS \times CVS)/QC, \tag{8.6}$$

where QC is the cardiac output. For the calculation of arterial blood concentration, CA, assumptions that a steady state in the lung is quickly reached upon inhalation, that the exhaled concentration is in equilibrium with CA, and that the chemical absorbed in the alveolar region are involved. In the blood flowing through the lung, the amount of change over time can be expressed as

$$\frac{dABlood}{dt} = QC \times (CV - CA) + QP \times \left(CIN - \frac{CA}{PB} \right), \tag{8.7}$$

where QP is pulmonary ventilation rate, CIN is the concentration inhaled, PB is blood:air partition coefficient, and CA/PB is the concentration exhaled. At steady state, dABlood/dt = 0, thus Equation 8.7 is reduced to

$$QC \times (CV - CA) + QP \times \left(CIN - \frac{CA}{PB} \right) = 0. \tag{8.8}$$

Solving Equation 8.8 for CA,

$$CA = \frac{QC \times CV + QP \times CIN}{QC + \frac{QP}{PB}}. \tag{8.9}$$

Now that the exposure conditions, model structure, and mass balance equations are clarified, let us turn to the Berkeley Madonna code for this case. Like a typical PBPK model code, the 1,1,1-trichloroethane code includes documentation, integration method, parameters, mass balance equations, and error-check equations. We will go through it line by line. For ease to read, the code contents are in highlighted text boxes, followed by explanations. Please note that our explanations are relatively brief to avoid the formation of a lengthy chapter; they are not meant to replace a PBPK modeling course/workshop.

{1,1,1-Trichloroethane code originally supplied by Dr. Reitz. Converted into a Berkeley Madonna form for the 2005 Colorado State University Beginner's PBPK Workshop by Yasong LU and Ray Yang. 7/16/2005. Reference: Reitz, R.H., McDougal, J.N., Himmelstein, M.W., Nolan, R.J., Schumann, A.M. 1988 Physiologically based pharmacokinetic modeling with methylchloroform: Implications for interspecies, high dose/low dose, and dose route extrapolations. *Toxicol. Appl. Pharmacol.* 95:185–199}

These sentences are a part of the documentation of this code. Different from the other components, documentation is not essential for code execution. However, it records important information pertinent to the code, e.g., the purpose(s) of the modeling, experimental conditions being simulated, date and author(s) of the code, history of the modifications to the code, rationale of the modeling structure and parameter value selections, and explanation of the terminology in the code. Documentation is critical for model code maintenance. Therefore, it is always a good practice to provide documentation as thoroughly as possible. In a Berkeley Madonna code, documentation is composed of the text strings confined in paired curly brackets or preceded by semicolons (see the following section).

METHOD STIFF

The METHOD statement defines the numerical integration method for model calculation. For PBPK modeling, STIFF is a frequently used method that automatically finds the appropriate integration intervals over time. See the section titled "Numerical Integration" for more details on numerical integration methods.

STARTTIME = 0
STOPTIME=12

The STARTTIME and STOPTIME statements define the starting and ending times of the simulation. The former is usually 0; the latter varies depending on the experimental duration.

```
{Physiological Parameters}
{Constants set for the rat}

  BW = 0.233                    ;Mean body weight (kg); Reitz code.
  QCC = 15.                     ;Cardiac output constant [L/(hr*kg^0.74)]; Reitz 1988.
  QPC = 15.                     ;Alveolar ventilation constant [L/(hr*kg^0.74)]; Reitz 1988.

{Blood flow fractions}
  QLC = 0.24                    ;Fractional blood flow to liver; Reitz 1988.
  QFC = 0.05                    ;Fractional blood flow to fat; Reitz 1988.
  QSC = 0.18                    ;Fractional blood flow to slowly perfused; Reitz 1988.
  QRC = 1.0-(QFC+QSC+QLC)       ;Fractional blood flow to rapidly perfused; Reitz 1988.

{Volume fractions}
  VLC = 0.04                    ;Fraction liver tissue; Reitz 1988.
  VFC = 0.07                    ;Fraction fat tissue; Reitz 1988.
  RC = 0.05                     ;Fraction richly perfused tissues; Reitz 1988.
  VSC = 0.91-VLC-VFC-VRC        ;Fraction slowly perfused; Reitz 1988.
```

This block defines the physiological parameters necessary for the modeling. Each parameter statement is followed by a semicolon and text string (documentation) explaining the meaning of the parameter symbol and the source of the parameter value. These statements, either following a semicolon or in between curly brackets, are for our own record or information, and they are ignored by Berkeley Madonna. The relatively strange-looking unit L/(hr*kg^0.74) for QCC and others is for allometric extrapolation between different species, usually following a power function (indicated here by ^0.74) of the body weight.

```
{Chemical specific parameters}
{Partition coefficients}
  PB = 5.76                     ;Blood/air; Reitz 1988.
  PLA = 8.6                     ;Liver/air; Reitz 1988.
  PFA = 263.                    ;Fat/air; Reitz 1988.
  PRA = 8.6                     ;Richly perfused/air; Reitz 1988.
  PSA = 3.15                    ;Slowly perfused/air; Reitz 1988.
```

```
PL=PLA/PB
PF=PFA/PB
PR=PRA/PB
PS=PSA/PB
```

The tissue:air partition coefficients were experimentally measured; they are divided by blood:air partition coefficient to convert to tissue:blood partition coefficients, which govern the distribution of the chemical in each compartment.

```
{Metabolism; saturable; estimated from Schumann data and Reitz drinking water study}
VMAXC = 0.419        ;Capacity of saturable metabolism [mg/(hr*kg^0.7)]; Reitz 1988.
KM = 5.75            ;Affinity of saturable metabolism (mg/L); Reitz 1988.
```

These lines define the Michaelis-Menten kinetic parameters for 1,1,1-trichloroethane metabolism in the liver.

```
{Scaled parameters}
QC = QCC*BW^0.74       ;Cardiac output (L/hr); Reitz 1988.
QP = QPC*BW^0.74       ;Alveolar ventilation (L/hr); Reitz 1988.
VF = VFC*BW            ;Fat volume (L)
VL = VLC*BW            ;Liver volume (L)
VR = VRC*BW            ;Richly Perfused volume (L)
VS = VSC*BW            ;Slowly Perfused volume (L)
QL = QLC*QC            ;Liver blood flow (L/hr)
QF = QFC*QC            ;Fat blood flow (L/hr)
QR = QRC*QC            ;Richly Perfused blood flow (L/hr)
QS = QSC*QC            ;Slowly Perfused blood flow (L/hr)
VMAX = VMAXC*BW^0.7    ;Capacity of saturable metabolism (mg/hr); Reitz 1988.
```

In this block, the physiological parameters and maximum metabolic velocity are scaled by the body weight.

```
{Exposure conditions: oral dosing}
BDOSE = 14.2          ;Oral bolus dose rate (mg/kg)
KA = 1.25             ;Rat GI absorption rate constant (/hr); Reitz 1988.
ODOSE = BDOSE*BW      ;Oral bolus dose (mg)
```

These statements define the oral exposure dose and the GI absorption rate constant.

```
{Exposure conditions: inhalation}
TCHNG = 6.                              ;Length of inhalation exposure (hrs)
   ;Unit conversion: from ppm to mg/L; often necessary for inhalation exposure scenarios.
MW = 133.5                              ;Molecular weight (g/mol)
CONC = 0.0                              ;Inhaled concentration (ppm)
CIN0 = CONC*MW/24450.                   ;Convert ppm to mg/L
CIN = IF TIME<TCHNG THEN CIN0 ELSE 0    ;Turn off inhalation after exposure
                                         interval
```

The inhalation exposure conditions are defined in this block. Two features here deserve some elaboration: (1) Unit conversion. In inhalation experiments, chemical concentrations are frequently expressed in parts per million (ppm), which must be converted to mg/L or the like for further calculations. The theoretical basis of the unit conversion is the ideal gas law. (2) The IF-THEN-ELSE statement. This statement is used to change a parameter under certain condition(s). In this case, the inhalation exposure is turned off when the TIME hits six hours. Please note that although this code accommodates both oral and inhalation exposure, they do not coexist unless there is a specific experiment with double-dosing by both oral gavage and inhalation routes. Thus, the inhaled concentration (CONC) is set as 0 here to avoid the undesirable double-dosing; when running the code for inhalation, we can turn off the oral dosing and give CONC an appropriate value.

At this point, all parameters have been defined in the code. The following sections demonstrate how the chemical amount and/or concentration in each compartment are calculated. For each compartment, there is a mass balance differential equation coupled with a statement (INIT) defining the initial value of the amount in the compartment, as well as commanding Berkeley Madonna to perform integration from this initial value. The notation AS' is one way in Berkeley Madonna to express dAS/dt. When necessary, the concentration in a compartment is calculated as the ratio of the amount therein over the compartment volume.

```
{Chemical distribution - mass balances}
;AS = Amount in Slowly Perfused (mg)
  AS' = QS*(CA-CVS)         ;Mass balance differential equation.
  INIT AS = 0.             ;Initial amount in slowly perfused.
  CS = AS/VS              ;Concentration in slowly perfused, mg/L.
  CVS = CS/PS             ;Effluent blood conc, in equilibrium with tissue conc, mg/L.
```

These lines calculate the amount and concentration in the slowly perfused compartment and the concentration in the venous blood flowing out of that compartment.

```
;AR = Amount in Rapidly Perfused (mg)
  AR' = QR*(CA-CVR)        ;Mass balance in rapidly perfused
  INIT AR = 0.            ;Initial amount in rapidly perfused
  CR = AR/VR             ;Conc in rapidly perfused, mg/L
  CVR = CR/PR            ;Effluent blood conc, mg/L

;AF = Amount in fat (mg)
  AF' = QF*(CA-CVF)        ;Mass balance in fat
  INIT AF = 0.            ;Initial amount in fat
  CF = AF/VF             ;Conc in fat, mg/L
  CVF = CF/PF            ;Effluent blood conc, mg/L
```

The chemical amount and concentration in the fat and the rapidly perfused compartment are calculated in the same way as for the slowly perfused compartment.

```
;AL = Amount in liver (mg)
  AL' = QL*(CA-CVL) - AM' + AO'  ;Mass balance in liver
  INIT AL = 0.            ;Initial amount in liver
  CL = AL/VL             ;Conc in fat, mg/L
  CVL = CL/PL            ;Effluent blood conc, mg/L

;AM = Amount metabolized (mg)
  AM' = VMAX*CVL/(KM+CVL)   ;Rate of metabolism, mg/L
  INIT AM = 0.            ;Initial amount metabolized, mg
```

```
;AO' = Rate of input to liver from stomach after oral bolus (mg)
   AO' = KA*MR                    ;Rate of GI absorption, mg/L
   INIT AO = 0.                   ;Initial value of absorbed amount, mg
```

This block shows the calculations for the liver compartment. Different from the fat and the rapidly and slowly perfused compartments, the mass balance in the liver includes metabolism and absorption from the GI compartment. To avoid confusion for beginners, it is prudent to point out that while we use KA to denote absorption rate constant, in an earlier equation (Equation 8.5) KAB was used. As long as the constants are clearly defined, and within one model all constants are consistent, a modeler is free to write his/her code. However, it is always a good idea to follow a clear, consistent "penmanship" and writing format in computer coding as well.

```
;MR = Amount remaining in stomach after oral bolus (mg)
;First-order absorption
   MR' = -KA*MR                   ;Absorption rate, mg/L
   INIT MR = ODOSE                ;Initial value of the amount in stomach = given dose, mg
```

These lines demonstrate the calculation of the amount in the GI compartment.

```
;Blood concentrations (mg/L)
   CV = (QL*CVL+QS*CVS+QF*CVF+QR*CVR)/QC  ;Venous blood conc, mg/L
   CA = (QC*CV+QP*CIN)/(QC+QP/PB)         ;Arterial blood conc, mg/L
   CEX = CA/PB                            ;Conc leaving the alveolar region, mg/L
   CEXMGL=0.667*CEX+0.333*CIN             ;Conc in exhaled air, mg/L
   CEXPPM = CEXMGL*24450./MW              ;mg/L converted to ppm, for
                                             comparing with data
```

The venous and arterial blood concentrations are calculated algebraically. By convention, alveolar respiration has been assumed to account for two-thirds of total respiration (Ramsey and Andersen 1984), hence the concentration in the exhaled air is a weighted average of the inhaled concentration (CIN) and the concentration leaving the alveolar region (CEX).

```
Error check
;Total amount of chemical delivered should equal to the amount calculated by the code.

   ;Amount inhaled
   AIN' = QP*CIN
   INIT AIN = 0.
   ;Amount exhaled
   AEX' = QP*CEX
   INIT AEX = 0.

   ;TOTAL = Total amount delivered
   TOTAL = ODOSE + AIN - AEX
   ;Calculated = Total amount calculated
   Calculated = AF+AL+AS+AR+AM+MR
   ERROR = (TOTAL - Calculated)/(TOTAL+1E-30)*100   ;ERROR should be close to 0.
```

This final block is set to check the potential error(s) in the code (i.e., Mass Balance Check). A small value (1E-30) is added to the denominator in the ERROR equation to avoid a situation where the denominator might end up being zero. If the total amount of chemical delivered experimentally is different from the summed amount in all compartments and eliminated, it would suggest that there is an error(s) in the code. This error-check tool, however, cannot uncover all errors in a code; thorough examination of a code is strongly encouraged.

Numerical Integration

Numerical integration is the basis for computer simulation in PBPK modeling, as opposed to finding an exact solution. In essence, it is an approach to approximate very closely the true solution of a calculation much the same way as we approximate an area under the curve (AUC) using the trapezoidal rule. In this latter case, the smaller the trapezoids (i.e., the step size), the more accurate the approximation of the AUC. For a more detailed discussion on the concept of "infinity" (e.g., using smaller and smaller stepsizes) in calculus, the readers are referred to Strogatz (2020). In Berkeley Madonna, there are six numerical integration methods available for use. They are Euler's Method, Runge-Kutta 2, Runge-Kutta 4, Auto-Stepsize, Rosenbrock (stiff), and Inverse Euler. Detailed explanation of these methods is beyond the scope of this chapter. We will simply point out two things here: First, a very popular method for approximating solutions to first-order initial value problems is the "fourth-order Runga-Kutta method" (i.e., Runge-Kutta 4 in Berkeley Madonna; Runga-Kutta refers to two German mathematicians). Second, for some differential equations, application of standard numerical integration methods such as the Euler and Runge-Kutta methods exhibit instability in the solutions. This "instability" or "difficult-behavior" in the equation is described as **stiffness** and is often caused by the presence of different time scales in the underlying problem. Stiff problems are ubiquitous in many areas of science, including biology. One of the methods in Berkeley Madonna, Rosenbrock (stiff), is specifically to be used for the stiff problems.

Sensitivity and Uncertainty

A PBPK model provides pharmacokinetic profiles of a chemical given physiological, biochemical, and thermodynamic parameters. For various reasons, it is valuable to identify the sensitivity of an output to the model parameters and to measure the effect of the variability or uncertainty in a parameter on model outputs. These evaluations involve sensitivity analysis and uncertainty analysis.

Sensitivity Analysis

The sensitivity analysis examines the influence of model parameters on outputs. Conceptually, there are two kinds of sensitivity analyses in mathematical modeling: local and global (Blower and Dowlatabadi 1994; Nestorov et al. 1997; Saltelli et al. 1999). The local sensitivity refers to the response of model outputs to the perturbation of a single parameter (i.e., the one-at-a-time sampling method), whereas the global sensitivity refers to the response of outputs to the simultaneous alterations in all parameters. The local sensitivity analysis is commonly used in the PBPK community (Clewell et al. 1994; Easterling et al. 2000; Emond et al. 2004; Evans and Andersen 2000; Evans et al. 1994; Sweeney et al. 2003). For a more recent discussion on local sensitivity analysis, please see Fisher et al. (2020). In recent years, several groups have started to apply global sensitivity analysis in PBPK models (Hsieh et al. 2018; Lumen et al. 2015; McNally et al. 2011).

The sensitivity of an output to a parameter can be quantitatively reflected by a sensitivity coefficient (SC). Considering an output R is a function of a parameter x, i.e., R = F(x), then

$$SC = \frac{F(x + \Delta x) - F(x)}{\Delta x}, \tag{8.10}$$

where Δx is a perturbation in x. When the Δx is sufficiently small, the SC is a partial derivative of R with respect to x, thus Equation (8.10) can be reformulated into

$$SC = \frac{\partial R}{\partial x}. \tag{8.11}$$

Since parameters and outputs have distinct units and magnitudes, the SC should be properly normalized for inter-parameter or inter-output comparisons. Thus,

$$SC = \frac{\dfrac{\partial R}{R}}{\dfrac{\partial x}{x}} = \frac{\partial \ln R}{\partial \ln x}, \tag{8.12}$$

where SC can be recognized as the sensitivity of the logarithm of an output R (lnR) to the logarithm of a parameter x (lnx); hence, it is also known as log-normalized sensitivity coefficient (LSC). Alternatively, SC can be presented as a normalized sensitivity coefficient (NSC) using Equation (8.13).

$$NSC = \frac{\frac{\Delta R}{R}}{\frac{\Delta x}{x}} = \left(\frac{\Delta R^*}{R} \frac{x}{\Delta x} \right) \tag{8.13}$$

An LSC or NSC identifies the percentage change in output due to a percentage change in a parameter. It has been suggested that LSCs and NSCs should be in the range of –1 to 1; a value substantially beyond the range indicates that the error in a parameter is greatly amplified in the output and hence implies undesirable feature(s) in the model (Clewell et al. 1994).

The utilities of sensitivity analysis include (1) identifying the most sensitive parameters for an output, which helps in understanding a pharmacokinetic behavior of interest (Emond et al. 2004; Evans and Andersen 2000); (2) evaluating the necessity of carefully measuring unknown parameters; if the output of interest is sensitive to an unknown parameter, precise measurement of this parameter is required; (3) directing targeted experimentation and improve study design. For example, sensitivity analysis may suggest optimal exposure conditions, necessary data to be collected, and the frequency of data collection (Evans et al. 1994; Schlosser 1994).

Uncertainty Analysis

The term "uncertainty" is often used along with variability although they are distinct concepts. Uncertainty is defined as the possible error in estimating a true value of a parameter; it is a defect in knowledge and can be reduced by improving experimental methods (Clewell and Andersen 1996; McLanahan et al. 2012). Variability, however, refers to the difference of a parameter among individuals; it is a fact that can be measured but not be changed (Clewell and Andersen 1996; McLanahan et al. 2012).

For the purpose of risk assessment, average pharmacokinetic information is not very useful because it does not take into account the uncertainty and variability of the parameters (Clewell and Andersen 1996). Uncertainty analysis measures the effects of uncertainty and variability in model parameters on predicted pharmacokinetics. Monte Carlo simulation is a common technique for uncertainty analysis. Prior to PBPK simulation, the statistical distributions of all parameters are determined. A set of the parameters is sampled from those distributions using Monte Carlo simulation. These parameters are then input into a PBPK model, which is executed and generates a set of outputs. Then another set of parameters is sampled, the PBPK model is re-executed, and the outputs are recorded. This process is repeated many times (e.g., 1,000) until many sets of outputs are generated. The outputs are statistically analyzed to get the means and variances. As such, the effects of the uncertainty and variability of parameters on outputs are measured (Blower and Dowlatabadi 1994; Chou and Lin 2021; Clewell and Andersen 1996; Hetrick et al. 1991; Li et al. 2018; Thomas et al. 1996b; Yang et al. 2021). Recently, a more advanced statistical approach, Bayesian analysis, has been applied in PBPK modeling to explore the effects of uncertainty and variability in model parameters (Bois 2001; Chou and Lin 2019; David et al. 2006; Jonsson 2001; Jonsson and Johanson 2001a; Marino et al. 2006; Weijs et al. 2013). This approach can separate uncertainty from variability. More information on the Bayesian approach is introduced later in the section titled "An Example of Application of PBPK Modeling in Dichloromethane Risk Assessment and Its Recent Development in Bayesian Population Approach."

PBPK MODELS FOR CHEMICAL INTERACTIONS (MULTIPLE CHEMICAL INTERACTIVE PBPK MODELS) IN CHEMICAL MIXTURES

Since humans are rarely, if ever, exposed to a single chemical, a key feature of PBPK modeling is that it can be used to integrate information on toxicological interactions. The most ideal and scientifically defensible data requirement for establishing an interactive PBPK model is that a validated PBPK model is available for each component chemical in the mixture. Furthermore, there should be many pharmacokinetic data sets in laboratory animals as well as in humans available for each of these component chemicals. We use the term "interactive PBPK model," which means a PBPK model that has the capability to simulate interactions between and among chemicals in a mixture. The interactive PBPK model is then built on the basis of known pharmacokinetic interactions. For instance, one chemical may inhibit the biotransformation of other mixture components and vice versa. The individual PBPK models may then be linked together at the liver compartment by introducing competitive (or other) inhibition terms in the mass balance differential equation. In our opinion, the application of PBPK modeling to toxicological interactions of chemical mixtures is necessary in cumulative risk assessment. However, this area is very complex and it is still an emerging field. For a more thorough discussion, the readers are referred to a chapter on PBPK modeling of chemical mixtures (Yang and Andersen 2005), the earlier version of this chapter, particularly on biochemical reaction network modeling (Yang and Lu 2007), as well as some of the more recent books and publications in the applications of computational methodologies to toxicology and risk assessment (Ekins 2007; Reisfeld and Mayeno 2012; Yang 2018; Yang et al. 2010). It should be emphasized here that PBPK modeling will only handle part of the chemical mixture issue in cumulative risk assessment; namely, the pharmacokinetic interactions at the whole body level. It is necessary to integrate PBPK modeling with other computational methodologies to more fully address the chemical mixture issue in cumulative risk assessment (Ekins 2007; Mayeno et al. 2005; Raies and Bajic 2016; Reisfeld and Mayeno 2012; Yang 2018; Yang et al. 2010).

Pioneering efforts in the PBPK modeling of more complex chemical mixtures were from a research group led by Professor Kannan Krishnan, Université de Montréal, Canada. Earlier work from this group concentrated on interactions and PBPK modeling between two chemicals (Pelekis and Krishnan 1997; Tardif et al. 1993; Tardif et al. 1995). As progress was made, these investigators began to build up the mixtures and devoted their effort to PBPK modeling of more and more complex chemical mixtures (Haddad et al. 1999; Haddad et al. 2000; Tardif et al. 1997). These investigators have successfully carried out PBPK modeling on the pharmacokinetic interactions on chemical mixtures involving up to five chemicals (Haddad et al. 2000; Krishnan et al. 2002); however, they advanced the hypothesis that pharmacokinetic interactions of complex chemical mixtures, regardless of the number of components, may be predicted based on the PBPK modeling of binary mixtures of the component chemicals (Haddad et al. 2000; Krishnan et al. 2002). According to their concept, thus, PBPK models for mixtures of any complexity can be created, as long as the quantitative information on the mechanism of interaction for each interacting pair (e.g., competitive inhibition rate constant) is available (Krishnan et al. 2002).

Applying the same approach created by Krishnan and coworkers, investigators at Colorado State University studied PBPK modeling of a ternary mixture of trichloroethylene (TCE), tetrachloroethylene (PERC), and 1,1,1-trichloroethane (methyl chloroform, MC) in rats and humans (Dobrev et al. 2001, 2002). Furthermore, Dennison et al. (2003) characterized the pharmacokinetics of gasoline, a very complex mixture, in rats using an integrated PBPK modeling and lumping approach. The PBPK model tracks selected target components with known toxicities (benzene, toluene, ethylbenzene, o-xylene, and n-hexane) and a lumped chemical group representing all non-target components. Competitive inhibition was the principal mechanism of pharmacokinetic interactions among these five selected target single chemicals and a pseudo-chemical from the lumped components. Computer simulation results from the six-chemical interaction model matched well with gas uptake pharmacokinetic experimental data from single chemicals, five-chemical mixture, and the two blends of gasoline. The PBPK model analyses indicated that metabolism of individual components was inhibited up to 27% during the six-hour gas uptake experiments of gasoline exposures.

The integration of pharmacokinetic and pharmacodynamic (or toxicokinetic or toxicodynamic) interactions based on known mechanisms into an interactive PBPK model or other biologically based computational models is an important contribution to risk assessment (Dennison et al. 2003; Dobrev et al. 2001, 2002; Fisher et al. 2020; Krishnan et al. 2002; Pelekis and Krishnan 1997; Peters 2012; Reddy et al. 2005; Tardif et al. 1993; Tardif et al. 1995) and probable clinical applications regarding combination therapy or polypharmacy (Lyons 2014; 2019). As science advances in toxicology and risk assessment, the integration of genomics and other omics, as well as high throughput in vitro assays coupled with in silico methods as advocated by Tox21 (NRC 2007), or as illustrated by the Halifax Project (Carcinogenesis 2015), would expand the complexity further in the area of toxicology and risk assessment of chemical mixtures and multiple stressors (House et al. 2017; Hsieh et al. 2021; Lin and Lin 2020). Along this line of thinking, the possible application of artificial intelligence (AI) as briefly discussed toward the end of this chapter would probably have a real potential to reduce the complexities for risk assessors interested in chemical mixtures/multiple stressors.

AN EXAMPLE OF APPLICATION OF PBPK MODELING IN DICHLOROMETHANE RISK ASSESSMENT AND ITS RECENT DEVELOPMENT IN BAYESIAN POPULATION APPROACH

Dichloromethane (DCM, methylene chloride) is a volatile organic solvent used in decaffeinated coffee, in the textile and pharmaceutical industries, as well as in paint stripping and metal degreasing. Animal studies in the early to mid-1980s implicated carcinogenic potentials of DCM in mice (NTP 1986; Serota et al. 1986a, 1986b). The initial cancer risk assessment, carried out by the US EPA, was based on the administered dose from drinking water studies in mice (Serota et al. 1986a, 1986b), and the exposure concentrations in inhalation studies (NTP 1986). In 1987, Andersen et al. calculated internal dose (i.e., target tissue dose) using PBPK modeling based on mechanisms of biotransformation and incorporated PBPK modeling into the cancer risk assessment process. Their conceptual PBPK model for DCM is shown in Figure 8.3 and it is quite similar to the PBPK models discussed earlier in Figures 8.1 and 8.2.

Two metabolic processes were considered for both the liver and the lungs: the oxidative pathway involving Cytochrome P450 (CYP) 2E1 (AM1L and AM1LU in Figure 8.3), which, being a high affinity and low capacity enzyme, follows Michaelis-Menten saturable (nonlinear) kinetics, and a glutathione S-transferase (GST) pathway (AM2L and AM2LU in Figure 8.3), which, being a low affinity but high capacity enzyme, follows first-order (linear) kinetics. Reactive metabolites formed from these respective processes were suggested to be formyl chloride and chloromethyl glutathione based on mechanistic understanding. The PBPK model was constructed and calibrated using data sets from a series of gas uptake pharmacokinetic studies conducted in their own laboratory (Andersen et al. 1987), and model validation was carried out using four different sets of data under a variety of experimental conditions, including human experiments, as well as studies published by different investigators (Angelo et al. 1984). Using the resulting DCM PBPK models for mice and humans, Andersen et al. (1987) did extensive computer simulations in mice under the experimental conditions of cancer bioassay studies, as well as extrapolations to humans under similar

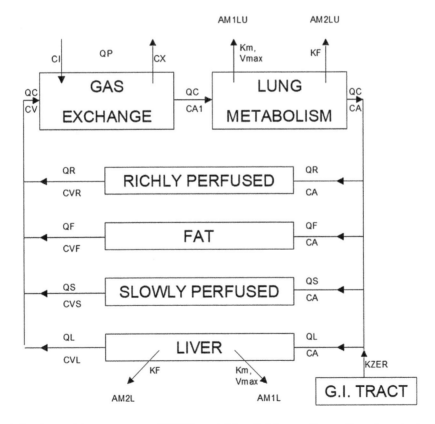

Figure 8.3 A graphic or conceptual PBPK model for dichloromethane. (based on Andersen et al., *Toxicol. Appl. Pharmacol.*, 87: 185–205, 1987.)

exposure conditions. Based on their calculated internal dose (target tissue dose) and in comparison with the tumor incidence data from the cancer bioassays (NTP 1986; Serota et al. 1986a, 1986b), they concluded that the GST pathway is the critical one producing carcinogenic metabolites. Furthermore, based on their analyses, they suggested that the conventional linear-extrapolation risk analyses conducted by the US EPA greatly overestimated (by about 140 to 170-fold) the risk of DCM in humans. In many ways, the Andersen et al. study (Andersen et al. 1987) created a scientific revolution in the risk assessment arena. Continued advancement of science in this area in the direction of considering populations led to the following important contributions: (1) genetic polymorphism of glutathione-S-transferase theta 1 (GSTT1) and extrahepatic CYP2E1 metabolism in different human populations in relation to risk assessment (El-Masri et al. 1999; Sweeney et al. 2004); (2) the application of Monte Carlo simulation with PBPK modeling to address the issue of variability, not only in DCM (Clewell 1995; Portier and Kaplan 1989; Thomas et al. 1996b) but also in other chemicals (El-Masri et al. 1996; Thomas et al. 1996a); (3) the advancement of Bayesian population PBPK modeling and the utilization of MCMC simulation and their integration into the human risk assessment (Bernillon and Bois 2000; Bois 2001; Bois et al. 1996a; Bois et al. 1996b; Bois et al. 2002; David et al. 2006; Jonsson 2001; Jonsson and Johanson 2001a, 2001b, 2003; Marino et al. 2006); and (4) the incorporation of the state-of-the-science into their Toxicology Review for DCM (US EPA 2011) for supporting their latest IRIS risk assessment of DCM. Details of the entire advancement of human risk assessment on DCM up to about 2015 are available in Yang et al. (2015). It is worth mentioning that recently a PBPK model for DCM has been applied to integrate with transcriptomics data to determine the role of hypoxia and altered circadian signaling in DCM carcinogenicity in mouse lungs and liver (Andersen et al. 2017). Recent advancement in the evaluation of carcinogenicity of DCM in mice, rats, hamsters, and humans has been summarized in Dekant et al. (2021).

For general knowledge on the Bayesian approach and decision-making, please consult McGrayne (2011) and Howson and Urbach (2006).

THE POTENTIAL APPLICATIONS OF AI TO PBPK MODELING

In the last ten years or so, the applications of AI in all areas, including medicine, have advanced at a rapid pace principally because of the development of deep learning artificial neural networks (de Ponteves 2019; Topol 2019). In the area of clinical applications of AI, for instance, successes have been reported in radiology/neurology, pathology, dermatology, ophthalmology, gastroenterology, and cardiology (Topol 2019). In many, if not all, clinical applications, comparisons were made between expert (i.e., doctors) diagnoses vs. computer (i.e., machine) diagnoses based on the vast amount of information available to them. As might be expected, the machines are overtaking the humans in terms of accuracy gradually (Topol 2019). Since the process of PBPK modeling is similar, in many ways, to clinical diagnoses involving expert opinions and decision-making, it is likely that machine learning and the development of layers of artificial neural network may be applied, sooner or later, to the area of PBPK modeling. We are aware of the "one-second" rule advocated by Andrew Ng in the feasibility of machine learning (online class on "AI for Everyone" by Coursera accessed by the lead author in January 2021). We believe that as the computational technology continues to advance, different layers of artificial neural networks will be developed for the steps of PBPK modeling, including search and review/evaluation of the literature, the building of the PBPK models based on the integration of physiology, anatomy, biochemistry, chemistry, physics, pharmacology, toxicology, etc., of the chemical(s) and biological systems of interest, as well as the computer simulations of the ADME of the chemical(s) in the bodies.

While direct applications of AI to develop PBPK models are still rare, AI technologies have been applied to predict chemical ADME properties, including solubility, clearance, permeabilities, metabolic stability, and drug-drug interactions (Bhhatarai et al. 2019; Göller et al. 2020; Wenzel et al. 2019; Wu et al. 2019). These ADME properties can, in turn, be incorporated into a PBPK model of the chemical to help develop a mechanistic PBPK model. For example, in a recent study, machine learning methods were used to construct a regression model to predict the time-dependent in vitro dissolution profiles based on a data set consisting of 674 dissolution profiles of various drugs in solid dispersion formulation (Gao et al. 2021). The predicted in vitro dissolution profile was input to a developed PBPK model to predict the in vivo pharmacokinetic profile of an amorphous solid dispersion formulation of the drug vemurafenib, and the model simulation results correlated with reported experimental data adequately. By integrating AI methods with QSAR modeling methods, ADME properties of a family of structurally similar chemicals or nanoparticles can also be predicted (Hessler and Baringhaus 2018; Singh et al. 2020), thereby facilitating the development of the so-called generic PBPK model for a group of chemicals or substances (i.e., read-across) to facilitate screening and evaluation of the pharmacokinetic profiles of compounds in a high-throughput manner.

Besides direct incorporation of ADME properties predicted with AI-assisted technologies into a PBPK model, AI methods can also be used to analyze plasma and tissue concentration data (either measured experimentally or predicted using a PBPK model) to get insights into the physicochemical or biochemical properties of the modeled substance with the target tissue dosimetry, thereby helping design the optimal drug formulation. For instance, Lazarovits et al. (2019) administered gold nanoparticles into mice via tail vein injection, and serum and tissue samples were collected at multiple time points (i.e., 1, 2, 4, 8, and 24 hours) following injection. In this study, concentrations of gold nanoparticles in serum and tissues were measured using inductively coupled plasma mass spectrometry (ICP-MS); proteins that were bound on the surface of gold nanoparticles at different time points were stripped off, and proteomic profiles were analyzed with liquid chromatography with tandem mass spectrometry (LC-MS/MS). The authors then built an artificial neural network model with the proteomic data as the input layers and the tissue concentrations of gold nanoparticles as the output layers. This study demonstrated the possibility of using AI technologies to help predict nanoparticle behavior in the body (Lazarovits et al. 2019). In a more recent study, a generic PBPK model was developed to simulate the delivery efficiency of different nanoparticles to the tumor tissue in mice (Cheng et al. 2020). The model was trained with 376 data sets of different types of nanoparticles. Traditional linear multivariate regression analysis was initially performed to identify the potential relationship between physicochemical properties of nanoparticles (e.g., size, shape, and Zeta potential) and the tumor deliver efficiency, but the results were suboptimal with determination coefficients between predicted versus observed data somewhere between 0.4 and 0.6 depending on the type of nanoparticles (Cheng et al. 2020). However, this data set provides a basis to apply AI approaches such as artificial neural network modeling to determine the relationship between physicochemical properties and tumor delivery efficiencies of nanoparticles, where the tumor delivery efficiencies were estimated from the generic PBPK model. This analysis is ongoing in the laboratory of Dr. Zhoumeng Lin, one of the authors of this chapter, at Kansas State University and, more recently, the University of Florida. For general knowledge about artificial neural network modeling, readers are referred to Baskin (2018).

The current applications of machine learning and AI methods to the area of PBPK modeling and analysis are mainly to support drug discovery and development. The authors believe that the same principles and technologies can be applied to PBPK modeling of environmental chemicals to support human health risk assessment.

BOX 8.1   BIOAVAILABILITY: AN INDEPENDENT VARIABLE IN RISK ASSESSMENT

Michael Gallo

Hazard of environmental xenobiotics is generally considered to be the function of toxicity of an agent and exposure. Risk is a hazard as a function of ameliorating factors. Bioavailability is one factor that is often overlooked or minimized in risk characterization.

Dioxin (2,3,7,8-tetrachlorodibenzo-p-dioxin) a by-product of the manufacture of the herbicide 2,4,5-T (a component of Agent Orange) and the antimicrobial hexachlorophene, is one of the most toxic man-made chemicals known. The toxicity of dioxin in laboratory animals varies by species (guinea pigs being most susceptible) and strains of mice (varying in susceptibility by three orders of magnitude), induces a TCDD syndrome that ranges from a wasting syndrome, immunotoxicity, and death in guinea pigs (most sensitive to dioxin toxicity) to asymptomatic induction of xenobiotic metabolizing enzymes in DBA mice (one of the least sensitive). Importantly, TCDD is a promoter of cancers in rats and mice in the ug/kg body weight range. The most prevalent sign of dioxin toxicity in chemical plant workers and Agent Orange–exposed Vietnam veterans is persistent chloracne.

Two of the most contaminated sites in the United States were in Times Beach, Missouri, and Newark, New Jersey. The Newark contamination resulted from the manufacturing of chlorinated phenolic compounds for decades. Contamination of soils occurred from the release of aqueous residue waste on the site, which was built on clean fill and road surface waste, while the Times Beach contamination resulted from a mixture of automobile waste oil and still bottoms from a hexachlorophene plant sprayed on a sandy loam soil followed by a flood that resulted in widespread surface contamination.

The initial risk assessments used the assumption of 85% bioavailability based on estimates from studies of Times Beach soil (McConnell et al. 1984). The 2,3,7,8-TCDD concentration in Newark (2,200 ppb) was ~2.5 times that of Times Beach (950 ppb) as measured after exhaustive Soxhlet extraction of soil samples while simple solvent extraction showed < 2.5 ppb from Newark and ~770 ppb from Times Beach. Based on these data, we hypothesized that soil matrix affects bioavailability of dioxin (Umbreit et al., 1986).

In a series of studies conducted in guinea pigs, we dosed animals (4m+4f/group) orally under light anesthesia via stomach tube as follows: corn oil control (a); decontaminated soil(b)** contaminated soil from Newark 3 ug/kg (c), 6 ug/kg (d), 12 ug/kg (e); decontaminated soil+6 ug/kg(f); and TCDD in corn oil 6 ug/kg (g). Signs for TCDD toxicity All animals were observed for signs of toxicity for 60 days. In the corn oil control group and decontaminated soil groups (a, b) and the contaminated soil groups (c–e), there were no signs of TCDD toxicity. However, in groups (f) and (g), most animals showed signs of toxicity, and 75% died within a month after dosing.

In a subsequent study, animals (4m+4f/group) were dosed with decontaminated soil +6 ug/kg (A), contaminated soil 12 ug/kg (B), or decontaminated soil (C) and observed for 60 days at which time all surviving animals were euthanized and livers taken for TCDD analysis (groups B and C). Livers from group (A) animals were collected at autopsy at time of death during the study. TCDD levels in livers samples for Groups A, B, and C were 18,000 ppt, 90 ppt, and 0 ppt, respectively.

The estimated bioavailability from Umbreit et al. (1986) is approximately 0.5% and from McConnell et al. (1984) is approximately 85%. This is a remarkable difference and emphasizes the point that *in determining bioavailability of nonvolatile chemicals from complex environmental matrices, one must consider (1)bioassays to determine potential toxic/pharmacologic effects of exposure, (2) tissue analyses for the compound of interest, (3) comparison of a simple solvent extraction to an exhaustive Soxhlet extraction (4) elucidating the constituents of the complex matrix and (5) determining the duration during which the chemicals have been absorbed within the matrix.*

T.H. Umbreit, E.J. Hesse, and M. A. Gallo. *Science* 232, 497–499 (1986).

E.E. McConnell et al., *Science* 223, 1077 (1984).

** *Decontaminated soil provided by US EPA, Edison, NJ*

ACKNOWLEDGMENTS

The earlier (1992–2005) development of research and concepts discussed in this chapter could not have been possible without the generous support of NIEHS (Superfund Basic Research Program Project P42 ES05949; R01 ES09655; T32 ES 07321; K25 ES11146; K25 ES012909), ATSDR/CDC (U61/ATU881475; RO1 OH07556), and US Air Force (F33615-91-C-0538; F49620-94-1-0304). The more recent thinking, for the lead author, is supported by Ray Yang Consulting, LLC.

REFERENCES

Andersen, M. E., Black, M. B., Campbell, J. L., Pendse, S. N., Clewell III, H. J., Pottenger, L. H., Bus, J. S., Dodd, D. E., Kemp, D. C., and McMullen, P. D. (2017). Combining Transcriptomics and PBPK Modeling Indicates a Primary Role of Hypoxia and Altered Circadian Signaling in Dichloromethane Carcinogenicity in Mouse Lung and Liver. *Toxicol Appl Pharmacol* 332:149–158. doi: 10.1016/j.taap.2017.04.002. Epub April 7, 2017. PMID: 28392392

Andersen, M. E., Clewell, H. J., 3rd, Gargas, M. L., Smith, F. A., and Reitz, R. H. (1987). Physiologically Based Pharmacokinetics and the Risk Assessment Process for Methylene Chloride. *Toxicol Appl Pharmacol* 87: 185–205.

Angelo, M. J., Bischoff, K. B., Pritchard, A. B., and Presser, M. A. (1984). A Physiological Model for the Pharmacokinetics of Methylene Chloride in B6C3F1 Mice following i.v. Administrations. *J Pharmacokinet Biopharm* 12: 413–436.

Baskin, I. I., (2018). Machine Learning Methods in Computational Toxicology. In O. Nicolotti (ed.), *Computational Toxicology: Methods and Protocols, Methods in Molecular Biology*, vol. 1800, Springer Science+Business Media, LLC, https://doi.org/10.1007/978-1-4939-7899-1_5. part of Springer Nature 2018 *Methods Mol Biol*, 1800: 119–139.

Bhhatarai, B., Walters, W. P., Hop, C. E. C. A., Lanza, G., and Ekins, S. (2019). Opportunities and Challenges Using Artificial Intelligence in ADME/Tox. *Nat Mater.*18(5): 418–422. doi: 10.1038/s41563-019-0332-5. PMID: 31000801 PMCID: PMC6594826 DOI: 10.1038/s41563-019-0332-5

Bernillon, P., and Bois, F. Y. (2000). Statistical Issues in Toxicokinetic Modeling: A Bayesian Perspective. *Environ Health Perspect* 108 (Suppl 5): 883–893.

Blower, S. M., and Dowlatabadi, H. (1994). Sensitivity and Uncertainty Analysis of Complex Models of Disease Transmission: An HIV Model, as an Example. *Int Stat Rev* 62: 229–243.

Bois, F. Y. (2001). Applications of Population Approaches in Toxicology. *Toxicol Lett* 120: 385–94.

Bois, F. Y., Gelman, A., Jiang, J., Maszle, D. R., Zeise, L., and Alexeef, G. (1996b). Population Toxicokinetics of Tetrachloroethylene. *Arch Toxicol* 70: 347–355.

Bois, F. Y., Jackson, E. T., Pekari, K., and Smith, M. T. (1996a). Population Toxicokinetics of Benzene. *Environ Health Perspect* 104 (Suppl. 6): 1405–1411.

Bois, F. Y., Maszle, D., Revzan, K., Tillier, S., and Yuan, Z. (2002). MCSim Version 5 Beta 2 http://toxi.ineris.fr/activites/toxicologie_quantitative/mcsim/article3/.

Brown, R. P., Delp, M. D., Lindstedt, S. L., Rhomberg, L. R., and Beliles, R. P. (1997). Physiological Parameter Values for Physiologically Based Pharmacokinetic Models. *Toxicol Ind Health* 13: 407–484.

Carcinogenesis (2015) Special volume 36(Supple 1) consisted of 12 review articles.

Cheng, Y., He, C., Riviere, J. E., Monteiro-Riviere, N. A., and Lin, Z. (2020). Meta-analysis of Nanoparticle Delivery to Tumors Using a Physiologically Based Pharmacokinetic Modeling and Simulation Approach. *ACS Nano* 14: 3075–3095.

Chou, W. C., and Lin, Z. (2019). Bayesian Evaluation of a Physiologically Based Pharmacokinetic (PBPK) Model for Perfluorooctane Sulfonate (PFOS) to Characterize the Interspecies Uncertainty between Mice, Rats, Monkeys, and Humans: Development and Performance Verification. *Environ Int* 129: 408–422. [PMID: 31152982] https://doi.org/10.1016/j.envint.2019.03.058

Chou, W. C., and Lin, Z. (2021). Development of a Gestational and Lactational Physiologically Based Pharmacokinetic (PBPK) Model for Perfluorooctane Sulfonate (PFOS) in Rats and Humans and Its Implications in the Derivation of Health-Based Toxicity Values. *Environ Health Persp* 129(3), March 2021: 037004-1–037004-22. DOI: 10.1289/EHP7671

Clewell, H. J., 3rd (1995). The Use of Physiologically Based Pharmacokinetic Modeling in Risk Assessment: A Case Study with Methylene Chloride. In S. Olin, W. Farland, C. Park, L. Rhomberg, R. Scheuplein, T. Starr and J. Wilson (eds.), *Low-Dose Extrapolation of Cancer Risks: Issues and Perspectives*, pp. 199–221. Washington, DC: ILSI Press.

Clewell, H. J., 3rd, and Andersen, M. E. (1996). Use of Physiologically Based Pharmacokinetic Modeling to Investigate Individual versus Population Risk. *Toxicology* 111: 315–329.

Clewell, H. J., 3rd, Lee, T. S., and Carpenter, R. L. (1994). Sensitivity of Physiologically Based Pharmacokinetic Models to Variation in Model Parameters: Methylene Chloride. *Risk Anal* 14: 521–531.

David, R. M., Clewell, H. J., Gentry, P. R., Covington, T. R., Morgott, D. A., and Marino, D. J. (2006). Revised Assessment of Cancer Risk to Dichloromethane II. Application of Probabilistic Methods to Cancer Risk Determinations. *Regul Toxicol Pharmacol* 45(1), June 2006: 55–65

Dekant, W., Jean, P., and Arts, J. (2021). Evaluation of the Carcinogenicity of Dichloromethane in Rats, Mice, Hamsters and Humans. *Regul Toxicol Pharmacol* 120: 104858. doi: 10.1016/j.yrtph.2020.104858. Epub December 31, 2020. •PMID:33387565 •DOI: 10.1016/j.yrtph.2020.104858

Dennison, J. E., Andersen, M. E., and Yang, R. S. (2003). Characterization of the Pharmacokinetics of Gasoline Using PBPK Modeling with a Complex Mixtures Chemical Lumping Approach. *Inhal Toxicol* 15: 961–986.

de Ponteves, H. (2019) *AI Crash Course*. Birmingham – Mumbai: Packt.

Dobrev, I. D., Andersen, M. E., and Yang, R. S. (2001). Assessing Interaction Thresholds for Trichloroethylene in Combination with Tetrachloroethylene and 1,1,1-Trichloroethane Using Gas Uptake Studies and PBPK Modeling. *Arch Toxicol* 75: 134–144.

Dobrev, I. D., Andersen, M. E., and Yang, R. S. (2002). In Silico Toxicology: Simulating Interaction Thresholds for Human Exposure to Mixtures of Trichloroethylene, Tetrachloroethylene, and 1,1,1-Trichloroethane. *Environ Health Perspect* 110: 1031–1039.

Easterling, M. R., Evans, M. V., and Kenyon, E. M. (2000). Comparative Analysis of Software for Physiologically Based Pharmacokinetic Modeling: Simulation, Optimization, and Sensitivity Analysis. *Toxicol Method* 10: 203–229.

Ekins, S. (2007) *Computational Toxicology. Risk Assessment for Pharmaceutical and Environmental Chemicals.* Hoboken, NJ: John Wiley & Sons, Inc.

El-Masri, H. A., Bell, D. A., and Portier, C. J. (1999). Effects of Glutathione Transferase Theta Polymorphism on the Risk Estimates of Dichloromethane to Humans. *Toxicol Appl Pharmacol* 158: 221–230.

El-Masri, H. A., Thomas, R. S., Sabados, G. R., Phillips, J. K., Constan, A. A., Benjamin, S. A., Andersen, M. E., Mehendale, H. M., and Yang, R. S. (1996). Physiologically Based Pharmacokinetic/Pharmacodynamic Modeling of the Toxicologic Interaction between Carbon Tetrachloride and Kepone. *Arch Toxicol* 70: 704–713.

Emond, C., Birnbaum, L. S., and DeVito, M. J. (2004). Physiologically Based Pharmacokinetic Model for Developmental Exposures to TCDD in the Rat. *Toxicol Sci* 80: 115–133.

Evans, M. V., and Andersen, M. E. (2000). Sensitivity Analysis of a Physiological Model for 2,3,7,8-Tetrachlorodi benzo-P-Dioxin (TCDD): Assessing the Impact of Specific Model Parameters on Sequestration in Liver and Fat in the Rat. *Toxicol Sci* 54: 71–80.

Evans, M. V., Crank, W. D., Yang, H. M., and Simmons, J. E. (1994). Applications of Sensitivity Analysis to a Physiologically Based Pharmacokinetic Model for Carbon Tetrachloride in Rats. *Toxicol Appl Pharmacol* 128: 36–44.

Fisher, J. W., Gearhart, J. M., and Lin, Z. (2020) *Physiologically Based Pharmacokinetic (PBPK) Modeling. Methods and Applications in Toxicology and Risk Assessment.* San Diego, CA: Academic Press.

Gao, H., Wang, W., Dong, J., Ye, Z., and Ouyang, D. (2021). An Integrated Computational Methodology with Data-Driven Machine Learning, Molecular Modeling and PBPK Modeling to Accelerate Solid Dispersion Formulation Design. *Eur J Pharm Biopharm* 158: 336–346. doi: 10.1016/j.ejpb.2020.12.001. Epub December 7, 2020. PMID: 33301864

Göller, A. H., Kuhnke, L., Montanari, F., Bonin, A., Schneckener, S., Laak, A. T., Wichard, J., Lobell, M., and Hillisch, A. (2020). Bayer's In Silico ADMET Platform: A Journey of Machine Learning over the Past Two Decades. *Drug Discov Today* 25(9): 1702–1709. doi: 10.1016/j.drudis.2020.07.001. Epub July 9, 2020. PMID: 32652309 DOI: 10.1016/j.drudis.2020.07.001

Haddad, S., Charest-Tardif, G., Tardif, R., and Krishnan, K. (2000). Validation of a Physiological Modeling Framework for Simulating the Toxicokinetics of Chemicals in Mixtures. *Toxicol Appl Pharmacol* 167: 199–209.

Haddad, S., Tardif, R., Charest-Tardif, G., and Krishnan, K. (1999). Physiological Modeling of the Toxicokinetic Interactions in a Quaternary Mixture of Aromatic Hydrocarbons. *Toxicol Appl Pharmacol* 161: 249–257.

Hessler, G., and Baringhaus, K. (2018). Artificial intelligence in Drug Design. *Molecules* 23(10): 2520. PMCID: PMC6222615 PMID: 30279331

Hetrick, D. M., Jarabek, A. M., and Travis, C. C. (1991). Sensitivity Analysis for Physiologically Based Pharmacokinetic Models. *J Pharmacokinet Biopharm* 19: 1–20.

House, J. S., Grimm, F. A., Jima, D. D., Zhou, Y. H., Rusyn, I., and Wright, F. A. (2017). A pipeline for High-Throughput Concentration Response Modeling of Gene Expression for Toxicogenomics, *Front Genet.* 8: 168. Published online November 1, 2017. doi: 10.3389/fgene.2017.00168 PMCID: PMC5672545 PMID: 29163636

Howson, C. and Urbach, P. (2006). *Scientific Reasoning. The Bayesian Approach.* Third Edition, Open Court, Chicago and La Salle, Illinois.

Hsieh, N. H., Chen, Z., Rusyn, I., and Chiu, W. A. (2021). Risk Characterization and Probabilistic Concentration–Response Modeling of Complex Environmental Mixtures Using New Approach Methodologies (NAMs) Data from Organotypic In Vitro Human Stem Cell Assays. *Environ. Health Perspect.* 129(1): 17004-1–17004-13. Research Open Access Published: January 4, 2021CID: 017004. https://doi.org/10.1289/EHP7600

Hsieh, N. H., Reisfeld, B., Bois, F. Y., and Chiu, W. A. (2018). Applying a Global Sensitivity Analysis Workflow to Improve the Computational Efficiencies in Physiologically-Based Pharmacokinetic Modeling. *Front. Pharmacol.* 9: 588. doi: 10.3389/fphar.2018.00588

Jonsson, F. (2001). Physiologically Based Pharmacokinetic Modeling in Risk Assessment. Development of Bayesian Population Methods. Ph.D. thesis. Division of Pharmacokinetics and Drug Therapy, Uppsala University, Stockholm, Sweden. p. 52.

Jonsson, F., and Johanson, G. (2001a). A Bayesian Analysis of the Influence of GSTT1 Polymorphism on the Cancer Risk Estimate for Dichloromethane. *Toxicol Appl Pharmacol* 174, 99–112.

Jonsson, F., and Johanson, G. (2001b). Bayesian estimation of variability in adipose tissue blood flow in man by physiologically based pharmacokinetic modeling of inhalation exposure to toluene. *Toxicology* 157: 177–193.

Jonsson, F., and Johanson, G. (2003). The Bayesian population approach to physiological toxicokinetic-toxicodynamic models--an example using the MCSim software. *Toxicol Lett* 138: 143–150.

Krishnan, K., Haddad, S., Beliveau, M., and Tardif, R. (2002). Physiological modeling and extrapolation of pharmacokinetic interactions from binary to more complex chemical mixtures. *Environ Health Perspect* 110 Suppl 6: 989–994.

Lazarovits, J., Sindhwani, S., Tavares, A. J., Zhang, Y., Song, F., Audet, J., Krieger, J. R., Syed, A. M., Stordy, B., Chan, W. C. W. (2019). Supervised learning and mass spectrometry predicts the in vivo fate of nanomaterials. *ACS Nano.* 13(7): 8023–8034. doi: 10.1021/acsnano.9b02774. Epub July 3, 2019. PMID: 31268684

Li, M., Cheng, Y.H., Chittenden, J.T., Baynes, R.E., Tell, L.A., Davis, J.L., Vickroy, T.W., Riviere, J.E., Lin, Z. (2019). Integration of Food Animal Residue Avoidance Databank (FARAD) empirical methods for drug withdrawal interval determination with a mechanistic population-based interactive physiologically-based pharmacokinetic (iPBPK) modeling platform: Example for flunixin meglumine administration. *Arch Toxicol* 93(7):1865–1880. [PMID: 31025081] https://doi.org/10.1007/s00204-019-02464-z

Li, M., Gehring, R., Riviere, J.E., Lin, Z.. (2018). Probabilistic physiologically based pharmacokinetic model for penicillin G in milk from dairy cows following intramammary or intramuscular administrations. *Toxicol Sci* 164(1):85–100. [PMID: 29945226]

Li, M., Wang, Y.S., Elwell-Cuddy, T., Baynes, R.E., Tell, L.A., Davis, J.L., Maunsell, F.P., Riviere, J.E., and Lin, Z. (2021). Physiological parameter values for physiologically based pharmacokinetic models in food-producing animals. Part III: Sheep and goat. *J Vet Pharmacol Therap* 44: 456–477. [PMID: 33350478] https://doi.org/10.1111/jvp.12938

Leung, H. W., Ku, R. H., Paustenbach, D. J., and Andersen, M. E. (1988). A physiologically based pharmacokinetic model for 2,3,7,8-tetrachlorodibenzo-p-dioxin in C57BL/6J and DBA/2J mice. *Toxicol Lett* 42, 15–28.

Lin, Z., Jaberi-Douraki, M., He, C., Yang, R. S. H., Fisher, J. W., and Riviere, J. E. (2017). Performance assessment and translation of physiologically based pharmacokinetic models from acslX™ to Berkeley Madonna™, MATLAB®, and R language: Oxytetracycline and gold nanoparticles as case examples. *Toxicol. Sci.* 158: 23–35. DOI: https://doi.org/10.1093/toxsci/kfx070.

Lin, Z., Li, M., Wang, Y.S., Tell, L.A., Baynes, R.E., Davis, J.L., Vickroy, T.W., Riviere, J.E.. (2020). Physiological parameter values for physiologically based pharmacokinetic models in food-producing animals. Part I: Cattle and Swine. *J Vet Pharmacol Therap* 43(5): 385–420. [PMID: 32270548] https://doi.org/10.1111/jvp.12861

Lin, Y. J., and Lin, Z. (2020). Probabilistic risk assessment of combined exposure to bisphenol a and its analogues by integrating toxcast high-throughput in vitro assays with In Vitro to In Vivo Extrapolation (IVIVE) via Physiologically Based Pharmacokinetic (PBPK) modeling. *J Hazard Mater*, 399, 122856. https://doi.org/10.1016/j.jhazmat.2020.122856

Lindstedt, S. L. (1987). Allometry: Body Size Constraints in Animal Design. In *Pharmacokinetics in Risk Assessment, Drinking Water and Health*, Vol. 8, pp. 65–79. National Academy Press, Washington, DC.

Lu, Y., Lohitnavy, M., Reddy, M. B., Lohitnavy, O., Ashley, A., and Yang, R. S. (2006). An updated PBPK model for hexachlorobenzene: Incorporation of pathophysiological states following partial hepatectomy and hexachlorobenzene treatment. *Toxicol Sci* 91: 29–41.

Lu, Y., Reith, S., Lohitnavy, M., Dennison, J., El-Masri, H., Barton, H. A., Bruckner, J., and Yang, R. S. H. 2008. Application of PBPK modeling in support of the derivation of toxicity reference values for 1,1,1-trichloroethane. *Reg Toxicol Pharmacol* 50: 249–260 [E-publication, December 14, 2007].

Lumen, A., McNally, K., George, N., Fisher, J. W., and Loizou, G. D. (2015). Quantitative global sensitivity analysis of a biologically based dose-response pregnancy model for the thyroid endocrine system. *Front Pharmacol* 6:107. doi: 10.3389/fphar.2015.00107.

Lyons, M. A. (2014) Computational pharmacology of rifampin in mice: An application to dose optimization with conflicting objectives in tuberculosis treatment. *J Pharmacokinet Pharmacodyn* 41: 613–623.

Lyons, M. A. (2019) Modeling and simulation of pretomanid pharmacodynamics in pulmonary tuberculosis patients. *Antimicrob Agents Chemother* 63: 1–24

Marino, D. J., Clewell, H. J., Gentry, P. R., Covington, T. R., Hack, C. E., David, R. M., and Morgott, D. A. (2006). Revised assessment of cancer risk to dichloromethane: Part I Bayesian PBPK and dose-response modeling in mice. *Regul Toxicol Pharmacol* 45(1), June 2006: 44–54.

Mayeno, A. N., Yang, R. S. H., and Reisfeld, B. (2005). Biochemical reaction network modeling: A new tool for predicting metabolism of chemical mixtures. *Environ Sci Tech* 39: 5363–5371.

McGrayne, S. B. (2011) *The Thoery That Would Not Die, How Bayes' Rule Crack the Enigma Code, Hunted Down Russian Submarines & Emerged Triumphant from Two Centuries of Controversy*. Yale University Press.

McLanahan, E. D., El-Masri, H. A., Sweeney, L. M., Kopylev, L. Y., Clewell, H. J., Wambaugh, J. F., and Schlosser, P. M. (2012). Physiologically based pharmacokinetic model use in risk assessment--Why being published is not enough. *Toxicol Sci.* 126(1): 5–15. doi: 10.1093/toxsci/kfr295. Epub November 1, 2011. PMID: 22045031 DOI: 10.1093/toxsci/kfr295

McNally, K., Cotton, R., and Loizou, G. D. (2011). A workflow for global sensitivity analysis of PBPK models. *Front. Pharmacol.* 2: 31. doi:10.3389/fphar.2011.00031

Mills, J. J., and Andersen, M. E. (1993). Dioxin hepatic carcinogenesis: Biologically motivated modeling and risk assessment. *Toxicol Lett* 68: 177–189.

Nestorov, I. A., Aarons, L. J., and Rowland, M. (1997). Physiologically based pharmacokinetic modeling of a homologous series of barbiturates in the rat: A sensitivity analysis. *J Pharmacokinet Biopharm* 25: 413–447.

NRC (2007) *Toxicity Testing in the 21st Century. A Vision and a Strategy*. National Academy Press

NTP (1986). Toxicology and Carcinogenesis Studies of Dichloromethane (Methylene Chloride) (CAS No. 75-09-2) in F344/N Rat and B6C3F1 Mice (Inhalation Studies). NTP-TR-306.

OECD, 2021. Guidance Document on the Characterization, Validation and Reporting of PBK Models for Regulatory Purposes. Organisation for Economic Co-operation and Development (OECD) Environment, Health and Safety Publications Series on Testing and Assessment no. 331. Available at: http://www.oecd.org/officialdocuments/publicdisplaydocumentpdf/?cote=ENV-CBC-MONO(2021)1%20&doclanguage=en

Paini, A., Leonard, J. A., Kliment, T., Tan, Y. M., and Worth, A. (2017). Investigating the State of Physiologically Based Kinetic Modelling Practices and Challenges Associated with Gaining Regulatory Acceptance of Model Applications. *Reg Toxicol Pharmacol* 90: 104–115.

Pelekis, M., and Krishnan, K. (1997). Assessing the Relevance of Rodent Data on Chemical Interactions for Health Risk Assessment Purposes: A Case Study with Dichloromethane-Toluene Mixture. *Regul Toxicol Pharmacol* 25: 79–86.

Peters, S. A. (2012). *Physiologically-Based Pharmacokinetics (PBPK) Modeling and Simulations. Principles, Methods, and Applications in the Pharmaceutical Industry*, John Wiley & Sons, Hoboken, New Jersey.

Portier, C. J., and Kaplan, N. L. (1989). Variability of Safe Dose Estimates When Using Complicated Models of the Carcinogenic Process. A Case Study: Methylene Chloride. *Fundam Appl Toxicol* 13: 533–544.

Raies, A. B., and Bajic, V. B. (2016). In Silico Toxicology: Computational Methods for the Prediction of Chemical Toxicity. *WIREs Comput Mol Sci* 6: 147–172.

Ramsey, J. C., and Andersen, M. E. (1984). A Physiologically Based Description of the Inhalation Pharmacokinetics of Styrene in Rats and Humans. *Toxicol Appl Pharmacol* 73: 159–175.

Reddy, M. B., Yang, R. S. H., Clewell, H. J., 3rd, and Andersen, M. E. (2005). *Physiologically Based Pharmacokinetics: Science and Applications*. John Wiley & Sons, Hoboken, NJ.

Reitz, R. H., McDougal, J. N., Himmelstein, M. W., Nolan, R. J., and Shumann, A. M. (1988) Physiologically Based Pharmacokinetic Modeling with Methylchloroform: Implications for Interspecies, High Dose/Low Dose, and Dose Route Extrapolations. *Toxicol Appl Pharmacol* 95: 185–199.

Reisfeld, B., and Mayeno, A. N. (2012) *Computational Toxicology. Vol. 1, Methods in Molecular Biology 929*, Humana Press, New York.

Robson, M. G., and Toscano, W. A. (2007). *Risk Assessment for Environmental Health*, John Wiley & Sons, Hoboken, New Jersey.

Rowland, M., Balant, L., and Peck, C. (2004). Physiologically Based Pharmacokinetics in Drug Development and Regulatory Science: A Workshop Report (Georgetown University, Washington, DC, May 29–30, 2002). *AAPS PharmSci* 6: 1–12.

Saltelli, A., Tarantola, S., and Chan, K. P. S. (1999). A Quantitative Model-Independent Method for Global Sensitivity Analysis of Model Output. *Technometrics* 41: 39–56.

Schlosser, P. M. (1994). Experimental Design for Parameter Estimation through Sensitivity Analysis. *J Toxicol Environ Health* 43: 495–530.

Serota, D. G., Thakur, A. K., Ulland, B. M., Kirschman, J. C., Brown, N. M., Coots, R. H., and Morgareidge, K. (1986a). A Two-Year Drinking-Water Study of Dichloromethane in Rodents. I. Rats. *Food Chem Toxicol* 24: 951–958.

Serota, D. G., Thakur, A. K., Ulland, B. M., Kirschman, J. C., Brown, N. M., Coots, R. H., and Morgareidge, K. (1986b). A Two-Year Drinking-Water Study of Dichloromethane in Rodents. II. Mice. *Food Chem Toxicol* 24: 959–963.

Singh, A. V., Ansari, M. H. D., Rosenkranz, D., Maharjan, R. S., Kriegel, F. L., Gandhi, K., Kanase, A., Singh, R., Laux, P., and Luch, A. (2020). Artificial Intelligence and Machine Learning in Computational Nanotoxicology: Unlocking and Empowering Nanomedicine. *Adv Healthc Mater.* 9(17): e1901862. doi: 10.1002/adhm.201901862. Epub July 6, 2020.

Strogatz, S. (2020) *Infinite Powers. The Story of Calculus, The Language of the Universe.* London: Atlantic Books.

Sweeney, L. M., Gargas, M. L., Strother, D. E., and Kedderis, G. L. (2003). Physiologically Based Pharmacokinetic Model Parameter Estimation and Sensitivity and Variability Analyses for Acrylonitrile Disposition in Humans. *Toxicol Sci* 71: 27–40.

Sweeney, L. M., Kirman, C. R., Morgott, D. A., and Gargas, M. L. (2004). Estimation of Interindividual Variation in Oxidative Metabolism of Dichloromethane in Human Volunteers. *Toxicol Lett* 154: 201–216.

Tardif, R., Charest-Tardif, G., Brodeur, J., and Krishnan, K. (1997). Physiologically Based Pharmacokinetic Modeling of a Ternary Mixture of Alkyl Benzenes in Rats and Humans. *Toxicol Appl Pharmacol* 144: 120–134.

Tardif, R., Lapare, S., Charest-Tardif, G., Brodeur, J., and Krishnan, K. (1995). Physiologically-Based Pharmacokinetic Modeling of a Mixture of Toluene and Xylene in Humans. *Risk Anal* 15: 335–342.

Tardif, R., Lapare, S., Krishnan, K., and Brodeur, J. (1993). A Descriptive and Mechanistic Study of the Interaction between Toluene and Xylene in Humans. *Int Arch Occup Environ Health* 65: S135–S137.

Thomas, R. S., Lytle, W. E., Keefe, T. J., Constan, A. A., and Yang, R. S. (1996a). Incorporating Monte Carlo Simulation into Physiologically Based Pharmacokinetic Models Using Advanced Continuous Simulation Language (ACSL): A Computational Method. *Fundam Appl Toxicol* 31: 19–28.

Thomas, R. S., Yang, R. S., Morgan, D. G., Moorman, M. P., Kermani, H. R., Sloane, R. A., O'Connor, R. W., Adkins, B., Jr., Gargas, M. L., and Andersen, M. E. (1996b). PBPK Modeling/Monte Carlo Simulation of Methylene Chloride Kinetic Changes in Mice in Relation to Age and Acute, Subchronic, and Chronic Inhalation Exposure. *Environ Health Perspect* 104: 858–865.

Topol, E. J. (2019) High-Performance Medicine: The Convergence of human and Artificial Intelligence. *Nature Med* 25: 44–56.

US EPA (2005). Approaches for the Application of Physiologically Based Pharmacokinetic (PBPK) Models and Supporting Data in Risk Assessment. Report number: EPA/600/R-05/043A. U.S. Environmental Protection Agency, Washington, DC.

US EPA (2011). Toxicological Review of Dichloromethane (Methylene Chloride) (CAS No. 75-09-2) in Support of Summary Information on the Integrated Risk Information System (IRIS). EPA/635/R-10/003F. U.S. Environmental Protection Agency, Washington, DC.

van de Waterbeemd, H., and Gifford, E. (2003). ADMET In Silico Modelling: Towards Prediction Paradise? *Nat Rev Drug Discov* 2: 192–204.

Wang, Y.S., Li, M., Tell, L.A., Baynes, R.E., Davis, J.L., Vickroy, T.W., Riviere, J.E., Lin, Z.. (2021). Physiological Parameter Values for Physiologically Based Pharmacokinetic Models in Food-Producing Animals. Part II: Chicken and Turkey. *J Vet Pharmacol Therap* 44(4), July 2021: 423–455. [PMID: 33289178] https://doi.org/10.1111/jvp.12931

Weijs, L., Yang, R. S. H., Das, K., Covaci, A., and Blust, R. (2013). Application of Bayesian Population Physiologically Based Pharmacokinetic (PBPK) Modeling and Markov Chain Monte Carlo Simulations to Pesticide Kinetics Studies in Protected Marine Mammals: DDT, DDE, and DDD in Harbor Porpoises, *Environ Sci Technol.* 47(9): 4365–4374. doi: 10.1021/es400386a. Epub April 18, 2013.

Wenzel, J., Matter, H., and Schmidt, F. (2019). Predictive Multitask Deep Neural Network Models for ADME-Tox Properties: Learning from Large Data Sets. *J Chem Inf Model.* 59(3):1253–1268. doi: 10.1021/acs.jcim.8b00785. Epub January 24, 2019. PMID: 30615828 DOI: 10.1021/acs.jcim.8b00785

Wu, Z., Lei, T., Shen, C., Wang, Z., Cao, D., and Hou, T. (2019). ADMET Evaluation in Drug Discovery. 19. Reliable Prediction of Human Cytochrome P450 Inhibition Using Artificial Intelligence Approaches. *J Chem Inf Model.* 59(11): 4587–4601. doi: 10.1021/acs.jcim.9b00801. Epub November 5, 2019. PMID: 31644282 DOI: 10.1021/acs.jcim.9b00801

Yang, F., Yang, F., Wang, D., Zhang, C. S., Wang, H., Song, Z. W., Shao, H. T., Zhang, M., Yu, M. L., and Zheng, Y. (2021). Development and Application of a Water Temperature Related Physiologically Based Pharmacokinetic Model for Enrofloxacin and Its Metabolite Ciprofloxacin in Rainbow Trout. *Front Vet Sci.* 7: 608348. doi: 10.3389/fvets.2020.608348. eCollection 2020. PMID: 33585600 PMCID: PMC7874017 DOI: 10.3389/fvets.2020.608348

Yang, R. S. H., and Andersen, M. E. (2005). Physiologically Based Pharmacokinetic Modeling of Chemical Mixtures. In M. B. Reddy, R. S. H. Yang, H. J. Clewell, 3rd and M. E. Andersen (eds.) *Physiologically Based Pharmacokinetics: Science and Applications.* New York: John Wiley and Sons, Inc.

Yang, R. S. H., and Lu, Y. The Application of Physiologically Based Pharmacokinetic (PBPK) Modeling to Risk Assessment. In M. G. Robson and W. A. Toscano (eds.), *Risk Assessment for Environmental Health.* John Wiley & Sons, Inc., San Francisco, 2007.

Yang, R. S. H., Weijs, L., McDougall, R., Housand, C. The Application of PBPK Modeling, the Bayesian Approach, and the Utilization of Markov Chain Monte Carlo Simulation in Risk Assessment. In A. M. Fan, E. M. Khan, and G. V. Alexeeff (eds.), *Toxicology and Risk Assessment*, Pan Stanford Publishing Pte. Ltd., Singapore, 2015.

Yang, R. S. H., Mayeno, A. N., Lyons, M. A., and Reisfeld, B. (2010) The Application of Physiologically Based Pharmacokinetics, Bayesian Population PBPK Modeling, and Biochemical Reaction Network Modeling to Chemical Mixture Toxicology. In M. Mumtaz (ed.), *Principles and Practice of Mixture Toxicology.* Wiley-VCH: Weinheim.

Yang, R. S. H. (2018) Toxicology and Risk Assessment of Chemical Mixtures and Multiple Stressors. In C. A. McQueen (ed.), *Comprehensive Toxicology*, Third Edition. Vol. 1, Oxford: Elsevier Ltd..

9 Adverse Outcomes Pathways (AOPs)

Elizabeth V. Wattenberg
School of Public Health University of Minnesota, Minneapolis, United States

CONTENTS

Introduction to Adverse Outcome Pathways 179
Basic Principles for the Development and Assessment of AOPs...180
Application of AOPs to Environmental Health Risk Assessment 182
Future Directions and Challenges 184
Literature Cited 184

LEARNING OBJECTIVES

Students who complete this chapter will be able to

1. Understand the basic principles for the development of Adverse Outcome Pathways,
2. Understand how Adverse Outcome Pathways are assessed, and
3. Learn about the application of Adverse Outcome Pathways.

INTRODUCTION TO ADVERSE OUTCOME PATHWAYS

Adverse outcome pathways (AOPs) provide a framework for organizing existing scientific evidence into plausible biological pathways, starting from the molecular and progressing to the organism level, which can be used to help predict whether chemicals or other environmental agents are likely to perturb such pathways resulting in toxicity (Villeneuve et al. 2014a; Vinken et al. 2017). AOPs that are designed for ecological risk assessment organize evidence up through the level of population health in an ecosystem. The application of AOPs for environmental health risk assessment described in this chapter, however, focuses only on human health. This chapter reviews the concept of AOPs, basic principles for the development and assessment of AOPs, the application of AOPs to environmental health risk assessment, and future directions and challenges. A major reference for definitions, information, and examples of AOPs is the AOP-Wiki (AOP-Wiki 2021g).

An AOP typically begins with the initial interaction of a chemical or another type of environmental agent with a critical molecular target. This interaction stimulates a sequence of biochemical and physiological events that typically lead to a toxicological endpoint that is observed in traditional safety assessment studies (see Figure 9.1) (Villeneuve et al. 2014a, 2014b). The key

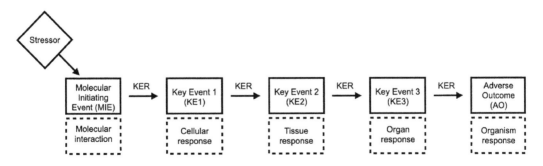

Figure 9.1 Graphical depiction of the components of an AOP. A stressor, such as a chemical, activates the MIE, which triggers a cascade of downstream biological effects called KE, which occur at increasingly complex biological levels, and ultimately result in an AO. Upstream and downstream KEs are linked by a KER. **Adapted from SW Edwards et al. (2016).**

components of an AOP include the following: stressor(s), a molecular initiating event (MIE), key events (KEs), key event relationships (KERs), and the adverse outcome (AO). The stressors are chemicals or other types of environmental agents that activate the AOP. The MIE represents the initial interaction of a stressor with the critical molecular target that triggers the subsequent biological effects in the AOP. The KEs are the series of linked biological effects that lead from the MIE to the AO. The KEs are typically organized according to the following order of biological and physiological complexity: biochemical/molecular, cellular, tissue level, organ level, organism level. The MIE and the AO can be considered specialized types of KEs. The KERs establish the links between upstream and downstream key events.

KEs, which represent changes in the biological system, have two major qualities: (1) they can be measured, and (2) they are required, but are not necessarily sufficient, for the AO to occur (Villeneuve et al. 2014b). The description of a KE typically includes the level of biological organization in which it occurs (e.g., molecular, cellular, organ), and the methods that can be used to measure the KE (Villeneuve et al. 2014b). The description may also include information on whether the KE is conserved across species, and if its function depends on a specific biological context such as cell type, life stage, or sex.

MIEs are the first step in the AOP, which makes them the most upstream KE in the AOP. MIEs represent the point of interaction between the stressor and a critical molecule, such as a receptor, DNA, enzyme, or lipids. The description of an MIE should include a list of stressors that can interact with the molecular target. Importantly, AOPs essentially describe the toxicodynamic processes of stressor action, which focus on how the stressor affects the biological systems. AOPs do not address the toxicokinetic processes that govern how much of the bioactive stressor reaches the site of the MIE following exposure (i.e., absorption, distribution, excretion, metabolism). Like other KEs, the description of an MIE provides information on how it is measured. The description may also provide information on whether the molecule is conserved across species. This can be useful for extrapolating from different types of model systems to humans. For example, a protein that is required for the MIE may have isoforms that have been detected across multiple species. The MIE description may also explain whether the target function depends on the cell type, life stage, or sex. An example of an MIE is inhibition of the enzyme acetylcholinesterase (AOP-Wiki 2021b). Stressors include the active metabolites of organophosphate and carbamate pesticides. Acetylcholinesterase is conserved across species, including insects and humans. It is present at all life stages and sexes.

The KEs that follow the MIE typically represent a cascade of effects that start at the biochemical/molecular level and then progress through increasingly complex biological and physiological levels that can include the cell, tissue, organ, and, ultimately, organ systems. For example, the KEs of "AOP 38 Protein Alkylation leading to Liver Fibrosis" (AOP-Wiki 2021f) are as follows: MIE: protein alkylation, KE1: cell injury/death, KE2: tissue-resident cell activation, KE3: increased proinflammatory mediators, KE4: activation of stellate cells, KE5: accumulation of collagen, AO: liver fibrosis.

The AO represents the final KE and typically occurs at the organ or organ systems level. For the purposes of risk assessment, the AO is typically a toxicological endpoint that is recognized as significant from a regulatory perspective. Examples of AOs include skin sensitization, organ toxicity, cancer, and neurological effects such as impairment of learning and memory.

KERs establish how upstream KEs are linked to proximate downstream KEs. Examples of KERs include the following: decreased mitochondrial adenosine triphosphate (ATP) production leads to increased necrosis (AOP-Wiki 2021d); inhibition of cyclooxygenase activity leads to reduced concentration of prostaglandin E2 (AOP-Wiki 2021e); abnormal morphogenesis leads to increased developmental defects (AOP-Wiki 2021a).

BASIC PRINCIPLES FOR THE DEVELOPMENT AND ASSESSMENT OF AOPS

The development of AOPs aligns with the major concepts described in the National Research Council (NRC) report "Toxicity Testing in the 21st Century: A Vision and a Strategy," published in 2007 (Krewski et al. 2010). The NRC report highlighted the need for a framework that could establish how mechanistic *in vitro* data could be used to predict toxicity in humans (Andersen et al. 2010; Krewski et al. 2009). In particular, this report emphasized the importance of taking advantage of the growing scientific knowledge and evidence emerging from molecular toxicology studies to map the biological pathways that underlie the adverse outcomes typically assessed by traditional *in vivo* toxicology studies. The NRC report was driven in part by the need to find alternatives to the traditional animal studies used for safety assessment. The reasons for seeking alternatives to animal testing include the prohibitive expense and amount of time required to conduct traditional *in vivo* safety assessment studies for the increasing number of chemicals in use, concerns about the ethics of animal testing, and persistent questions regarding the validity of animal studies to predict toxicity in humans. The overall idea was to reduce the use of traditional animal studies by applying high-throughput *in vitro* assays, in combination with computational toxicology, to predict which chemicals were likely to perturb key biological pathways leading to harmful toxic effects. In brief, there was a call to increase the efficiency and accuracy of predictive toxicity testing while reducing the cost and use of animals (Andersen et al. 2010; Edwards et al. 2016; Krewski et al. 2009). This led to the launching of an AOP Development Program by the Organisation for Economic Co-operation and Development in 2012, which then led to the establishment of the AOP-Wiki, a repository for collaboratively developed AOPs, along with information and knowledge for developing AOPs (AOP-Wiki 2021g; Edwards et al. 2016).

The basic principles of AOP development were established through a series of workshops (Edwards et al. 2016). The overarching concept of AOPs is that they are a plausible series of measurable changes in biological systems that are linked by causal relationships and supported by scientific evidence (Villeneuve et al. 2014a, 2014b). Like many practices of environmental health risk assessment, AOP development relies on the application of existing information (Vinken et al. 2017). Accordingly, one of the basic principles of AOP development is that AOPs are dynamic; they continue to evolve as new evidence becomes available (Villeneuve et al. 2014a). Another basic principle of AOPs is that they are not narrowly designed to explain the mechanisms of a specific chemical (Villeneuve et al. 2014a). Rather, they define an MIE that serves as the activation point of the AOP by stressors. An assay for the MIE could be used to screen chemicals to identify a range of stressors that are likely to perturb the AOP leading to the AO. As discussed earlier, AOPs describe a toxicodynamic process; they do not account for the toxicokinetic processes that govern the steps between exposure and delivery of the ultimate stressor to the site of the MIE. In other words, they focus on how the stressor affects the biological system, not how the biological system affects the stressor. This is in contrast to the mode-of-action (MOA) concept applied by the United States Environmental Protection Agency (US EPA), which is similar to AOPs, except that MOAs can be developed for specific chemicals, and they incorporate toxicokinetic processes (Meek et al. 2014; Vinken et al. 2017).

Another principle of AOP development is that AOPs are modular in the sense that each KE represents a building block. The KEs are not unique to a specific AOP. Rather, they can be shared by multiple AOPs. In other words, KEs represent a biological state that may be the result of different upstream events. The AOPs themselves are typically designed as a linear sequence of a limited number of KEs linked by KERs. A single AOP is not intended to be a comprehensive map of the complex networks of biological systems that can be modulated by a stressor. Instead, each AOP respresents a well-defined segment that could be used to construct such a map. KEs in the segment may serve as points of convergence for other AOPs. This idea aligns with two other major principles. First, AOPs represent a practical segment of a biological network that can be thoroughly evaluated. Second, the application of AOPs to predict the complexity of how biological systems respond to stressors involves mapping networks of AOPs.

There are several different approaches that can be used to develop AOPs (Villeneuve et al. 2014a; Vinken et al. 2017). One approach is to start with an AO and work backward to investigate pathways that, if perturbed by a stressor, could lead to the AO. This is referred to as top-down because it starts at the most complex biological level and works back through decreasing biological complexity to ultimately identify the key target molecule required for the MIE. This approach may be used by investigators who seek to understand biological pathways through which environmental exposures can cause the AO. Another approach is to start with a well-defined MIE and work forward to identify the pathways leading from the MIE to AOs. This is referred to as bottom-up because it begins at a basic biological level of molecules and proceeds through increasingly complex biological levels. This approach can be useful for developing predictive screening methods if a well-developed assay is available for the MIE and downstream KEs. AOP development can also start with a well-defined KE. This is referred to as middle-out development. For example, a KE may be recognized as an important step in a biological process that if disrupted could result in an AO, such as an important step involved in fetal development. Starting in the middle, the AOP be can developed both to identify preceding KEs and subsequent KEs leading to the AO.

There are also several approaches to developing AOPs that do not require a specific KE as a starting point, in contrast to those described earlier. For example, although AOPs are not intended to be chemical specific, a case study on the mechanistic pathways of a specific chemical may be used to identify an MIE that could be activated by stressors other than the chemical used in the case study. AOPs can also be developed by analogy. This approach starts with an AOP that has been developed and thoroughly evaluated in a particular organism. The AOP can be used as a basis to determine whether the KEs and KERs are conserved in other organisms. Rather than starting with a pathway that has been established through a case study or by analogy, AOPs may also be developed based on data mining. This approach involves taking advantage of different types of databases and using computational approaches to develop hypotheses regarding KERs, which can be confirmed by experiments.

Finally, an important part of AOP development is assessment, which involves establishing biological plausibility and providing a transparent discussion of the strengths and limitations of each KE and KER, as well as addressing uncertainties and important data gaps (Villeneuve et al. 2014b). The assessment of the biological plausibility of AOPs is based on the Bradford-Hill criteria, which were developed to evaluate causality in epidemiological studies (Hill 1965; Meek et al. 2014; Vinken et al. 2017). A weight of evidence approach is used to rate the available scientific evidence that supports a KER as either weak, moderate, or strong. The first criterion is biological plausibility. This involves evaluating whether, based on established biological knowledge, it is likely that the upstream KE will result in the downstream KE. The second criterion is essentiality. As mentioned earlier, it is important to establish that each KE is required for the AO to occur. For example, chemical inhibitors or genetic modifications can be used in experimental models to determine if blocking a given KE prevents the downstream KE from occurring, and consequently prevents the AOP from proceeding. Conversely, the KE must occur for the AOP to proceed. The third criterion is empirical support. The weight of evidence evaluation of KERs should include an analysis of dose-response and temporal data to confirm that the dose response for the upstream KE is consistent with the dose response for the downstream KE, and the upstream KE occurs prior to the downstream KE.

APPLICATION OF AOPS TO ENVIRONMENTAL HEALTH RISK ASSESSMENT

Currently, AOPs are best suited for qualitative assessments, such as hazard identification, rather than quantitative assessments, which are required for dose-response assessment (Becker et al. 2015; Delrue et al. 2016; Patlewicz et al. 2015; Vinken et al. 2017). For example, AOPs can be used to facilitate the use of mechanistic data to make regulatory decisions. AOPs provide a graphical depiction of how existing knowledge about biological mechanisms supports the likelihood that a chemical will cause a specific AO. The weight of evidence analysis provides a transparent evaluation of the strength of the mechanistic data for prediction.

AOPs can also be applied to address different types of uncertainty and data gaps in the risk assessment and regulatory process (Patlewicz et al. 2015). For example, AOPs may be used to enhance read-across approaches for hazard identification. Read across involves predicting the toxicity of chemicals for which limited data are available based on similarities of the chemical to others for which there are abundant data. Read-across approaches are typically based on similarities in chemical structure. AOPs can be used to group chemicals by similar biological action based on mechanistic data, instead of grouping chemicals based on structure alone. This type of application can be used to generate a hypothesis or support hazard prediction for chemicals for which data are available for upstream KEs, but not for AOs. AOPs can also be used to prioritize chemicals for a more thorough assessment by *in vivo* studies. For example, screening chemicals for MIEs may indicate which chemicals require further *in vivo* testing to determine if they can cause an AO as predicted by the AOP. Priorities for testing may also be based on the potency of chemicals to activate the MIE (Patlewicz et al. 2015). AOPs can also be used to identify data gaps that need to be addressed by new research. For example, the weight of evidence assessment of each KE and KER can identify critical biological effects that require more data to shift the weight of evidence assessment from weak or moderate to strong. Finally, AOPs may also indicate where assays need to be developed to screen chemicals for modulation of KEs.

Well-defined AOPs may serve as the bases for developing testing strategies for the safety assessment of chemicals that do not rely on animal data. One example of this application is a testing scheme proposed for predicting the potential of chemicals to cause skin sensitization (AOP-Wiki 2021c; Bauch et al. 2012; MacKay et al. 2013). Skin sensitization is the toxicology endpoint of concern for chemicals that cause allergic contact dermatitis. It is a common response in the general population from exposures to consumer products, including cosmetics and cleaning products, and in workers who experience occupational exposure to chemicals. The traditional method for the assessment of skin sensitization involves animal studies, including the murine local lymph node assay, the Guinea Pig Maximization Test, and the Buehler Test (Bauch et al. 2012). The incentive to develop methods for testing for skin sensitization that do not involve animal testing was based in part on amendments to the European Union Cosmetics Directive, which prohibited animal testing for cosmetic products and ingredients. The proposed testing approach developed by Bauch et al. aligns with "AOP 40 Covalent Protein Binding Leading to Skin Sensitisation" (AOP-Wiki 2021c; Bauch et al. 2012): MIE: covalent binding to protein, KE1: activation of kerationcytes, KE2: activation of dendritic cells, KE3: activation/proliferation of T-cells, AO: skin sensitization (AOP-Wiki 2021c). The testing strategy focuses on the MIE, KE1, and KE2. *In silico* methods were proposed for testing chemicals for protein reactivity, which measures the MIE, and *in vitro* methods were proposed for testing activation of the Keap-1/Nrf2 signaling pathway and activation of dendritic cells, which measure KE1 and KE2, respectively (Bauch et al. 2012).

AOPs may also be used to generate hypotheses about the types of AOs specific stressors might cause. The hypotheses can then be tested with the intent of identifying important health effects caused by specific environmental exposures. This approach was discussed by Leem and Chung to help determine AOs associated with widespread exposure to humidifier disinfectants in South Korea; the disinfectants contained the bacteriocidal agent polyhexamethylene guanidine (PHMG)-phosphate (Leem and Chung 2016). Between 1995 and 2011, millions of people in South Korea were exposed to disinfectants that they added to their humidifiers, which resulted in lung injury and death (Choi et al. 2016; Leem and Chung 2016; Paek et al. 2015). The potential for toxicity from inhalation of PHMG-phosphate had been considered low because of its high molecular weight and low vapor pressure (Song et al. 2014). Humidifiers, however, may release particles that can penetrate deep into the lung (Kim et al. 2016). An epidemiological study was conducted to determine the association between exposure to disinfectants and different types of lung injury (Paek et al. 2015). The source of the data included reports of suspected lung injury associated with exposure to the humidifier disinfectant submitted by clinicians and the general public (Paek et al. 2015). A committee classified the cases as definite, probable, possible, or unlikely. The original study reviewed 374 cases. The committee unanimously classified 329 of these as follows: 117 definite, 34 probable, 38 possible, and 140 unlikely; 62 of the definite and probable cases died. Two subsequent investigations added 334 more reports (Leem and Chung 2016). A major concern has been raised that the extent of injury throughout the population resulting from this exposure is much larger than was estimated by the epidemiological studies (Choi et al. 2016; Leem and Chung 2016; Paek et al. 2015). In particular, by focusing on lung injury to deep parts of the lung, these studies may have missed a much broader range of adverse health effects, including cardiovascular, renal, developmental, musculoskeletal, and effects on the eyes and skin (Choi et al. 2016). Applying the AOP framework to organize existing toxicological data on PHMG-phosphate could generate hypotheses and provide mechanistic support regarding different types of AOs that could be caused by this bacteriocide; people who have experienced a range of toxicities from exposure could then get proper support (Choi et al. 2016; Leem and Chung 2016). *In vivo* and *in vitro* data are already available to indicate important KEs, such as production of reactive oxygen species, induction of inflammatory mediators, and changes in levels of proteins involved in wound healing, and also AOs, including lung fibrosis and effects on the spleen and thymus (Kim et al. 2016; Song et al. 2014).

A data mining approach has been used to develop AOPs to help predict the toxicity of microplastics (Jeong and Choi 2019). Microplastics have been detected throughout the environment (Jeong and Choi 2019; Kosuth et al. 2018). The hazards from exposure to microplastics can result from both chemicals that adsorb onto the plastics and additives to the plastics themselves. Jeong and Choi used a data mining and computational approach to focus on the hazards associated with additives to the plastics. First, they identified 50 of the most common additives. Next, they mined animal testing from the database ChemID plus and mined mechanistic data using the toxicity forecaster developed by the US EPA called ToxCast™ (ChemIDplus 2021; US EPA 2021). ToxCast™ has data on at least 1,800 chemicals that have undergone high-throughput screening using over 700 types of assays (US EPA 2021). They used a computational approach to identify the 15 most relevant mechanisms of toxicity for the additives, which together with a systematic review of mechanisms of toxicity served as the basis for AOP development. AOPs begin with the formation of reactive oxygen species and lead to changes in lipid metabolism, inflammation, changes in energy metabolism, and cancer.

Several other potential applications of AOPs are also being explored. For example, AOPs have been proposed as a framework for organizing existing *in vivo* and *in vitro* data to help predict if food proteins are likely to cause an allergic reaction (van Bilsen et al. 2017). There is also an interest in developing AOPs for the evaluation of food additives, which could be used to develop *in silico* and *in vitro* testing strategies to screen new chemicals for potentially hazardous effects

(Kramer et al. 2019; Vinken et al. 2020). Another application of AOPs is to help clarify the mechanisms through which environmental exposure to chemicals causes different types of neurotoxicity, such as Parkinson's disease and developmental effects that result in impairment of learning and memory, which can then be used to develop testing strategies to help predict if chemicals are likely to be neurotoxic (Bal-Price and Meek 2017). Finally, an AOP was developed for peroxisome proliferator-activated receptor gamma antagonism leading to pulmonary fibrosis (Jeong et al. 2019). ToxCast™ data was then used to identify possible chemical stressors that could activate the AOP, for subsequent validation of the AOP.

FUTURE DIRECTIONS AND CHALLENGES

As discussed in this chapter, the major strengths of AOPs are providing a framework for the thorough and transparent evaluation of mechanistic data that is organized to depict a plausible biological pathway leading from a molecular interaction of a stressor through a cascade of biological effects, which lead to a toxicological endpoint that is relevant to risk assessment and regulation. AOPs take advantage of mechanistic data generated by molecular toxicology studies, including an evaluation of conservation of mechanisms across species, to support the plausibility of human health outcomes identified both through animal studies and epidemiological studies (Leist et al. 2017; Sewell et al. 2018). AOPs can also support the movement to reduce animal testing by helping to identify important data gaps through the weight of evidence evaluation and indicating how the development and application of specific *in silico* and *in vitro* tests can be used to help predict toxicity (Leist et al. 2017; Sewell et al. 2018). Broader applications of AOPs to environmental health risk assessment will require determining how AOPs can more fully address the complex reality of how biological systems respond to chemicals and other environmental stressors (Leist et al. 2017; Sewell et al. 2018). For example, stressors often perturb a network of biological pathways, each of which may be modulated by feedback loops and other compensatory responses, including repair systems (Leist et al. 2017; Sewell et al. 2018).

To move beyond hazard identification, AOPs will also need to be developed to address quantitative assessment. For example, it will be important to consider the relationship between exposure assessment, toxicokinetics, and AOPs. These conditions determine the concentration of the stressor that reaches the molecular target described by the MIE. Another important consideration is determining how the duration of exposure affects the ability of the AOP to proceed from the MIE to other KEs and ultimately the AO. Accordingly, the threshold for each step in the AOP needs to be determined, which, as discussed earlier, requires an understanding of feedback loops and compensatory mechanisms (Leist et al. 2017; Sewell et al. 2018).

In brief, AOPs currently serve as well-defined and thoroughly evaluated segments of biological pathways. The major challenge for the future is how AOPs can evolve to more fully represent the complexity of biological systems.

LITERATURE CITED

Andersen, M. E., M. Al-Zoughool, M. Croteau, M. Westphal, and D. Krewski. 2010. The Future of Toxicity Testing. *J Toxicol Environ Health B Crit Rev* 13 (2–4): 163–96. https://doi.org/10.1080/10937404.2010.483933.

AOP-Wiki. 2021a. Abnormal, Morphogenesis Leads to Increased, Developmental Defects. Edited by https://aopwiki.org/relationships/1025.

AOP-Wiki. 2021b. Acetylcholinesterase (AchE) Inhibition. Edited by https://aopwiki.org/events/12.

AOP-Wiki. 2021c. Covalent Protein Binding Leading to Skin Sensitisation. Edited by https://aopwiki.org/aops/40.

AOP-Wiki. 2021d. Decrease, Mitochondrial ATP Production Leads to Increase, Necrosis. Edited by https://aopwiki.org/relationships/1873.

AOP-Wiki. 2021e. Inhibition, Cyclooxygenase Activity Leads to Reduction, Prostaglandin E2 Concentration. Edited by https://aopwiki.org/relationships/95.

AOP-Wiki. 2021f. Protein Alkylation Leading to Liver Fibrosis. Edited by https://aopwiki.org/aops/38.

AOP-Wiki. 2021g. Welcome to the Collaborative Adverse Outcome Pathway Wiki (AOP-Wiki). Edited by https://aopwiki.org/.

Bal-Price, A., and M. E. B. Meek. 2017. Adverse Outcome Pathways: Application to Enhance Mechanistic Understanding of Neurotoxicity. *Pharmacol Ther* 179: 84–95. https://doi.org/10.1016/j.pharmthera.2017.05.006.

Bauch, C., S. N. Kolle, T. Ramirez, T. Eltze, E. Fabian, A. Mehling, W. Teubner, B. van Ravenzwaay, and R. Landsiedel. 2012. Putting the Parts Together: Combining In Vitro Methods to Test for Skin Sensitizing Potentials. *Regul Toxicol Pharmacol* 63 (3): 489–504. https://doi.org/10.1016/j.yrtph.2012.05.013.

Becker, R. A., G. T. Ankley, S. W. Edwards, S. W. Kennedy, I. Linkov, B. Meek, M. Sachana, H. Segner, B. van der Burg, D. L. Villeneuve, H. Watanabe, and T. S. Barton-Maclaren. 2015. Increasing Scientific Confidence in Adverse Outcome Pathways: Application of Tailored Bradford-Hill Considerations for Evaluating Weight Of Evidence. *Regul Toxicol Pharmacol* 72 (3): 514–37. https://doi.org/10.1016/j.yrtph.2015.04.004.

ChemID*plus*. 2021. https://chem.nlm.nih.gov/chemidplus/.

Choi, J. E., S. B. Hong, K. H. Do, H. J. Kim, S. Chung, E. Lee, J. Choi, and S. J. Hong. 2016. Humidifier Disinfectant Lung Injury, How Do We Approach the Issues? *Environ Health Toxicol* 31: e2016019. https://doi.org/10.5620/eht.e2016019.

Delrue, N., M. Sachana, Y. Sakuratani, A. Gourmelon, E. Leinala, and R. Diderich. 2016. The Adverse Outcome Pathway Concept: A Basis for Developing Regulatory Decision-Making Tools. *Altern Lab Anim* 44 (5): 417–429. https://doi.org/10.1177/026119291604400504.

Edwards, S. W., Y. M. Tan, D. L. Villeneuve, M. E. Meek, and C. A. McQueen. 2016. Adverse Outcome Pathways-Organizing Toxicological Information to Improve Decision Making. *J Pharmacol Exp Ther* 356 (1): 170–181. https://doi.org/10.1124/jpet.115.228239.

Hill, A. B. 1965. The Environment and Disease: Association or Causation? *Proc R Soc Med* 58 (5): 295–300.

Jeong, J., and J. Choi. 2019. Adverse Outcome Pathways Potentially Related to Hazard Identification of Microplastics Based on Toxicity Mechanisms. *Chemosphere* 231: 249–255. https://doi.org/10.1016/j.chemosphere.2019.05.003.

Jeong, J., N. Garcia-Reyero, L. Burgoon, E. Perkins, T. Park, C. Kim, J. Y. Roh, and J. Choi. 2019. Development of Adverse Outcome Pathway for PPARγ Antagonism Leading to Pulmonary Fibrosis and Chemical Selection for Its Validation: Toxcast Database and a Deep Learning Artificial Neural Network Model-Based Approach. *Chem Res Toxicol* 32 (6): 1212–1222. https://doi.org/10.1021/acs.chemrestox.9b00040.

Kim, H. R., K. Lee, C. W. Park, J. A. Song, D. Y. Shin, Y. J. Park, and K. H. Chung. 2016. Polyhexamethylene Guanidine Phosphate Aerosol Particles Induce Pulmonary Inflammatory and Fibrotic Responses. *Arch Toxicol* 90 (3): 617–632. https://doi.org/10.1007/s00204-015-1486-9.

Kosuth, M., S. A. Mason, and E. V. Wattenberg. 2018. Anthropogenic Contamination of Tap Water, Beer, and Sea Salt. *PLoS One* 13 (4): e0194970. https://doi.org/10.1371/journal.pone.0194970.

Kramer, N. I., Y. Hoffmans, S. Wu, A. Thiel, N. Thatcher, T. E. H. Allen, S. Levorato, H. Traussnig, S. Schulte, A. Boobis, Imcm Rietjens, and M. Vinken. 2019. Characterizing the Coverage of Critical Effects Relevant in the Safety Evaluation of Food Additives by AOPs. *Arch Toxicol* 93 (8): 2115–2125. https://doi.org/10.1007/s00204-019-02501-x.

Krewski, D., D. Acosta, Jr., M. Andersen, H. Anderson, J. C. Bailar, 3rd, K. Boekelheide, R. Brent, G. Charnley, V. G. Cheung, S. Green, Jr., K. T. Kelsey, N. I. Kerkvliet, A. A. Li, L. McCray, O. Meyer, R. D. Patterson, W. Pennie, R. A. Scala, G. M. Solomon, M. Stephens, J. Yager, and L. Zeise. 2010. Toxicity Testing in the 21st Century: A Vision and a Strategy. *J Toxicol Environ Health B Crit Rev* 13 (2–4): 51–138. https://doi.org/10.1080/10937404.2010.483176.

Krewski, D., M. E. Andersen, E. Mantus, and L. Zeise. 2009. Toxicity Testing in the 21st Century: Implications for Human Health Risk Assessment. *Risk Anal* 29 (4): 474–479. https://doi.org/10.1111/j.1539-6924.2008.01150.x.

Leem, J. H., and K. H. Chung. 2016. Combined Approaches Using Adverse Outcome Pathways and Big Data to Find Potential Diseases Associated with Humidifier Disinfectant. *Environ Health Toxicol* 32: e2017003. https://doi.org/10.5620/eht.e2017003.

Leist, M., A. Ghallab, R. Graepel, R. Marchan, R. Hassan, S. H. Bennekou, A. Limonciel, M. Vinken, S. Schildknecht, T. Waldmann, E. Danen, B. van Ravenzwaay, H. Kamp, I. Gardner, P. Godoy, F. Y. Bois, A. Braeuning, R. Reif, F. Oesch, D. Drasdo, S. Höhme, M. Schwarz, T. Hartung, T. Braunbeck, J. Beltman, H. Vrieling, F. Sanz, A. Forsby, D. Gadaleta, C. Fisher, J. Kelm, D. Fluri, G. Ecker, B. Zdrazil, A. Terron, P. Jennings, B. van der Burg, S. Dooley, A. H. Meijer, E. Willighagen, M. Martens, C. Evelo, E. Mombelli, O. Taboureau, A. Mantovani, B. Hardy, B. Koch, S. Escher, C. van Thriel, C. Cadenas, D. Kroese, B. van de Water, and J. G. Hengstler. 2017. Adverse Outcome Pathways: Opportunities, Limitations and Open Questions. *Arch Toxicol* 91 (11): 3477–3505. https://doi.org/10.1007/s00204-017-2045-3.

MacKay, C., M. Davies, V. Summerfield, and G. Maxwell. 2013. From Pathways to People: Applying the Adverse Outcome Pathway (AOP) for Skin Sensitization to Risk Assessment. *Altex* 30 (4): 473–486. https://doi.org/10.14573/altex.2013.4.473.

Meek, M. E., C. M. Palermo, A. N. Bachman, C. M. North, and R. Jeffrey Lewis. 2014. Mode of Action Human Relevance (Species Concordance) Framework: Evolution of the Bradford-Hill Considerations and Comparative Analysis of Weight of Evidence. *J Appl Toxicol* 34 (6): 595–606. https://doi.org/10.1002/jat.2984.

Paek, D., Y. Koh, D. U. Park, H. K. Cheong, K. H. Do, C. M. Lim, S. J. Hong, Y. H. Kim, J. H. Leem, K. H. Chung, Y. Y. Choi, J. H. Lee, S. Y. Lim, E. H. Chung, Y. A. Cho, E. J. Chae, J. S. Joh, Y. Yoon, K. H. Lee, B. Y. Choi, and J. Gwack. 2015. Nationwide Study of Humidifier Disinfectant Lung Injury in South Korea, 1994–2011. Incidence and Dose-Response Relationships. *Ann Am Thorac Soc* 12 (12): 1813–1821. https://doi.org/10.1513/AnnalsATS.201504-221OC.

Patlewicz, G., T. W. Simon, J. C. Rowlands, R. A. Budinsky, and R. A. Becker. 2015. Proposing a Scientific Confidence Framework to Help Support the Application of Adverse Outcome Pathways for Regulatory Purposes. *Regul Toxicol Pharmacol* 71 (3): 463–477. https://doi.org/10.1016/j.yrtph.2015.02.011.

Sewell, F., N. Gellatly, M. Beaumont, N. Burden, R. Currie, L. de Haan, T. H. Hutchinson, M. Jacobs, C. Mahony, I. Malcomber, J. Mehta, G. Whale, and I. Kimber. 2018. The Future Trajectory of Adverse Outcome Pathways: A Commentary. *Arch Toxicol*. 1657–1661.

Song, J. A., H. J. Park, M. J. Yang, K. J. Jung, H. S. Yang, C. W. Song, and K. Lee. 2014. Polyhexamethyleneguanidine Phosphate Induces Severe Lung Inflammation, Fibrosis, and Thymic Atrophy. *Food Chem Toxicol* 69: 267–275. https://doi.org/10.1016/j.fct.2014.04.027.

US EPA. 2021. Toxicity Forecasting. Edited by https://www.epa.gov/chemical-research/toxicity-forecasting.

van Bilsen, J. H. M., E. Sienkiewicz-Szłapka, D. Lozano-Ojalvo, L. E. M. Willemsen, C. M. Antunes, E. Molina, J. J. Smit, B. Wróblewska, H. J. Wichers, E. F. Knol, G. S. Ladics, R. H. H. Pieters, S. Denery-Papini, Y. M. Vissers, S. L. Bavaro, C. Larré, K. C. M. Verhoeckx, and E. L. Roggen. 2017. Application of the Adverse Outcome Pathway (Aop) Concept to Structure the Available In Vivo and In Vitro Mechanistic Data for Allergic Sensitization to Food Proteins. *Clin Transl Allergy* 7: 13. https://doi.org/10.1186/s13601-017-0152-0.

Villeneuve, D. L., D. Crump, N. Garcia-Reyero, M. Hecker, T. H. Hutchinson, C. A. LaLone, B. Landesmann, T. Lettieri, S. Munn, M. Nepelska, M. A. Ottinger, L. Vergauwen, and M. Whelan. 2014a. Adverse Outcome Pathway (AOP) Development I: Strategies and Principles. *Toxicol Sci* 142 (2): 312–320. https://doi.org/10.1093/toxsci/kfu199.

Villeneuve, D. L., D. Crump, N. Garcia-Reyero, M. Hecker, T. H. Hutchinson, C. A. LaLone, B. Landesmann, T. Lettieri, S. Munn, M. Nepelska, M. A. Ottinger, L. Vergauwen, and M. Whelan. 2014b. Adverse Outcome Pathway Development II: Best Practices. *Toxicol Sci* 142 (2): 321–330. https://doi.org/10.1093/toxsci/kfu200.

Vinken, M., D. Knapen, L. Vergauwen, J. G. Hengstler, M. Angrish, and M. Whelan. 2017. Adverse Outcome Pathways: A Concise Introduction for Toxicologists. *Arch Toxicol* 3697–3707.

Vinken, M., N. Kramer, T. E. H. Allen, Y. Hoffmans, N. Thatcher, S. Levorato, H. Traussnig, S. Schulte, A. Boobis, A. Thiel, and Imcm Rietjens. 2020. The Use of Adverse Outcome Pathways in the Safety Evaluation of Food Additives. *Arch Toxicol* 94 (3): 959–966. https://doi.org/10.1007/s00204-020-02670-0.

10 Epigenetics in Risk Assessment

Carmen Marsit and Jinze Li
Emory University Rollins School of Public Health, Atlanta, GA, United States

CONTENTS

Developmental Origins and Critical Periods of Epigenetic Effects 190
Interpreting Epigenetic Variation and Its Relation to the Environment 191
Assessing Epigenetics..192
Applying Epigenetics in Risk Assessment 194
Challenges and Opportunities in Using Epigenetics in Risk Assessment...194
Literature Cited 196

LEARNING OBJECTIVES

Students who complete this chapter will be able to

1. Define epigenetics and the forms of epigenetic regulation,
2. Understand how epigenetic features are evaluated,
3. Consider critical period of exposure and potential epigenetic consequences, and
4. Apply epigenetic evaluation is applied to risk assessment.

Humans, like all multicellular organisms, begin as a single cell and progress through a series of cellular divisions and differentiation events resulting in a mature organism. In the case of humans, from that single cell, over 200 different types of cells are formed, contributing to the 78 organs which make up a human body. Yet, each of these different types of cells contains the same genetic material, the human genome, which provides the blueprint for the RNA and proteins that build those cells and tissues and allow them to function. The question then is, how does a single genome, identical in practically every cell of the body allow for such variety in form and function?

In 1952, Conrad Waddington, a British geneticist and embryologist, coined the term epigenetics, defined as "science concerned with the causal analysis of development" (Waddington 1952). In this same work, he introduced his epigenetic landscape model, depicted as a ball on the top of a hill, with a series of bifurcating valleys through which it can roll, as a metaphor for the cell fate decisions that a cell makes as it undergoes the differentiation process of a pluripotent cell to its final differentiated state. We can similarly describe this like a Plinko board (Figure 10.1) where a token is dropped at the top of the board and at each peg can fall in different directions until it reaches its final state within a slot at the bottom. Much like genetics prior to the discovery of the DNA double helix, this early understanding of epigenetics laid out the concept that there are mechanisms by which cells differentiate, but the actual mechanisms themselves were still unclear.

Epigenetics today can be defined as the heritable control of gene expression or gene expression potential beyond the coding of DNA sequencing. In this case, heritable means that the regulation can remain through cellular division (mitosis) and that the mechanism invoked works with transcriptional machinery to control if and how RNA is transcribed from the DNA sequence. Thus, epigenetics describes a *persistent* cellular memory that allows for specific DNA sequences to be activated or silenced and can underlie cell fate. This concept of persistence and role in cellular differentiation is critical, as it guides the interpretation of epigenetic changes that are observed in response to an environmental exposure or disease process.

Fundamentally, epigenetic regulation drives the structure and accessibility of DNA to undergo transcription. DNA in the cell is exquisitely packaged in order to condense its size and control its function. The double helix of DNA wraps around nucleosomes, which consist of a dimer of tetramers of histone proteins H3 and H4 with H2A and H2B. Around this nucleosome core, 146bp of DNA wraps, and additional histones operate outside of the nucleosome to link nucleosomes together in a successive coiling structure forming chromatin.

DOI: 10.1201/9780429291722-10

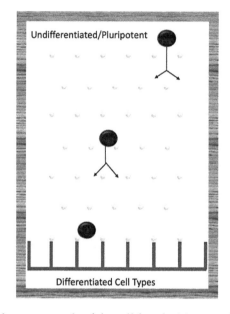

Figure 10.1 Plinko board as an example of the cell fate decisions made as a cell moves from an undifferentiated to a fully differentiated state.

In addition to playing a role in creating a structure for condensing DNA, the histone proteins also serve as critical proteins in the regulation of DNA accessibility and function. The histones of the nucleosome have tails of peptides that extend outside of the nucleosome core structure and which can undergo a variety of post-translational modifications. These modifications commonly include methylation, phosphorylation, acetylation, and ubiquitylation and are placed onto histones by a variety of histone-modifying enzymes. These modifications can serve a variety of functions, leading to changes in the nucleosome structure and DNA accessibility, and acting as signals for transcriptional activation and repression machinery to bind and operate. Thus, chromatin modification is a key epigenetic regulatory process, as these histone modifications can be perpetuated through cell divisions and maintain the activation or inactivation state of genes or gene regulatory elements on the DNA.

At the level of the DNA itself occurs the most widely studied form of epigenetic regulation, DNA cytosine methylation. DNA methylation is the addition of a methyl group to the 5'position of a cytosine residue in the context of a cytosine-guanine dinucleotide (referred to as CpG sites). This methylation is catalyzed by specific DNA methyltransferase enzymes with specific affinity for CpG sites and which utilize the cellular methylation donor, S-adenosylmethionine as a cofactor (Figure 10.2A). Across the genome, CpG sites occur less often than would be expected by chance, and where they do occur, they regularly occur as regions with a high frequency of CpG sites, known as CpG islands. These CpG islands are often found in the promoter region of genes, where transcriptional regulation takes place. Canonically, CpG islands in gene promoters lacking DNA methylation are co-incident with histone modifications that signal for transcriptional activity or potential, while those demonstrating DNA methylation co-occur with histones modified for transcriptional repression or silencing (Figure 10.2B). Yet, CpG DNA methylation can be identified in other regions of the genome, where this pattern is not maintained. For example, within gene bodies, CpG sites are often methylated, and this serves as a marker of transcriptionally active genes, likely playing a role in transcriptional processivity. In nongenic regions of the genome, DNA methylation may alter long-distance chromatin interactions, allowing for transcriptional enhancers and their associate protein complexes to interact with gene promoter regions, altering transcriptional control. In all cases, DNA methylation is working in concert with histone modifications to signal for various proteins to interact and functionally mediate the results of these signals.

The patterns of DNA methylation and their co-incident histone modifications are unique to individual cell types and are set during the differentiation process of a cell from its pluripotent state to its final differentiated form. So, for many cells and tissues of the body, this occurs in embryonic and fetal development through a carefully orchestrated series of events. Following fertilization

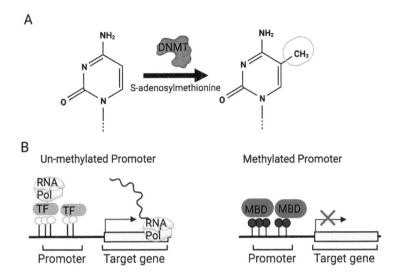

Figure 10.2 Overview of DNA methylation. (A) Methylation of DNA occurs as an enzymatically catalyzed process by DNA Methyltransferase (DNMT) with the cofactor S-adenosylmethione, which acts as the methyl donor. (B) A gene promoter that is devoid of DNA methylation (left) allows for the binding of Transcription Factors (TF) and the recruitment of an RNA polymerase (RNA Pol) to allow for the transcription of that gene's mRNA. When the promoter region is methylated (right), methyl-binding domain MBD) proteins bind to the promoter region and inhibit transcription. (Created with BioRender.com).

and during the initial cellular divisions and cleavages of the zygote, DNA methylation across most of the genome is lost. The cells of the inner cell mass of the blastocyst, pluripotent stem cells, lack the majority of DNA methylation, allowing them to take on pathways of differentiation to form every type of cell in the body. As those cells divide and differentiate, de novo DNA methylation and histone modifications occur, creating the cell-specific patterns that will identify each of the somatic cells. Similarly, the trophoblast lineages, which will form the placenta and membranes of the fetus undergo their own differentiation and de novo methylation process. Finally, during the process of gonadal differentiation, the primordial germ cells take on their initial epigenetic features. While the majority of these differentiation processes and their epigenetic programming events occur during in utero development, there are also terminal differentiation processes that can occur later in life. For example, puberty represents an additional period where sex organs mature and additional epigenetic programming occurs as those cells differentiate to their final forms. Additionally, pathologic processes that involve differentiation events, such as those found in carcinogenesis, are an additional opportunity for epigenetic programming to occur.

The critical role that epigenetic mechanisms play in cellular differentiation, and ultimately cellular function, provides an impetus to understand if and how environmental exposures can

BOX 10.1   ENDOCRINE-DISRUPTING COMPOUNDS (EDCS) AND EPIGENETICS

Endocrine Disruption: A Challenge for Risk Assessment

John A. McLachlan and Christopher A.B. McLachlan

Endocrine disruption refers to the alteration of the endocrine or reproductive system by environmental chemicals that mimic or block natural hormones. It has come to be associated with various agents effecting infertility, obesity, or other metabolic changes, often following exposure early in development.

Much of what we know about endocrine disruption derives from observations following prenatal exposure to the potent synthetic estrogen, diethylstilbestrol, or DES. Close to five million pregnant women were treated with DES in the 1950s and 1960s with subsequent findings of rare genital tract cancers in some of the daughters after they reached puberty. The dose and developmental time of exposure were well documented. The DES cohort has been studied for 50 years, revealing the long-term results of developmental estrogen exposures with effects on subsequent fertility, menopause, and other endocrine disorders. Findings in laboratory animals have replicated and, in some cases, predicted, those in humans, using similar doses and developmental windows. Animal studies have provided mechanistic insights into the actions of DES during development including the importance of epigenetic changes; that is, the imprinting of genes in development that change the function of cells or organs later. DES is associated with persistent long-term developmental changes in multiple species that have been studied in addition to humans. An example of congruity between animal models and human experience is seen with the recent findings of hypospadias (abnormal opening of the penile urethra) in sons and grandsons of both humans and mice treated in utero with DES. There have also been reports of reproductive defects in granddaughters of DES-exposed women.

The discovery that numerous environmental chemicals exhibited estrogenic activity spurred interest in the risk to humans for DES-like actions known as endocrine disruption. Synthetic chemicals (plastics, pesticides, persistent organic pollutants), plant compounds (phytoestrogens), and fungal products are among the sources of hormonal activity in the environment. While usually weak acting, these compounds demonstrate DES-like effects in animal models. An additional concern for human risk to *EDCs* is that numerous species of wildlife (mammals, fish, reptiles, birds, amphibians) exhibit estrogenic effects (feminization) when exposed to ambient levels of estrogenic environmental compounds adding credence to the concept of risk for human exposure at environmental levels of hormonally active compounds.

An important component of risk assessment involves hazard identification. The molecular mechanisms underlying the actions of endocrine-disrupting chemicals are especially useful since the chemicals in this class work through known mechanisms involving hormone receptors. A recent expert consensus statement uses key characteristics of EDCs as a strategy to understand and predict hazards based on mechanisms (La Merrill et al., 2020). The authors utilized ten key molecular characteristics of DES and an estrogenic environmental agent, bisphenol A (BPA), a ubiquitous chemical used to make plastics. This approach demonstrated multiple hazard identities between the well-known drug and the lesser-known environmental contaminant. Endocrine disruption is particularly well suited for this type of hazard identification since the molecular and cellular mechanisms of endocrine active chemicals are well-known. The value of this approach to hazard identification provides useful information to assess risk.

Considering the challenges facing risk assessment of endocrine disruption, the position taken by the Endocrine Society on behalf of basic and clinical research in 2009 and again in 2015 is "that the evidence for adverse reproductive outcomes is strong and mounting.". Given the current debate regarding the importance of reports of decreases in human sperm counts to overall fertility, the challenges are there to address. This may require a mechanism-based approach to risk assessment.

LITERATURE CITED

La Merrill, M. A. H., L. N. Vandenberg, M. T. Smith, W. William Goodson, P. Browne, H. B. Patisaul, V. J. Cogliano, T. J. Woodruff, K. S. Korach, A. C. Gore, K. Z. Guyton, A Kortenkamp, L. Rieswijk, H. Sone, L. Zeise, and R. T. Zoelle. 2020. Consensus on the Key Characteristics of Endocrine-Disrupting Chemicals as a Basis for Hazard Identification." *Nat. Rev. Endocrinol.* 16: 45–57. https://doi.org/10.1038/s41574-019-0273-8.

impact these features. Such data could be used, then, as an additional piece of evidence regarding the potential risk of an environmental exposure.

DEVELOPMENTAL ORIGINS AND CRITICAL PERIODS OF EPIGENETIC EFFECTS

The Developmental Origins and Health and Disease (DOHaD) hypothesis emerged from a series of landmark studies that demonstrated that birth size is associated with long-term chronic disease risk. Most of these studies have focused on cardiovascular disease and metabolic syndromes (Barker 1988; Barker 1998; Barker and Osmond 1988) and have linked environmental stressors during in utero development, including diet, xenobiotic exposures, and stress, to altered fetal growth. It is generally accepted that birth size is not causal to these downstream sequelae and serves as a proxy for complex underlying etiologic mechanisms that influence intrauterine growth as well as program adult physiological systems (Welberg and Seckl 2001). This fetal programming effect is likely an evolutionary mechanism allowing the organism an opportunity to adapt on a more proximal time scale to prepare for the environment it is about to experience. Given the essential role of epigenetic mechanisms in development and in the programming of cell differentiation and fate, much attention has been paid to examining if these mechanisms serve as the underlying mediators of DOHaD.

Considered seminal to the development of DOHaD are studies on the Dutch Famine of World War II. Due to Nazi occupation of Amsterdam, food supplies were limited to the population, and rationing was instituted for a defined period of time. A birth cohort of children born around this period was developed and has served as an opportunity to examine the timing and impact of an extreme stressor, in this case famine, on lifelong health programming. In addition, more recent research on these individuals has identified persistent epigenetic changes and has linked those to specific time periods of exposure during gestation as well as to adverse health outcomes in adulthood (Heijmans et al. 2009). This evidence has been critical in demonstrating a potential role for epigenetics in developmental programming and has been expanded to consider various nutritional and metabolic environments, as well as other xenobiotic exposures during in utero development, and their epigenetic impacts, both in human observational studies, as well as in experimental models (Bansal and Simmons 2018; El Hajj et al. 2014; Eriksson 2016; Goyal, Limesand, and Goyal 2019; Joss-Moore, Albertine, and Lane 2011; Safi-Stibler and Gabory 2020).

The literature now abounds with observational studies of epigenetic changes or variations identified in children, at birth, associated with exposures prenatally. The most robust and reproducible findings, thus far, have been linking maternal smoking during pregnancy and altered DNA methylation in the cord blood of offspring (Kaur et al. 2019). In a large international consortium-wide meta-analysis (Ramakrishnan et al. 1981), over 6,000 individual CpG sites were identified to exhibit either increased or decreased DNA methylation associated with sustained maternal smoking in pregnancy, and many of these changes to the methylation state could still be observed in the children at later ages. The most reproducible of those findings was in the aryl-hydrocarbon receptor repressor (AHRR) gene, demonstrating reduced DNA methylation associated with smoking, with such confidence that this site has been evaluated as a clinically relevant biomarker of maternal smoking in pregnancy (Lee et al. 2017).

INTERPRETING EPIGENETIC VARIATION AND ITS RELATION TO THE ENVIRONMENT

There are at least two potential and overlapping ways in which environmental stressors during development could be contributing to observed epigenetic changes. First, as noted earlier in the chapter, the differentiation of somatic cells from pluripotent progenitors requires specific epigenetic reprogramming, including DNA methylation and histone modifications into cell-type specific patterning. Environmental stressors or exposures that could alter the mechanisms of that patterning, could lead to changes in the epigenetic features and thus changes to cellular function. In one possible scenario, these environmental impacts could occur during initial cell divisions and differentiation events and thus be observable consistently within any somatic tissue of an individual but show variation between individuals. Known as metastable epialleles, this phenomenon has been observed in the settings of nutritional deficits (Silver et al. 2015), as well as with various environmental exposures, including endocrine disruptors (Dolinoy et al. 2007; Faulk et al. 2016). If the impacts occur at other critical developmental windows, they may lead to more cell-type or tissue-specific epigenetic disruption, which may be more difficult to observe unless these alterations contribute to a specific pathologic process and samples can be obtained.

The second explanation for an observed epigenetic change, which is not mutually exclusive of the first, is that environmental exposure or stressors lead to the selective pressure of or direct stimulation of a differentiation event, which because of the role of epigenetic mechanisms in differentiation, is observed as an epigenetic change. As an example, there is substantial evidence that 2,3,7,8-tetrachlorodibenzo-p-dioxin, i.e., dioxin, can impact immune function through impacts on CD4+ T cell and T regulatory cell differentiation (Marshall and Kerkvliet 2010) in adult studies. Developments in DNA methylation analyses now allow for the estimation of such effects, at least, in regards to immune cells. These methods make use of references panels of DNA methylation from isolated immune cells, and deconvolution methodologies to estimate the proportions of different cell types in mixed peripheral blood samples, thereby allowing for comparison of changes to these cellular compositions based on exposures (Houseman et al. 2012; Kelsey and Wiencke 2018; Salas et al. 2018).

Similar impacts on immune cells or other cells and tissues would also be possible during the developmental period, including in utero and early childhood, as developmental plasticity provides an opportunity for cells to adapt to their experienced environment as they continue to mature and grow. This makes the in utero developmental period and early childhood some of the most important critical windows for an impact of environmental exposures to demonstrate epigenetic effects and highlights, particularly, vulnerabilities that must be considered in risk assessment and reduction strategies.

ASSESSING EPIGENETICS

As mentioned earlier, the most widely studied of the epigenetic features is that of DNA methylation, due to its stability as a covalent modification to DNA and the corresponding availability of tools and techniques that can be availed for its examination.

The most common technique used in the study of DNA methylation is bisulfite modification. Treatment of genomic DNA with a sodium bisulfite solution leads to the deamination of cytosine nucleotides to uracil (C→U) unless that cytosine is methylated, in which case it is protected from deamination and remains a cytosine. Polymerase chain reaction (PCR) amplification of the resulting DNA can replace the uracil with thymine, and lead to a template DNA that is devoid of cytosines except for those sites exhibiting DNA methylation (Figure 10.3). This template DNA can then be subjected to a variety of methods to determine the location of those cytosines, the most comprehensive of which would be whole genome sequencing. Due, though, to the loss of much of the specificity of the DNA with the sodium bisulfite conversion, whole genome sequencing remains an expensive proposition for most research applications, as the high read depths required for accurate alignment to the source genome sequence require long extensive sequencing at a high cost. Array-based methods, such as Illumina's Methylation EPIC array, which interrogates over 850,000 CpG sites for DNA methylation across the genome, have become more widely adopted, particularly in human population applications, as these methods provide reproducible data on a near genomic scale. More recently, a murine array from Illumina has been introduced, which will allow for interrogation of DNA methylation in animal models of exposures. For more gene or genomic region targeted applications, methods based on short read sequencing, such as pyrosequencing or mass spectrometry-based analyses, can be used, and for specific CpG sites, quantitative real-time PCR-based methods are utilized.

In all cases, these methods result in a quantitative output representing the proportion of methylated alleles at a CpG site within each sample, given that any one CpG on DNA can only be either methylated or not. As described in the prior section, this is consistent with the interpretation of epigenetic variation in denoting differences in functional cell types within a given sample (Figure 10.4).

Histone modifications and the accessibility of chromatin can also be examined, more often in experimental systems, due to the challenges inherent in their quantification. In general, to examine specific histone modifications and their location requires the use of a technique known as chromatin immunoprecipitation, wherein cells are treated with a cross-linking agent such as formalin, DNA is sheared, and an antibody is used to precipitate a specifically modified histone cross-linked to the genomic DNA where it was located. That DNA is then released and can be identified through sequencing or PCR-based approaches. Although this allows for comprehensive detailing of sites of histone modification, the challenges in the sample preparation and required DNA mass needs for examination often making applying these studies outside of a laboratory experiment more difficult.

Assay for Transposase Accessible Chromatin using sequencing (ATAC-seq) is a technique that is growing more widely used in human clinical or population contexts in order to examine genome-wide chromatin accessibility. This method utilizes the activity of Tn5 Transposase, a bacterial enzyme that when mutated can act as an integrase, capable of inserting DNA sequences in the genome. For ATAC-seq, isolated chromatin is treated with the hyperactive Tn5 Transposase, which inserts sequencing adapters into open regions (lacking silencing histone structures) of the genome. The tagged DNA is then isolated, amplified, and sequenced, and through bioinformatic tools, it is used to infer regions of accessibility or inaccessibility of the genome. This provides an additional level of evaluation of epigenetic changes related to environmental exposures both in experimental models and in human population studies.

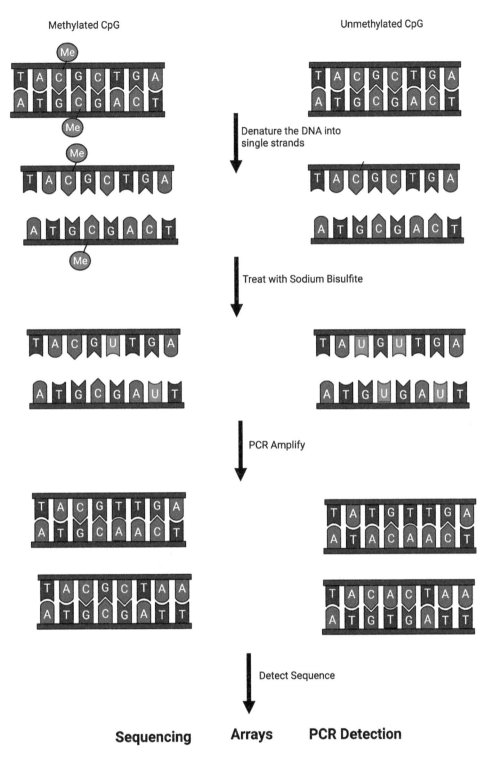

Figure 10.3 Overview of the process of DNA bisulfite modification allowing the assessment of DNA methylation in genomic DNA. (Created with BioRender.com).

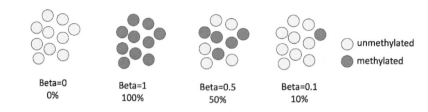

Figure 10.4 The quantitative assessment of DNA methylation using arrays or sequencing-based approaches results in a beta value between 0 and 1, representing the proportion of DNA methylation of a specific CpG site across the cells in the sample.

APPLYING EPIGENETICS IN RISK ASSESSMENT

Given the critical role that epigenetic mechanisms play in cellular development, differentiation, and function, it is attractive to consider epigenetics when thinking about the potential risk of an environmental agent. There is clear evidence, for example, that altered DNA methylation patterns and histone modifications are widespread in cancers, and in fact, epigenetic mechanisms are considered drivers of all of the phenotypic and functional "hallmarks" of a cancer (Flavahan et al. 2017). Similarly, specific regions of DNA methylation and its associated chromatin conformation are critical in defining the identity and function of a variety of immune effector cells, whose presence or absence can be contributing to or indicative of a disease process (Calle-Fabregat et al. 2020). Taken together with the growing body of evidence linking differences or changes in epigenetic features with environmental exposures, there is an obvious opportunity to see epigenetics mechanism as an additional consideration in risk evaluation.

There is growing interest in applying the adverse outcome pathway (AOP) framework to the consideration of epigenetic mechanisms as evidence for causal relationships between an exposure and disease process or outcome. An AOP (Figure 10.5) is a conceptual model which identifies a series of events at the molecular, cellular, tissue, system, and population level that bring about a toxic effect when an organism is exposed (Ankley et al.).

To successfully utilize this framework requires the incorporation of experimental and observational data at various levels. Epigenetic evaluations, though, may not all be equally valid or appropriate for examination at all biological levels, and so considerations need to be made in both designing the research needed for addressing risk and in evaluating the existing evidence for its relevance and authority. For example, in examining the impacts of an endocrine-disrupting compound on a hormone responsive cell, some of the initial steps in the pathway will involve interactions with receptors and biochemical signaling events, which themselves will not be captured by epigenetic assessments. Instead, the downstream impacts of those initial events, related to activation of specific genes in a stable fashion will be observable using assessments of histone modifications and chromatin access, while DNA methylation may or may not demonstrate alteration depending on the stability of these responses. Only once a cell's overt function(s) is being altered and leading to differentiation events indicative of cellular reprogramming might altered DNA methylation be observed. In general, this is likely the observations made in human clinical or population studies or within animal models, where the system dynamics of cellular interactions can allow for more complete reprogramming to occur. Then, as we move to a population-level response, the examination of epigenetic impacts becomes much less relevant, as the cellular responses are minor compared to major ecological effects on population dynamics.

CHALLENGES AND OPPORTUNITIES IN USING EPIGENETICS IN RISK ASSESSMENT

The application of epigenetic research in risk assessment strategies does hold potential, particularly in considering the impacts of exposures in development and during key windows of susceptibility such as childhood, puberty, and pregnancy, which are often less incorporated in traditional risk assessment frameworks. For example, examining epigenetic variation associated with a novel chemical exposure and comparing it to previously characterized exposure could allow for earlier identification of potential toxicity, and earlier regulatory action, than waiting for health phenotypes to develop. This could be particularly useful in studies during development, where not only could toxic effects be identified but also offspring could be at risk so that interventions employed prior to later life health impacts.

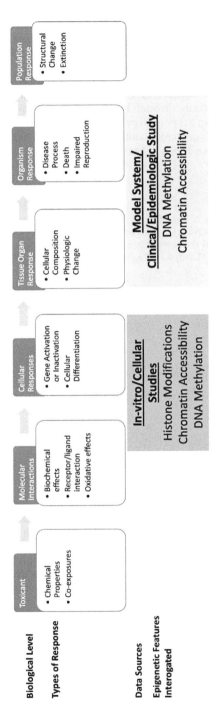
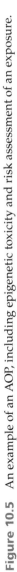

Figure 10.5   An example of an AOP, including epigenetic toxicity and risk assessment of an exposure.

Certainly, though, there are limitations to the application of epigenetics in risk assessment as well. Given the role of epigenetic mechanisms in cellular differentiation, the interpretation of any identified variation associated with an exposure from human population studies must be made carefully. This variation represents changes in cellular function and phenotype, but given that not all potential variants of cells have been characterized epigenetically, what that exact cell is or may be doing may not be fully understood. With the development of epigenomic editing tools based on CRISPR technology, there are opportunities to characterize the cellular impacts of any identified epigenetic variation and to gain a more complete understanding of the potential health impacts.

The other limitation has been a lack of integrated studies across the AOP continuum, where data from in-vitro and in-vivo research is then translated into human populations. This type of comprehensive analysis occurs only through multidisciplinary and collaborative research efforts, as this research requires an array of expertise and approaches. As research programs in environmental epigenetics and epigenomics continue to build and as the approaches mature, the data on epigenetic impacts of exposures will become more reliable and useful in risk assessment strategies.

LITERATURE CITED

Ankley, G. T., R. S. Bennett, R. J. Erickson, D. J. Hoff, M. W. Hornung, R. D. Johnson, D. R. Mount, J. W. Nichols, C. L. Russom, P. K. Schmieder, J. A. Serrrano, J. E. Tietge, and D. L. Villeneuve. 2010. Adverse Outcome Pathways: A Conceptual Framework to Support Ecotoxicology Research and Risk Assessment. *Environ Toxicol Chem* 29 (3): 730–741. https://doi.org/10.1002/etc.34. https://www.ncbi.nlm.nih.gov/pubmed/20821501.

Bansal, A., and R. A. Simmons. 2018. Epigenetics and Developmental Origins of Diabetes: Correlation or Causation? *Am J Physiol Endocrinol Metab* 315 (1): E15–E28. https://doi.org/10.1152/ajpendo.00424.2017. https://www.ncbi.nlm.nih.gov/pubmed/29406781.

Barker, D. J. 1988. Childhood Causes of Adult Diseases. *Arch Dis Child* 63 (7): 867–869. https://doi.org/10.1136/adc.63.7.867. https://www.ncbi.nlm.nih.gov/pubmed/3415312.

Barker, D. J. 1998. In Utero Programming of Chronic Disease. *Clin Sci (Lond)* 95 (2): 115–128. https://www.ncbi.nlm.nih.gov/pubmed/9680492.

Barker, D. J., and C. Osmond. 1988. Low Birth Weight and Hypertension. *BMJ* 297 (6641): 134–135. https://doi.org/10.1136/bmj.297.6641.134-b. https://www.ncbi.nlm.nih.gov/pubmed/3408942.

Calle-Fabregat, C., O. Morante-Palacios, and E. Ballestar. 2020. Understanding the Relevance of DNA Methylation Changes in Immune Differentiation and Disease. *Genes (Basel)* 11 (1). https://doi.org/10.3390/genes11010110. https://www.ncbi.nlm.nih.gov/pubmed/31963661.

Dolinoy, D. C., R. Das, J. R. Weidman, and R. L. Jirtle. 2007. Metastable Epialleles, Imprinting, and the Fetal Origins of Adult Diseases. *Pediatr Res* 61 (5 Pt 2): 30R–37R. https://doi.org/10.1203/pdr.0b013e31804575f7. https://www.ncbi.nlm.nih.gov/pubmed/17413847.

El Hajj, N., E. Schneider, H. Lehnen, and T. Haaf. 2014. Epigenetics and Life-Long Consequences of an Adverse Nutritional and Diabetic Intrauterine Environment. *Reproduction* 148 (6): R111–120. https://doi.org/10.1530/REP-14-0334. https://www.ncbi.nlm.nih.gov/pubmed/25187623.

Eriksson, J. G. 2016. Developmental Origins of Health and Disease – from a Small Body Size at Birth to Epigenetics. *Ann Med* 48 (6): 456–467. https://doi.org/10.1080/07853890.2016.1193786. https://www.ncbi.nlm.nih.gov/pubmed/27268105.

Faulk, C., J. H. Kim, O. S. Anderson, M. S. Nahar, T. R. Jones, M. A. Sartor, and D. C. Dolinoy. 2016. Detection of Differential DNA Methylation in Repetitive DNA of Mice and Humans Perinatally Exposed to Bisphenol A. *Epigenetics* 11 (7): 489–500. https://doi.org/10.1080/15592294.2016.1183856. https://www.ncbi.nlm.nih.gov/pubmed/27267941.

Flavahan, W. A., E. Gaskell, and B. E. Bernstein. 2017. Epigenetic Plasticity and the Hallmarks of Cancer. *Science* 357 (6348). https://doi.org/10.1126/science.aal2380. https://www.ncbi.nlm.nih.gov/pubmed/28729483.

Goyal, D., S. W. Limesand, and R. Goyal. 2019. Epigenetic Responses and the Developmental Origins of Health and Disease. *J Endocrinol* 242 (1): T105–T119. https://doi.org/10.1530/JOE-19-0009. https://www.ncbi.nlm.nih.gov/pubmed/31091503.

Heijmans, B. T., E. W. Tobi, L. H. Lumey, and P. E. Slagboom. 2009. The Epigenome: Archive of the Prenatal Environment. *Epigenetics* 4 (8): 526–531. https://doi.org/10.4161/epi.4.8.10265. https://www.ncbi.nlm.nih.gov/pubmed/19923908.

Houseman, E. A., W. P. Accomando, D. C. Koestler, B. C. Christensen, C. J. Marsit, H. H. Nelson, J. K. Wiencke, and K. T. Kelsey. 2012. DNA Methylation Arrays as Surrogate Measures of Cell Mixture Distribution. *BMC Bioinformatics* 13: 86. https://doi.org/10.1186/1471-2105-13-86. https://www.ncbi.nlm.nih.gov/pubmed/22568884.

Joss-Moore, L. A., K. H. Albertine, and R. H. Lane. 2011. Epigenetics and the Developmental Origins of Lung Disease. *Mol Genet Metab* 104 (1–2): 61–66. https://doi.org/10.1016/j.ymgme.2011.07.018. https://www.ncbi.nlm.nih.gov/pubmed/21835665.

Kaur, G., R. Begum, S. Thota, and S. Batra. 2019. A Systematic Review of Smoking-Related Epigenetic Alterations. *Arch Toxicol* 93 (10): 2715–2740. https://doi.org/10.1007/s00204-019-02562-y. https://www.ncbi.nlm.nih.gov/pubmed/31555878.

Kelsey, K. T., and J. K. Wiencke. 2018. Immunomethylomics: A Novel Cancer Risk Prediction Tool. *Ann Am Thorac Soc* 15 (Suppl 2): S76–S80. https://doi.org/10.1513/AnnalsATS.201706-477MG. https://www.ncbi.nlm.nih.gov/pubmed/29676642.

Lee, D. H., S. H. Hwang, M. K. Lim, J. K. Oh, D. Y. Song, E. H. Yun, and E. Y. Park. 2017. Performance of Urine Cotinine and Hypomethylation of AHRR and F2RL3 as Biomarkers for Smoking Exposure in a Population-Based Cohort. *PLoS One* 12 (4): e0176783. https://doi.org/10.1371/journal.pone.0176783. https://www.ncbi.nlm.nih.gov/pubmed/28453567.

Marshall, N. B., and N. I. Kerkvliet. 2010. Dioxin and Immune Regulation: Emerging Role of Aryl Hydrocarbon Receptor in the Generation of Regulatory T Cells. *Ann N Y Acad Sci* 1183: 25–37. https://doi.org/10.1111/j.1749-6632.2009.05125.x. https://www.ncbi.nlm.nih.gov/pubmed/20146706.

Ramakrishnan, V. R., S. Yabuki, I. Y. Sillers, D. G. Schindler, D. M. Engelman, and P. B. Moore. 1981. Positions of Proteins S6, S11 and S15 in the 30 S Ribosomal Subunit of Escherichia Coli. *J Mol Biol* 153 (3): 739–760. https://doi.org/10.1016/0022-2836(81)90416-2. https://www.ncbi.nlm.nih.gov/pubmed/7040690.

Safi-Stibler, S., and A. Gabory. 2020. Epigenetics and the Developmental Origins of Health and Disease: Parental Environment Signalling to the Epigenome, Critical Time Windows and Sculpting the Adult Phenotype. *Semin Cell Dev Biol* 97: 172–180. https://doi.org/10.1016/j.semcdb.2019.09.008. https://www.ncbi.nlm.nih.gov/pubmed/31587964.

Salas, L. A., J. K. Wiencke, D. C. Koestler, Z. Zhang, B. C. Christensen, and K. T. Kelsey. 2018. Tracing Human Stem Cell Lineage during Development Using DNA Methylation. *Genome Res* 28 (9): 1285–1295. https://doi.org/10.1101/gr.233213.117. https://www.ncbi.nlm.nih.gov/pubmed/30072366.

Silver, M. J., N. J. Kessler, B. J. Hennig, P. Dominguez-Salas, E. Laritsky, M. S. Baker, C. Coarfa, H. Hernandez-Vargas, J. M. Castelino, M. N. Routledge, Y. Y. Gong, Z. Herceg, Y. S. Lee, K. Lee, S. E. Moore, A. J. Fulford, A. M. Prentice, and R. A. Waterland. 2015. Independent Genomewide Screens Identify the Tumor Suppressor VTRNA2-1 as a Human Epiallele Responsive to Periconceptional Environment. *Genome Biol* 16: 118. https://doi.org/10.1186/s13059-015-0660-y. https://www.ncbi.nlm.nih.gov/pubmed/26062908.

Waddington, C. H. 1952. *The Epigenetics of Birds. Cambridge Biological Studies.* Cambridge: University Press.

Welberg, L. A., and J. R. Seckl. 2001. Prenatal Stress, Glucocorticoids and the Programming of the Brain. *J Neuroendocrinol* 13 (2): 113–128. https://doi.org/10.1046/j.1365-2826.2001.00601.x. https://www.ncbi.nlm.nih.gov/pubmed/11168837.

197

11 Probabilistic Models for Characterizing Aggregate and Cumulative Risk

Qingyu Meng
California Department of Toxic Substances Control, Sacramento, CA, United States
Desert Research Institute, Reno, NV, United States

CONTENTS

Introduction 199
Aggregate and Cumulative Risks...200
    Basic Risk Assessment Equations for Cancer and Noncancer Assessments 200
    Aggregate Assessment of Exposure and Risk...202
    Cumulative Assessment of Exposure and Risk 204
    Characterizing Aggregate and Cumulative Risks 205
        Measurement Studies...205
        Modeling Studies...209
Probabilistic Models for Characterizing Aggregate and Cumulative Risks.................211
    Probability and Probability Distributions...211
        Probability and Risk Assessment 211
        Common Probability Distributions in Risk Assessment......................................212
    Probabilistic Models for Exposure and Risk Assessment...215
        Scoping for Probabilistic Modeling...215
        Fundamental Approach for Probabilistic Modeling...216
        Critical Issues in Probabilistic Modeling...220
Thought Questions 223
Disclaimers..223
References..223

LEARNING OBJECTIVES

Students who complete this chapter will be able to

1. Calculate cancer risk and hazard quotient using the fundamental deterministic models for risk and exposure assessment,
2. Demonstrate the concept of aggregate and cumulative exposures and risks, and
3. Understand the rationale and describe the procedure for probabilistic exposure and risk assessments.

INTRODUCTION

Humans are constantly exposed to multiple environmental chemicals from various sources and via different exposure pathways. Common daily activities, such as eating, drinking, personal hygiene, commuting, working, and recreating, bring everyone in contact with many of the 86,000 chemicals in commerce today, present in air, drinking water, breast milk, soil and dust, and consumer products (NRC 2014). Park et al. (2012) measured 3,221 chemicals in human plasma and found that more than two-thirds of these chemicals are exogenous. The nationwide body burden of environmental chemicals has been monitored by the Centers for Disease Control and Prevention (CDC) since the 1970s, under the National Health and Nutrition Examination Survey (NHANES) program. More than 200 environmental chemicals and their metabolites, including pesticides, plasticizers, per- and polyfluoroalkyl substances (PFAS), and flame retardants, have been observed in the US population (CDC 2021).

Some of these chemicals are persistent organic pollutants, such as PFAS and dichlorodiphenyltrichloroethane (DDT), which remain in our bodies for many years (ATSDR 2019, 2021); other chemicals are nonpersistent, such as 1,4-dioxane, a widespread contaminant in drinking water,

DOI: 10.1201/9780429291722-11

and the half-life of which is in hours in our body (ATSDR 2012). Both persistent and nonpersistent chemicals may have adverse impacts on human health.

To evaluate the health impacts of the total body burden of environmental chemicals, both aggregate exposure and cumulative exposure need to be considered. Aggregate exposure refers to a person's total exposure to a chemical through all exposure pathways, and cumulative exposure refers to a person's total exposure through all pathways to multiple chemicals sharing similar mechanisms of action or contributing to similar adverse health end points (US EPA 2019b).

Indeed, evaluating aggregate and cumulative exposure is required explicitly or inexplicitly by some federal laws and state regulations. For example, the Food Quality Protection Act (FQPA) of 1996 requires that exposure to pesticides be evaluated for all potential pathways, including both dietary pathways (i.e., consumption of food and beverages) and nondietary pathways (i.e., intake of pesticides in air, water, and soil or dust). The FQPA codified the need for more and better exposure data to help in the process of risk-based decision-making and mandated aggregate and cumulative assessments (*Food Quality Protection Act of 1996, PUBLIC LAW 104–170* 1996). The FQPA was one of the first acts to explicitly require a regulatory agency to conduct aggregate assessments of exposure to pesticides from multiple routes – namely, exposures by inhalation of airborne compound, dermal absorption of chemicals in contact with the skin, and ingestion of chemicals in both food and other materials that young children ingest, such as soil and house dust. The Frank Lautenberg Chemical Safety for the 21st Century Act, passed in 2016, also directs the US Environmental Protection Agency (US EPA) to protect "potentially exposed or susceptible sub-populations," i.e.,

> a group of individuals within the general population identified by the [US EPA] Administrator who, due to either greater susceptibility or greater exposure, may be at greater risk than the general population of adverse health effects from exposure to a chemical substance or mixture, such as infants, children, pregnant women, workers, or the elderly.
> (*The Frank R. Lautenberg Chemical Safety for the 21st Century Act*, 2016)

The Minnesota Water Guidance requires that the Minnesota Department of Health evaluate cumulative exposures and impacts of multiple chemicals in drinking water (Minnesota Department of Health 2020). Similarly, the California Safer Consumer Product Regulations directs the Department of Toxic Substances Control to evaluate "[t]he chemical's cumulative effects with other chemicals with the same or similar hazard trait(s) and/or environmental or toxicological end point(s)" (*CCR, Title 22, Sections 69502.2* 2008).

The process to quantify aggregate or cumulative risks is complex. However, it is a useful and necessary exercise because quantitative methods allow us to make informed decisions and discriminate between important and trivial exposures and risks, evaluate trade-offs, set priorities, and allocate resources. Quantitative risk assessment methods also allow us to address members of susceptible and vulnerable populations (e.g., children and people living in environmental justice communities) who are likely to experience a disproportionately high risk for environmental diseases.

In this chapter, the fundamental concepts for quantitative risk assessment and the governing equations used in cancer and noncancer risk assessment will be reviewed first. Then the methods used for quantitative aggregate and cumulative risk assessment will be introduced. Next, fundamental concepts of probability and commonly used probability distributions will be presented. Finally, the key issues and the procedure for conducting probabilistic modeling for characterizing aggregate and cumulative risks will be demonstrated with examples.

AGGREGATE AND CUMULATIVE RISKS
Basic Risk Assessment Equations for Cancer and Noncancer Assessments

Human health risk assessments can be classified into two categories: those assessing cancer or those assessing noncancer (or systemic) risks. Today, many international (e.g., World Health Organization (WHO)), federal (e.g., EPA, Food and Drug Administration), and state agencies (e.g., Cal EPA) use quantitative risk assessment as a basis for regulatory decisions about single chemicals and chemical mixtures.

Cancer risks are assessed based on the assumption that thresholds do not exist for carcinogens. Cancer risk is typically estimated by developing estimates of "excess lifetime cancer risk," which is the increased probability of developing cancer as a result of the exposure in question. Excess lifetime cancer risk is commonly calculated using the following equation:

$$R = LADD \times SF,$$ (11.1)

where

- R is excess lifetime cancer risk, a unitless probability (e.g., 10^{-5} = 1 in 100,000);
- $LADD$ is lifetime average daily dose (defined in Equation 11.2), typically in the unit of mg/kg-day (mg of chemical per kg of body weight per day); and
- SF is the slope factor that is an upper-bound estimate of carcinogenic potency, developed from human or animal data, and typically, in the unit of $[mg/kg\text{-}bw/day]^{-1}$.

$$LADD = \frac{C \times IR \times EF \times ED}{BW \times LT},$$ (11.2)

where

- $LADD$ is the lifetime average daily dose specified in Equation 11.1;
- C is the average chemical concentration in exposure media during the exposure period, typically in the unit of $\mu g/m^3$ for air pollutants, mg/L for water contaminants, or mg/kg for contaminants in soil or food;
- IR is the average intake rate during the exposure period, which is the product of the contact rate of exposure media (e.g., the amount of water a person drinks each day [L/day] or the amount of air a person breathes each day $[m^3/day]$) and the exposure frequency (number of days per year);
- EF is exposure frequency, in the unit of days/year;
- ED is exposure duration, in the unit of year;
- BW is body weight, in the unit of kg; and
- LT is lifetime, in the unit of day.

Given that some parameters in Equation 11.1 (e.g., SF) and Equation 11.2 (e.g., C and IR) vary with age. LADD and R can be calculated separately for each designated age segment and then summed up across age segments for a total LADD or R (US EPA 2004). The output of Equation 11.1 is the upper-bound estimate of the increase in cancer risk resulting from the exposure in question, typically reported as "X in a million." This is the likelihood that up to X additional people out of one million equally exposed people would contract cancer. This estimated risk is in addition to the baseline cancer cases that would occur more or less spontaneously over a lifetime in an unexposed population of one million people. A number of conservative assumptions are associated with both the exposure estimate (i.e., LADD) and the slope factor (i.e., SF) for the purpose of public health protection. Some default values and assumptions (e.g., a person's lifetime of 70 years) can be obtained in guidelines published by regulatory agencies. A few examples include *Guidelines for Carcinogen Risk Assessment* (US EPA 2005a), *Supplemental Guidance for Assessing Susceptibility from Early-Life Exposure to Carcinogens* (US EPA 2005b), and *Guidelines for Human Exposure Assessment* (US EPA 2019b).

Noncancer risk assessments are conducted based on the assumption that a threshold exists for each toxicant – if the exposure level is below the threshold, there is no adverse effect. For a single chemical, the hazard for noncancer health effects is typically expressed as hazard quotient (HQ), which is the ratio of a potential exposure to a health benchmark. This may be mathematically defined as

$$HQ = ADD/HB,$$ (11.3)

where

- HQ is a unitless hazard quotient;

- *ADD* is the average daily dose (defined in Equation 11.4), typically in the unit of mg/kg-day (mg of chemical per kg of body weight per day); and

- *HB* is a health benchmark, such as the Reference Dose (RfD) developed by the US EPA, or some other point of departure, such as a LED10 (lower limit on the effective dose, 10th percentile).

$$ADD = \frac{C \times IR \times EF \times ED}{BW \times AT}, \tag{11.4}$$

where

- *ADD* is the average daily dose as specified in Equation 11.3;

- *C* is the average chemical concentration in exposure media during the exposure period, typically in the unit of $\mu g/m^3$ for air pollutants, mg/L for water contaminants, or mg/kg for contaminants in soil or food;

- *IR* is the average intake rate during the exposure period, which is the product of the contact rate of exposure media (e.g., the amount of water a person drinks each day [L/day] or the amount of air a person breathes each day [m^3/day]) and the exposure frequency (number of days per year);

- *EF* is exposure frequency, in the unit of days/year;

- *ED* is exposure duration, in the unit of year;

- *BW* is body weight, in the unit of kg; and

- *AT* is the time period over which the dose is averaged, in the unit of day.

Similar to LADD and *R*, *ADD* and *HQ* can also be calculated for different age groups (US EPA 2004). In addition, *HQ* can be calculated for specific target organ systems, such as respiratory system or hematologic system (OEHHA 2015). An HQ less than 1 means that no adverse health effects are expected as a result of exposure, and an HQ greater than 1 indicates that adverse health effects are possible. The practical upshot of this is that an HQ exceeding 1 does not necessarily mean that adverse effects will occur, especially if the population of exposed individuals is small or the range of human susceptibility is limited.

Alternatively, hazards for noncancer health effects can be characterized by margin of exposure (MOE), which is essentially the reciprocal of the HQ, as defined in Equation 11.5.

$$MOE = HB/ADD \tag{11.5}$$

An MOE is calculated by dividing the health benchmark by the actual or projected environmental exposure of interest. "Margin" here can be deemed as a "safety buffer" between exposure and health benchmark. As a rule of thumb, the larger the MOE, the lower the concern about that particular chemical exposure. When the no-observed-adverse-effect level (NOAEL) or the lowest-observed-adverse-effect level (LOAEL) is used as the health benchmark for MOE calculation, uncertainty factors accounting for interspecies and intraspecies extrapolations are commonly applied to determine the acceptable MOE. For example, the minimum acceptable MOE is 100 if NOAEL is used as the HB, considering an uncertainty factor of 10 for animal-to-human extrapolation and another uncertainty factor of 10 for human-to-sensitive human extrapolation.

Because of the way most health benchmarks are developed, HQs and MOEs are single numbers and cannot be translated to a probability that adverse health effects will occur, although unifying cancer and noncancer risk assessment has received increasing attention (NRC 2009) and methods have been proposed to calculate probabilities of noncancer hazards (Chiu and Slob 2015). In the practice of calculating an HQ or R, some required parameters (e.g., RfDs or cancer slope factors) are developed by regulatory agencies such as the US EPA, or transnational bodies such as the WHO. The other parameters, such as ADDs or LADDs, are typically developed on a case-specific basis for each assessment. The exposure assessment process is key to developing aggregate and cumulative risks.

Aggregate Assessment of Exposure and Risk

Aggregate exposure assessment combines exposures to a single agent across all relevant routes, pathways, and sources, and aggregate risk refers to the risk resulting from aggregate exposure to a single agent (US EPA 2003b).

Aggregate risk assessment is conducted to assess health impacts associated with chemical exposures with a multimedia and multipathway nature. One classic example of multimedia and multipathway exposure is environmental lead (Pb) exposure. Pb is present in multiple environmental media, including ambient and indoor air, water, soil and dust, food, and consumer products. After being released into the environment, Pb moves between environmental media as it moves from its point of release to human contact with it. For instance, Pb can be released from a smelter into the air and then deposits on leafy vegetable plants, followed by consumption by animals or humans. To study the body burden of Pb, it is critically important to aggregate and differentiate Pb exposures across all pathways and routes.

Another example of aggregate exposure and risk assessment can be illustrated by assessing human exposure to chlorpyrifos, an organophosphate pesticide (OP). The Food Quality and Protection Act requires the consideration of aggregate exposure and risk for pesticide assessments. Chlorpyrifos is semivolatile, meaning that if it is sprayed on a surface indoors, it can remain on the surface where it is applied, or it can volatilize and become airborne and thus be available for inhalation or dermal absorption if it is deposited on a new surface with which a child has frequent contact. To investigate all possible exposures to this compound, one needs to have estimates of the presence of the OP pesticide chlorpyrifos in all relevant environmental media.

To estimate aggregate exposure to any chemical across multiple exposure pathways requires a lot of information, including chemical concentrations in all relevant exposure media, exposure media intake rates, and the frequency and duration of exposure. Aggregate risk for cancer can be estimated using Equation 11.6:

$$R_A = \sum_{j=1}^{m} LADD_j \times SF_j, \tag{11.6}$$

where

- R_A is the cancer risk (defined in Equation 11.1) due to aggregate exposures;

- j is the jth exposure route, and m is the number of exposure routes (inhalation, ingestion, and dermal absorption);

- $LADD_j$ is the lifetime average daily dose (defined in Equation 11.1) for the jth exposure route; and

- SF_j is the slope factor (defined in Equation 11.1) for the jth exposure route.

For noncancer end points, a hazard index (HI) can be calculated using Equation 11.7:

$$HI_A = \sum_{j=1}^{m} ADD_j / HB_j, \tag{11.7}$$

where

- HI_A is a unitless hazard index due to aggregate exposures;

- j is the jth exposure route, and m is the number of exposure routes (inhalation, ingestion, and dermal absorption);

- ADD_j is the average daily dose (defined in Equation 11.3) for the jth exposure route; and

- HB_j is a health benchmark (defined in Equation 11.3) for the jth exposure route.

Aggregate assessments aim to estimate risk or hazard by combining all relevant exposure routes. In aggregate risk assessment, it is critically important to match a health benchmark and estimated exposure. It is preferred to have a health benchmark derived from the same exposure route as that in exposure assessment. For example, while assessing hazards or risks associated with ingestion exposure, it would be preferred to have a health benchmark derived from oral exposure. Otherwise, route-to-route extrapolation might be needed. It is also important to match a health benchmark for each exposure route by the anticipated exposure frequency and duration – a health benchmark derived from short-term exposure studies might not be useful to evaluate long-term chronic health impacts.

Cumulative Assessment of Exposure and Risk

In contrast to aggregate exposure and risk assessment, which focuses on a single agent across all relevant exposure routes, cumulative exposure refers to the "total exposure to multiple agents that causes a common toxic effect(s) on human health by the same, or similar, sequence of major biochemical events," i.e., multiple chemical and multiple route exposures (US EPA 2019b). Cumulative risk refers to the risks induced by cumulative exposures (US EPA 2003b).

People are constantly exposed to multiple chemicals on a daily basis. Some substances cause similar health effects, and cumulative exposure and risk assessment might be appropriate to evaluate the overall health impacts caused by these substances. For example, PFAS is a chemical class containing more than 5,000 species (US EPA 2019a). PFASs are widely and substantially used in consumer products (e.g., carpets, food packaging materials, electronics, and nonstick cookware), and in industrial, commercial, and military applications (e.g., PFAS manufacturing and the application of firefighting foam). PFASs are released into the environment throughout the whole lifecycle of a consumer or commercial product. PFASs in air, drinking water, food, soil, and dust directly contribute to human exposure. Some of the PFAS species, if co-exposed, can contribute to similar adverse effects, such as hepatotoxicity and reproductive toxicity, and cumulative impacts could be estimated for these PFAS species (e.g., PFBS and PFHxS) (Borg et al. 2013).

The basic equations for calculating cumulative risk assessment are represented by extensions of the equations presented earlier. For example, a cumulative assessment of excess lifetime cancer risk can be calculated by summing the calculated risk for each compound across all relevant exposure routes (Equation 11.8):

$$R_C = \sum_{i=1}^{n}\sum_{j=1}^{m} LADD_{ij} \times SF_{ij}, \tag{11.8}$$

where

- R_C is the cancer risk (defined in Equation 11.1) due to cumulative exposures;

- i is the ith chemical, n is the number of chemicals included in the cumulative assessment, j is the jth exposure route, and m is the number of exposure routes (inhalation, ingestion, and dermal absorption);

- $LADD_{ij}$ is the lifetime average daily dose (defined in Equation 11.1) for the ith chemical and the jth exposure route; and

- SF_j is the slope factor (defined in Equation 11.1) for the ith chemical and the jth exposure route.

Equation 11.8 is simply the summing of risks imposed by different chemicals. In a more refined assessment, the target tissues and mechanism of carcinogenic action, as well as the upper-bound nature of many cancer slope factors, would need to be considered.

For noncancer end points, a HI is calculated for cumulative assessment using Equation 11.9:

$$HI_C = \sum_{i=1}^{n}\sum_{j=1}^{m} ADD_{ij}/HB_{ij}, \tag{11.9}$$

where

- HI_C is a unitless hazard index due to cumulative exposures;

- i is the ith chemical, n is the number of chemicals included in the cumulative assessment, j is the jth exposure route, and m is the number of exposure routes (inhalation, ingestion, and dermal absorption);

- ADD_{ij} is the average daily dose (defined in Equation 11.3) for the ith chemical and the jth exposure route; and

- HB_{ij} is a health benchmark (defined in Equation 11.3) for the ith chemical and the jth exposure route.

As a screening exercise, hazard quotients for single chemicals may be added to form a HI_C to approximate the potential magnitude of a problem, but in a typical situation, only chemicals "causes a common toxic effect(s) on human health by the same, or similar, sequence of major biochemical events" (US EPA 2019b) are included in a refined assessments (e.g., OP pesticides). An HI_C of less than 1.0 will likely not result in health effects over a lifetime of exposure, but an HI_C greater than 1.0 does not necessarily mean that adverse effects will occur but rather indicates an increased probability of adverse effects. HI is not used to characterize the overall health impacts of the mixture under consideration but to measure the total hazard based on the individual components. Similarly, a MOE Index could be calculated.

It should also be pointed out that a cumulative risk assessment is not just combining a series of aggregate exposure and risk assessments across different chemicals. A few fundamental issues in toxicology and exposure assessment need to be addressed for cumulative risk assessment. First, cumulative assessments consider the synergistic or antagonistic interactions among agents, and it doesn't necessarily mean that risks from individual agents should be "added" through either independent action or concentration addition. Second, the common health end points and the mechanisms underlying the adverse effects across single chemicals need to be addressed, and the most sensitive toxic effect needs to be defined in cumulative risk assessment. Third, relative potency factors or toxicity equivalency factors, if available, could be used for cumulative assessment for certain groups of chemicals (e.g., polycyclic aromatic hydrocarbons, dioxin and dioxin-like compounds, pesticides, and certain PFAS species), assuming concentration addition, i.e., each individual chemical within a group acts via a similar mechanism of action (US EPA 2003a, 2009, 2010; RIVM 2018). Fourth, the frequency of the co-occurrence of exposures to chemicals needs to be considered. Finally, although the emphasis of this textbook is on chemical exposure, the "agents" considered in cumulative exposure and risk assessments are not limited to chemical agents, and other biological or physical agents and social stressors could also be considered in the assessment. Some commonly used tools for cumulative risk assessment are summarized by MacDonell et al. (2013). Approaches, data needs, and examples for characterizing aggregate and cumulative exposure and risk will be presented in the next section.

Characterizing Aggregate and Cumulative Risks
Measurement Studies

Aggregate and cumulative assessments can quantify the contributions of chemicals and exposure routes to the combined exposures and risks, and identify risk and exposure drivers. Aggregate or cumulative exposures and risks can be characterized according to Equations 11.6–11.9 through measurements or modeling. In either case, measurements or modeling, developing an aggregate or cumulative exposure and risk assessment is a data-intensive process, and it requires specific data for contaminant concentrations in each exposure media (e.g., air, drinking water, soil and dust, and food), personal activities (e.g., frequency and amount of drinking water), and physiological parameters (e.g., age, gender, and body weight).

The complexity of a measurement study can be demonstrated with a large field study of pesticide exposure in children, the Minnesota Children's Pesticide Exposure Study (MNCPES) (Adgate et al. 2000). MNCPES simultaneously collected all the various measurements needed to quantify aggregate exposure to several OP pesticides. In the study, investigators and participants collected samples and other information needed to estimate aggregate exposure from all routes in a representative sample of 102 urban and rural children between ages 3 and 13 over four summer months. Using measurements of the OP chlorpyrifos from air, food, beverages, drinking water, surface dust, and soil, it was possible to aggregate across pathways by developing potential dose rates using the general equations presented earlier (Clayton et al. 2003). Since chlorpyrifos is not considered a human carcinogen, ADD for each individual could be calculated following Equation 11.4 for each exposure route and compared with the corresponding health benchmark (RfD). Finally, a HI can be developed for aggregate risk following Equation 11.7.

Table 11.1 illustrates the amount of effort for measuring chlorpyrifos in different environmental and exposure media, which is the first step for aggregate exposure and risk assessment. For each medium, the percentiles of chlorpyrifos concentration as well as the percentage of samples above detection limits are listed. To convert the measured chlorpyrifos concentrations into ADDs, a few other personal activities and physiological parameters need to be obtained either from existing guidelines or from measurements for each study participant. For example, to calculate the ADD for inhalation exposure, an inhalation rate could be obtained from the US EPA's Exposure Factors Handbook (US EPA 2011), and the participant's body weight could be obtained

Table 11.1: Number and Type of Environmental and Personal Samples, Measurement Durations, and Analytical Results for Chlorpyrifos Aggregate Exposure Assessment

Medium	Type of Sample	Units	N	Percentage Measurable	Median	90th Percentile
Personal air	6-day average	ng/m	60	95	1.58	11.7
Solid food	4-day average	μg/kg	96	57	0.53	1.26
Beverage	4-day average	μg/kg	101	0	NA*	NA
Drinking water	Grab sample	μg/L	55	2	NA	NA
Surface dust	Wipe, one time	ng/cm	99	62	1.15	1.33
Soil	Surface soil, grab sample	μg/kg	102	3	NA	NA

Note: Not available.

from a questionnaire survey or measurement. Similarly, the ADD for dietary ingestion could be calculated by multiplying the measured chlorpyrifos concentrations in food and beverage by the measured mass of food and beverage each participant consumed and then dividing by each participant's body weight. Comparing the calculated ADD could be used to evaluate the relative importance of different exposure routes.

In this MNCPES example, the dermal pathway was not assessed because no dermal loading measurements were available to convert the surface-dust-loading values, and it was judged that exposure via this pathway for these children was relatively small compared to ingestion and inhalation sources. Similarly, the low percentage of detectable concentrations in the soil and drinking water samples meant that estimates were not derived from these potential sources.

The concept of cumulative risk assessment is illustrated below using PFAS exposures. Borg et al. (2013) conducted a cumulative risk assessment of 17 PFAS species for the general and an occupational Swedish population. Borg et al. (2013) identified six studies, in which blood or serum PFAS species were measured as a biomarker of exposure to quantify the body burden of PFAS exposures. All these studies were small scale, with the number of participants ranging from 8 to 80. Borg et al. (2013) identified two common health end points, i.e., hepatotoxicity and reproductive toxicity, across the 17 PFAS species. RfDs, as a health benchmark, associated with hepatotoxicity and reproductive toxicity for each PFAS species were either derived from the literature using NOAEL (or LOAEL) or obtained using read-across extrapolation, which is a technique used to predict missing physicochemical or toxicological properties for one chemical by using data from another chemical (another PFAS species in this case). HQs were calculated for both hepatotoxicity and reproductive toxicity for each PFAS species, and the HI for each health end point was calculated by adding HQs across the PFAS species. The resulting HIs for the general population were 0.27 and 0.18 for hepatotoxicity and reproductive toxicity, respectively, and PFOS was the risk driver. For the occupational population (professional ski waxers), the HIs were 5.5 and 1.7, for hepatotoxicity and reproductive toxicity, respectively, and PFOA was the risk driver. Figure 11.1 illustrates the serum concentrations and the resulting HQs of the 17 species for both the general and the occupational populations. Data for generating Figure 11.1 were obtained from Tables 7 and 8 in Borg et al. (2013).

The cumulative risk assessment conducted by Borg et al. (2013) used serum PFAS species (i.e., internal PFAS exposures or biomarkers of PFAS exposure) to quantify total PFAS exposures. Serum PFAS concentrations reflect the body burden of PFAS exposures, but cannot differentiate contributions from different exposure routes and pathways. Linking internal exposures and external exposure routes and pathways is critically important for identifying dominant exposure sources and pathways, which can be used for exposure and risk mitigation.

Poothong et al. (2020) conducted a study to link external PFAS exposures to internal serum PFAS concentrations. In this study, Poothong et al. (2020) estimated the exposure to 18 perfluoroalkyl acids (PFAAs) and 12 PFAA precursors through different exposure pathways, including diet ingestion, dust ingestion, inhalation, and dermal absorption, for 61 adults in Oslo, Norway. PFAAs and their precursors were measured in diet, hand wiping, indoor dust, and indoor and personal air samples. Serum PFAS samples were also measured for each study participant. Daily intake of PFAAs was estimated for each exposure route and pathway using equations similar to Equation 11.4. The total estimated PFAA intake was then converted to serum PFAA concentrations

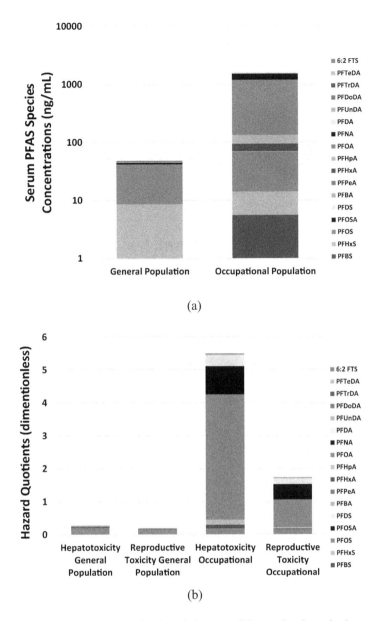

Figure 11.1 Serum PFAS species levels (a) and the overall hazard indices for hepatotoxicity and reproductive toxicity (b).

with a pharmacokinetic model. The estimated and the measured serum PFAA concentrations were within the same order of magnitude. PFOA was the dominant contributor to the estimated daily PFAA intake, and the predominant exposure pathway contributing to PFAA exposures was dietary ingestion, followed by dust ingestion, indoor air inhalation, and dermal absorption. Figure 11.2 illustrates the relative contributions of various exposure pathways to the estimated PFAA intake for PFAA species. Data for generating Figure 11.2 were obtained from Table 2 in Poothong et al. (2020).

The chlorpyrifos and PFAS examples illustrated earlier demonstrate that measurement studies can generate valuable data for aggregate or cumulative exposure and risk assessments. For a small population and limited number of chemicals, it is possible to gain exposure measurements from the most relevant pathways. In the OP chlorpyrifos aggregate assessment, the researcher developed ranges of children's exposures to chlorpyrifos due to drinking water, eating food, or

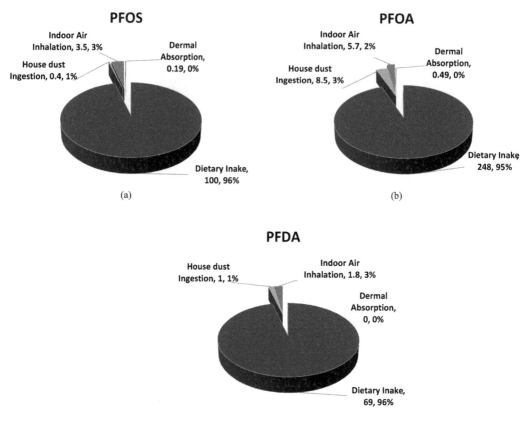

Figure 11.2   Relative importance of different exposure pathways contributing to the estimated daily intakes for PFOS (a), PFOA (b), and PFDA (c), the top three contributors to the estimated total PFASs intake. For each slice in the pie chart, the first number is the estimated daily intake in the unit of pg/kg-day, and the second number is the percent contribution of the associated exposure pathway.

breathing air. In the PFAS cumulative assessment, the investigator measured the exposure to multiple PFAS species through multiple exposure pathways.

However, we need to keep in mind that measurement studies become quickly challenging or even infeasible for a large population's exposure to multiple chemicals through various exposure pathways. For example, although measurements are available for widely used compounds such as chlorpyrifos, the process becomes more difficult and uncertain if assessments consider less frequently used compounds. As there are 40 OP compounds in commerce and thousands of chemicals in use, it quickly becomes impossible to measure all routes and pathways.

Generalizability is another limitation for these small-scale measurement studies based on convenient samples. Measurements obtained from one study might not be able to be extrapolated to other populations with different behaviors, ages, or living in different climates. The variability in exposures and risks observed in a measurement study might not be representative of a broader population.

In addition, human observational studies depend on the willingness of the child participants and their caretakers to perform certain activities (i.e., wear a personal air sampler or provide duplicate diet samples). Participants could refuse to participate in the collection of any sample type, so the number of measurements would be unequal across media. For example, in the chlorpyrifos exposure study (Table 11.1), investigators collected a soil sample in each home, but personal air sampling results are available for only 60 children.

Although measurement studies can generate valuable data used for aggregate or cumulative assessments, given the previously listed limitations, exposure and risk modeling is much needed as a complementary and equally important approach to exposure and risk assessment. Modeling approaches could be used to address population variability, generalizability, and uncertainty issues in exposure and risk assessment, and could also be used to answer "what if" questions to provide evidence and support for public health regulations.

Modeling Studies

A model is defined as "a simplification of reality that is constructed to gain insights into select attributes of a particular physical, biological, economic, or social system" by the National Research Council (NRC 2007). This definition is also adopted by the US EPA (US EPA 2019b). A computational model, which is usually developed based on conceptual models, could be a useful tool to assemble different types of data (e.g., pollutant concentrations, personal activities, and dose-response parameters) for exposure and risk estimation and prediction.

Models can be classified in different ways, such as mechanistic models and empirical models or exposure models, pharmacokinetic models, and dose-response models. For the purpose of exposure and risk assessment, models are commonly classified as deterministic models and probabilistic (or stochastic) models.

Deterministic Models. Deterministic models use a single set of fixed values as input for model parameters, and the output is a fixed single exposure or risk prediction (WHO 2005; US EPA 2019b). A deterministic model could be a mechanistic model (i.e., models based on physical or chemical processes) or an empirical model (e.g., empirical or statistical relationships between two variables).

Equations 11.1–11.9 could be deterministic models if a single set of fixed input parameters are used. For example, a single ADD (Equation 11.4) could be calculated based on a single set of chemical concentrations, intake rates, exposure duration, body weight, and averaging time. One legitimate question is which set of input parameters should be used to estimate exposure or risk. In risk assessment, deterministic models are usually applied to estimate the central tendency (e.g., mean) and the high-end (e.g., 95th percentile or maximum) exposure and risk (US EPA 2001). If the input parameter reflects the average value across a population (i.e., the average concentration and intake rate), the deterministic will yield an average estimate of risk. However, if the input parameters reflect high-end exposures (e.g., maximum concentrations), the model will generate a high-end or conservative risk estimate.

Deterministic models have been widely accepted as exposure and risk screening tools in risk assessment for a few reasons. First, many input parameters for deterministic models can be obtained from various risk assessment guidelines published by government agencies. Second, the calculations based on deterministic models are straightforward and require fewer computational skills. Third, the model output is simple and easy to communicate to decision-makers and the public. Examples of deterministic models include the US EPA's Exposure and Fate Assessment Screening Tool (E-FAST) developed to estimate chemical release and exposures from consumer products and the US EPA's Regional Screening Levels (US EPA 2021) used for exposure and risk screening for multipathway exposures at contaminated sites (e.g., Superfund sites).

Although deterministic models are most useful for screening-level assessment, i.e., assessing the likelihood of health risk under default or conservative assumptions, deterministic models don't provide a full range of exposures and risks for a given population. Neither do deterministic models adequately and explicitly address variabilities and uncertainties of model input and output parameters (US EPA 2014), which might be critical for decision-making, particularly under the scenarios of low MOE. These limitations of deterministic models can be addressed by probabilistic models.

Probabilistic Models. Probabilistic models use probability distributions, as opposed to single values, as model input parameters for one or multiple variables, and quantify the distribution of exposures and risks across a population. Similar to deterministic models, a probabilistic model could be a mechanistic model or an empirical model (WHO 2005).

Although both deterministic models and probabilistic models are based on the same sets of fundamental exposure and risk equations (e.g., Equations 11.1–11.9), probabilistic models leverage the variability and uncertainty of the input parameters and characterize the variability and uncertainty of the outcome exposure or risk estimates. In the example of calculating ADD based on Equation 11.4, the distributions of chemical concentration, intake rate, exposure duration, body weight, and averaging time could be used as input parameters for probabilistic models, which would generate a distribution of ADD across the population. In addition, if the uncertainties of the model input variables are characterized, the probabilistic model can estimate the uncertainty in

ADD. The probability distributions for input variables can be obtained from measurement studies or from exposure and risk assessment guidelines, such as the US EPA's *Exposure Factors Handbook* (US EPA 2011). In a probabilistic model, some variables could be treated as a fixed value, such as an Reference Concentration (RfC) or RfD, and in some references, those models using both fixed values and probability distributions as model input are referred to as hybrid models (WHO 2005).

Probabilistic models cannot eliminate uncertainties but can better characterize uncertainties in exposure and risk estimates. Probabilistic models can also be used to examine relative contributions of each input variable or distribution parameter on the variability or uncertainty in exposure and risk estimates. Examples of probabilistic models include the US EPA's Stochastic Human Exposure and Dose Simulation (SHEDS) models and the Dutch National Institute for Health and Environment's (RIVM) ConsExpo model.

Probabilistic models generally require more skills, input data, and resources, but it is not necessary to model exposure and risk using probabilistic models in every situation. Multiple guidelines recommend using a "tiered approach" for exposure and risk assessment, which will be articulated next (US EPA 2014, 2019b; WHO 2005).

Tiered Approach. As noted, it is not necessary to apply probabilistic models in every situation. The level of model complexity should be consistent with the purpose of the assessment, which should be developed during the problem formulation or scoping stage of a risk assessment. For exposure and risk prioritization or screening, a screening-level model (typically a deterministic model) is likely to be sufficient. However, for assessment with increasing regulatory significance, such as setting National Ambient Air Quality Standards, a probabilistic model with the capability to quantify variability and uncertainty in exposure and risk estimates might be required. In such a case for making significant and sensitive decisions, a risk manager can benefit from the output of sophisticated probabilistic models, which can fully quantify risks and associated uncertainties for each decision alternative.

A tiered approach for exposure and risk modeling has been recommended in a few guidelines (US EPA 2001, 2014, 2019b; WHO 2005) and is illustrated in Figure 11.3.

The US EPA's Risk Assessment Forum White Paper summarizes the scenarios when probabilistic models are particularly useful (US EPA 2014). A few major scenarios are listed here, and the rest can be found in the reference (US EPA 2014). Probabilistic models are particularly useful when a deterministic model determines a low level of MOE when interindividual variability is a concern for environmental justice communities, when there is a need to rank the contribution of various exposure pathways or environmental agents to the overall risk, and when expert judgment needs to be incorporated into the model to characterize uncertainty. Probabilistic models are probably not necessary when a deterministic model determines a large level of MOE even under very conservative conditions. In addition, model complexity and data quality are different but related

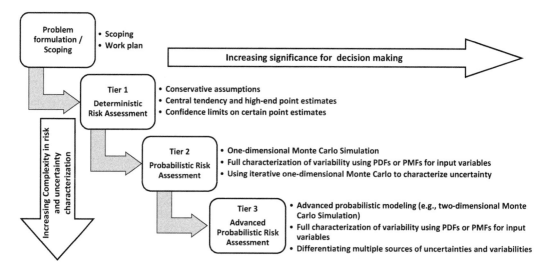

Figure 11.3 Tiered approach for modeling exposure and risk. (Adapted from US EPA 2014 and US EPA 2001).

issues – a sophisticated model wouldn't generate reliable results without high-quality input data. Therefore, probabilistic models could be less reliable if reliable input data are not available or accessible (WHO 2005).

Although two approaches, i.e., measurements and modeling, have been presented here for characterizing aggregate and cumulative exposures and risks, these two approaches are not mutually exclusive. Measurement studies provide valuable input data for various exposure and risk models, and measurement results can be used to calibrate models or evaluate modeling results. Exposure and risk models can guide measurements, can examine risk drivers (e.g., exposure pathways or certain agents), and can identify vulnerable and susceptible populations. Based on modeling results, researchers can conserve resources to measure and investigate those potentially most significant exposure pathways and agents or the most susceptible populations.

PROBABILISTIC MODELS FOR CHARACTERIZING AGGREGATE AND CUMULATIVE RISKS

As stated in the previous section, probabilistic models can be employed to better understand variabilities and uncertainties in exposure and risk estimates. Probabilistic models require probability distributions as model input for one or multiple variables and yield probability distributions for exposures and risks. To better understand the process of conducting risk assessment using probabilistic models, we next briefly review some fundamental concepts of probability and probability distributions, and discuss these concepts in the context of aggregate and cumulative assessments.

Probability and Probability Distributions
Probability and Risk Assessment

In the fundamental exposure and risk equations (Equations 11.1–11.9), each fixed set of input variable values will generate one fixed output exposure or risk estimate. However, most input variables in those equations can take multiple values depending on exposure scenarios. For example, in Equation 11.4 for ADD calculation, chemical concentration (C) comes from multiple measurements. One could use the mean, median, maximum, or any other measured values as the input concentration. Similarly, intake rate (IR) varies from person to person, and different values can be assigned to it. The variation in chemical concentration or intake rate reflects the natural variability of C or IR across the population. In addition, we usually do not have precise measurements of the input variables, due to uncertainties, including measurement errors. For example, the measured chemical concentration is not the reality but a proxy of the reality due to the representativeness of a sample and measurement errors. Consequently, the variabilities and uncertainties of model input variables transmit to model output, leading to the variability and uncertainty in exposure or risk estimates.

To account for the variability and uncertainty of a model input in probabilistic models, that model input needs to be treated as a random variable. Three fundamental concepts, i.e., random variable, the distribution of a random variable, and probability, lay the groundwork for propagation of variability and uncertainty in aggregate and cumulative risk models.

A *random variable* is "a variable that may assume any value from a set of values according to chance" (US EPA 2001). A random variable could be discrete or continuous. A discrete random variable takes "values [that] either constitute a finite set or else can be listed in an infinite sequence in which there is a first element, a second element, and so on," and a continuous random variable takes "values [that] consists of an entire interval on the number line" (Devore 2000). In the context of human health risk assessment, examples of discrete random variables include gender, race, building characteristics (e.g., attached vs. detached house), and drinking water source (e.g., groundwater, tap water, and bottled water). Examples of continuous random variables include environmental pollutant concentration, inhalation rate, and daily ingestion of water.

The *probability distribution* of a random variable describes the distribution of probabilities (or the allocation of the total probability) across different values or intervals of a random variable (Devore 2000). A probability distribution can be mathematically described as a *probability mass function* (PMF) for a discrete random variable or as a *probability density function* (PDF) for a continuous random variable. A PMF describes the *probability* of each value a discrete random variable can take. A PDF does not show the probability of a specific value a continuous random variable can take because a continuous variable can theoretically have an infinite number of values, and it is meaningless to develop a probability for a specific number assigned to the variable. Instead, the integral of a PDF over a given interval shows the *probability* of the continuous variable taking a

211

value within that interval. The mathematical formula for PMF is presented in Equations 11.10 and Equation 11.11 for PDF.

$$p(x) = P(X = x), \tag{11.10}$$

where

- p(x) is the PMF, and
- P is the probability for a discrete random variable X taking the value of x.

$$P(a \leq X \leq b) = \int_a^b f(x)dx, \tag{11.11}$$

where

- P is the probability for a continuous random variable X taking a value in the interval [a, b], and
- f(x) is the probabilistic density function of the continuous variable X.

The probability distribution of a random variable conveys some key information in human health risk assessment. For example, the distribution of ADD (see Equation 11.4) across a population can tell us the most likely exposure values across the population (e.g., modes), high-end or low-end exposures (e.g., skewness), and the variability of the exposure (e.g., skewness and kurtosis). Different values can be sampled from a PDF or PMF using numerical techniques, such as Monte Carlo simulation, to generate model input for a probabilistic model. A few commonly used PDFs and PMFs in human health risk assessment are summarized in the next section.

Alternatively, a probability distribution can be presented as a cumulative distribution function (CDF), F(x), defined in Equation 11.12 for a discrete variable and Equation 11.13 for a continuous variable.

$$F(x) = P(X \leq x) = \sum_{t \leq x} p(t) \tag{11.12}$$

$$F(x) = P(X \leq x) = \int_{-\infty}^{x} f(t)dt \tag{11.13}$$

A CDF calculates the cumulative probability by summing the PMF for a discrete variable or integrating the PDF for a continuous variable. In human health risk assessment, a CDF is particularly useful to demonstrate the risk levels at each percentile of the risk distribution, which is the output from a probabilistic model. For example, it might show that the one-in-a-million risk is associated with the 99th percentile of the distribution.

It should be noted that some probability distributions used as model input are not generated based on real-world measurement (e.g., environmental media sampling) but based on expert judgment or some other published data. In this case, while we may be able to provide a range of values that we think are a likely or even most likely value, they are subjective descriptions of our state of knowledge about media concentrations. This is a subjective, personal view of probability that is often applied as professional judgment in risk assessment but is often not sufficiently acknowledged. It is important to remember that even though such probabilities are somewhat subjective, the probability assignments are not completely arbitrary.

Next, we will briefly review some commonly used probability distributions in human health risk assessment.

Common Probability Distributions in Risk Assessment

Some probability distributions commonly encountered in human health risk assessment are summarized in this section, followed by a brief description of how to fit and select a distribution. The PDFs and PMFs of these distributions are presented in Table 11.2.

Table 11.2: Probability Distributions and Their Probability Density (or Mass) Functions

Distribution Name	PDF or PMF	Example PDF or PMF Shape
Normal distribution	$f(x;\mu,\sigma^2)=\dfrac{1}{\sigma\sqrt{2\pi}}e^{-\frac{1}{2}\left(\frac{x-\mu}{\sigma}\right)^2}\ (-\infty<x<\infty)$	
Lognormal distribution	$f(x;\mu,\sigma^2)=\begin{cases}\dfrac{1}{x\sigma\sqrt{2\pi}}e^{-\frac{1}{2}\left(\frac{\ln(x)-\mu}{\sigma}\right)^2}&(x\ge 0)\\[2mm]0&(x<0)\end{cases}$	
Gamma distribution	$f(x;\alpha,\beta)=\begin{cases}x^{\alpha-1}\dfrac{\beta^\alpha e^{-\beta x}}{\Gamma(\alpha)}&(x>0)\\[2mm]0&(x\le 0)\end{cases}$	
Weibull distribution	$f(x;\alpha,\beta)=\begin{cases}\dfrac{\alpha}{\beta^\alpha}x^{\alpha-1}e^{-\left(\frac{x}{\beta}\right)^\alpha}&(x\ge 0)\\[2mm]0&(x<0)\end{cases}$	
Exponential distribution	$f(x;\lambda>0)=\begin{cases}\lambda e^{-\lambda x}&(x\ge 0)\\0&(otherwise)\end{cases}$	
Beta distribution	$f(x;\alpha>0,\beta>0)=\begin{cases}\dfrac{\Gamma(\alpha+\beta)}{\Gamma(\alpha)\Gamma(\beta)}x^{\alpha-1}(1-x)^{\beta-1}&(0<x<1)\\[2mm]0&(otherwise)\end{cases}$	

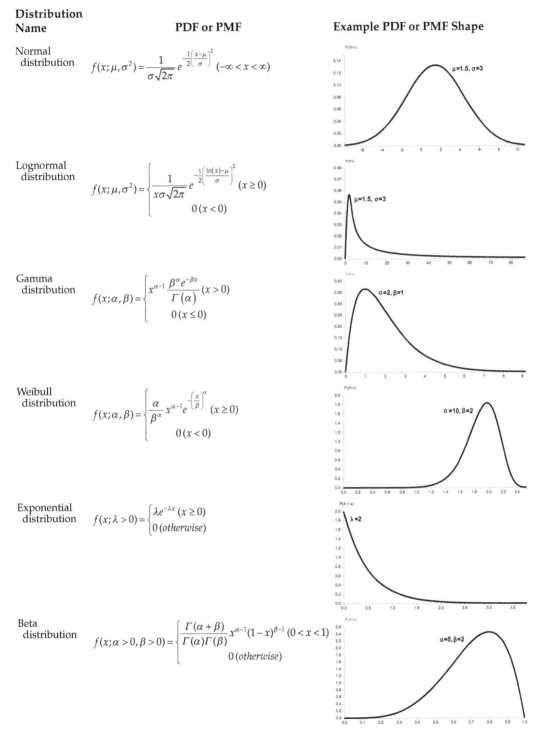

(Continued)

Table 11.2 (Continued)

Distribution Name	PDF or PMF	Example PDF or PMF Shape

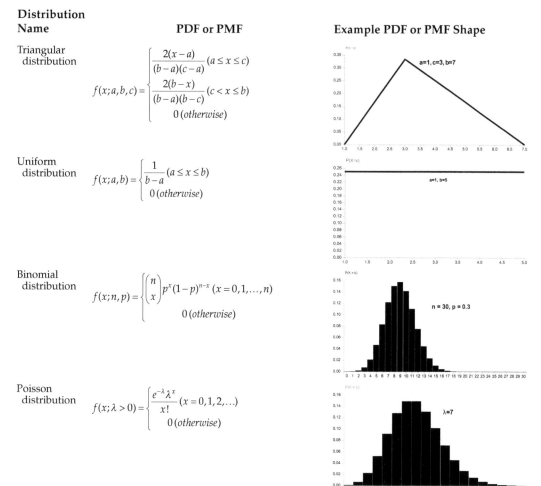

Triangular distribution

$$f(x;a,b,c) = \begin{cases} \dfrac{2(x-a)}{(b-a)(c-a)} & (a \le x \le c) \\[2mm] \dfrac{2(b-x)}{(b-a)(b-c)} & (c < x \le b) \\[2mm] 0 & (otherwise) \end{cases}$$

Uniform distribution

$$f(x;a,b) = \begin{cases} \dfrac{1}{b-a} & (a \le x \le b) \\[2mm] 0 & (otherwise) \end{cases}$$

Binomial distribution

$$f(x;n,p) = \begin{cases} \binom{n}{x} p^x (1-p)^{n-x} & (x = 0,1,\dots,n) \\[2mm] 0 & (otherwise) \end{cases}$$

Poisson distribution

$$f(x;\lambda > 0) = \begin{cases} \dfrac{e^{-\lambda}\lambda^x}{x!} & (x = 0,1,2,\dots) \\[2mm] 0 & (otherwise) \end{cases}$$

Normal Distribution. This distribution arises in many applications and is probably the most well-known distribution. If a measurement is subject to many small sources of random error and negligible systematic error, then the distribution of the measured values is described by a symmetric, bell-shaped curve that is centered on the true value of the variable. Random errors are equally likely to result in readings above or below the true value. If we have only random errors, then after many measurements the number of readings above and below the true value will be the same, and our distribution of results will be centered around the true value. The PDF takes on values over the entire range of real numbers. The mathematical function that describes this curve is called the normal distribution or the Gaussian distribution.

Lognormal Distribution. If a random variable is lognormally distributed, then the logarithm of the random variable is described by a normal distribution. This distribution is a good representation of quantities that are constrained to being nonnegative and are positively skewed. It is appropriate for representing large uncertainties that are expressed on a multiplicative or order-of-magnitude basis. lognormal distribution can fit well with environmental pollutant concentrations or estimated risks.

Exponential Distribution. A random variable follows an exponential distribution if the variable describes the time interval between two major events or the distances between two impacted locations in a Poisson process. Exponential distribution is closely related to Gamma distribution and Weibull distribution described later in this section. The time interval between exposures might follow an exponential distribution. It is the basis for survival analysis and has been applied in dose-response research.

Gamma Distribution. A random variable follows an exponential distribution if the variable describes the time that elapses until an event. Gamma distribution is very flexible and can assume a variety of shapes by varying its parameters. A gamma distribution can be reduced to an exponential distribution by adjusting the parameters of its density function. Gamma distributions have been used in dose-response research. Gamma distribution has also been used to fit water intake data and food ingestion data (Parsons 2012; US EPA 2003c).

Weibull distribution. Weibull distribution originated from reliability tests, describing time to failure. Similar to gamma distribution, a Weibull distribution is also very flexible and can model a variety of shapes. A Weibull distribution can be reduced to an exponential distribution by adjusting the parameters of its density function. In public health research, Weibull distribution has been applied in survival analysis and dose-response assessment. The incubation time distribution has also been fitted with the Weibull distribution for COVID-19 (Qin et al. 2020).

Beta Distribution. If a random variable is bounded within a finite range (e.g., between 0 and 1), it might follow a beta distribution. Beta distribution is flexible in shape and commonly used to model ratio and percentage variables, such as the fraction of time spent indoors.

Triangular Distribution. This describes a situation where the minimum, maximum, and values most likely to occur are known. This distribution can be constructed for a random variable with limited information. It might be acceptable to model a random variable with triangular distribution under "data-poor" conditions.

Uniform Distribution. The use of uniform distribution is appropriate when we are able and willing to identify a finite range of possible values for some variable, but unable to decide which values within this range are more likely to occur than others. Uniform distribution might also be assigned as a noninformative prior in Bayesian modeling.

Binomial Distribution. Binomial distribution is a discrete distribution, and it models the number of successes in a repeated finite trial with a fixed probability of success for each trial. Binomial distribution is particularly useful to model a binary situation, such as whether or not to use air conditioning and whether or not to use certain consumer products.

Poisson Distribution. Poisson distribution describes the number of independent events taking place during a period of time. In exposure assessment, Poisson distribution can be used to model exposure frequency, such as the number of times a person smokes each day and the number of times a person consumes fish each month.

There are other distributions that are also useful for risk assessment purposes, but these distributions presented in Table 11.2 are most commonly encountered in exposure and risk assessments. Information on the mathematical properties of other distributions and their use can be found in the references at the end of this chapter.

Various approaches, including histograms and box-and-whisker plots, can be applied to visualize the distribution of an existing data set (e.g., concentration of a pollutant or ingestion rate). A Q-Q plot can also be used to examine the distribution of an existing data set against a theoretical distribution. In addition, goodness-of-fit tests, including the Chi-Square test, Kolmogorov-Smirnov test, and Shapiro-Wilk test, can be employed to test whether the collected data follow a theoretical distribution. Once a probability distribution is determined, data can be sampled from the distribution as input for probabilistic models. It should be noted that not all data sets can be fitted with a theoretical distribution. In that case, one could define an empirical distribution based on the collected data (US EPA 2001).

Probabilistic Models for Exposure and Risk Assessment
Scoping for Probabilistic Modeling

The level of complexity in probabilistic modeling should be consistent with the assessment goal and the nature of decision-making. Before conducting probabilistic modeling, the scope of the assessment should be articulated by communicating with risk managers and other stakeholders in the problem formulation stage of the risk assessment. The problem formulation stage should articulate the scope of the assessment and the decision-making process and criteria. For example, a risk assessor needs to understand (1) which populations will be evaluated for what health end points under which scenarios, (2) what level of quantifying variability and uncertainty would meet the needs for decision-making, and (3) how important evaluating the relative contribution of different exposure pathways or contaminants would be for risk management decisions. Once the assessment objectives become clear, a risk assessor needs to evaluate the availability, accessibility, assumptions, and quality of models and input data, according to which, the assessment objectives may need to be adjusted or refined. This could be an iterative process until a consensus is reached for assessment goals. A risk assessor then needs to develop a plan to make the assessment transparent and clear by documenting the assessment goal, model tiers (see Figure 11.3) and assumptions, data source and data quality, the procedure for assessing variability and uncertainty, the procedure for sensitivity analysis, and the methods for model and results evaluation. Some of these aspects will be discussed in the following sections.

Fundamental Approach for Probabilistic Modeling

As stated in previous sections, probabilistic models use probability distributions as model input parameters for one or multiple variables and quantify the distribution of exposure or risk across a population.

For example, assuming X is a random variable following a normal distribution with a mean of 0 and a variance of 1, i.e., N(0, 1), and Y is another random variable following a normal distribution N(10, 5), then what is the distribution of the random variable Z, given that $Z = X + Y$? In this simple case, the distribution of the random variable Z can be obtained analytically, i.e., Z following a normal distribution with a mean of 10 and a variance of 6. However, not all probability distributions can be solved analytically, and numerical simulation plays a critical role in probabilistic modeling. The following hypothetical example regarding electronic cigarette (e-cigarette) vaping will be used to demonstrate how numerical simulations are employed in probabilistic modeling.

All parameters presented in Table 11.3 for this e-cigarette example are defined in Equations 11.1 and 11.2, except for C and N, which are equivalent to C and IR in Equation 11.2, but their units are modified for this exposure scenario. The amount of formaldehyde in each puff (C) is calculated based on Son et al. (2020); the number of puffs per day (N) is obtained from Dautzenberg and Bricard (2015); the cancer slope factor is published by the California Office of Environmental Health Hazard Assessment (OEHHA 2011). All the other input parameters in Table 11.3 are consistent with the assumptions commonly applied in environmental risk assessments. The distribution of excess lifetime cancer risk will be developed based on Equations 11.1 and 11.2. In this example, solving the distribution of R analytically based on the distributions of the input parameters is not straightforward. Therefore, numerical simulations will be employed to derive the distribution of R.

Monte Carlo simulation is the most commonly used numerical simulation method in probabilistic modeling for risk assessment. Monte Carlo simulation is an iterative process. For each iteration, a set of plausible values of input variables for a risk equation (e.g., Equations 11.1–11.9) are generated from each variable's respective probability distribution, producing an exposure or risk estimate. The process repeats thousands of times, repeatedly selecting values for model input and producing model output, and eventually derives an exposure or risk distribution. Figure 11.4 illustrates Monte Carlo simulation.

Monte Carlo simulation can be applied to characterize the variability in risk across a population by sampling from distributions reflecting the variability of model input variables. This is the traditional Monte Carlo approach, aka one-dimensional Monte Carlo simulation. In the e-cigarette example, the formaldehyde concentration (C) follows a lognormal distribution ($\mu = 1.0$, $\sigma = 0.4$), which reflects the variability in formaldehyde generation across the population. Similarly, the number of puffs per day (N) follows a Poisson distribution ($\lambda = 132$), which reflects the variability

Table 11.3: Input Parameters for Calculating Cancer Risk Associated with Formaldehyde Exposure Due to E-cigarette Vaping

Parameter	Explanation	Value	Unit
C	The amount of formaldehyde in each puff	Lognormal distribution ($\mu = 1.0$, $\sigma = 0.4$)	μg/puff
N	The number of puffs an e-cigarette user vapes	Poisson distribution ($\lambda = 132$)	puffs/day
EF	Exposure frequency	365	days/year
ED	Exposure duration	30	year
BW	Body weight	70	kg
LT	Lifetime	25,550	days
SF	Cancer slope factor	0.021	$(\text{mg/kg-day})^{-1}$
R	Excess lifetime cancer risk	A distribution to be solved numerically	Unitless

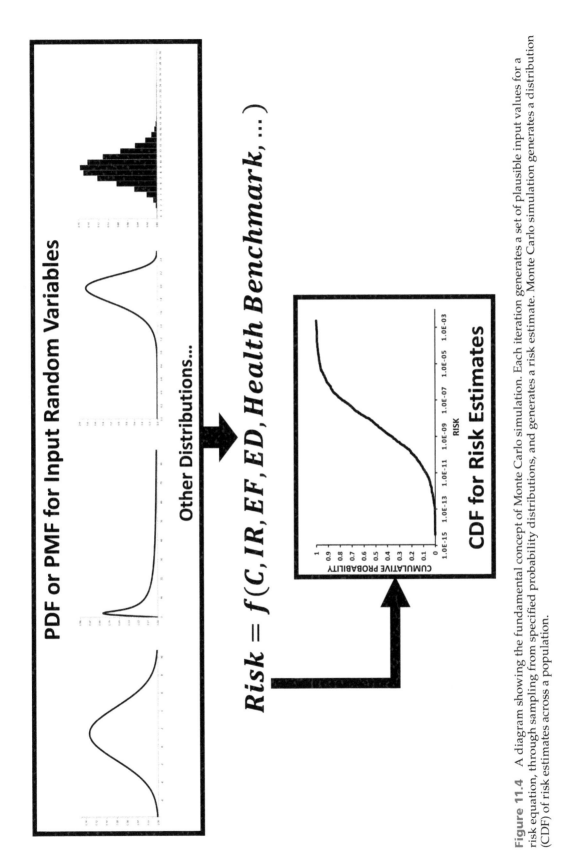

Figure 11.4 A diagram showing the fundamental concept of Monte Carlo simulation. Each iteration generates a set of plausible input values for a risk equation, through sampling from specified probability distributions, and generates a risk estimate. Monte Carlo simulation generates a distribution (CDF) of risk estimates across a population.

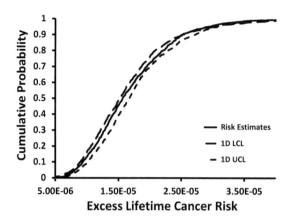

Figure 11.5 The cumulative distribution of the excess lifetime cancer risk, calculated through a one-dimensional Monte Carlo simulation (N = 1,000 iterations). The solid curve reflects the variability under μ = 1.0 for the lognormal distribution of formaldehyde concentration. The dash lines reflect the variabilities under μ = 0.96 and μ = 1.04 for the lognormal distribution of formaldehyde concentration.

in e-cigarette use across the population. For the purpose of demonstration, all the other parameters are set to be fixed in this example. During each iteration of a one-dimensional Monte Carlo simulation, a random number of C is generated from the specified lognormal distribution, and a random number of N is generated from the specified Poisson distribution. A value of the excess lifetime cancer risk is calculated based on the generated numbers and the other fixed values through Equations 11.1 and 11.2. The solid curve in Figure 11.5 illustrates the distribution of the calculated excess lifetime cancer risk after 1,000 iterations. One-dimensional Monte Carlo simulation has limited capability to characterize the impact of uncertainties in input variables on model output. In this example, the mean formaldehyde emission is 1.0 µg/puff, and the upper and lower 95% confidence limits (UCL and LCL) associated with the mean are 1.04 µg/puff and 0.96 µg/puff, respectively. The impact of the uncertainty in the mean formaldehyde emission on the calculated risk can be estimated by repeating the same Monte Carol simulation twice with UCL and LCL as input parameters, respectively. The resulting risk distributions are illustrated in Figure 11.5 with dash lines. The estimated median risk (i.e., cumulative probability = 50%) is 1.6×10^{-5}, with a 95% confidence interval between 1.5×10^{-5} and 1.7×10^{-5}. If a risk model has multiple uncertainties in input parameters, a one-dimensional Monte Carlo simulation will not be a convenient tool to characterize those uncertainties, which, however, can be characterized with two-dimensional Monte Carol simulations.

In a two-dimensional Monte Carlo simulation, probability distributions for model input are differentiated into two categories, distributions characterizing variability and distributions characterizing uncertainty. These two types of distributions are sampled separately in two-dimensional Monte Carlo simulations. In the e-cigarette example, formaldehyde emission (C) follows a lognormal distribution (μ = 1.0, σ = 0.4). However, this lognormal distribution itself might have a certain degree of uncertainty. For example, we may have adequate evidence showing that the parameter μ is not a fixed value but is a random variable following a normal distribution of $N(1.0, 0.11)$. Similarly, the parameter λ for the Poisson distribution of the variable N might follow a uniform distribution between 120 and 140.

A two-dimensional Monte Carlo simulation starts with sampling parameter uncertainty – in this e-cigarette example, sampling a value for μ from $N(1.0, 0.11)$ and a value for λ from a uniform distribution between 120 and 140. Second, the sampled μ value will be assigned as the mean for the lognormal distribution to generate a value for C, and the sampled λ value will be plugged into the Poisson distribution to generate a value for N. The third step is to calculate R based on the sampled values of C and N, along with the other fixed input constants (EF, ED, BW, LT, and SF). The second and the third steps will be repeated, similar to a one-dimension Monte Carlo simulation, until a distribution of R is generated. Then the process resumes again by sampling parameter uncertainty to generate another distribution of R. The whole process repeats (e.g., 1,000 iterations)

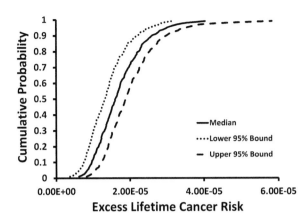

Figure 11.6 The cumulative distribution of the excess lifetime cancer risk calculated through a two-dimensional Monte Carlo simulation. The solid curve reflects the median distribution of R across 100 simulated CDFs of R based on different input values of μ and λ. The dash lines are the 5th and the 95th percentiles of the 100 simulated CDFs, corresponding to the 95% lower and upper bounds of the simulated distributions.

until the variability and uncertainty of R could be sufficiently characterized. The two-dimensional Monte Carlo simulation results are illustrated in Figure 11.6. The central tendency (cumulative probability = 50%) of the estimated excess lifetime cancer risk is 1.6×10^{-5}, and the 90% confidence interval for the estimate of the 50th percentile is (1.3×10^{-5}, 1.9×10^{-5}). The high-end risk estimate (cumulative probability = 95%) is 3.0×10^{-5} with a 90% confidence interval of (2.6×10^{-5}, 3.5×10^{-5}).

A two-dimensional Monte Carlo simulation accounts for parameter uncertainty and allows both variable variability and parameter uncertainty to be included in a risk model. Therefore, a two-dimensional Monte Carlo simulation is a useful tool to model multiple parameter uncertainties and evaluate the impact of both variability and uncertainty on risk estimates.

Commercially available software packages for conducting one-dimensional or two-dimensional Monte Carlo simulations include Crystal Ball®, @Risk®, and many others. Monte Carlo simulations can also be implemented with programming packages, such as R (*mc2d* package), SAS, Python, or Excel. Some existing exposure models developed by the US EPA, including the SHEDS model and the Air Pollutants Exposure model (APEX), have integrated one-dimensional and two-dimensional Monte Carlo simulation techniques in exposure prediction.

The level of complexity of a Monte Carlo simulation is associated with the tier of a probabilistic model, illustrated in Figure 11.3. One-dimensional Monte Carlo simulation is often applied in Tier 2 models to account for the variability of input variables and characterize the variability of exposure and risk estimates. Tier 2 models quantify uncertainties in input parameters in a limited way by repeating one-dimensional Monte Carlo simulations a few times. In the e-cigarette example, three simulations are conducted based on the mean, the UCL, and the LCL of the parameter μ to characterize the uncertainty. In contrast, two-dimensional Monte Carlo simulation is often applied in Tier 3 models, with the full capability to quantify uncertainties and characterize the confidence interval in risk estimates. As illustrated in the e-cigarette example, a two-dimensional Monte Carlo simulation separates probability distributions for variability and for uncertainty. For example, the variability of formaldehyde emission follows a lognormal distribution, and uncertainty of the input parameter μ of the lognormal distribution follows a normal distribution. A Tier 3 model allows for multiple sources of parameter uncertainties and can separate variability and uncertainty through nested computational loops.

It should be noted that there are many sources of uncertainties in exposure and risk assessments. Parameter uncertainty is only one of the many uncertainties. Other sources of uncertainty and variability will be further discussed in the next section. In addition, the e-cigarette example demonstrates the fundamental concepts of Monte Carlo simulation, without introducing overwhelmingly complicated assumptions. In reality, a Monte Carlo simulation could be more complicated, and a few critical issues need to be considered while conducting a simulation. These issues are briefly discussed in the next section.

Critical Issues in Probabilistic Modeling

Censored Data. Some model input data follow a censored distribution, which refers to a probability distribution with thresholds above or below which data are not available. For example, pollutant concentrations with data below the limit of detection are considered left-censored data (e.g., formaldehyde concentration in the e-cigarette study). Similarly, pollutant concentrations with data above the measurement limit of an instrument are considered right-censored data. Censored data could be estimated with detection limits, half detection limits, or imputed numbers. Detailed approaches to handling censored data are discussed by Helsel (2004).

Truncated Distribution. Each value assigned to a model input parameter must reflect realistic exposure conditions. For this purpose, sometimes a threshold is imposed on a distribution to make the input parameters plausible. In the e-cigarette example, if we know it is unrealistic for an e-cigarette user to vape more than 200 puffs per day, a maximum value of 200 can be imposed on the Poisson distribution. The impact of a threshold value on the risk outcome can be estimated with a two-dimensional Monte Carlo simulation by treating the threshold value as a random variable or with other sensitivity analysis approaches to be specified in the section of Sensitivity Analysis (US EPA 2001).

Correlated Input Parameters. In the e-cigarette example, all input variables are assumed to be mutually independent, which means the value generated for one variable is not affected by another variable. However, the relationship between input variables could be more complicated in reality. For example, the number of puffs per day could be positively associated with exposure frequencies, and the associations between the two variables could be linear or nonlinear. In addition, the input parameters for a variable's probability distribution could also be correlated. For example, the mean of the lognormal distribution for formaldehyde emission could be correlated with the standard deviation of the distribution. If the correlations are strong or might have a significant impact on model output, the probability model needs to be modified to reflect the correlation; alternatively, data can be generated from joint distributions with Monte Carlo simulation (US EPA 2014).

Numerical Stability. In a Monte Carlo simulation, it is legitimate (actually very important) to ask how many iterations are needed. To answer this question, a margin of error needs to be set before conducting a simulation. For example, the goal of the simulation is to have the variation in central tendency estimate less than 5%. Then a sufficient number of iterations will be explored/tested to achieve this goal or to achieve the predetermined "numerical stability." It should be noted that the concept of "numerical stability" is associated with the percentile of cumulative distribution of risk estimates. The number of iterations sufficient for the central tendency estimate might be insufficient for a high-end risk estimate (US EPA 2001).

Sensitivity Analysis. A sensitivity analysis is a systematic approach to evaluating how model output varies with different model input values. Detailed guidance on how to conduct a sensitivity analysis is beyond the scope of this chapter. The role of sensitivity analysis in probabilistic modeling and commonly used methods are briefly discussed in this section. Details are documented in the US EPA's *Risk Assessment Guidance for Superfund* (US EPA 2001) and the US EPA's *Risk Assessment Forum White Paper* (US EPA 2014).

The primary purpose of a sensitivity analysis is to identify the most influential model input variables or distribution parameters on model output. In the e-cigarette example, assuming both formaldehyde and tobacco-specific N-nitrosonornicotine (NNN) are evaluated, and we observe that a small change in NNN leads to a large variation in the cumulative risk estimate, then we need to study more on the distribution of NNN to better quantify its variability and reduce its uncertainty. Similarly, if primary, secondary, and tertiary vapor exposures are evaluated, and we find that the tertiary vapor exposure contributes the most to the variation in the cumulative risk estimate, we probably need to focus more on the tertiary vapor exposure as an influential pathway. In addition, a sensitivity analysis can address a certain aspect of model uncertainty. For example, if formaldehyde emission in the e-cigarette example can be equally plausibly characterized by a gamma distribution or a lognormal distribution, a sensitivity analysis could address this uncertainty and assess the impact of distribution selection on risk estimation.

Common methods used to identify influential variables or parameters include sensitivity ratio, sensitivity score, Pearson or Spearman correlation coefficient, and regression analysis (US EPA 2001).

Uncertainty. Addressing uncertainty and variability is a critical component of risk assessment. Uncertainty and variability are different concepts. Uncertainty will be discussed in this section and variability in the following section. Uncertainty refers to a lack of knowledge about the exposure and toxicological properties of a chemical. In probabilistic modeling, uncertainty occurs because of unknowns in models, input variables, and variable distributions. Uncertainty may be reduced by obtaining more information.

Uncertainty occurs throughout the risk assessment process, including toxicity assessment and exposure assessment (NRC 2009). The classification of a chemical into a certainty category in the hazard identification step, such as carcinogens, mutagens, or endocrine disruptors, has inherent uncertainty. Deriving RfCs, RfDs, or cancer slope factors in dose-response assessment contains many layers of uncertainties, including inter- and intraspecies extrapolations, high-dose to low-dose extrapolation, route-to-route extrapolation, chemical-to-chemical extrapolation, and data quality. Exposure assessment and dose estimation also contain inherent uncertainties, such as exposure scenarios and exposure concentrations. In a modeling framework, these uncertainties can be classified into three categories, i.e., scenario uncertainty, model uncertainty, and parameter uncertainty.

Scenario uncertainty refers to the mischaracterization of risks (either overestimation or underestimation) due to the incomplete description of exposure or risk scenarios. Scenario uncertainty includes the omission of certain chemical agents in cumulative assessments, the exclusion of certain exposure pathways or sources in aggregate assessments, or the ignorance of certain exposed populations. The omission of tertiary exposure to NNN in the e-cigarette example is a scenario uncertainty.

In probabilistic modeling, mathematical and statistical models are used to describe chemical, physical, exposure, toxicokinetic, and toxicodynamic processes. A model usually contains assumptions, has its own application domain, and simplifies the reality. Model uncertainty refers to the uncertainty in using a mathematical model to estimate the real-world exposure and risk. Model uncertainty arises from the deviation of model assumptions from reality, the limitation of a model's application domain, and the exclusion of key physical, chemical, and biological processes. A model lacking the capability to process the partitioning of semivolatile organic compounds (SVOC) between phases would mischaracterize SVOC exposures.

Parameter uncertainty refers to the uncertainty in numerical values used as model input. Parameter uncertainty originates from measurement errors, sampling errors, and the use of default or extrapolated values. The e-cigarette example contains a few parameter uncertainties: Formaldehyde concentration values contain measurement uncertainties, the number of puffs per day might not be derived from a representative sample of e-cigarette users, and the default body weight of 70 kg might be biased high or low for a certain population. Another example is shown in the PFAS cumulative risk assessment: Points of departure of PFOSA for hepatotoxicity and reproductive toxicity are derived from PFOS based on read-across extrapolation.

All types of the aforementioned uncertainties need to be characterized either qualitatively or quantitatively. Uncertainty analysis is an integral part of risk assessment. Characterizing uncertainty can increase the transparency and the credibility of probabilistic risk assessment (NRC 2009). Decision-makers and the public can also benefit from uncertainty analysis in terms of understanding major knowledge gaps and the accuracy of the assessment. WHO (2008) provides ten principles for uncertainty analysis. Although these principles are proposed in the context of exposure assessment, they are applicable in risk assessment. The extent and nature of an uncertainty analysis should be addressed in the scoping stage of a risk assessment and should match the complexity of the risk assessment and the needs of decision-making (NRC 2009).

A tiered approach for uncertainty analysis is documented by the US EPA (2001) and WHO (2008), and this approach is reiterated by NRC (2009) and European Chemicals Agency (ECHA; 2012). There are four levels in this approach for uncertainty analysis with increasing refinement, which matches the complexity and needs of a risk assessment. At the most fundamental level, conservative default values and assumptions are applied in the risk assessment and are documented in the uncertainty analysis. At the next level, a qualitative assessment of uncertainty is applied in a systematic way to characterize the uncertainty for all significant model input parameters. Then, a quantitative approach using bounding values is applied to quantify the uncertainty, which has been illustrated in the e-cigarette example of a one-dimensional Monte Carlo simulation to characterize the uncertainty associated with the central tendency risk estimate. At the highest level, a probabilistic approach is employed to quantify the uncertainty for multiple variables, which has been also illustrated in this chapter with a two-dimensional Monte Carlo simulation to characterize the uncertainties associated with formaldehyde emission and e-cigarette use pattern. Lower-tier uncertainty analyses are usually performed to meet the needs for screening-leveling regulatory or research needs, and a high-tier uncertainty analysis are performed to meet the needs for regulatory compliance (WHO 2008).

Although Monte Carlo simulation has been widely applied to quantify uncertainties in probabilistic model outcomes, it is most useful in characterizing parameter uncertainty (US EPA 2001).

Other types of uncertainties may or may not be quantified by Monte Carlo. A qualitative assessment could be applied to characterize scenario uncertainty or model uncertainty. In addition, model uncertainty could be characterized by quantitative methods, including Bayesian model averaging and evaluating likelihood functions (US EPA 2014). In a broader sense, sensitivity analysis could be regarded as part of uncertainty analysis to characterize various uncertainties and their impact on risk and exposure assessment.

Sensitivity analysis is used to identify the most influential model input parameter and examine the impact of model input on model output. WHO (2008) regards sensitivity analysis as an integral component of uncertainty analysis. The results of a sensitivity analysis highlight key variables and parameters, which should be focused on more data collection or uncertainty reduction. The impact of different exposure scenarios and different models on risk estimates could be integrated into the framework of a sensitivity analysis.

Variability. Variability is different from uncertainty. Variability refers to the inherent heterogeneity of a system, which cannot be reduced but can be better characterized through further investigation (ECHA 2012; US EPA 2001).

There are many examples of variability in exposure and risk assessments. In the e-cigarette example, formaldehyde emission is different from device to device and from person to person, and the number of puffs per day also varies from day to day and from person to person. Similar to uncertainty, variability exists throughout the whole process of a risk assessment, such as inter- and intraspecies variability in toxicity assessment, and variability in personal activity and pollutant concentration in exposure assessment. Of particular concern in human health risk assessment are human variability, spatial variability, and temporal variability (US EPA 2019b; 2014). Human variability includes inter- and intrapersonal (or population) variations in factors related to exposure (e.g., activity pattern and physiological characteristics), toxicokinetics (e.g., uptake rates), and toxicodynamics (e.g., effective dose). Spatial variability refers to spatial variation in factors directly or indirectly affecting exposures and risks (e.g., pollutant concentrations in air or water, climate zones, and proximity to highways). Temporal variability refers to temporal variation in factors directly or indirectly affecting exposures and risks (e.g., seasonal variations and diurnal variations). All these variabilities are related to differences in exposures or susceptibility across a population and are affected by age, gender, ethnicity, genetic background, lifestyle, and socioeconomic status. Assessing variability in exposure and risk enables us to focus on vulnerable or susceptible populations and people in environmental justice communities.

In probabilistic modeling, the variability of a variable is described with a distribution, which is used as risk model input. The output of a probabilistic model is also a distribution, reflecting the distribution of risk or exposure across a population. This concept has been illustrated in the e-cigarette example with one-dimensional and two-dimensional Monte Carlo simulations. It should be noted that variability and uncertainty should be separated in probabilistic modeling, i.e., avoiding a distribution intermingled with variability and uncertainty. In the e-cigarette example, the variability of formaldehyde emission follows a lognormal distribution, but the uncertainty of the lognormal mean follows a normal distribution. Similarly, the variability of vaping frequency follows a Poisson distribution, but the uncertainty of the distribution parameter (λ) is described with a uniform distribution. Separating variability and uncertainty in probabilistic modeling can better inform risk assessors and risk managers about different sources and scales of variability and uncertainty in the risk characterization stage.

Expert Elicitation. In probabilistic risk assessment, it is critical to quantify uncertainties. However, there are situations where data are not available or not sufficient to develop an empirical distribution for uncertainty estimates. In such cases of lacking data, expert elicitation is a promising approach to filling knowledge gaps and estimating uncertainties (NRC 2009).

Expert elicitation is a process involving "asking a set of carefully selected experts a series of questions related to a specific array of potential outcomes and usually providing them with extensive briefing material, training activities, and calibration exercises to help in the determination of confidence intervals" (NRC 2009). In the process, probability is quantified based on expert judgment.

Expert judgment can be incorporated into probabilistic modeling as nonempirical information under a Bayesian inference framework (Kelly and Smith 2011). Bayesian statistical methods require prior distribution and empirical data as model input and generate a posterior distribution. Expert judgment or "subjective probability distributions" serves as the initial estimate, or a prior distribution, based on the state of knowledge. This prior distribution is updated or refined continuously based on emerging evidence. Under the Bayesian framework, expert judgments and empirical evidence (e.g., objective measurements) are synthesized and generate a refined estimate.

THOUGHT QUESTIONS

1. What are the similarities and differences in cumulative and aggregate assessment of exposures and risks?
2. What are the major sources and types of uncertainties in exposure and risk assessment?
3. What are the differences between variability and uncertainty?
4. How are uncertainties and variabilities characterized in risk assessment?
5. What are the advantages of using probabilistic models in exposure and risk assessment?

DISCLAIMERS

The findings and conclusions in this chapter are those of the author and do not necessarily represent the official position of the California Department of Toxic Substances Control.

REFERENCES

Adgate, John L., C. Andrew Clayton, James J. Quackenboss, Kent W. Thomas, Roy W. Whitmore, Edo D. Pellizzari, Paul J. Lioy, et al. 2000. Data Collection Issues: Measurement of Multi-Pollutant and Multi-Pathway Exposures in a Probability-Based Sample of Children: Practical Strategies for Effective Field Studies. *Journal of Exposure Science & Environmental Epidemiology* 10 (S6): 650–661. https://doi.org/10.1038/sj.jea.7500126.

ATSDR. 2012. *Toxicological Profile for 1,4-Dioxane*. Atlanta, Georgia: ATSDR.

ATSDR. 2019. *Toxicological Profile for DDT*. Atlanta, Georgia: ATSDR.

ATSDR. 2021. *Toxicological Profile for Perfluoroalkyls*. Atlanta, Georgia: ATSDR.

Borg, Daniel, Bert-Ove Lund, Nils-Gunnar Lindquist, and Helen Håkansson. 2013. Cumulative Health Risk Assessment of 17 Perfluoroalkylated and Polyfluoroalkylated Substances (PFASs) in the Swedish Population. *Environment International* 59 (September): 112–123. https://doi.org/10.1016/j.envint.2013.05.009.

CCR, Title 22, Sections 69502.2. 2008. Vol. CCR, Title 22, Chapter 55. Safer Consumer Products.

CDC. 2021. *Fourth National Report on Human Exposure to Environmental Chemicals Update*. Atlanta, Georgia: CDC.

Chiu, Weihsueh A., and Wout Slob. 2015. A Unified Probabilistic Framework for Dose–Response Assessment of Human Health Effects. *Environmental Health Perspectives* 123 (12): 1241–1254. https://doi.org/10.1289/ehp.1409385.

Clayton, Andrew, Edo D. Pellizzari, Roy W. Whitmore, James J. Quackenboss, John Adgate, and Ken Sefton. 2003. Distributions, Associations, and Partial Aggregate Exposure of Pesticides and Polynuclear Aromatic Hydrocarbons in the Minnesota Children's Pesticide Exposure Study (MNCPES). *Journal of Exposure Science & Environmental Epidemiology* 13 (2): 100–111. https://doi.org/10.1038/sj.jea.7500261.

Dautzenberg, Bertrand, and Damien Bricard. 2015. Real-Time Characterization of E-Cigarettes Use: The 1 Million Puffs Study. *Journal of Addiction Research & Therapy* 06 (02). https://doi.org/10.4172/2155-6105.1000229.

Devore, Jay. 2000. *Probability and Statistics for Engineering and the Sciences*. 5th Edition. Pacific Grove, CA: Duxbury.

ECHA. 2012. "Guidance on Information Requirements and Chemical Safety Assessment Chapter R.19: Uncertainty Analysis. ECHA-12-G-25-EN. Helsinki, Finland: ECHA.

Food Quality Protection Act of 1996, PUBLIC LAW 104–170. 1996. 7 USC 136.

Helsel, Dennis. 2004. *Nondetects and Data Analysis: Statistics for Censored Environmental Data*. Hoboken, NJ: John Wiley & Sons, Inc.

Kelly, Dana, and Curtis Smith. 2011. *Bayesian Inference for Probabilistic Risk Assessment*. Springer Series in Reliability Engineering. London: Springer London. https://doi.org/10.1007/978-1-84996-187-5.

MacDonell, Margaret M., Lynne A. Haroun, Linda K. Teuschler, Glenn E. Rice, Richard C. Hertzberg, James P. Butler, Young-Soo Chang, et al. 2013. Cumulative Risk Assessment Toolbox: Methods and Approaches for the Practitioner. *Journal of Toxicology* 2013: 1–36. https://doi.org/10.1155/2013/310904.

Minnesota Department of Health. 2020. *Evaluating Concurrent Exposures to Multiple Chemicals*. St. Paul, MN: Minnesota Department of Health.

NRC. 2007. *Models in Environmental Regulatory Decision Making*. Washington, DC: National Academies Press. https://doi.org/10.17226/11972.

NRC. 2009. *Science and Decisions: Advancing Risk Assessment*. Washington, DC: National Academies Press. https://doi.org/10.17226/12209.

NRC. 2014. *Identifying and Reducing Environmental Health Risks of Chemicals in Our Society: Workshop Summary.* Washington, DC: National Academies Press. https://doi.org/10.17226/18710.

OEHHA. 2011. *Air Toxics Hot Spots Program Risk Assessment Guidelines, Appendix B.* Sacramento, CA: OEHHA.

OEHHA. 2015. *Air Toxics Hot Spots Program Risk Assessment Guidelines.* Sacramento, CA: OEHHA.

Park, Youngja H., Kichun Lee, Quinlyn A. Soltow, Frederick H. Strobel, Kenneth L. Brigham, Richard E. Parker, Mark E. Wilson, et al. 2012. High-Performance Metabolic Profiling of Plasma from Seven Mammalian Species for Simultaneous Environmental Chemical Surveillance and Bioeffect Monitoring. *Toxicology* 295 (1–3): 47–55. https://doi.org/10.1016/j.tox.2012.02.007.

Parsons, David. 2012. Probabilistic Modelling for Assessment of Exposure via Drinking Water. Defra WT1263, DWI 70/2/273. Cranfield University.

Poothong, Somrutai, Eleni Papadopoulou, Juan Antonio Padilla-Sánchez, Cathrine Thomsen, and Line Småstuen Haug. 2020. Multiple Pathways of Human Exposure to Poly- and Perfluoroalkyl Substances (PFASs): From External Exposure to Human Blood. *Environment International* 134 (January): 105244. https://doi.org/10.1016/j.envint.2019.105244.

Qin, Jing, Chong You, Qiushi Lin, Taojun Hu, Shicheng Yu, and Xiao-Hua Zhou. 2020. Estimation of Incubation Period Distribution of COVID-19 Using Disease Onset Forward Time: A Novel Cross-Sectional and Forward Follow-up Study. *Preprint. Infectious Diseases (except HIV/AIDS).* https://doi.org/10.1101/2020.03.06.20032417.

RIVM. 2018. Cleaning Products Fact Sheet: Default Parameters for Estimating Consumer Exposure – Updated Version 2018. RIVM Report 2016-0179. National Institute for Public Health and the Environment, The Netherlands: Ministry of Health, Welfare and Sport.

Son, Yeongkwon, Clifford Weisel, Olivia Wackowski, Stephan Schwander, Cristine Delnevo, and Qingyu Meng. 2020. The Impact of Device Settings, Use Patterns, and Flavorings on Carbonyl Emissions from Electronic Cigarettes. *International Journal of Environmental Research and Public Health* 17 (16): 5650. https://doi.org/10.3390/ijerph17165650.

The Frank R. Lautenberg Chemical Safety for the 21st Century Act. 2016. *15 USC Ch. 53: Toxic Substances Control.*

US EPA. 2001. Risk Assessment Guidance for Superfund: Volume III - Part A, Process for Conducting Probabilistic Risk Assessment. EPA 540-R-02-002. Washington, DC: US EPA.

US EPA. 2003a. Developing Relative Potency Factors for Pesticide Mixtures: Biostatistical Analyses of Joint Dose-Response. EPA/600/R-03/052. Cincinnati, OH: US EPA.

US EPA. 2003b. Framework for Cumulative Risk Assessment. EPA/630/P-02/001F. Washington, DC: US EPA.

US EPA. 2003c. Multimedia, Multipathway, and Multireceptor Risk Assessment (3MRA) Modeling System. EPA530-D-03–001a. Washington, DC: US EPA.

US EPA. 2004. Example Exposure Scenarios. Washington, DC: US EPA.

US EPA. 2005a. Guidelines for Carcinogen Risk Assessment. EPA/630/P-03/001F. Washington, DC: US EPA.

US EPA. 2005b. Supplemental Guidance for Assessing Susceptibility from Early-Life Exposure to Carcinogens. EPA/630/R-03/003F. Washington, DC: US EPA.

US EPA. 2009. *Recommended Toxicity Equivalency Factors (TEFs) for Human Health Risk Assessments of Dioxin and Dioxin-Like Compounds.* Washington, DC: US EPA.

US EPA. 2010. Development of a Relative Potency Factor (RPF) Approach for Polyclic Aromatic Hydrocarbon (PAH) Mixtures. EPA/635/R-08/012A. Washington, DC: US EPA.

US EPA. 2011. Exposure Factors Handbook. EPA/600/R-090/052F. Washington, DC: US EPA.

US EPA. 2014. Risk Assessment Forum White Paper: Probabilistic Risk Assessment Methods and Case Studies. EPA/100/R-14/004. Washington, DC: US EPA.

US EPA. 2019a. EPA's Per- and Polyfluoroalkyl Substances (PFAS) Action Plan. EPA 823R18004. US EPA.

US EPA. 2019b. Guidelines for Human Exposure Assessment. EPA/100/B-19/001. Washington, DC: US EPA.

US EPA. 2021. *Regional Screening Levels (RSLs) – User's Guide.* Washington, DC: US EPA. https://www.epa.gov/risk/regional-screening-levels-rsls-users-guide.

WHO. 2005. *Harmonization Project Document. 3: Principles of Characterizing and Applying Human Exposure Models/ International Programme on Chemical Safety.* Inter-Organization Programme for the Sound Management of Chemicals. Geneva: World Health Organization.

WHO, ed. 2008. *Uncertainty and Data Quality in Exposure Assessment.* IPCS Harmonization Project Document, no. 6. Geneva: World Health Organization.

12 Occupational Risk Assessment

Adam M. Finkel
Health Science at the University of Michigan, Ann Arbor, MI, United States

Douglas O. Johns
Spokane Mining Research Division, National Institute for Occupational Safety and Health, Centers for Disease Control and Prevention, Spokane, WA, United States

Christine Whittaker
Division of Science Integration, National Institute for Occupational Safety and Health, Centers for Disease Control and Prevention, Cincinnati, OH, United States

CONTENTS

Background 226
    Acute Fatal and Nonfatal Injuries 227
    Occupational Disease 232
    Occupational Exposures 233
    Assessing and Managing Workplace Risks: NIOSH, OSHA, and EPA 235
        NIOSH 235
        OSHA 235
        Role of the EPA in Occupational Risk Management 236
Overview of Occupational Risk Assessment Methodology and Policy 239
    Court Decisions Affecting Risk Assessment 242
    The Mechanics of Occupational Risk Assessment 244
    Dose-Response Analysis 247
    Case Study: Methylene Chloride 249
Control of Hazards 253
    Elimination 253
    Substitution 253
    Engineering Controls 254
    Administrative Controls 255
    Personal Protective Equipment 256
The Evolution of Industrial Hygiene and the Role of New Professionals 258
Emerging Hazards 258
    Nanotechnology 258
    Impact of Climate on Workers 258
    New Industrial Processes 259
    Exposure to Mixtures 261
    Technological Change 261
Thought Questions 261
Disclaimers 261
References 262

LEARNING OBJECTIVES

Students who complete this chapter will be able to

1. Understand the scope, magnitude, distribution, and changes during the past half-century in the major safety and health hazards workers face on the job, both in absolute terms and relative to analogous risks in the community or ambient environment;
2. Become familiar with the institutions (primarily Occupational Safety and Health Administration, National Institute for Occupational Safety and Health, and Mine Safety and Health Administration) set up in the United States to evaluate and control these

DOI: 10.1201/9780429291722-12

hazards and with the major legal, scientific, and political challenges these agencies have faced over the past 50 years;

3. Understand how quantitative risk assessment (QRA) for occupational hazards has developed, how it differs from QRA as applied to similar hazards in the general environment, and which aspects of methodology remain the least well developed; and

4. Appreciate the complex interplay of science and policy involved in controlling occupational risks – in particular, the limited role of formal cost-benefit balancing in managing workplace risks – and be able to discuss some of the innovative approaches government, industry, and labor are contemplating to reduce risks through means other than command-and-control regulation.

BACKGROUND

Just as the nature of work has changed throughout the history of the human species, so too have the health and safety risks to which workers are exposed. Though occupational hazards have long been recognized (for example, there are detailed references in the history of Herodotus, circa 450 BC, to how to safely construct trenches so as to protect workers; even earlier, the Old Testament (Deuteronomy 22:8) instructed the faithful to "make a parapet around your roof so that you may not bring the guilt of bloodshed if someone falls from the roof"), there is little documented evidence of the study of occupational health as a distinct discipline prior to the eighteenth century (Gochfeld 2005). The Industrial Revolution brought with it new and widespread risks of work-related injury, illness, and death, which resulted in organized labor demands and public outcry for better working conditions, ultimately resulting in the passage of laws designed to protect the health and safety of workers (Rosner and Markowitz 2020). Occupational risks have evolved over time, and despite considerable progress in reducing work-related risks in the United States, American workers continue to be exposed daily to persistent and emerging hazards (Schulte 2017; Tamers et al. 2020).

Approximately 60% of the US civilian noninstitutional population ages 16 and over are employed, totaling more than 158 million persons working either full or part time (83.3% and 16.7% of the employed population, respectively) in more than 10 million separate establishments (BLS 2022; US Census Bureau 2022). These people face many of the same hazards on the job as those who do not work full or part time face in their daily lives, including hazards in the ambient environment, the community, the home, and in transportation. As we will see, however, workers almost invariably are exposed to these hazards at a much higher frequency, intensity, or concentration than nonworkers are. In addition, of course, workers are exposed to various unique hazards that are not found outside the occupational setting. A central irony in considering occupational risk assessment in the context of the broad field of risk assessment is that many environmental health standards were motivated by discoveries of human disease in the workplace (see Table 12.1) and are based quantitatively on scientific studies of worker populations. For that matter, quantitative estimates of the value of averting a "statistical fatality" are also derived from economic studies in the workplace (see, e.g., Viscusi 2013) – but too often the protections that have resulted from these inquiries have failed to adequately protect workers. Traditionally, hazards in the ambient environment have captured much greater attention than similar or identical hazards faced to a greater degree by workers.

This chapter focuses on occupational illness, where risk assessment methods have of necessity become relatively well developed, but we need to recognize at the outset that occupational injury was the first workplace problem area to gain national attention. Events such as the Triangle Shirtwaist Fire of 1911, which claimed 146 victims in New York City (Von Drehle 2003), the 1947 explosion in Texas City, in which at least 580 workers died when a docked ship carrying ammonium nitrate exploded (Pandanell 2005), and landmark books such as Upton Sinclair's *The Jungle* ([1906] 1985, detailing working conditions in the meatpacking plants around Chicago) focused some attention on occupational injury events and led finally to the passage of the Occupational Safety and Health (OSH) Act of 1970, which created both the Occupational Safety and Health Administration (OSHA) and the National Institute for Occupational Safety and Health (NIOSH). OSHA, along with the Mine Safety and Health Administration (MSHA), which was created by the Federal Mine Safety and Health Act of 1977, is responsible for developing and enforcing workplace regulations and standards. NIOSH, on the other hand, is an agency within the Centers for Disease

Table 12.1: Diseases First Noted in Occupational Settings That Impelled Environmental Standards

Disease	Cause	References
Asbestosis	Asbestos exposure	Selikoff et al. (1965); Selikoff et al. (1967); Selikoff and Greenberg (1991).
Silicosis	Exposure to silica-containing rock dust	For a historical overview, see Bufton and Melling (2005).
Black lung	Exposure to coal mine dust	Black lung disease was recognized in the early part of the 20th century. For an overview of the subject, see Smith (1981).
Byssinosis	Exposure to cotton dust	Corn (1981).
Various malignant and other diseases	Radiation exposure, including radon in mines	For an overview, see Upton (1987).
Lead poisoning	Lead dust exposure	Lead poisoning was known to the ancients; several more recent papers review its effects. See Baker Jr. et al. (1979); Winegar et al. (1977).
Neurological symptoms	Pesticide exposure, solvent exposure	Landrigan et al. (1980); Baker Jr. et al. (1985).
Dermatitis, hyper- pigmentation, keratoses, blackfoot disease	Arsenic exposure	Landrigan et al. (1980).
Leukemia	Benzene exposure	Landrigan (1987).

Control and Prevention (CDC) mandated to conduct occupational health and safety research, train occupational health professionals, and make recommendations for the prevention of work-related injury, illness, and death. While generally considered a nonregulatory agency, NIOSH is directly responsible for the administration of a number of occupational safety and health regulatory programs, including the approval of respiratory equipment and the implementation of the World Trade Center Health Program.

Acute Fatal and Nonfatal Injuries

The most fundamental measure of the risk of occupational fatalities, of course, is the national death toll and the related measure of the death rate. Table 12.2 shows the number of workplace fatalities since the OSH Act was passed more than 50 years ago, along with the number of US civilian employees in each year and the crude death rate (in fatalities per 100,000 workers). Note the current population fatality rate of about 3 per 100,000 per year yields a working-lifetime risk of roughly 1.4×10^{-3} (1 chance in about 750) of suffering a fatal workplace injury during a career. This probability will be put in context later in the chapter when we discuss the various definitions of "acceptable risk" in the workplace and elsewhere.

Figure 12.1.A shows that most of the 4,764 fatalities in 2020 occurred in the construction, transportation, and agricultural sectors of the economy, though as shown in Figure 12.1.B, the fatality rate (per 100,000 workers) is very similar between the construction and mining sectors. Interestingly, total injuries and injury rate are highest in the healthcare and social assistance sectors, as depicted in Figures 12.1.A and 12.1.B, respectively. Figure 12.2 shows general decreases over the past 30 years of the four most frequent work-related fatal and nonfatal events. However,

BOX 12.1 ASSESSING TRENDS IN WORKPLACE POPULATION RISK

Adam M. Finkel

The most striking aspect of these statistics is the rather steady decline in total deaths and the (almost) inevitable decrease in death rate over the 50-year period. Some critics of OSHA (Kniesner and Leeth, 1995) assert that the slope of the downward trend was actually steeper before 1970 than after (which, if true, would not necessarily be an indication of OSHA's ineffectiveness, since we might expect continued decrements in the fatality rate to be harder and harder to achieve as the absolute rate decreased).

Table 12.2: **Workplace Fatalities Since the Passage of the OSH Act**

Year	Employment Work Deaths Counts	Total Employment (Thousands)	Work Deaths per 100,000 FTE Workers	Employment Work Injury Counts (Private Industry)	Work Injuries per 100 FTE Workers (Private Industry)
1970	13,800	77,700	18.0		
1971	13,700	78,500	17.0		
1972	14,000	81,300	17.0		10.9
1973	14,300	84,300	17.0	6,078,700	11.0
1974	13,500	86,200	16.0	5,915,800	10.4
1975	13,000	85,200	15.0	4,983,100	9.1
1976	12,500	88,100	14.0	5,163,700	9.2
1977	12,900	91,500	14.0	5,460,300	9.3
1978	13,100	95,500	14.0	5,799,400	9.4
1979	13,000	98,300	13.0	6,105,700	9.5
1980	13,200	98,800	13.0	5,605,800	8.7
1981	12,500	99,800	13.0	5,404,400	8.3
1982	11,900	98,800	12.0	4,856,400	7.7
1983	11,700	100,100	12.0	4,854,100	7.6
1984	11,500	104,300	11.0	5,419,700	8.0
1985	11,500	106,400	11.0	5,507,200	7.9
1986	11,100	108,900	10.0	5,629,000	7.9
1987	11,300	111,700	10.0	6,035,900	8.3
1988	10,800	114,300	9.0	6,440,400	8.6
1989	10,400	116,700	9.0	6,576,300	8.6
1990	10,500	117,400	9.0	6,753,000	8.8
1991	9,900	116,400	9.0	6,345,700	8.4
1992	6,217	119,583	5.0	6,799,400	8.9
1993	6,331	120,791	5.0	6,737,400	8.5
1994	6,632	124,469	5.0	6,766,900	8.4
1995	6,275	126,248	5.0	6,575,400	8.1
1996	6,202	127,997	4.8	6,238,900	7.4
1997	6,238	130,810	4.7	6,145,600	7.1
1998	6,055	132,684	4.5	5,922,800	6.7
1999	6,054	134,666	4.5	5,707,200	6.3
2000	5,920	136,377	4.3	5,650,100	6.1
2001[a]	5,915	136,252	4.3	5,215,600	5.7
2002	5,534	137,700	4.0	4,700,600	5.3
2003	5,575	138,928	4.0	4,365,200	5.0
2004	5,764	140,411	4.1	4,257,300	4.8
2005	5,734	142,894	4.0	4,214,200	4.6
2006	5,840	145,501	4.0	4,085,400	4.4
2007	5,657	147,215	3.8	4,002,700	4.2
Year	Employment Work Deaths Counts	Total Hours Worked (millions)	Work Deaths Per 100,000 FTE Workers	Employment Work Injuries Counts (All Industries)	Work Injuries Per 100 FTE Workers (All Industries)
2008	5,214	271,958	3.7	4,634,100	4.2
2009	4,551	254,771	3.5	4,140,700	3.9
2010	4,690	255,948	3.6	3,883,600	3.8
2011	4,693	258,293	3.5	3,857,700	3.8
2012	4,628	264,374	3.4	3,820,800	3.7
2013	4,585	268,127	3.3	3,753,300	3.5
2014	4,821	272,663	3.4	3,675,800	3.4
2015	4,836	277,470	3.4	3,658,500	3.3
2016	5,190	283,101	3.6	3,534,600	3.2
2017	5,147	285,977	3.5	3,475,900	3.1

(Continued)

Table 12.2: **(Continued)**

Year	Employment Work Deaths Counts	Total Hours Worked (millions)	Work Deaths Per 100,000 FTE Workers	Employment Work Injuries Counts (All Industries)	Work Injuries Per 100 FTE Workers (All Industries)
2018	5,250	292,528	3.5	3,544,400	3.1
2019	5,333	296,600	3.5	3,496,700	3.0
2020	4,764	269,900	3.4	3,229,200	2.9

Note: Data for injuries and illnesses are first published for survey year 1972. However, due to the lack of a national system for tracking occupational illnesses, it is likely that these numbers reflect solely injuries. In fact, beginning in 1992, the Bureau of Labor Statistics (BLS) reported these data as injuries only and did not mention "illnesses." In 2007, BLS changed its methods for reporting fatality rates and also changed the reporting for injuries from private sector to all sectors. Therefore, caution must be taken in comparing data from before and from after 2007.

[a] *Excludes fatalities from the events of September 11, 2001.*

Sources: *Data from 1970 to 1991 is from National Safety Council Accident Facts, 2022.Data from 1992 to 2020 is from the BLS, 2022. In 1994, the National Safety Council [NSC] changed their reporting method for workplace fatalities and adopted the BLS count. The earlier NSC numbers are based on an estimate; the BLS numbers are based on an actual census.*

within that time span, there have been extended periods in which the trends in these work-related fatalities and injuries have remained flat or even increased.

Table 12.3 provides further detail on the racial composition of workers killed on the job, showing a clear decline in total fatalities and injuries over the past 30 years. However, it is concerning that the death toll has increased among some groups of workers, particularly Hispanics, over the past five to ten years.

For every fatal injury in the United States, nearly 1,000 other nonfatal injuries also occur. In 2020, the BLS reported a total of 2.7 million workplace injuries and illnesses; all but roughly 500,000 of these were injuries; of the illnesses recorded, nearly half were skin conditions or occupational hearing loss, and it is unclear to what extent *any* chronic work-related illnesses such as cancer,

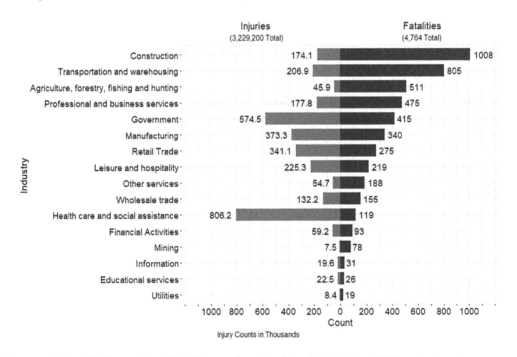

Figure 12.1 (A) Occupational fatalities and nonfatalities by industry, 2020: private sector, government, and self-employment. (Continued)

Source: BLS (2020).

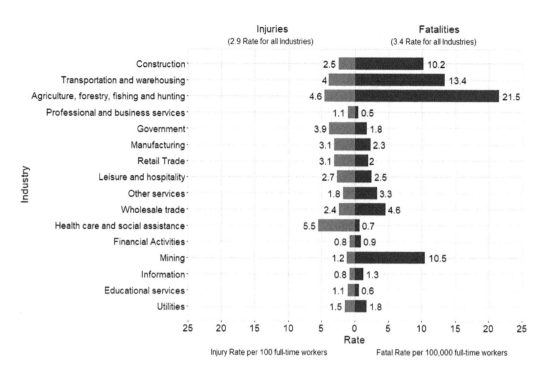

Figure 12.1 (Continued) (B) Occupational fatality and nonfatality rate by industry, 2020: private sector, government, and self-employment.

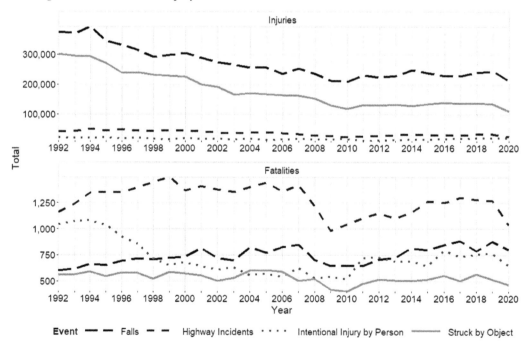

Figure 12.2 The four most frequent work-related fatal and nonfatal events, 1992–2020.

Sources: **Bureau of Labor Statistics (2020).**

Table 12.3: Fatal and Nonfatal Injuries Involving Days Away from Work by Race, 1992–2020

	Total Fatalities	Total Injuries[a]	White Fatalities	White Injuries[a]	Black or African American Fatalities	Injuries[a]	Hispanic or Latino Fatalities	Injuries[a]	Asian or Pacific Islander Fatalities	Injuries[a]	American Indian or Alaskan Native Fatalities	Injuries[a]	Other Races or Not Reported Fatalities	Injuries[a]
1992	6,217	2,331,098	4,711	1,252,527	618	190,616	533	198,022	169	30,554	36	8,289	150	651,090
1993	6,331	2,252,591	4,665	1,250,071	649	195,780	634	192,304	190	33,230	46	9,156	147	572,051
1994	6,632	2,236,639	4,954	1,234,065	695	197,449	624	189,719	179	33,915	39	7,218	141	574,272
1995	6,275	2,040,929	4,599	1,070,115	684	196,751	619	191,665	161	28,594	27	8,646	185	545,157
1996	6,202	1,880,525	4,586	1,001,424	615	165,700	638	169,300	170	27,010	35	7,316	158	509,775
1997	6,238	1,833,380	4,576	966,289	661	163,823	658	187,221	195	30,969	34	7,551	114	477,528
1998	6,055	1,730,534	4,478	882,428	583	157,435	707	179,399	148	26,782	28	7,431	111	477,058
1999	6,054	1,702,470	4,410	859,591	616	155,149	730	182,896	180	25,328	54	6,812	63	472,693
2000	5,920	1,664,018	4,244	827,455	575	139,280	815	186,028	185	25,857	33	6,955	68	478,442
2001[b]	5,915	1,537,567	4,175	765,228	565	133,785	895	191,959	182	25,317	48	5,661	50	415,616
2002	5,534	1,436,194	3,926	688,009	491	114,453	841	180,419	140	22,099	40	8,225	96	422,989
2003	5,575	1,315,920	3,988	617,160	543	108,470	794	161,330	158	20,400	42	6,910	50	401,770
2004	5,764	1,259,320	4,066	591,570	546	103,820	902	164,920	180	20,690	28	5,140	42	373,180
2005	5,734	1,234,680	3,977	567,790	584	101,170	923	164,600	163	17,950	50	5,830	35	377,480
2006	5,840	1,183,500	4,019	523,320	565	94,370	990	159,440	159	19,170	46	5,190	61	382,020
2007	5,657	1,158,870	3,867	519330	609	94200	937	158,140	172	20,510	29	6130	43	360,560
2008	5,214	1,078,140	3,663	464,500	533	83,970	804	146,800	152	18,010	32	4,230	30	360,630
2009	4,551	964,990	3,204	412,730	421	78,840	713	126,310	148	15,740	33	3,950	32	327,440
2010	4,690	933,200	3,363	391,850	412	73,140	707	123,710	149	14,750	32	4,630	27	325,140
2011	4,693	918,140	3,323	380,740	440	71,740	749	120,340	124	14,730	30	4,340	27	326,260
2012	4,628	918,720	3,177	367,380	486	71,200	748	123,700	154	16,360	37	4,240	26	335,850
2013	4,585	917,090	3,125	363,220	439	70,500	817	125,270	132	15,190	35	4,850	37	338,100
2014	4,821	916,440	3,332	358,210	475	72,280	804	125,250	142	17,390	34	4,020	34	339,300
2015	4,836	902,160	3,241	347,200	495	73,590	903	125,820	123	17,020	36	4,040	38	334,500
2016	5,190	892,270	3,481	325,760	587	73,460	879	128,630	167	15,680	38	3,900	38	344,850
2017	5,147	882,730	3,449	308,610	530	69,900	903	123,510	161	15,870	38	3,640	66	361,230
2018	5,250	900,380	3,405	298,030	615	71,600	961	124,450	163	15,050	42	3,270	64	388,000
2019	5,333	888,220	3,297	295,340	634	73,930	1,088	125,160	195	15,120	30	3,110	89	375,600
2020	4,764	1,176,340	2,898	367,280	541	106,730	1,072	161,890	158	25,290	32	4,130	63	511,030

a   Injury counts based on the number of nonfatal occupational injuries involving days away from work by selected worker characteristics and number of days away from work, and median number of days away from work, private industry, 1992–2020.
b   Data from 2001 exclude fatalities from September 11, 2001, terrorist attacks.

Source: BLS (2022).

heart disease, or neurological damage are recorded. The injury rate for the entire population was roughly 4.8 cases per 100 workers in 2004, with rates of 10 per 100 or more (that is, 1 chance in 10 of being injured during the year) in especially risky occupations such as primary metal manufacturing, wood products manufacturing, air transportation, courier services, and nursing home care. More than half of the injuries in 2004 were serious enough to involve one or more days away from work and/or a change of working conditions (i.e., transfer to a different job or restrictions placed on work activities) dictated by the injury; nearly 25% of these lost-workday injuries were serious enough to result in one month or more of an absence from work.

Work-related fatalities can be enumerated rather precisely, with the annual number of deaths attributable to occupational injuries in the United States placed in the 5,000 to 8,000 range (Pratt et al. 1996; Stout and Linn 2002). The national recording systems doubtless fail to count some nonfatal injuries occurring at work, either because of exemptions to the required reporting or the failure of some employers to file reports. A recent article (Rosenman et al. 2006) found that the BLS data accounted for only about 32% of work-related injuries that occurred in Michigan during 1999–2001, suggesting a substantial underestimate.

Occupational Disease

The total number of deaths attributed to occupational exposures is more difficult to quantify. Inspection of Table 12.1 reveals the potential for numerous occupationally related diseases. Research in this area often focuses on a single disease or a single industry; compendia of data are not available. However, the number is certainly much greater than the numbers for injury fatalities. Neurodegenerative diseases, lung diseases, and various forms of cancer suggest a much higher total likely in the 50,000 to 75,000 deaths-per-year range. The true numbers may be even higher since the effects of occupational exposures to physical and chemical stressors are not completely understood. Perhaps the most sophisticated estimates of the number of occupational diseases in the United States were derived by Leigh et al. (1997), who developed an estimate of "the incidence, the mortality, and direct and indirect costs associated with occupational injuries and illnesses in the United States" for the year 1992 using a complex methodology (see also Takala et al. (2014) for similar estimates worldwide and more recent estimates for the United States). They took data from several government agencies and made use of an attributable risk proportion argument whereby the fraction of risk directly attributable to occupational exposures is applied to general morbidity and mortality statistics. They estimated that roughly 60,000 deaths and 850,000 illnesses annually can be attributed to chronic diseases caused by workplace exposures.

BOX 12.2   OCCUPATIONAL SAFETY *OR* HEALTH? RESOURCE ALLOCATION AT OSHA

Adam M. Finkel

In comparing the magnitude of the national problem of fatal occupational injuries with that of premature deaths due to occupational disease, there is no doubt that the latter number is far greater than the former. As many as ten times more workers die prematurely from occupational disease than from acute occupational injury, as evidenced by the previously cited studies and the galvanizing examples of worker disease in the past (e.g., Hawk's Nest, black lung, brown lung, and vinyl chloride; see Cherniack 1986; Young Jr. and Rachal 1996; Annas 1981; Jones 1981). Nevertheless, OSHA continues to devote a very large and arguably a growing per centage of its staff, budget, and enforcement resources to the problem of worker injury. OSHA claims (Cordaro 2015) that roughly 20% of its inspections are "health inspections," implying that while inspections looking for safety violations dominate, a substantial minority of OSHA inspections are designed to find and fix chronic disease hazards. However, it turns out that OSHA tallies as a "health inspection" any investigation where the lead inspector is an industrial hygienist, even if the inspection involves no chemical sampling or attempts to find violations of OSHA health standards. Finkel (2008) testified that based on OSHA's own affidavits in a Freedom of Information Act case he litigated, only about 3% of OSHA's inspections involve any air, wipe, or bulk chemical sampling. Examination of the complete data file for OSHA sampling in the calendar year 2019 (OSHA 2019) reveals that samples were taken at 2,093 unique establishments; this figure indeed represents 2.7% of the 75,463 inspections (federal OSHA plus all state-plan states) conducted in that year.

Occupational Exposures

Unfortunately, it is virtually impossible to produce a predictive (as opposed to the epidemiology-based estimates discussed earlier in the chapter) estimate of the aggregate risk of occupational exposures to toxic substances due to a lack of historical measurements of exposures in workplaces. There has never been a comprehensive survey of what substances US workers are exposed to and at what concentrations. Two attempts to survey a representative sample of workplaces for certain substances were carried out by NIOSH in the mid- to late-1980s: a 1983 study of exposure measurements in approximately 4,500 workplaces in over 500 industries and an analogous mining-specific 1989 study in 431 metal-nonmetal mines and 60 coal mines. Since 1989, though, the CDC has conducted nearly 20 separate National Health and Nutrition Examination Surveys (NHANES) to gauge the nutritional status of US residents, several of which have included extensive survey questions to estimate exposures to chemicals in the home and extensive measurements of the body burdens (i.e., the total amount in the body) of various substances in residents.

The largest database of nonrandom samples of contaminant concentrations in US workplaces is the result of OSHA compliance inspections (note that while some observers insist that because these samples are taken during inspections, they are biased high, toward facilities with the worst concentrations, it is also quite possible that because OSHA often conducts its sampling only as incidental to safety-focused inspections, these readings are not systematically biased). Since 1979, when the agency began collecting inspection information in a single database, OSHA inspectors have collected more than two million air, wipe, and bulk samples. OSHA has never published reports analyzing trends in these data, and only a handful of journal articles have done so for various single substances (Gomez 1991; Lavoue et al. 2013; Yassin et al. 2005). These data are now available on a public website (https://www.osha.gov/opengov/health-samples), allowing access to and searches among these data.

Another source of occupational chemical exposure data is the NIOSH Health Hazard Evaluations (https://www2a.cdc.gov/hhe/search.asp), which summarize NIOSH investigations at individual facilities and often include measured exposure data. However, these data sources are not comprehensive, and thus even the most basic questions about the average contaminant levels workers are exposed to across multiple establishments can only be roughly estimated. It is worth noting that a preliminary investigation concludes that for some substances, workers face concentrations up to one *millionfold* higher than citizens face in the ambient environment (Finkel 2005).

With regard to *criteria pollutants*, occupational settings typically display higher concentrations of airborne pollutants than are allowed in communities or ambient air, but perhaps not on the order of 3 to 6 orders of magnitude that are seen in the case of toxic air pollutants. Table 12.4 compares the allowable values for several air contaminants. *Permissible exposure limits* (PELs) are occupational standards OSHA sets that supply a degree of protection for workers exposed to such compounds in their work environments. They represent time-weighted, eight-hour exposure levels. For example, in the case of sulfur dioxide, a worker could be exposed to 5 ppm of SO_2 for an entire eight-hour shift without a violation of the PEL. Similarly, a worker could be exposed to 10 ppm for four

Table 12.4: A Comparison of Occupational Standards and Ambient Air Quality Standards

Compound	PEL[a]	NAAQS[b]	Notes[c]
NO_2	5 ppm[d]	100 ppb	1-hour average
SO2	5 ppm	75 ppb	1-hour average
O_3	0.1 ppm	0.07 ppm	8-hour average
CO	50 ppm	9 and 35 ppm	8-hour and 1-hour averages
Lead	0.05 mg/m^3	0.00015 g/m^3	Quarterly average[e]
Dust	15 mg/m^3	0.035 and 0.012 mg/m^3	24-hour and annual averages[f]

[a] *Permissible exposure limit (PEL)*: eight-hour time-weighted average allowed values in occupational settings.
[b] *National ambient air quality standards (NAAQS)*: allowable outdoor concentrations; designed to protect health and supply a margin of safety.
[c] NAAQS often have multiple standards with different averaging times for the same contaminant. The longer the averaging time, the lower the allowed concentration.
[d] The OSHA PEL for NO_2 is a ceiling limit not to be exceeded at any time.
[e] Rarely violated since the removal of lead from gasoline.
[f] NAAQS listed for $PM_{2.5}$.

hours, and there would be no violation of the standard if no further exposure were experienced during the eight-hour shift. Note that for some substances, OSHA establishes short-term limits (STEL) not to be exceeded over a short averaging time (typically 15 minutes) or ceiling limits that cannot be exceeded for any length of time. National Ambient Air Quality Standards set by EPA are generally much lower than PELs, as they are required to protect the general population (including sensitive subpopulations) and supply an adequate margin of safety for such individuals. Note that Table 12.4 involves a comparison of regulatory limits, whereas the preceding discussion of toxic air pollutants involves a comparison of measured or modeled concentration values – therefore, the ratios of occupational to environmental values must be interpreted separately in light of the different sorts of comparisons being made here.

An exception to this general trend is found for ozone exposure. Allow able ozone exposure in the occupational environment does not differ substantially from what is allowable in the

BOX 12.3   ASBESTOS IN THE WORKPLACE

Jeffery Mandel

"Asbestos" is the name given to a group of six different fibrous silicates, five of which are considered amphiboles (amosite, crocidolite, tremolite, actinolite, anthophyllite) and one belongs to the serpentine family of minerals (chrysotile). All of these minerals occur naturally in the environment and have found their way into a multitude of manufacturing processes because of their inert properties, particularly as heat insulators and fire protectors. Each type may exist in fibrous (asbestiform) and non-fibrous forms, depending on their ability to cleave along parallel planes (fibrous). The ability to cleave results in greater exposure and pathogenicity. As a rule, the amphibole types are considered more pathogenic, although all types have the potential to cause respiratory disease. Currently, chrysotile is the predominant mineral fiber in use and is still mined and used legally in some countries.

Generally, the amphibole types are longer and thinner, with dimensional characteristics typically greater than 5 microns in length and 0.25 microns in width. Toxicity in humans is related to these fiber dimensions, likely due to the inability of the immune system (e.g., macrophages) to clear these fibers. The pathogenicity is also related to the ability of the fiber to penetrate into the deeper parts of the lungs, the concentration of exposure and the length of time exposed. These factors result in an accumulation of fibers and subsequently increased risk for lung pathology. Shorter and thicker fibers are considered less pathogenic. Non-fibrous, shorter fibers are considerably less pathogenic.

In terms of human disease, excessive fibrous exposure primarily results in lung disease characterized by one or more of the following: plaque (scarring) formation around the lining of the lungs, fibrous scarring of the lung substance (pneumoconiosis), lung cancer (all types) and mesothelioma, a rare cancer of the mesothelial lining surrounding the lungs. This same risk of smoking does not apply to mesothelioma. As a general rule, the lung cancer risk associated with fibrous asbestos exposure is in the range of four to five times higher than those not exposed. In the presence of heavy cigarette smoking and fibrous asbestos exposure, the risk of lung cancer increases in a multiplicative way. Fibrous asbestos-related diseases are all related to the amount and length of exposure and, typically, require a prolonged latency before the disease manifests.

For regulatory purposes, the time-weighted average (TWA) that has been adopted by OSHA for fibrous asbestos is 0.1 fibers per cubic centimeter of air. The TWA is used in combination with the length of exposure in years to provide a cumulative exposure estimate. OSHA also uses the aspect ratio (length:width ratio) greater than 3:1 for counting significant fibers. Specific microscopic methods are employed to make this measurement, including phase contrast and transmission electron microscopy. As a point of reference, cumulative occupational exposure to the above metrics, in the range of 5–1,200 fiber years per cubic centimeter has resulted in pneumoconiosis and lung cancer. Exposure to fibrous asbestos also occurs to the GI tract. Accordingly, concern has been expressed for the development (and risk) for GI cancers to occur in the setting of this exposure. However, epidemiologic investigation into non-respiratory cancer risk has not been definitive.

community, since health effects are found at only modestly elevated concentrations of this irritating air contaminant.

Together, all these injuries (fatal and nonfatal) and illnesses exact a huge cost on the nation, albeit one that is hard to estimate or even to define precisely. In particular, less severe impairment – ranging from minor hearing loss to full disability – increases the social cost of occupational disease substantially (Leigh et al. 2004). Considering only some of these costs (e.g., medical expenses and lost earnings) and explicitly ignoring other costs that are even harder to quantify (e.g., pain and suffering and effects on the families of the victims), Leigh et al. (1997) estimated that occupational injuries and illnesses cost approximately $171 billion annually (roughly 2% of the entire US gross domestic product). A report by Islam and Anderson (2006) estimated the cost of work-related injuries and disease to be $176 billion annually in the United States.

Controlling exposures to workplace hazards also involves substantial costs, although the amount already spent on the controls that currently exist may bear no relationship to the amount that would be needed to avert the injuries and illnesses that still occur. One such cost estimate comes from Johnson (2001), who estimated that OSHA regulations cost the economy roughly $40 billion annually. However, evidence supports the view that the costs of occupational regulations are generally overestimated, partly due to economies of scale or technological learning after promulgation. In the workplace, the most comprehensive study (OTA 1995) suggested that costs predicted before regulations are implemented often exceed actual costs by a factor of two or more; a more recent study found even greater bias (Ruttenberg 2004). A well-known case example is OSHA's vinyl chloride regulation, where dire predictions of oppressive costs evaporated within weeks of the final issuance of the standard; it turned out that reducing workplace concentrations of vinyl chloride also *saved* companies money, as they wasted less of the valuable product into the atmosphere (Chemical Week 1976).

Assessing and Managing Workplace Risks: NIOSH, OSHA, and EPA

NIOSH

Research and Recommendations. NIOSH is organized into divisions, laboratories, and offices located throughout the United States covering a broad range of research and programmatic areas, including occupational health and safety surveillance, exposure assessment, workplace health and hazard assessments, laboratory and basic etiological research, and control of workplace hazards, among others. Integrating findings from these efforts, NIOSH conducts qualitative and quantitative occupational risk assessments, develops policy and technical documents, and develops and disseminates educational occupational safety and health information. Through the OSH Act, NIOSH has the authority to recommend occupational health and safety standards to protect workers from toxic substances and physical agents that are "safe for various periods of employment, including but not limited to the exposure levels at which no employee will suffer impaired health or functional capacity or diminished life expectancy as a result of [their] work experience" (Pub. L. 91-596, Sec 20(a)(3)). Such recommended exposure limits (RELs) are typically published in criteria documents and finalized in response to internal and external peer reviews and public comments.

In addition to criteria documents, NIOSH develops and publishes guidance on assessing risks to workers. Two notable documents of relevance to this discussion are the *NIOSH Chemical Carcinogen Policy* (2016a) and *NIOSH Practices in Occupational Risk Assessment* (2020). The first document describes how NIOSH classifies chemical carcinogens in the workplace, sets a target risk for occupational carcinogen risk assessments of 1 excess cancer case per 10,000 workers exposed to a carcinogen over a working lifetime, and describes how NIOSH considers the ability to detect and quantify airborne concentrations of chemicals in developing its guidance. The second document provides guidance on how NIOSH conducts occupational risk assessments and includes information on data selection, hazard identification, exposure-response modeling methods, use of uncertainty factors, and other topics related to occupational risk assessment.

OSHA

Regulation and Enforcement. OSHA is the federal agency responsible for promulgating and enforcing regulations to protect US workers from hazards that cause injuries and disease. Counting both those employed by the federal agency and those who work for the roughly 25 state OSH agencies that conduct their own inspections, OSHA employs roughly 1,800 inspectors, responsible for over 10 million establishments. These inspectors, called "CSHOs" for "compliance safety and health officers," visit worksites and look for violations of specific OSHA safety and health standards or breaches of the "general duty clause" of the OSH Act, which allows OSHA to issue citations against employers who knowingly fail to abate "recognized hazards that are causing or are likely to cause death or serious physical harm" (even in the absence of a specific standard). In 2021, federal OSHA conducted about 24,300 inspections, and the state agencies with delegated authority conducted about 31,000 more: roughly one-third of these were programmed inspections of companies whose injury rates the previous year were among the highest in the nation. Roughly one-quarter of the inspections were in response to complaints filed by employees, or to accidents that caused fatalities or multiple hospitalizations, and roughly one-quarter were in response to referrals from other local, state, or federal organizations or follow-up inspections to verify satisfactory abatement of hazards previously identified. Nearly 60% of all inspections now involve construction sites, although that percentage may appear higher than expected because OSHA records multiple inspections at the same construction site when it examines the work of different contractors.

When OSHA inspectors find violations at the worksite, they can recommend various levels of monetary penalty; about 60% of all violations are deemed *serious*, meaning that they cause a substantial probability of death or serious physical harm, with an average penalty of roughly $3,000 per violation (generally, most OSHA penalties are negotiated downward by 50% or more during discussions with employers). Another 3% are repeat violations of the same standard by the same employer (roughly $13,000 average penalty), and about 0.5% are *willful*, meaning that they are committed knowingly by an employer who either intentionally disregards the standard or is "plainly indifferent to its requirements," with an average penalty of $60,000. A Pulitzer prize-winning series in the *New York Times* (Barstow 2003) documented that although over 1,200 cases between 1982 and 2002 involved willful violations that had led to worker deaths, OSHA sought criminal charges against the employers in only about 80 of those cases (7%).

If OSHA was provided the personnel and budget to conduct more on-site inspections, recent scholarship indicates that inspections are not only a way to recognize (and, it is hoped, avert) dangerous workplace conditions, but that they have a significant, lasting, and economically reasonable effect on reducing worker injuries themselves. Writing in the journal *Science*, researchers from the business schools at Berkeley and Harvard (Levine et al. 2012) found that establishments in California that Cal/OSHA randomly chose for inspection saw their workplace injury rate decline by almost 10% more than a matched group of California firms that were not inspected. The researchers concluded that this harm reduction persisted for at least five years after the initial inspections and that the inspected firms experienced no measurable declines in sales, employment, or credit rating.

The OSH Act empowers OSHA to set mandatory standards to govern specific safety and health risks. Congress gave OSHA special authority during the first two years of the agency's existence (1970–1972) to "inherit" existing national consensus standards such as those developed by the American National Standards Institute (ANSI), the American Society for Testing and Materials, the National Fire Protection Association, and other organizations, as well as those that were issued under the Walsh-Healey Public Contracts Act of 1936, and adopt them as mandatory regulations. Also, during this period, OSHA adopted roughly 400 threshold limit values (TLVs®) that had been recommended before 1968 by the American Conference of Governmental Industrial Hygienists (ACGIH), establishing them as mandatory PELs. Since 1972, however, OSHA has had to promulgate standards under a lengthy (and increasingly complex) process. Due to the lengthy and complex nature of the standard-setting process and the small number of staff assigned to develop standards, OSHA has only promulgated about 40 safety standards and 25 health standards since 1972. For only 18 substances (see Table 12.5) has OSHA established mandatory exposure limits and only roughly half of those were based on risk assessment. Two of OSHA's most far-reaching standards were promulgated but never took effect. In 1989, OSHA attempted to modernize its list of over 400 PELs to keep up with changes (almost exclusively more stringent changes) to the TLVs between 1970 and that date. A federal judge invalidated the new list, however, on the grounds that OSHA had failed to undertake any of the quantitative risk assessment (QRS) the Supreme Court had deemed essential in the 1980 *Benzene* decision (see p. 242). In 2001, in the first use of the 1996 Congressional Review Act, both houses of Congress repealed OSHA's new ergonomics standard that would have required controls to reduce repetitive stress injuries at work.

Role of the EPA in Occupational Risk Management

While the primary role of the EPA has focused on the protection of the health of individuals in the community setting, the agency has also been involved periodically with occupational health protection from chemical exposures.

Table 12.5: Substances with a Permissible Exposure Limit Set by OSHA Since 1971

Substance	Year Final Standard Issued (after Subsequent Revisions, if Any)
Vinyl chloride	1974
Coke oven emissions	1976
Dibromochloropropane	1978
Arsenic	1978
Cotton dust	1978
Acrylonitrile	1978
Lead	1978 (general industry); 1993 (construction)
Ethylene oxide	1984
Benzene	1987
4,4'-Methylenedianiline	1992
Cadmium	1992
Formaldehyde	1992
Asbestos	1992
1,3-Butadiene	1996
Methylene chloride	1997
Chromium (hexavalent)	2006
Respirable Crystalline Silica	2016
Beryllium	2017

Toxic Substances Control Act. The Toxic Substances Control Act (TSCA) of 1976 provided EPA with the authority to require reporting, record keeping, testing, and restrictions relating to chemical substances and mixtures. TSCA applies to almost all chemicals in the environment with the exception of food, drugs, cosmetics, and pesticides, which are covered under different laws. Under TSCA, EPA has the authority to

- require premanufacture notification for new chemical substances before manufacture;
- require testing of chemicals by manufacturers, importers, and processors;
- issue Significant New Use Rules (SNUR) when a significant new use was identified that could result in exposures or releases of concern;
- maintain an inventory of existing chemicals;
- require certification of importing and exporting of chemicals;
- require record keeping and reporting by manufacturers, importers, processers, and distributors of chemicals; and
- require manufacturers, importers, processors, and distributors of chemicals to immediately report to EPA information that reasonably supports the conclusion that a chemical substance or mixture presents a substantial risk of injury to health or the environment.

Although EPA's focus was typically on community and environmental exposures to chemicals, in implementing the new chemical provisions of TSCA, EPA frequently assessed risks to workers during the premanufacture and SNUR evaluations. This is in contrast to how EPA typically handled existing chemicals, where EPA focused almost exclusively on community and environmental exposures.

On June 22, 2016, the first major update to TSCA was signed into law. The Frank R. Lautenberg Chemical Safety for the 21st Century Act amended the TSCA. This update had far-reaching implications for how EPA assesses and regulates both new chemicals and existing chemicals. Some of the major updates include

- a requirement for EPA to evaluate existing chemicals with clear and enforceable deadlines,
- comprehensive risk evaluations for existing chemicals,

- increased public transparency for chemical information, and

- a consistent source of funding for EPA to implement the provisions of the law.

The most impactful change with regard to occupational risk assessment was the addition of workers to EPA's scope. In the definitions, Sec.3 (12) is the following:

> The term "potentially exposed or susceptible subpopulation" means a group of individuals within the general population identified by the Administrator who, due to either greater susceptibility or greater exposure, may be at greater risk than the general population of adverse health effects from exposure to a chemical substance or mixture, such as infants, children, pregnant women, *workers,* or the elderly.

This addition expanded EPA's role in evaluating workers' risks beyond consideration of new chemicals to risks from exposure to existing chemicals. In its risk evaluation under the amended TSCA, EPA determines whether substances present an unreasonable risk of injury to health or the environment, without consideration of costs or other nonrisk factors. This includes a determination of unreasonable risks to potentially exposed or susceptible populations, such as workers. EPA has not defined specific risk probabilities that are identified as unreasonable risk because they determined that it would be "inappropriate to capture the broad set of health and environmental risk measures and information that might be relevant to chemical substances." Instead, EPA considers specific factors that the agency uses in making its risk determinations. According to the EPA *Procedures for Chemical Risk Evaluation Under the Amended Toxic Substances Control Act*, these factors include

- the effects of the chemical substance on health and human exposure to such substance under the conditions of use (including cancer and noncancer risks),

- the effects of the chemical substance on the environment and environmental exposure under the conditions of use,

- the population exposed (including any susceptible populations),

- the severity of hazard (the nature of the hazard, the irreversibility of hazard), and uncertainties.

For carcinogens, the risk probability EPA considers unreasonable is becoming clearer. As of this writing, several TSCA risk evaluations have now been finalized, and for carcinogenic hazards, EPA has repeatedly cited the *NIOSH Chemical Carcinogen Policy* target risk level of 1 excess cancer case per 10,000 workers exposed to a carcinogen over a working lifetime as its guidance for *unreasonable risk*. When EPA determines that exposures may lead to unreasonable risk, the agency is required to develop risk mitigation strategies to eliminate those risks. These may include banning the chemical; development of restrictions on handling and use, including implementation of engineering controls, work practices, and selection and use of personal protective equipment; and development of occupational (or environmental) exposure limits.

While TSCA confers broad authority to EPA to conduct occupational risk assessment and develop chemical regulations for the workplace, it is not the only statutory authority that EPA has that impacts worker health.

Development of Acute Exposure Guidelines. EPA has an ongoing program designed to assess risks and develop guidelines for short-term or *acute* exposure to environmental contaminants. These Acute Exposure Guideline Levels (AEGLs; Environmental Protection Agency 2006a) focus on exposures that occur very infrequently, and that might be caused by a spill, a train crash, or another catastrophic event. According to EPA (2006a), AEGLs are threshold exposure limits for airborne contaminants applicable to the general public that occur over acute time scales, usually defined as ten minutes to eight hours. Such exposures are likely to produce toxic effects. Airborne concentrations below the AEGL-1 represent exposure levels that can produce mild and progressively increasing, but transient and nondisabling, effects. AEGL-1 levels are airborne concentrations above which most individuals, including sensitive individuals, are likely to experience discomfort but which are transient and not likely to disable the individual. The next level, AEGL-2, may result in long-lasting or permanent effects and may result in impairing the individual's ability to escape from the exposure. The highest AEGL is AEGL-3, a level that, if exceeded, is likely to cause life-threatening effects or even death. While AEGLs are written to apply to all members of the public, workers, such as first responders, are most likely to experience such exposures and are at higher risk because of this.

It is of interest to examine how such standards are developed. In developing AEGLs, EPA works with both national authorities, such as OSHA, and local authorities, including county public health offices. Typically, EPA makes use of a Federal Advisory Committee (2006) that consists of scientists, physicians, and stakeholders drawn from the community at large and who act as special government employees in developing these standards for exposure. The process is iterative, with reviews by two different external committees before the final AEGL is finalized, with the National Academies serving as the final peer reviewer. As can be seen from this development, the AEGL process is designed to afford input from many different groups of scientists and stakeholders in developing these important standards. Further, the iterative process ensures that up-to-date information from the published literature as well as ancillary information from other sources is used to afford protections to those likely to be exposed. However, we hasten to emphasize that the public process for developing OSHA standards and NIOSH recommendations is also quite rigorous. In addition to all of the opportunities for public written and oral comment during public meetings on the topic, OSHA is unusual among federal agencies in that it is required to conduct rulemaking hearings in which OSHA staff are made available for cross-examination by members of the public and the regulated communities. Also, OSHA and EPA are two of the three federal agencies (the Consumer Financial Protection Bureau being the third) that must conduct a separate round of comment before it proposes a regulation, limited to representatives from the small business community who were given special access via the 1996 Small Business Regulatory Enforcement Fairness Act (SBREFA).

Agriculture. EPA controls the impact of agricultural chemicals, including pesticides and fertilizers, through the Federal Insecticide, Fungicide, and Rodenticide Act (FIFRA), the Safe Drinking Water Act, and the Clean Air Act Amendments of 1990. EPA's role is to ensure that the air we breathe and the water available for public consumption are safe and unlikely to cause harm. EPA also takes a secondary role in ensuring that our food supply is safe by enforcing regulations on pesticide application and registration; only certain pesticides may be used on agricultural products destined for the food supply, and only specified amounts may be used.

The risks experienced by farmers and farmworkers are affected by these regulations. Control of the kinds and amounts of pesticides used on agricultural crops reduces the exposure experienced by workers. Further, EPA regulates the *reentry time*, the time workers must wait before returning to a field onto which pesticides were applied. In conjunction with controls placed by other agencies (e.g., OSHA, on work practices), such controls reduce the adverse health impact on the worker. Although worker exposure to pesticides would seem to be squarely within OSHA's purview, a federal court decision in 1974 ruled that EPA's initial reentry rules preempted OSHA. Since then, EPA became the only agency with meaningful enforcement authority for worker exposure to pesticides in many situations.

"Risk Transfer" from the Environment to the Workplace. EPA and OSHA, and a few visionaries in the academic community (see especially Lowell Center for Sustainable Production 2006), have begun to explore the intriguing (and daunting) possibility that compliance with environmental regulations may tend to exacerbate worker exposures. In theory, this problem was recognized decades ago, in special cases such as the attempts to protect ecosystems from lead by encapsulating bridge-repainting projects in large enclosures, which had the side-effect of increasing lead inhalation hazards to the workers within them. In 1999, EPA and OSHA cosponsored a conference (Environmental Protection Agency 1999) to examine whether "risk transfer" was a more general phenomenon, especially as EPA continued to promulgate "maximum available control technology" (MACT) standards for industrial processes under the Clean Air Act. One obvious way to comply with emission limitations from point sources is simply to increase the fraction of a toxic air pollution that remains within the workplace, as apparently has happened in several of the cases detailed in that conference (see, e.g., Piltingsrud et al. 2003).

OVERVIEW OF OCCUPATIONAL RISK ASSESSMENT METHODOLOGY AND POLICY

QRA for environmental exposures, as described in Chapters 2, 3, 4, and 11, shares many of the same fundamental principles with occupational risk assessment. Some of the commonalities and divergences between these two subdisciplines may simply mirror aspects of the risks themselves. Some obvious differences between the two types of risk include the following:

- *Population size.* Whereas many environmental contaminants (e.g., ground-level ozone, fine particulate matter) expose nearly all US citizens to some degree, most of the health hazards OSHA considers affect less than 1% of the national population, and some (see Table 12.6) affect as few as several thousand workers. Therefore, this disparity of a factor of 10^2 to 10^4 in affected

Table 12.6: **Lifetime Excess Cancer Risks Associated with All the OSHA Substance-Specific PELs (Set Subsequent to the 1980 *Benzene* Decision)**

Substance (Year)	Species Used for Extrapolation	Number of Workers Exposed	Risk at Old PEL	Risk at Average Exposure Level (at Time of Promulgation)	Risk at New PEL
Ethylene Oxide (1984)	Rat	71,000 (directly exposed) 69,000 (indirectly exposed)	(50 ppm) $63–109 \times 10^{-3}$	??	(1 ppm) $1.2–2.3 \times 10^{-3}$
Benzene (1987)	Rat/mouse/ human	238,000	(10 ppm) 95×10^{-3}	??	(1 ppm) 10×10^{-3}
4,4'-Methylene-dianiline (1992)	Mouse	4,000	(no prior PEL)	(70 ppb) 6×10^{-3}	(10 ppb) $8 \times 10^{-4}*$ $9 \times 10^{-4}**$
Asbestos (1992)	Human	1,316,000	(2 fibers/cm^3) 64×10^{-3}	??	(0.2 fibers/cm^3) 6.7×10^{-3}
Formaldehyde (1992)	Rat	2,160,000 (at > 0.1 ppm)	(3 ppm) $8.3 \times 10^{-3}**$ $0.07 \times 10^{-3}*$	??	(0.75 ppm) $0.006 \times 10^{-3}*$ $2.6 \times 10^{-3}**$
Cadmium (1992)	Rat/human	525,000	(100 µg/m^3) 58×10^{-3} 157×10^{-3}	??	(5 µg/m^3) $3 \times 10^{-3} – 15 \times 10^{-3}$
1,3-Butadiene (1996)	Mouse	9,700	(1000 ppm) ?? (note: 60 ppm ≈ 99th percentile of exposure)	(1.25 ppm)	(1 ppm) 1.3×10^{-3} to 8.1×10^{-3} (multiple assessments)
Methylene Chloride (1997)	Mouse	240,000	(500 ppm) 126×10^{-3}	(43 ppm) $6.2 \times 10^{-3}**$ $2.1 \times 10^{-3}*$	(25 ppm) $3.6 \times 10^{-3}**$ $1.2 \times 10^{-3}*$
Chromium (VI) (2006)	Human	558,000	(52 µg/m^3) $100–350 \times 10^{-3}$	(2.75 µg/m^3) $≈ 5.5–25 \times 10^{-3}$	(5 µg/m^3) $10 – 45 \times 10^{-3}$
Respirable Crystalline Silica (2016)	Human	2,312,000	(100 µg/m^3 in general industry, GI; 250 µg/m^3 in construction/ shipyards, CS) Lung cancer: $11–54 \times 10^{-3}$ (GI); $33–231 \times 10^{-3}$ (CS) Silicosis: 85×10^{-3} (GI); 192×10^{-3} (CS)	??	Lung cancer: $5–23 \times 10^{-3}$ Silicosis: 44×10^{-3}
Beryllium (2017)	Human	61,750	(2 µg/m^3) Beryllium sensitization (BeS): 64×10^{-3} Chronic beryllium disease (CBD): 204×10^{-3} Lung cancer: 140×10^{-3}		(0.2 µg/m^3) BeS: 9.3×10^{-3} CBD: 7.2×10^{-3} Lung cancer: 15×10^{-3}

* = maximum likelihood estimate.
** = 95th percentile upper confidence limit.

population size may counteract or exceed the disparity in average concentration, which of course cuts in the opposite direction (occupational exceeding environmental).

- *Population characteristics.* By and large, the general population exposed to environmental hazards is more diverse than the working population. Workers, especially those exposed to chronic health hazards, are generally between ages 18 and 65 and so do not exhibit some special sensitivities to exposures that are peculiar to infants, children, or the very old. Workers are also healthier than many in the general population simply by virtue of being fit enough to perform moderate or strenuous physical labor; hence, epidemiologists are well aware of the "healthy worker effect" that complicates the interpretation of disease rates in occupational cohorts when background rates from the general population are the basis for comparison (McMichael 1976). On the other hand, the fact that workers may have a longer-than-average life expectancy in the absence of additional risk factors does not necessarily mean they are any less susceptible than the general population to these incremental stresses. Although no studies to date have resolved this issue, first principles suggest that many important genetic and other determinants of risk (e.g., variation in enzymes that activate or detoxify carcinogens and other substances) bear no relationship to age or the ability to do work. This observation supports the argument that the occupational population is, on average, no less susceptible than the general population, to say nothing of individuals within either population whose sensitivities may fall anywhere along the spectrum.

- *Exposure patterns.* Occupational exposures are generally confined to 40 of the 168 hours in a week and generally do not extend for much more than 45 years, whereas some environmental exposures approach the theoretical maximum of continuous lifetime exposure, variously assumed to be 70 or 72 years (resulting in an exposure adjustment factor of 45/72). Depending on the mode of action of the substance(s) involved, the intermittent nature of occupational exposures, in addition to extended or other unusual work schedules, can call for a quantitative adjustment (as when bioassay data are adjusted by 5/7 and 8/24 to account for the workweek) or a qualitatively different assessment. Sporadic high exposures can be riskier when compared to continuous lower exposures of a similar TWA exposure that does not exceed a biological threshold; the converse pattern can apply, as when the intermittent exposures allow for physiologic recovery and hence have little chronic adverse effect.

- *Exposure concentrations.* Workplace concentrations of chemical contaminants are often much higher than environmental concentrations. This means that contaminants may cause a range of health effects in workers that are not experienced by the general population exposed to much lower concentrations of the same chemical. For example, workers may be exposed to concentrations that cause acute adverse health effects, whereas the general population may only be exposed to trace levels of the same contaminant. Despite these differences, however, the fact is that most of the agents of particular concern in environmental risk management emerge from workplaces or stem from choices that citizens make both in the workplace and the general environment (e.g., environmental tobacco smoke, which for some people is a fairly constant exposure during the workday and then at home). On the other hand, to the extent that residents and white-collar workers have suffered health effects from exposures to contaminants at and around the World Trade Center site, for example, it was because they essentially experienced occupational levels and patterns of exposure not much different from those encountered by the responders (especially to the extent that some in the latter group, but not the former, had access to respiratory protective devices).

Several persistent differences separate the methods and orientations that environmental and occupational perspectives bring to the *assessment* of the related risks within their own domains. Of note, occupational risk assessment often concerns human exposures within a factor of ten or less of exposures that cause statistically significant increases in adverse health effects in populations of laboratory animals and humans. This is contrasted with a factor of 10,000 or more that is frequently required in environmental assessments. Even more concerning, as an example, the average measured exposure (in the OSHA sampling database) of workers to the neurotoxin and presumed human carcinogen 1-bromopropane was slightly *greater* than the concentration (62.5 ppm) that rodents were exposed to in the National Toxicology Program bioassay of the substance; this concentration caused an 800% increase in tumor incidence in the animals so exposed. The important point here is not only that worker risks are large but also that concerns about the possible errors of overestimation caused by having to extrapolate from "high" to "low" doses simply don't apply in many occupational situations, where little or no extrapolation is needed. It is not possible that a threshold exists between the (harmful) exposure in a bioassay and the exposure humans face when the latter equals or exceeds the former.

One decision that has impacted how OSHA conducts risk assessment was the Supreme Court's *Benzene* decision (*Industrial Union Department, AFL-CIO v. American Petroleum Institute*; see Vig and Faure 2004). This decision required OSHA to quantify risk rather than merely assert that only the lowest feasible limit was acceptable. OSHA also attempted to update its PELs in its most ambitious health standard of all, the 1989 rule that sought to change over 420 PELs to reflect the current science and to track changes in the TLVs between 1970 and 1989. A federal court struck down all of these limits in 1992 on the grounds that OSHA had not assessed the risk of any of the substances at the old or new PELs (and so OSHA can now enforce only the PELs based on the TLVs as they existed in 1970 plus the relatively few comprehensive standards promulgated since then). OSHA issued four more risk-based health standards in the 1990s and in at least one case pioneered some computational methods and codified evidentiary criteria for replacing a default assumption with a more sophisticated biologic model (see the methylene chloride case study on p. 249).

Court Decisions Affecting Risk Assessment

In two landmark decisions reached less than one year apart, the US Supreme Court concluded first that OSHA must perform QRA and use those results to guide how and how strictly it regulates health hazards. In a separate decision, the Supreme Court clarified that OSHA is not permitted to base its regulations on a quantitative comparison of the monetary value of these risk-reduction benefits to the cost of reducing the risks. Both decisions hinged on the interpretation of Section 6(b)(5) of the Occupational Safety and Health Act of 1970 – that in regulating "toxic materials or harmful physical agents," OSHA must

> Set the standard which most adequately assures, to the extent feasible, on the basis of the best available evidence, that no employee will suffer material impairment of health or functional capacity even if such employee has regular exposure to the hazard dealt with by such standard for the period of his working life.

In its 1980 *Benzene* decision, the Supreme Court (by a narrow 5–4 vote, with the five justices in the majority issuing four separate opinions explaining their decision) made QRA the cornerstone of OSHA regulation of occupational health hazards and issued the most detailed language to date about the high court's interpretation of several fundamental aspects of risk assessment and management. OSHA issued a final standard governing worker exposure to benzene in April 1977, lowering the PEL from 10 ppm to 1 ppm. At 10 ppm or slightly above, workers exposed to benzene can experience central nervous system effects and diseases of the blood-forming organs (including aplastic anemia, an often-fatal disease); even in the 1970s, there was substantial evidence from human studies that levels of benzene exposure at or below 10 ppm increase the risk of various forms of leukemia. OSHA, however, in line with its Cancer Policy (which it had published in proposed form in 1976), declined to quantify the possible cancer risk either at 10 ppm or 1 ppm; rather, it set the PEL at the lower number on the grounds that while an exposure limit of zero was appropriate for a carcinogen, 1 ppm was the lowest feasible level. OSHA acknowledged that various industrial sectors that use benzene could achieve levels lower than 1 ppm but made a policy judgment that a uniform limit was appropriate. Both the AFL-CIO and the American Petroleum Institute filed petitions seeking to strengthen or weaken the 1977 standard, respectively.

The five justices who voted to invalidate the benzene standard objected on two basic grounds to the central precept of OSHA's Cancer Policy – that carcinogens should be controlled to the lowest feasible level, irrespective of the extent of exposure, the strength of the dose-response relationship, or other factors. First, the Court concluded that Congress did not intend terms such as "a safe and healthful workplace" to mean absolutely risk-free, a condition that literally could only apply if workplaces were shut down. Second, it concluded that a federal agency like OSHA has the responsibility to demonstrate the need for a regulation and cannot shift the burden to the regulated industry to show that the rule is not needed – that in setting the benzene standard, OSHA had "relied squarely upon a special policy [the Cancer Policy] for carcinogens that imposed a burden on industry of proving the existence of a safe level of exposure."

Together, the Court's requirements that OSHA not seek to eliminate all risk (however trivial its magnitude) and that it must marshal evidence to determine a regulation is necessary to "assure that no employee will suffer material impairment of health" add up to a recipe for QRA, as expressed in the heart of the *Benzene* decision: "[T]he burden [is] on the agency to show that long-term exposure to 10 ppm of benzene presents a *significant risk* of material health impairment" (emphasis added). This conclusion, as the following case studies will demonstrate, immediately changed OSHA from an agency that repudiated QRA to one that had to embrace it as the primary tool for justifying new regulations and for setting the level of stringency.

The *Benzene* decision was much more than a statement that risk must be quantified, however. The Court delved into some of the details about *how* QRA could be undertaken and used, and generally provided OSHA with its blessing to fashion agency risk assessments according to its own policy judgments and scientific interpretations, with the explicit goal of avoiding putting the agency into a "mathematical straitjacket." First, the Court made clear that OSHA could decide for itself what level of risk was large enough to be "significant" and what level was so small it had to be deemed "insignificant." It provided specific (but extremely broad) guidance as to what risks it thought were "plainly acceptable" and which ones were "plainly unacceptable" by stating that an individual risk of one in a billion (10^{-9}) "could not be considered significant," while "a reasonable person might well consider" a risk of one in a thousand (10^{-3}) to be significant. *As Congress has generally instructed EPA (see, e.g., the Clean Air Act Amendments of 1990, and the Safe Drinking Water Act) to regulate risks down to a level of one in a million (10^{-6}), OSHA has thus for the past 40 years been permitted to set standards that match EPA in stringency, but OSHA has rarely if ever come within a factor of 1,000 of this level of protection, often for reasons of technical or economic feasibility of the standard.*

Not only did the *Benzene* decision give OSHA the authority to declare a risk within that broad range "acceptable," but the Court also allowed OSHA to choose a numerical estimate of risk according to its own science-policy judgments and even signaled that it understood that those judgments might be intentionally precautionary:

> So long as they are supported by a body of reputable scientific thought, the agency is free to use conservative assumptions in interpreting the data with respect to carcinogens, risking error on the side of over-protection rather than under-protection.

At least in theory, therefore, OSHA could set a PEL for a carcinogen so that the risk to a highly susceptible worker might, even using conservative assumptions, be almost as low as 10^{-9}, so long as it could show that industry could feasibly meet that extremely strict level.

In 1987, OSHA promulgated a revised benzene standard at the same exposure limit (1 ppm) as it had proposed 10 years earlier. In the revised standard, OSHA estimated that the lifetime excess leukemia risk at 10 ppm was approximately 95 per thousand, or 9.5×10^{-3} at the new PEL (OSHA concluded that no lower limit was feasible, even though "significant risk" remained at the newly permissible level). The four justices who dissented from the *Benzene* decision were very concerned that by requiring OSHA "to 'quantify' the risk in order to satisfy a court that it is 'significant,'… [the Court] seems to require [OSHA] to do the impossible." The history of OSHA standard setting over the subsequent 25 years provides ample evidence that using QRA to set risk-based standards is far from impossible. But neither is it easy.

The following year, by a 5–3 vote (one justice did not participate in this case), the Court upheld OSHA's standard limiting the allowable amount of cotton dust in US workplaces (American Textile Manufacturers Institute v. Donovan 1981; see Ashford and Caldart 1996), rejecting the argument of the textile industry that OSHA must weigh the benefit of reductions in health risks against the costs to industry of achieving them. As early as the 1820s, cotton dust was recognized as associated with a progressive obstructive lung disease now known as byssinosis, or brown lung disease. In the United States, roughly 100,000 workers had developed byssinosis by 1970. It should be noted that within a few years of the Court upholding OSHA's regulation, the number of new cases of byssinosis plummeted to less than 25 per year nationwide, although the gradual decline of the US domestic textile industry certainly contributed to this positive development. In 1974, the TLV for cotton dust was lowered to 200 µg/m³, and four years later, OSHA promulgated a less stringent set of standards that varied by the industrial process involved, ranging from 200 µg/m³ in yarn manufacturing to 750 µg/m³ in weaving operations. OSHA performed a thorough QRA of the risk of lung disease from cotton dust at the exposures prevailing at that time and at the proposed new limits and calculated the costs of complying with the standard, but it did not monetize the health benefits and compare them to their costs. The Court said that it "is difficult to imagine what else the agency could do to comply with this Court's decision in [*Benzene*])." OSHA also rejected the petition of the Textile Workers Union of America that the PEL be set at 100 µg/m³, on the grounds that the lower limit was not "within the technological capability of the industry."

The Supreme Court emphasized the phrase "to the extent feasible" in the OSH Act, and concluded that Congress did not intend that OSHA engage in cost-benefit analysis, but rather must reduce worker risks "limited only by the extent to which this is capable of being done" – now limited further, of course, by the Court's recent instruction in *Benzene* that OSHA cannot further reduce risks that have become too small to be "significant." Interestingly, the Court described the OSH Act as embracing rather than rejecting cost-benefit thinking, but embracing a brand of cost-benefit balancing that "place[s] the benefit of worker health above all other considerations save those making attainment of this benefit unachievable." In a parallel to *Benzene*, the justices also carved out an interpretation of "significant cost," to clarify when controls that *can* be adopted are nevertheless too expensive to truly be "feasible." They concluded that when OSHA can reasonably show (as it did here) that the industry involved can comply with the regulation and "maintain long-term productivity and competitiveness," it has met its congressional test of feasibility. In fact, the Court explicitly left open the possibility that in the future it might also conclude that OSHA regulation that did threaten the profitability of industry might yet be regarded as "feasible." Therefore, *Benzene* and *Cotton Dust* read together make it clear that OSHA can promulgate health regulations that impose high costs and reduce risks down to small (but not "insignificant") levels.

In practice, over the past decades, OSHA has been prodded, mostly via executive orders enforced by the Office of Information and Regulatory Affairs, to provide all of the detailed information about cost and benefit that an agency that had to compare them quantitatively *would* provide. So whether OSHA ultimately ends up choosing the level of stringency of each standard so as to maximize net benefit, or so as to eliminate significant risk to the extent feasible, these are merely two different ways of considering costs and benefits, and may lead to an identical or similar regulatory decision.

The Mechanics of Occupational Risk Assessment

Occupational risk assessment, as is the case with environmental risk assessment, is generally viewed as consisting of several steps: hazard identification, occupational exposure assessment, exposure-response analysis, and risk characterization, a framework first codified in 1983 (NAS 1983) and still used today. At NIOSH, the institute has developed *NIOSH Practices in Occupational Risk Assessment* (https://www.cdc.gov/niosh/docs/2020-106/default.html), which describes in detail how NIOSH selects the data, conducts QRA, and addresses uncertainty and variability in the resulting risk estimates. The underlying assumptions that NIOSH makes with regard to risk assessment are also described in that document. OSHA generally conducts risk assessment in similar ways as does NIOSH; in promulgating and justifying its regulations, OSHA sometimes makes explicit reference to a NIOSH risk assessment for a given substance, but always also conducts its own independent analysis, which it subjects to rigorous public comment via the public hearings it is required to conduct. The basic steps in occupational risk assessment are described here.

Hazard Identification. As the name would suggest, *hazard identification* is the qualitative association of an activity, location, or pollutant with a hazard. Historically, much of the knowledge that we have on the health effects of certain activities, or that are associated with exposure to environmental contaminants, comes from the occupational setting since in these settings hazards are frequently abundant and exposures are substantial. For example, exposures experienced by uranium mine workers have led to a better understanding of the effect of radiation exposure in the general population. Similarly, repetitive strain injuries were first noticed in manufacturing settings, where repeated motion is common. Later, it was noticed in office workers and in the general community. However, it is unlikely that study of nonoccupationally exposed individuals alone would have led to the insight obtained from those exposed in workplace settings. Exposures are generally greater, and for a longer duration, making the hazard more readily identifiable in the occupation exposed.

Hazard identification alone does not indicate anything quantitative about the risks of chemical exposure. In the case of carcinogens, several agencies and organizations classify chemicals with regard to their carcinogenicity without necessarily conducting a quantitative analysis (exposure-response analysis) to estimate risks. The National Toxicology Program, the EPA, and the International Agency for Cancer Research routinely assess the evidence for carcinogenicity and make a hazard determination for chemicals of interest (and sometimes for industrial processes and even occupations). These organizations classify carcinogens as "known to cause cancer in humans" or "reasonably anticipated to" (EPA further divides the category below "known" into "probable" and "possible" carcinogens. NIOSH uses the information from these three organizations to make a determination whether a chemical is an occupational carcinogen, and OSHA requires manufacturers to report on their Safety Data Sheets the results of NTP, EPA, or IARC hazard identification determinations. In making its assessment, in addition to the carcinogen classifications, NIOSH takes into consideration the occupational relevance of the evidence supporting carcinogenicity (NIOSH 2016a).

Occupational Exposure Assessment. Industrial hygiene (also called occupational hygiene) focuses on the exposures experienced by individuals who work in industrial or occupational settings and may be viewed as a branch of the larger science of exposure assessment. Some definitions are needed to start. These include the *concentration* of pollutants in an environmental medium, the *exposure* experienced by an individual, and the *dose* received by the individual.

1. *Concentration, exposure, and dose differentiated.* An important distinction to be made is between the related concepts of concentration, exposure, and dose. Consider the following scenario: A worker is required to enter an enclosed space that formerly was filled with a volatile solvent. The atmosphere in the enclosed space is saturated with the vapor of the solvent.

   In order to assess the experience of the worker, we must consider three different concepts: concentration, exposure, and dose. The concentration in the tank (i.e., space) is relatively simple to understand: it is the saturation vapor pressure of the organic solvent. It can be readily measured using appropriate instrumentation or estimated from the physical and chemical properties of the solvent. This is the concentration that the worker experiences in the enclosed space. But what is her exposure? Exposure, defined as the amount of hazardous substance delivered to some body boundary, can come from one of three different *routes*: inhalation, for which the lung epithelium is the boundary of interest; ingestion, for which the gut epithelium is the boundary of interest; and body-surface contact, for which a body surface, usually the skin, is the boundary of interest. Dose, on the other hand, is the quantity of chemical that crosses the boundary and enters the body. Estimation of dose frequently depends on the mode of toxicity. If a chemical is direct-acting at the exposure interface, dose and exposure would be identical. However, if a chemical must be absorbed through the lung, gut, or skin, and then metabolized to an active agent before being distributed to the organ of interest, the dose (sometimes called effective dose or toxic dose) may be quite different from the exposure. For example, if the chemical must be absorbed through the lung into the blood stream, distributed to the liver, where it is metabolized and then the active metabolite distributed to the brain to produce the health effect, the actual effective dose would be very different from the exposure. For most chemicals, we don't know enough about the critical steps in absorption, metabolism, distribution, and elimination of the chemical to precisely determine the effective dose, so, in many cases, exposure and dose are used interchangeably in the scientific literature.

2. *Pathways.* The specific ways the pollutant moves through the environment can be many and varied and should be distinguished from *routes* of exposure. Here is a simple example to distinguish these two concepts better. One may be exposed to sulfur dioxide in various ways, the majority of which lead to exposure through the inhalation route. One particular pathway is the generation of sulfur dioxide through the combustion of sulfur-containing coal, followed by the concomitant release of this gas from the combustion facility, and advection and dispersion in the air. An alternative pathway in an industrial setting might arrive from the use of sulfurous acid in a manufacturing process with the concomitant release of sulfur dioxide at an individual workstation. The worker at his workstation is then exposed directly to sulfur dioxide via the inhalation route. These two pathways differ substantially and would require entirely different control strategies to reduce exposure. However, since both exposures are through the inhalation route, the risk assessment process would be similar. At this point, the determination of exposure requires us to gather much more information about the scenario. In the exposure scenario where a worker is entering a tank with saturated vapor, the worker should be provided with a respirator that supplies air from outside the tank, as it would be much too dangerous to send an individual into such an enclosed space without such a device. For a saturated vapor in an enclosed tank, the primary concern would be inhalation exposure. If the respirator was fitted perfectly and functioning properly, the worker's inhalation exposure would be close to zero. However, respirators may be used improperly or not at all, resulting in inhalation exposure greater than expected under this ideal scenario. However, the worker would also receive exposure through the skin; thus dermal exposure may be an important route and potentially could result in health effects. We must be careful to consider all potential routes and attempt to identify all pathways of exposure.

3. *Magnitude, frequency, and exposure duration.* It is also important in understanding exposure to look at the time course of the exposure, sometimes referred to as the *exposure profile*. The definition of exposure requires averaging over time that, in turn, results in a great deal of lost information. Intuitively, we may imagine that exposure to a very high concentration of contaminant for a short duration followed by exposure to no concentration at all for the remainder of, say, a work shift may have different consequences from exposure to a modest concentration over the entire work shift. The total would be the same, but the duration and concentration of exposure would be different. For example, one worker may be welding for 15 minutes in a relatively enclosed space and be subjected to a concentration of metal fumes of 40 mg/m^3. He thus receives an exposure of 40 mg/m^3 × 0.25 h = 10 mg/m^3 × 1.0h. After welding, he goes on to different activities in a different part of the facility in which he experiences no concentration of welding fumes and thus receives no further exposure during the shift. His coworker, working in the same area but not exposed directly to the fumes, remains for the entire eight-hour shift. Measurement of metal fume concentrations over the course of the day in the location of the second worker gives 1.25 mg/m^3. The worker in this location receives an identical exposure: 1.25 mg/m^3 × 8 h = 10 mg/m^3 × 1.0 h, but the pattern is different. Depending on the chemical exposure, the health consequences may also be different. To account for such differences, it is important for the exposure assessor to be cognizant of the magnitude, frequency, and duration of the exposure. One should always ask, what is the peak concentration experienced during the monitoring period? Does it differ significantly from the mean concentration? How frequently are high-concentration peaks found? Are the concentrations relatively stable, or is there a good deal of variability from minute to minute or hour to hour? Do the peaks recur regularly or episodically? What is the duration of the exposure? Is it short followed by no exposure, or does it occur at moderate levels for a long period? Such information can prove invaluable in both assessing the risks of chemical exposure and in addressing potential effects and control strategies.

4. *Methods of exposure assessment.* Exposure assessors typically undertake exposure assessment investigations in one of two ways: (1) direct exposure assessment methods and (2) indirect exposure assessment methods. Direct exposure assessment methods involve outfitting an individual with some type of monitor that measures pollutant concentrations experienced by the individual as he goes about his daily activities. This is most easily visualized for airborne contaminants. In this case, an air monitor collects a sample of the air breathed by the individual over a period of time. That air sample is then analyzed for the contaminant of interest either on a real-time or time-integrated basis (both are commonly used in occupational settings). Similar monitors may be envisioned for exposures occurring via the ingestion or dermal pathways as well. By the direct method, actual exposures experienced by an individual can be observed. This is a major strength in assessing exposure and is generally desirable. However, portable monitors may not exist for the particular contaminant under investigation, or may unduly influence the activity patterns of the individual; that is to say, the normal activities that are undertaken in the workplace. They also may be bulky, require an electrical connection, or otherwise interfere with job duties.

An alternative strategy involves indirect exposure assessment, in which microenvironments, or areas, or activities likely to give similar and relatively homogeneous exposures are monitored using, perhaps, more sophisticated monitoring equipment and where the movement of the individual within and between such microenvironments is noted. Again, the inhalation route is most easily visualized. In this case, air pollution monitors are placed in various locations (e.g., workstations) to determine concentrations found in these locations. Exposure is then determined by having the individual note the amount of time spent in each of the microenvironments, multiplying the concentration measured by the amount of time spent in the microenvironment, and adding all such values together. For other routes of exposure, a similar approach can be used.

Yet another strategy, one not involving any direct measurement, can also be envisioned. With this strategy, an activity pattern for an individual can be assumed, perhaps through a large data-gathering effort addressing the locations where individuals typically spend their time. An example is the job-exposure matrix in which certain job titles are assumed to have homogenous and known exposures. Such an approach is used often in occupational epidemiology. An example might include distinguishing between two groups of workers (e.g., manufacturing-line workers and office workers) at the same location. Office workers might be assumed to have low (or even no) exposure, while manufacturing-line workers receive high (or perhaps even quantified) exposures.

5. *Biological markers of exposure.* Exposure to environmental contaminants requires the simultaneous presence of a contaminant concentration and a human subject to receive the exposure. Both the direct and indirect methods described previously assume that the exposure occurs if these two components exist. However, the only way to be sure is to use the response of the human subject as a measure. This is what exposure assessors do when they use biological markers (sometimes referred to as *biomarkers*) of exposure. Biological markers of exposure to a given contaminant make use of biological material (e.g., exhaled breath, urine, blood or blood components, fecal samples, or tissues). These samples are analyzed for the contaminant in question, called the *parent compound*, or a metabolite or biological by-product to determine the exposure. Occupational exposure to trichloroethylene, an important industrial solvent, offers a good example. Urine samples can be taken from individuals and analyzed both for trichloroethylene and for its metabolites (e.g., trichloroacetic acid) to ascertain exposure to this class of compound. Using measures of these two compounds, we can infer the magnitude of the initial exposure and, through analysis of the metabolic processes involved, the timing of such exposure.

6. *Other exposure-related issues.* Unlike the technology-based standards that the EPA sometimes sets, which require the estimation of exposures once the required controls are installed, OSHA PELs fix the maximum post-regulatory concentration. In other words, there is no need to estimate future exposures, as the regulation itself determines what is allowable. OSHA standards are compared to the actual exposures of individuals, rather than the environments they live or work in; an employer is deemed to be out of compliance if a personal air sampling device attached to a worker shows a concentration above (with statistical significance) a PEL.

Occupational PELs assume that a worker is employed over a 45-year *working lifetime* (essentially from age 20 through age 65) and that risk is accumulated during this period. Contrast this to the full 70-year lifetime assumed by the EPA when projecting cancer risk. Some have suggested that since individual industries and worksites are regulated, exposure – and thus risk – should only be accumulated during the time that the average worker remains with a single employer, perhaps 10 to 15 years (see, e.g., Burmaster 2000). This argument is weak in that workers normally change jobs within the same industry and are likely to continue accumulating exposure during their next job as well, if not to the identical substances then to similar ones that act via a common toxicologic mechanism. Workers should be protected for their entire working lifetimes.

OSHA is required to perform exposure assessment when promulgating a regulation. It must, for example, account for the exposures experienced prior to the regulation being put in place and for likely compliance discrepancies. That may result in an over- or underexposure experienced by the workers themselves. This is especially noteworthy because, in practice, working facilities are normally considered to be in compliance if measured concentrations of contaminants at the site are less than 125% of the PEL. Further, compliance requirements allow conversion of exposure measurements that take place over less-than-full to full-shift exposures assuming zero exposure during the remaining shift time, biasing inferred exposures. In addition, no allowance is made for previous exposures; exposures are assumed to be fresh each day with no accumulated effects.

Dose-Response Analysis

In occupational risk assessment, dose-response analysis can be used with epidemiological data or animal bioassay data to predict health impacts on workers. Data collected as part of an occupational epidemiology study are generally regarded as the ideal data for dose-response (also called exposure-response) analysis because there is by definition no need to analogize across species to estimate human risk. Ideally, if sufficient exposure data have been collected or estimated, measurements can be linked to individual work histories and health (or death) records to permit dose-response estimation for the working population. Occupational epidemiological studies, however, are typically conducted for only a small fraction of a working lifetime, so even when these data are available, assumptions must be made to estimate health effects from exposure over a working lifetime. This requires understanding the disease process, the mode of action of the chemical exposures, and sophisticated statistical modeling of the available data. One example of an occupational epidemiologically-based risk assessment is the NIOSH risk assessment for diacetyl (a chemical found in butter flavoring). In that assessment, NIOSH modeled the change in lung function in workers exposed to diacetyl in popcorn manufacturing. Statistical modeling of the exposure data collected and measurements of lung function led to NIOSH recommendations for a REL for diacetyl (NIOSH 2016). For more information on how to use epidemiological data in occupational risk assessment, see *NIOSH Practices in Occupational Risk Assessment* (NIOSH 2020).

In contrast, animal bioassays require interspecies extrapolation for human risk assessment, but they do allow assessors to consider carefully controlled exposures rather than concentrations workers happen to have already encountered. In animal studies, generally, a relatively small number of animals are exposed to the compound of interest at several levels, up to (and often including) a significant fraction of the *maximum tolerated dose (MTD)*. The MTD is defined as the highest dose of the test agent during the chronic study that can be predicted not to alter the animals' longevity from effects other than carcinogenicity. In many cases, cancer is the outcome of interest, and tumor development in the animal is the way such an outcome is quantified. The number of dose groups in such an investigation is quite limited, often consisting of no more than three or four; these may include a control group receiving no exposure, an MTD/2 group that receives a high dose, and another group (or two) at lesser fractions of the MTD. In general, but not always (see 1-bromopropane example on p. 252), these doses are higher than might be experienced in a normal, nonoccupational setting, even under the most adverse conditions.

A significant question then becomes, how do we extrapolate the effect seen at the high levels of exposure experienced by the animals to the low levels experienced by the human subjects facing the exposure in an environmental or occupational setting? This is not as simple as it seems; there are many ways to do the low-dose extrapolation, and unfortunately, they often give significantly different answers. One common procedure for estimating the effect of low concentrations is the mathematical modeling of the dose-response curve. When the exposure of interest is to a genotoxic carcinogen, a model known as the *linearized multistage model* (LMS) is often used. The models typically use the data for all of the dose groups to estimate the probability that an animal receiving a given dose would develop cancer. This approach may be used alone or in combination with the benchmark dose (BMD) approach, in which the dose response is modeled down to a pre-defined point of departure and then a linear extrapolation is applied to estimate the risk levels of interest. We will not discuss the details of the LMS or BMD analysis here, but we will point out that in both these approaches, there is an implicit assumption in the model that at low doses, the probability of an adverse health outcome increases with increasing doses (in other words, that there is no threshold).

Once the data are fit using the LMS or BMD, we must account for differences between human beings and the rodents who are exposed in order to determine an occupational exposure limit. Typically, to account for the differences in size between, say, mice and human beings, risk assessors scale the dose by a function of the body-weight (BW) ratio. $BW^{3/4}$ is typically used as metabolic processes scale approximately this way. Risk assessors often also typically look at the quality of the statistical fit to the dose-group data and use the *upper confidence limit* (UCL) on the linear slope value. That is, the statistical fit would give a number, called the *maximum likelihood estimate* (MLE), but to account for some uncertainty in the slope estimation, risk assessors frequently assume a larger slope based on the variability in the observed response. This assumption is slightly "conservative," but the UCL cannot be more than a factor of about 4 above the expected value of the slope (as can be seen in Hattis and Goble 1991).

Not all occupational risk assessments have followed this approach. For some occupational standards, BW extrapolation has been done in a linear fashion; that is, the scaling is BW^1. This is less protective, by roughly a factor of 4 (when rat data are used) or 7 (mouse data) than $BW^{3/4}$. Further, the MLE estimate is sometimes taken, rather than the UCL on the plausible slope of the dose-response function, again affording less protection.

For chemicals that have health effects other than cancer (for example, liver toxicity, neurological effects, or respiratory irritation), the dose-response analysis typically includes the assumption that there is a threshold below which the body either does not experience toxicity or can recover from that toxicity. Modeling animal toxicity data for those types of health effects has some similarities and some differences from modeling carcinogenicity data. Extrapolation of animal data to humans is often done similarly to cancer data. But, since a threshold of toxicity is assumed, the modeling may be a bit different. In the case of noncancer health endpoints, typically the statistical model that may best fit the data is unknown, so a BMD approach, in which several models are fit to the data, is used. Once the results are obtained, the model fits are compared and a best-fitting model is selected. This can be done by inspection of the model fits or by using a statistical procedure called Bayesian model averaging in which the statistical weight of each model is estimated based on how well the model fits the data. The result of this is a statistically weighted "average" model that represents an amalgam of the models used in the analysis based on their individual model fits. Often this provides a superior model fit to selecting a "best-fitting" model by inspection.

Once a best-fitting model is established, the BMD is estimated at a prescribed benchmark response (often 10% for incidence data). Adjustment factors (sometimes called uncertainty factors) are then applied to the benchmark dose to estimate a dose below the BMD that may also fall below the presumed biological threshold of toxicity. These factors account for interspecies variability in metabolism and susceptibility, interindividual variability in metabolism and susceptibility, differences in the experimental duration and the desired exposure duration (e.g., working lifetime), sufficiency of database, and other considerations. Rather than estimating a prescribed risk level (for example, 1 excess case of cancer per 10,000 workers exposed for a working lifetime), the final exposure value for noncancer health effects is one presumed to be unlikely to produce irreversible harm in more than a small portion of the more susceptible subpopulation – colloquially, a "safe" level.

Case Study: Methylene Chloride

OSHA's 1997 regulation imposing various restrictions on the industrial use of methylene chloride (MC) provides an unusually wide-ranging look at the scientific and science-policy issues that can arise in writing and implementing a risk-based regulation. QRA featured prominently in several of these issues and provided OSHA with an opportunity to innovate in ways that made the MC regulation a cutting-edge one for its time. MC is a very common chlorinated solvent (US production in 2016 was approximately 270 million pounds), with uses ranging from stripping paint to industrial degreasing to gluing together pieces of polyurethane foam (as in the manufacture of upholstered furniture). The paint-stripping process often involves immersing the object in a tank of liquid MC, as when stripping furniture, or by spraying an MC solution onto large objects, as when repainting airplanes. All of these processes give ample opportunity for occupational exposure. OSHA began considering a regulation for MC in the late 1980s when the United Auto Workers and other unions petitioned OSHA to that effect (during the same period, the FDA banned the use of MC in aerosol cosmetic products). At the time, OSHA estimated that approximately 250,000 US workers, employed at roughly 90,000 different establishments (many of them obviously very small businesses), were exposed to MC. Although OSHA adopted a PEL of 500 ppm for MC when the agency was created in 1970, its surveys suggested that almost all of those workers were exposed to concentrations lower than 500 ppm – but that an estimated 60,000 workers routinely encountered concentrations between 25 ppm and 200 ppm.

MC can cause a variety of adverse health effects in experimental animals and in humans. At roughly 2,000 ppm, MC can cause death by asphyxiation; between 1980 and 2018, one group of researchers (Hoang et al. 2021) found reports of 85 fatalities from accidental overexposures to MC, generally in confined spaces such as tank trucks, but also in larger enclosures as in the use of MC to strip paint from the floors of poorly ventilated rooms. In concentrations at or below the 500 ppm PEL, MC can cause central nervous system depression in humans and (because MC is metabolized to carbon monoxide) can increase blood carboxyhemoglobin concentration, raising concern about potential acute and chronic cardiovascular effects. The critical effect in the development of the PEL for MC, however, was its potential carcinogenicity: a well-conducted National Toxicology Program bioassay in male and female mice showed significant excesses of malignant lung and liver tumors in animals exposed by inhalation to roughly 2,000 ppm MC, only a factor of four above the prevailing PEL. Epidemiologic studies of workers exposed to MC did not provide clear evidence of carcinogenicity, although most of the studies involved relatively small populations in relatively well-controlled operations. For example, one prominent study examined 1,300 workers whose average MC exposure was only 26 ppm, a level that OSHA eventually concluded would have yielded an excess cancer risk of roughly 3 cases per thousand, essentially statistically indistinguishable in a cohort of this size, given the much higher natural background rate of lung and other cancers in the normal population.

In light of this evidence, OSHA ultimately promulgated regulations setting a PEL of 25 ppm and a STEL of 125 ppm (so that no exposure averaged over 15 minutes shall exceed the STEL). OSHA estimated that the excess lifetime cancer risk at the new PEL was approximately 3.6 per thousand, substantially higher than the 10^{-3} benchmark referenced by the Supreme Court in 1980 as clearly significant risk. OSHA determined, however, that 25 ppm was the lowest level that all affected industry sectors could feasibly meet (although in no case did OSHA estimate that the cost of complying with the standard would amount to more than 2% of the sales revenue of affected firms). Neither the labor unions nor the affected industries challenged the standard in court after OSHA agreed to make minor changes in one ancillary provision of the standard and to allow several additional months for certain industry sectors to come into compliance. OSHA also estimated, considering the number of workers then exposed to various concentrations of MC, that the new standard would prevent approximately 30 cancer deaths per year and would cost US industry roughly $100 million per year (over a ten-year period) to implement.

Although the general provisions in the MC standard deviated little from the template OSHA had used for its other substance-specific standards after the *Benzene* decision, OSHA's risk assessment for MC broke new ground in at least three major respects.

1. *Incorporation of a metabolic model for interspecies extrapolation.* By the early 1990s, MC had become perhaps the single most extensively studied industrial chemical with respect to the pathways and rates governing its metabolism in both rodents and humans. Various research groups had reached a consensus that both rodents and humans metabolize MC via two competing biochemical pathways: a mixed-function oxidase system that converts MC to carbon monoxide and a pathway involving the enzyme glutathione-S-transferase (GST), which produces at least two reactive intermediates known to interact with DNA and RNA. This information allowed the development of physiologically based pharmacokinetic (PBPK) models of the metabolism of MC in rodents and humans. PBPK modeling is a method for estimating the exposure to a metabolite of a chemical when there are data available on the absorption, distribution, metabolism, and excretion of the chemical in the body, *and* the metabolite that causes the toxicity of interest has been identified. An understanding of both the disposition of the chemical in the body and its toxic mode of action is necessary for PBPK modeling to be useful in risk assessment. In the case of MC, the data were available to support PBPK modeling.

   PBPK modeling offered an opportunity for OSHA to estimate risk in light of both the uncertainty in interspecies extrapolation (from mice to humans) and the variability in how different humans metabolize MC. With the help of scientists from two universities and a state health department, OSHA refined the basic PBPK model published in the scientific literature, incorporating quantitative measures of uncertainty in the 46 different parameters (23 in mice and a corresponding number in humans) needed to run the model, as well as measures of pairwise correlation between all relevant parameters. The thought process that led OSHA to conclude that the PBPK approach to assessing MC risk was superior to the default assumption also enabled OSHA to implement one of the major recommendations of both the 1983 and 1994 National Academy of Sciences risk assessment committees that agencies describe for the interested public the quantity and quality of information they deem necessary to depart from a generic default so that researchers can investigate specific questions productively and other stakeholders can gauge whether the agency followed its own advice in making such crucial science-policy decisions. As a result of this experience, OSHA developed a list of 11 scientific criteria to evaluate using these types of data in future chemical risk assessments (Exhibit 12.1) This decision represented the first time a US federal agency set a regulatory occupational exposure limit for a toxic substance using a PBPK model for interspecies extrapolation rather than an extrapolation method, such as a BW or surface-area ratio (see Kuempel et al. 2015 for a discussion of the 11 OSHA criteria in context of improving occupational risk assessment).

2. *Rejection of an alternative theory claiming that MC causes cancer in mice but not in humans.* As part of the rulemaking effort, OSHA also evaluated a series of journal articles, which postulated that humans are insensitive to the carcinogenic effects of MC seen in mice. A petition that OSHA reopen the hearing record to evaluate these articles claimed that

   This research, which is now complete, shows that mice ... are uniquely sensitive at high exposure levels to MC-induced lung and liver cancer, and that ... there are no foreseeable conditions of human exposure in which the carcinogenic effect seen in mice would be expected to occur in man.

   This assertion was based on several hypotheses, including (1) that MC produces lung tumors in a type of cell (the Clara cell) that may be relatively more abundant in mice than in humans, (2) that mouse liver and lung cells may be more susceptible than human cells to single-strand DNA breaks when exposed to MC, and (3) that the GST enzyme that metabolizes MC may be more abundant in mouse cells than in human cells and that it can be found in the nuclei of mouse cells but may tend to concentrate in the cytoplasm of human cells (i.e., not in as close

EXHIBIT 12.1   OSHA'S SCIENTIFIC CRITERIA FOR ACCEPTING A PBPK MODEL

1. The predominant and all relevant minor metabolic pathways must be well described in several species, including humans. (Two metabolic pathways are responsible for the metabolism of MC in humans, mice, rats, and hamsters.)
2. The metabolism must be adequately modeled. (Only two pathways are responsible for the metabolism of MC as compared to several potential routes of metabolism for other compounds, such as benzene and dioxins. This simplified the resulting PBPK models.)
3. There must be strong empirical support for the putative mechanism of carcinogenesis (e.g., genotoxicity), and the proposed mechanism must be plausible.
4. The kinetics for the putative carcinogenic metabolic pathway must have been measured in test animals in vivo and in vitro and in corresponding human tissues (lung and liver) at least in vitro, although in vivo human data would be the most definitive.
5. The putative carcinogenic metabolic pathway must contain metabolites that are plausible proximate carcinogens (e.g., reactive compounds such as formaldehyde or S-chloromethyl glutathione).
6. The contribution to carcinogenesis via other pathways must be adequately modeled or ruled out as a factor. For example, there must be a reasonable analysis of why reactive metabolites formed in a second pathway would not contribute to carcinogenesis (e.g., formyl chloride produced via the mixed-function oxidase (MFO) pathway is likely to be too short-lived to be important in MC carcinogenesis).
7. The dose surrogate in target tissues (lung and liver in the case of MC) used in PBPK modeling must correlate with tumor responses experienced by test animals (mice, rats, and hamsters).
8. All biochemical parameters specific to the compound, such as blood:air partition coefficients, must have been experimentally and reproducibly measured. This must be true especially for those parameters to which the PBPK model is most sensitive.
9. The model must adequately describe experimentally measured physiological and biochemical phenomena.
10. The PBPK models must have been validated with data (including human data) that were not used to construct the models.
11. There must be sufficient data, especially data from a broadly representative sample of humans, to assess uncertainty and variability in the PBPK modeling.

Source: Occupational Safety and Health Administration (1997, pp. 1533–1534).

proximity to the cell's genetic material). OSHA invited the scientific community and other interested parties to review the published studies on this topic. Various experts commented that mice and humans can differ *quantitatively* in their sensitivity to MC and that the PBPK approach accounted for such quantitative distinctions. Commenters also disputed the notion that mouse and human GST could only exist in fundamentally different portions of the cells of each species. By evaluating new and emerging science and by engaging experts in the process, OSHA demonstrated that this approach can significantly improve the quality of risk assessment.

3. *Estimating individual risk for a hypothetical person of above-average susceptibility to exposure-related disease.* When OSHA calculated the excess cancer risk of exposure to 25 ppm MC using the PBPK model, it arrived at a slightly lower average value of risk than it had predicted using a simple BW extrapolation several years previously (1.2×10^{-3} versus 2.3×10^{-3}). However, all of the information on uncertainty and interindividual variability needed to calibrate and run the PBPK model allowed OSHA to explore what the excess risk would be to workers with differing degrees of susceptibility to MC (at least those differences due to variation in individual metabolism) and with different assumptions about uncertainty.

Ultimately, OSHA determined that it would be more responsive to the spirit of the OSH Act language that "no employee shall suffer material impairment of health" if it estimated risk for a worker of above-average susceptibility. Due to either uncertainty or interindividual variability (or a combination of both), OSHA estimated there was approximately a 5% chance that the excess risk to a randomly selected worker would be at least threefold higher than the mean value of 1.2 × 10^{-3}, and so it based its final PEL on the basis of this 95th percentile estimate of 3.6 × 10^{-3}. To our knowledge, this was the first time that a US federal agency quantitatively analyzed interindividual variability in susceptibility to a toxic substance and explicitly estimated risk to consider persons of above-average susceptibility. Note that the PEL of 25 ppm did not meet the *Benzene* decision criterion that risk be reduced at least to 10^{-3} because OSHA determined that a lower level would not be economically feasible for all affected industry sectors.

In June 2020, EPA finalized its comprehensive risk evaluation of MC and found unreasonable risks to consumers from all consumer uses of MC and to workers from most commercial uses of MC. Additionally, EPA found unreasonable risks from most commercial uses of this chemical to workers nearby but not in direct contact with MC (which EPA refers to as "occupational non-users"). These determinations were based on consideration of both short- and long-term inhalation and dermal exposure. In response to determinations of unreasonable risks to workers and consumers, EPA banned sales of MC in paint and coating removers for consumer use and, as of this writing, is considering additional risk mitigation strategies for workers.

Frequently, when chemical regulations are promulgated, companies move to substitute different, less regulated, often less well-studied chemicals. This is called a risk-risk trade-off (Graham and Wiener 1995; Sunstein 1996). One example of this is the substitution of 1-bromopropane (synonym: *n*-propyl bromide), as an alternative to MC. At the time that the OSHA MC regulation was taking effect, both this compound and a more toxic contaminant (2-bromopropane) formed during its synthesis were known to cause both neurological and reproductive damage in laboratory animals, and the National Toxicology Program concluded in 2003 that at current occupational exposure levels, 1-bromopropane poses "serious concern for reproductive and developmental effects in humans" (NTP 2003). In addition, in 2004, Robinson reported (Robinson 2004) that six workers in a foam cushion factory in Utah developed chronic neuropathic pain and difficulty walking after being exposed to approximately 130 ppm 1-bromopropane over a period of several months (see also Urbina 2013). The National Toxicology Program conducted inhalation bioassays on 1-bromopropane and found there was clear evidence of carcinogenic activity of 1-bromopropane in female rats and female mice and some evidence of carcinogenicity of 1-bromopropane in male rats.

BOX 12.4   MORE RISK-RISK TRADE-OFFS IN OCCUPATIONAL HEALTH AND SAFETY

Adam M. Finkel

Although some trade-offs do seem inevitable (for example, that the benefits of reducing ground-level ozone will be offset to some extent by the additional skin cancers that will result from lower ozone concentration), questions remain about whether in general claims of dire secondary outcomes from reducing existing risks are wholly legitimate. Among other claims, various industries warned OSHA (and the Office of Information and Regulatory Affairs) during the final stages of OSHA's methylene chloride rulemaking that the MC standard would result in a rash of fires and explosions as companies that could not meet the standard were forced to switch to acetone – a flammable substitute – as a solvent, adhesive, and so on. Similarly, the trade association representing operators of general aviation aircraft warned that "without MC," repainting of these aircraft would have to be done using substitute paint strippers, which could lead to substandard or less frequent paint removal and "a major risk factor to the flying public" from corrosion and metal fatigue under the paint going undiscovered (House Subcommittee on Workforce Protections 2001). At the time, OSHA told both Office of Management and Budget (OMB) and the congressional oversight panel that it did not anticipate widespread substitution away from MC (that the new exposure limit could easily be met in these and other sectors) and that in any event, these industries were capable of handling substitutes safely and producing safe products. Now that ample time has elapsed in which any dire offsetting risks would have been evident, it appears that there has been at most one significant industrial fire or explosion involving acetone in processes where MC might possibly have been used (to be sure, that number was near zero prior to the issuance of the MC standard as well), and no reported general aviation accidents where improper paint stripping was a factor.

Although OSHA still does not have a PEL for 1-bromopropane, ACGIH set its TLV at 0.1 ppm in 2016, and in 2021, EPA made 1-bromopropane the first "new" addition to its list of 188 Hazardous Air Pollutants since the Clean Air Act Amendments became law in 1990 (based on petitions filed in 2010 and 2011 by a state environmental agency and an industry trade association).

CONTROL OF HAZARDS

In an effort to manage risk to the worker, several types of control strategies are recommended. Employers should follow the hierarchy of controls that OSHA, NIOSH, and EPA emphasize in their communication, pursuing each strategy from first to last before moving to the next one: elimination, substitution, implementation of engineering controls, administrative controls, and the use of personal protective equipment. This hierarchy is designed to encourage employers to make process changes that remove the risk entirely or, failing that, to reduce exposures through engineering controls and – only if these are not feasible – to resort to measures that place extra burden on workers themselves. Let us examine each of these controls (Figure 12.3).

Elimination

The first option for removal of hazards in the workplace is the elimination of the hazardous substance or process entirely. This, of course, eliminates the hazard once and for all and offers complete protection for the worker. Unfortunately, this is not always possible. Some activities, such as the operation of hazardous machinery, cannot be removed from the workplace. Some consumer products could be discontinued entirely, but this is often fraught given our market economy. Hence, alternative control strategies must be invoked.

Substitution

If a material, a process, or an individual piece of equipment is by its very nature hazardous, a reduction in risk for the worker may be efficiently achieved through the substitution of a less-hazardous process, equipment, or material. Workers would then no longer be exposed to the original hazard, but rather to a different and lesser one. This is an effective strategy and may offer long-run cost reduction in that lost worker time is reduced along with reduced workers' compensation costs. Initial capital outlays may be large, however, especially if a process must be revamped

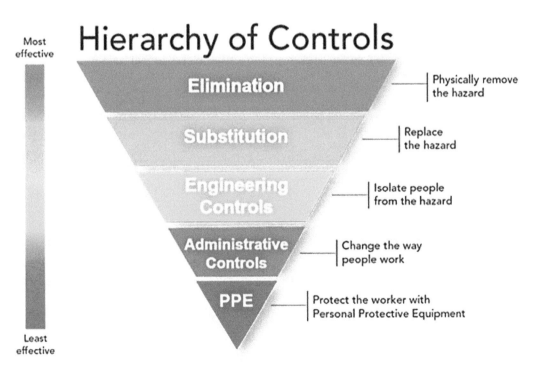

Figure 12.3 The NIOSH Hierarchy of Controls.

entirely. Development of an effective substitution strategy requires a good deal of thought as well as experience in developing the new procedures.

Process Substitution. The substitution option may be most clearly indicated using some examples. In automotive manufacturing, for example, painting may be accomplished using a spray bay in which aerosolized paint is applied to the metallic frame of the automobile. The potential for inhalation exposure is great in such a spray, and the hazard associated with inhalation of paint and solvent vapors is well understood. An effective substitute for this process, whereby the metallic frame of the vehicle is dipped into the paint, thereby reducing aerosolization and exposure, is readily envisioned and has been implemented. The implementation of such a substitution is not without difficulties, however. New paint formulations must be developed that afford good adhesion and attractive finished products. Even drying is problematic and requires a further change in the process. A significant retooling of the painting component of an assembly line for automaking is the indirect result of this hazard reduction.

Equipment Substitution. While modification of a process offers the best reduction in risk for the worker, the cost of such a modification may be prohibitive. The change of a single piece of equipment may be sufficient to reduce risk substantially at a much lower cost. The selection of replacement equipment often requires the expertise of both management and worker in that the financial investment will be supplied by the management side, while familiarity with the process and working environment will be better known to the worker.

Consider the case of solvent use in an occupational setting. Small quantities of solvents are often delivered in glass bottles ranging in size from 250 mL to 4 L or more. The larger bottles are relatively difficult to handle and may be dropped or dislodged from their storage area with the potential for significant exposure to the worker. Replacement of such bottles by safety storage cans that are unbreakable, or by enclosing the bottle in a plastic case, substantially reduces the risk of breakage. Such modification of storage equipment can be done at low cost and often offers a significant improvement in worker safety.

Material Substitution. In an industrial process, it is often necessary to use hazardous materials. However, the substitution of a less-hazardous material for a more hazardous one can often be affected without loss of efficiency in the process overall. Consider the following examples.

Historically, there are many examples of material substitutions with concomitant improvement in worker safety. Classic examples include the substitution of the red phosphorous allotrope for the white. The latter ignites on contact with air and is thus a hazard for both direct burns to the worker and fire within the facility. The red allotrope is much more easily handled and does not present the same safety concerns. Another example is the substitution of phosphors for radium on watch dials. One early use for radioactive materials was on watch dials to allow them to be visible in the dark. Unfortunately, the workers painting these dials suffered from a series of radiation-induced ailments. This substitution improved the health of these workers immensely by reducing radiation exposure risk. The substitution of chlorinated solvents for petroleum naphthas in industry substantially reduced the fire hazard in cleaning operations. We must be careful in the selection of substitution materials, however, to ensure that one hazard is not being replaced by another.

Engineering Controls

Engineering controls invoke the application of mechanical solutions in an effort to reduce exposure to hazards. Engineering controls can be broadly grouped into the following categories: isolation and ventilation.

Isolation. Some processes cannot be changed, nor can the intrinsic risk associated with the process be reduced. In these cases, the only real alternative is to remove the worker from direct contact with the process. This is called *isolation*. As the name would suggest, isolation involves placing some type of barrier between the workers and the hazard to which they might otherwise be exposed. These barriers can be *physical*, a wall or simply distance between the worker and the hazard, or *temporal*, a process that operates when the worker is not present until it is complete. Some equipment is inherently dangerous due to the need for large amounts of energy to run it. Examples include high-pressure hydraulic lines, rotating machinery, and cutting blades. Because of the nature of the processes involved (e.g., moving heavy machinery and cutting metals), there is a significant potential for severe injury. Isolation offers a major reduction in risk. A physical barrier, a fence, enclosing rotating parts in metal, or isolating high-pressure hydraulic lines offers a good solution. Workers are not afforded an opportunity to come into contact with the dangerous equipment.

Certain operations, such as heat treating or cutting and drilling, cannot be nonhazardous. A heat-treating process requires elevated temperatures at the site of the work. These temperatures may be sufficient to burn on contact or may simply raise the ambient temperature to levels that surpass the body's ability to cope. Similarly, noise levels associated with a specific activity may be sufficient to cause permanent hearing loss either instantaneously or through long exposure. Isolation of the process (or the worker) may be the only feasible solution to such a problem.

Perhaps the easiest example to understand involves isolation from radiological or biological hazards. Highly radioactive materials, such as those found in nuclear research facilities, power plants, and medicine, often require a thick shield to prevent workers from receiving dangerous levels of exposure. The process itself may be isolated in such cases and workers only allowed to interact by remote control or with robotic devices.

Ventilation. In many occupational settings, the principal hazard is air contamination. Examples have been discussed previously and include exposure to dusts, vapors, metal fumes, and biological contaminations. It is often most convenient to reduce the hazard to the worker by supplying fresh, clean air. This is a direct application of the old adage "the solution to pollution is dilution." Ventilation may be concisely defined as the removal of contaminated air, the introduction of clean air, or both, in an effort to dilute a physical or chemical hazard to some acceptable level. Ventilation systems are often divided into two large categories, though significant overlap exists between these two rubrics. These are (1) local exhaust and supply ventilation and (2) general exhaust ventilation.

1. *Local exhaust and supply ventilation.* Often in industrial facilities, sources of air contamination are somewhat isolated by the process itself. Dust may be generated by a sanding and grinding operation that is limited to a single department or even a single machine. Organic vapors may be associated with a single degreasing tank. A biological hazard may exist at only one laboratory bench. In such cases, it makes sense to treat the source of the contamination directly. If the source area could be partially enclosed (thus isolating the process) and the contaminating material removed before it permeates the area, risk to the workers in general could be substantially reduced. This solution is quite effective both in a risk-reduction sense and in an economic sense. Exhaust systems can be designed with capture efficiencies approaching 100% for small areas.

2. *General exhaust ventilation.* While local exhaust and supply ventilation can be very efficient if sources of contamination within a facility are relatively isolated, they are not an effective solution if sources are dispersed throughout the facility. For example, a foundry may have multiple sources of particulate matter of various types and indeterminate generation patterns. Local exhaust ventilation methods are not appropriate in such circumstances; it is necessary to rely on general ventilation within the entire faculty to reduce risk to workers. General exhaust ventilation works much the same way as local exhaust ventilation except that now the entire facility is viewed as the "local" source. Large air-moving devices actively exhaust the contaminated air from within the building and supply fresh, outdoor air in its place. Such systems are costly in terms of capital outlay and in terms of heating and air-conditioning needs for the facility. However, if this situation is as described with numerous dispersed sources of contamination, risk reduction for workers often cannot be effected in any simpler or more cost-effective way.

Administrative Controls

Administrative controls, in which policies and procedures are implemented that reduce worker risk, have historically been the purview of management, but more recently cooperation between management and workers has made these more effective. Administrative controls include education of both management and the workforce on the risks experienced by the worker. While the education of the worker may seem obvious, as he needs to be aware of hazards and take proper steps to reduce them, the role of management may seem less obvious. Yet the role of management may be even more important than the role of the worker in implementing and maintaining a safe working environment. One administrative control that requires an understanding of the mode of toxicity and careful thought about dose-response relationships is the notion of "employee rotation," in which the employer may seek to subject a greater number of workers to the hazard for a shorter amount of time by rotating different workers through the high-exposure task over time. For some hazards (some acute hazards and some physical hazards) this type of "spreading the risk" is appropriate. However, for carcinogens and other hazards for which the risk accumulates with exposure, OSHA and the occupational safety and health community generally oppose this strategy because if the toxicant has no threshold, all rotation does is spread the same amount of risk over more workers, widening the UCL of how many workers might be harmed. On the other hand, if the toxicant does have a true biological threshold, exposure-spreading might actually be sensible (assuming we could accurately estimate the threshold level and keep accurate track of each worker's cumulative exposure).

Personal Protective Equipment

Even when all of the above procedures are implemented, there may still be significant residual risk for workers. Some industrial processes, such as cleaning solvent tanks or handling radioactive material or chemical hazards, are intrinsically hazardous and cannot be made hazard-free. Under these conditions, one is forced to examine the use of *personal protective equipment* (PPE), a form of worker isolation, as a final choice in protecting the worker. Simple examples include the use of safety shoes to reduce foot injuries in occupational settings, and the use of hearing protection in settings where noise is excessive. In areas subject to high levels of air contamination, the use of respirators may be necessary. Respirators supply clean breathing air to the worker and range from simple filters that remove excess dust or organic vapors from the air to more complex apparatus that supply air to a worker entering an enclosed space that might not have sufficient oxygen to sustain life or that might be subject to concentrations of toxic gases high enough to cause injury. For extremely hazardous work in which any contact with the environment comes with substantial risk, full-body protection, sometimes referred to as moon suits, may be required. Such PPE protects the entire body from inhalation exposure, ingestion exposure, and dermal exposure. Such protection is used under the most hazardous of conditions – circumstances where biological, chemical, or other hazards are so great that any contact with the environment might prove harmful.

OSHA allows employers to control workers' exposures to chemicals by using respiratory protection when they can show that in a given operation, it is infeasible for engineering controls alone to

BOX 12.5   CONTROLS, PROFIT, EMPLOYMENT, AND HEALTH

Adam M. Finkel

With the advent of OSHA in the 1970s, the bottom-line operating costs for a facility could be markedly affected by fines and shutdowns. Management often took an adversarial position with respect to OSHA regulations, as well as with respect to organized workers or workers in general. This attitude has changed in the last 35 years. Astute managers have become aware of the potential to reduce workers' compensation premiums to increase productivity and to reduce training costs through the implementation of sensible workplace risk-reduction measures. It is now quite common to see a partnership between management and workers to develop education programs designed to make workers aware of the hazards in a workplace and to take ownership of their own safety and health. OSHA has taken a leadership role in this process as well through the implementation of its voluntary protection program (VPP), whereby facilities that go through rigorous training and evaluation procedures are allowed to reduce the likelihood and scope of OSHA inspections required. Such cooperative interaction is the hallmark of effective administrative control programs, ensuring safe workplaces and more productive facilities.

More broadly, the relationship between regulatory costs, especially the costs of OSHA regulations, and unemployment is controversial but important to consider as society seeks to further reduce occupational injury and illness. Unemployment and loss of income, after all, is itself risky and can lead to morbidity and mortality. However, in addition to the various studies (see above) suggesting that the costs of regulation are frequently exaggerated, recent scholarship tends to agree that regulations rarely "kill" significant net numbers of jobs (Coglianese et al. 2015). Regulations do, however, often create jobs in one sector while eliminating them in another, so it is important for policymakers to examine whether small net changes in employment mask significant economic and health effects on individuals who cannot find re-employment in the growing sectors of industry.

achieve a PEL (or when there is a TLV but no PEL, as part of the employer's General Duty). OSHA revised its respiratory protection standard (29 CFR 1910.134) in 1998, and in 2006 added a table of Assigned Protection Factors (APFs) based on the ability of each broad class of respirator (e.g., filtering facepiece or "dust mask," elastomeric cartridge respirator, powered air-purifying respirator or "PAPR," supplied-air hood) to reduce the concentration of a particle or vapor outside the respirator

BOX 12.6 INFORMATION DISCLOSURE: AN IMPORTANT AND FREE-STANDING PART OF THE HIERARCHY

Adam M. Finkel

Some controls to reduce occupational hazards rely on the simple power of knowledge. Information disseminated by the government, or disclosed by employers, can serve to empower workers to better understand and better protect themselves, or to help companies gauge and improve their performance, or in some cases to alert employers to the downsides of non-compliance with regulations and other norms. The power of information can be brought to bear at any level in the hierarchy of controls.

Perhaps the best example of the first type of information-as-solution involves OSHA's Hazard Communication Standard (29 CFR §1910.1200), often known as "HazCom," which since 1983 has given workers crucial understanding of the substances they may encounter in their workplaces, the health risks they pose, and the ways to reduce their exposures and risks. The cornerstone of the HazCom rule is the "Safety Data Sheet" (SDS; formerly known as the MSDS, or Material Safety Data Sheet), which is a resource for companies and workers that is supposed to fully disclose all of the health and safety hazards of a given substance, how to control them, and how to recognize and treat symptoms of acute or chronic overexposure. For much of the past 40 years, citations for not having SDSs accessible to workers have been among the most frequently issued OSHA citations, although the agency does not nearly as often cite manufacturers for disseminating incomplete or inaccurate data sheets. In 2012, OSHA amended HazCom to align with the newer United Nations Globally Harmonized System of Classification and Labeling of Chemicals, while retaining most or all of the substantive requirements of the existing rule.

OSHA often produces guidance documents and other informational material designed to help employers understand how (and why) to comply with workplace standards (for one listing of some of this voluminous material, see https://www.osha.gov/topics/text-index). But OSHA also requires in some cases that employers themselves disclose information that could help all companies better understand trends in workplace conditions. In particular, for several years, OSHA required large employers not only to post on-site annual summaries of the serious injuries that occurred at their facility (including calculating the injury rate per 100 employee-years of work) but also to electronically transmit the log and data to OSHA for analysis. That 2016 rule was rescinded in 2019 but was brought back into force in early 2022.

A third type of useful information relies on the power of deterrence. Beginning in the Obama administration (but again, rescinded in the subsequent administration), OSHA greatly increased its use of press releases, targeted at local media, explaining why a particular company had just received a major civil penalty for one or more violations of OSHA standards. OSHA had always issued occasional press releases for total fines of several hundred thousand dollars or more but began issuing them for total penalties of $40,000 or more, which increased the total number of releases nationwide from roughly 150 per year to nearly 500 per year. The rationale behind this initiative was that corporate leadership may well care much more about the possible effect on their stock price of documenting their lapses. However, the policy was also criticized for two main reasons: (1) in some cases, articles were written based on penalties proposed by OSHA that were later negotiated downward, and (2) using the dollar amount as the sole criterion means that a facility with one serious lapse would be publicized, while one with dozens of less serious ones might not. Ultimately, the deterrent effect of OSHA's policy received a major validation in a study by Johnson (2020), who demonstrated that after press releases were issued, future violations at all similar facilities within 5 km of the subject facility went down by more than 70%. Johnson concluded that a single press release could have a similar deterrent effect as more than 200 on-site OSHA inspections would have had.

to a lesser concentration. OSHA defines the "Maximum Use Concentration" as the APF multiplied by the PEL; for example, if the PEL for a given contaminant is 20 ppm, and the employer provides a respirator with an APF of 10, the employee can wear that respirator in an atmosphere containing 200 ppm of the substance and be in compliance with the OSHA standard.

THE EVOLUTION OF INDUSTRIAL HYGIENE AND THE ROLE OF NEW PROFESSIONALS

Historically, industrial hygiene (or occupational hygiene) has focused on worker exposures to a single contaminant such as specific solvents, nuisance dusts, or radiation. However, recent studies in epidemiology, toxicology, and pharmacokinetics indicate that such a focus may be too narrow. Health outcomes are likely associated with multiple exposures over a lifetime to compounds that may act as synergists or promoters of disease. To address the complex workplaces of today, the profession of industrial hygiene is changing. New professionals in the field must now have broad-based knowledge of the mechanisms of contaminant action. They must study biology, toxicology, epidemiology, and other related sciences. The "new industrial hygienist" must be aware of the compounding effects from, for example, exposure to various related solvents or classes of pesticides, some of which accumulate in the body over the lifespan of the worker. Thus, an understanding of the historical exposures experienced by workers is also necessary. The metabolism of compounds that enter the body must be understood as well; fast-metabolizing compounds may produce toxic metabolites, and slow-metabolizing compounds may accumulate in body-storage compartments and cause health problems years after exposure.

Those aspiring to become industrial hygienists in the twenty-first century must become more general in their education and in their work aspirations. In the coming years, industrial hygienists will still be required to "know their instrumentation" and be able to take samples in the field. But they will also need to be aware of secondary exposures experienced by workers in their nonwork activity, as well as the impact of the industrial environment on the surrounding community. Consistent with the NIOSH Total Worker Health® (TWH) model and program, changes to the workplace (e.g., nonstandard work arrangements and the gig economy), and the demographics of the workforce (e.g., older workers and an increasing prevalence of chronic disease among the employed) warrant a more comprehensive and holistic approach to protecting and promoting worker safety and health. The TWH approach integrates traditional occupational safety and health in the workplace with concerns about overall worker well-being, both within and outside of work. Through academic training, continued professional development, and collaboration across disciplines, current and future occupational health and safety professionals will greatly benefit from an expanded set of skills and knowledge to meet the demands of a changing working environment (Schulte et al., 2019).

EMERGING HAZARDS

Today, workers continue to experience many of the same historical hazards in the workplace, but there are also new hazards to contend with – engineered nanomaterials, the adverse effects of artificial intelligence, psychosocial hazards etc. And new and unanticipated hazards are still likely to emerge. Often, the hazards are not evident at first, as with radiation and asbestos, but come to light only after workers have received exposures long and significant enough to develop the clinically evident disease. We hope not to repeat some of the mistakes of the past. Let us examine some emerging concerns to make ourselves aware of the possibilities of worker injury and disease.

Nanotechnology

Nanotechnology, the use of very small, even molecular-scale, machines, may well be the principal advance of the 21st century and have a variety of uses across many industries – from food production, to coatings, to cosmetics and industrial processes. There is potential for worker harm from exposure to nanomaterials, which, if inhaled, tend to settle deeper in the lung and can be transported to remote areas of the body to cause health impacts. Now is the time to examine such exposures and refine methods of protecting workers from inadvertent injury and illness in the nanotechnology workplace (Service 2005).

Impact of Climate on Workers

There are many health and safety considerations associated with extreme weather events that have a significant impact on workers, particularly those who spend considerable time working outdoors. The effects can be direct, such as heat stroke or even death resulting from working in hot conditions for prolonged periods of time. Extreme weather can also indirectly affect the health and safety of workers, as changes in precipitation and temperature can impact the concentrations of ambient air pollution as well as the prevalence of biological hazards including vector-borne diseases.

Changes in climate have also contributed to an increase in the frequency and severity of wild-fires, resulting in a growing concern not just for the health and safety of wildland firefighters but for all outdoor workers potentially exposed to smoke from wildfires. Three states significantly impacted by wildfires – California, Oregon, and Washington – have recently issued rules to protect workers from wildfire smoke: https://www.cdc.gov/niosh/topics/firefighting/wffsmoke.html. These rules include requirements for employers to provide training, implement engineering or administrative controls, and provide or even require respirator use, depending on the level of the US Environmental Protection Agency's air quality index (AQI) for PM2.5, a primary component of wildfire smoke. As the AQI is linked to the National Ambient Air Quality Standards that are established to protect public health, the actions of these states would seem to constitute a tacit acknowledgment that occupational standards for respirable particulate matter, exposures to which rarely occur in isolation, do not adequately protect the health of workers.

New Industrial Processes

New industrial processes are being developed constantly. Consider that integrated circuits and the concomitant assembly technology have all been developed in the last 50 years. New processes such as genetic engineering, related biotechnologies, and advanced manufacturing techniques (e.g., 3D printing) are likely to be developed more fully in the next 25 years. We must consider the impact on the health of workers who engage in these industrial activities. Are they at risk for certain known diseases? Are there new diseases that will emerge from these new processes? Some industrial processes will be common 25 years from now that are not even known at this point. How will we set up a mechanism that affords adequate protection to evaluate the impact on workers of these new processes? For a very recent example of a modern hazard only becoming known as a cause of serious occupational disease years after exposures began, see the literature on the relationship between diacetyl (used in artificial butter flavoring) and "popcorn lung disease" (*bronchi olitis obliterans*) (see, e.g., Schneider 2006).

BOX 12.7   REPEATED HEAD TRAUMA

Adam M. Finkel

Evidence has emerged over the past decade (although the risk had been suspected and written about for more than a century) that multiple concussions, along with "subconcussive" impacts, are strongly associated with the development of a grave neurodegenerative disease now generally called chronic traumatic encephalopathy (CTE), for chronic traumatic encephalopathy (Baugh et al. 2012). Head trauma poses fascinating problems for occupational safety and health professionals: (1) it is both an injury and the apparent cause of a serious illness; (2) the illness can affect more than the worker (prominent reports exist of professional athletes who harmed others while suffering the cognitive and behavioral effects of CTE); (3) repetitive head trauma is both an occupational (professional sports, logging, military service, commercial driving, etc.) and a frequent nonoccupational exposure; (4) some of the entertainment and sports occupations where head trauma is most prominent are clearly under OSHA's jurisdiction but are not typical scenes of OSHA inspection or regulation; (5) PPE may not be helpful in this case, as the damage accrues when the human brain impacts the inside of the skull, not from the initial impact per se. The Harvard Football Players Health Study (Finkel et al. 2018) wrote a comprehensive analysis of how OSHA could help to reduce CTE risks in workplaces, discussing various informational, partnership, General Duty Clause enforcement, and standard-setting options that might provide some relief to workers, and by extension to college athletes et al not covered by OSHA. Interestingly, the most important court case further establishing that the OSH Act gives OSHA jurisdiction over sports and entertainment as well as manufacturing and service industries involved the 2014 case of *SeaWorld v. DOL*, where OSHA levied fines against a water park for allowing trainers to work in the water with an orca who had previously killed trainers at other parks.

BOX 12.8   NIGHT SHIFT WORK AND BREAST CANCER RISK
Mingzhu Fang

All types of organisms possess natural, internal circadian rhythms that are adjusted to the local environment by external cues, including light, nutrients, and temperature. In humans, the central clock, which is located at the suprachiasmatic nucleus of the hypothalamus, receives light signals through the eyes to adjust the internal circadian rhythm to the 24-hour light-dark cycle of the solar day. The central clock also synchronizes circadian rhythms across most peripheral organs and cells via endocrine (e.g., melatonin) and neural pathways. Therefore, our body systems are adapted to the 24-hour solar day at the behavioral, biochemical, physiological, and cellular and molecular levels.

Circadian disruption is defined as internally or externally induced acute or chronic temporal disorganization and misalignment of the time structure in living systems. Specifically, circadian disruption occurs when the daily circadian rhythms in our bodies are not adjusted to the environmental light-dark cycle and/or are no longer coordinated with each other. Excessive exposure to light at night (LAN), persistent night shift work, jet lag, and sleep deprivation can cause circadian disruption. Long-term circadian disruption causes chronic diseases, including cancer and metabolic syndrome.

Recent survey data indicate that greater than 27% of employees are working alternative shifts and that 7%–20% of workers in occupations, such as the protective services, healthcare, production, and transportation are working at night. Night shift work causes a complex exposure scenario, involving exposure to electric LAN, sleep disturbances, meal time changes, and social stressors. In most health outcome studies, exposure assessments of night shift work are mainly based on lifestyle and occupational surveys and/or daily activity diaries. The information provided in the surveys and diaries are reviewed, and the sleep time, amount, and quality are assessed for each subject. Outdoor LAN exposures are measured with time-varying satellite data analysis, whereas indoor LAN exposures are usually measured using light intensity data loggers. In contrast, only a limited number of studies have measured personal light exposures in shift workers in various exposure scenarios. Recently developed medical devices, such as Actigraph, can monitor light exposure and activity, which can be used to assess circadian rhythms accurately in individuals over an extended period of time.

Earlier epidemiological studies in shift workers indicate that nurses and pilots have an increased risk of cancer, especially in breast and prostate, respectively. Results from an occupational cohort study showed an increased risk of breast cancer among women who worked long-term (for 10 or more years) night shift, especially those who worked the night shift for more than 20 years. A similar conclusion has been made by an analysis of data from Nurses' Health Study cohorts with 24-year follow-up for total 9,541 incident cases of invasive breast cancer. These studies found a significantly increased risk of breast cancer in women with 20 years or more of night shift work, particularly among women who began night shift work in early adulthood (before age 30). In a pooled analysis of five European case-control studies of night shift work and breast cancer incidence, night shift work was positively associated with increased breast cancer risk in premenopausal women. In these studies, women who worked the night shift with high intensity (at least three times/week) for more than 20 years were at the highest risk, and the associations were strongest in women with hormone receptors positive (i.e., ER+ and ER+/HER2+) breast cancer subtypes.

Laboratory animal studies have also provided compelling evidence for the carcinogenicity of altered light-dark schedules in various organs (e.g., breast and liver) of rodents. Chronic exposure to constant light increased the incidence of carcinogen-induced mammary tumors in female rats. Moreover, long-term exposure to a jet-lag protocol mimicking rotating shift work, accelerated the growth of xenograft breast cancer in immune-deficient mice. Furthermore, chronic jet lag advanced tumor onset and accelerated tumor growth in breast cancer-prone transgenic mice and conditional p53 mutant mice.

These human and animal data together with mechanistic study results prompted the International Agency for Research on Cancer to classify night shift work as *probably carcinogenic to humans* (Group 2A) (IARC 2010; IARC 2020). A recent National Toxicology Program cancer hazard assessment report concluded that persistent night shift work that disrupts circadian rhythms can cause breast cancer in women and may cause prostate cancer in men (NTP 2021).

REFERENCES

International Agency for Research on Cancer (IARC). 2010. "Painting, Firefighting, and Shiftwork." IARC Monographs on the Identification of Carcinogenic Hazards to Humans Volume 98. IARC MONOGRAPHS ON THE IDENTIFICATION OF CARCINOGENIC HAZARDS TO HUMANS. Lyon, France. https://publications.iarc.fr/Book-And-Report-Series/Iarc-Monographs-On-The-Identification-Of-Carcinogenic-Hazards-To-Humans/Painting-Firefighting-And-Shiftwork-2010

International Agency for Research on Cancer (IARC). 2020. "Night Shift Work." *IARC Monographs on the Identification of Carcinogenic Hazards to Humans Volume 124.* IARC MONOGRAPHS ON THE IDENTIFICATION OF CARCINOGENIC HAZARDS TO HUMANS. Lyon, France. https://publications.iarc.fr/593

National Toxicology Program (NTP). 2021. "NTP Cancer Hazard Assessment Report on Night Shift Work and Light at Night." NTP Review of Shift Work at Night, Light at Night, and Circadian Disruption. https://ntp.niehs.nih.gov/ntp/results/pubs/cancer_assessment/lanfinal20210400_508.pdf

Exposure to Mixtures

Historically, risk assessors have focused on one hazard at a time, even though we know that workers are exposed to multiple hazards on the job. For example, pharmaceutical manufacturers use a variety of compounds in the synthesis of their products; electronics industries use a large amount of silicon but dope the surfaces with different trace elements to build circuitry with specific properties. Understanding the effects of these mixtures of compounds is the main need for future industrial hygienists (Fox et al. 2018; Lentz et al. 2015). The task is not easy. How will these mixtures be measured? How will the components be weighted with regard to health outcomes? Are there compounds that interact synergistically to produce a large effect on health while each individually produces none? This is the challenge of the future.

Technological Change

Overall, the role of the future hygienist is to adapt to the technological change that is certain to come, while "holding the fort" against hazards known for decades or more, where continued vigilance is necessary to provide workers with a fighting chance to return home safely each day.

THOUGHT QUESTIONS

1. What are the most important aspects of occupational risk assessment methodology that tend to make risk estimates *conservative* (prone to overestimation), and which aspects work in the opposite direction? On balance, do you think OSHA risk assessment errs on the side of precaution too much or not enough?
2. What are the most significant hazards identified in recent years that have been insufficiently characterized or addressed by the occupational safety and health community? What new hazards would you urge OSHA or NIOSH to pay more attention to in the immediate future?
3. How can society reliably assess the contribution of specific interventions (e.g., regulations, enforcement, partnerships) to observed changes in measured results (fatalities, injuries, illnesses) given the difficulty in knowing what changes might have occurred in the absence of the interventions?
4. Given the many procedural and analytic challenges inherent in researching and regulating occupational safety and health risks, and the considerable overlap between community and workplace exposures, what would the merits and pitfalls be of creating a single agency with jurisdiction over both environmental and occupational risks?

DISCLAIMERS

The findings and conclusions in this chapter are those of the authors and do not necessarily represent the official position of the National Institute for Occupational Safety and Health, Centers for Disease Control and Prevention. Throughout this chapter, particularly in the online interactive version, additional material is provided in boxes. This material was assigned by the editors and does not necessarily represent the views of the chapter authors or of NIOSH.

Some material in the 2007 version of this chapter was originally contributed by P. Barry Ryan.

REFERENCES

American Textile Manufacturers Institute et al. v. Donovan, Secretary of Labor et al., No. 79-1429 (1981).

Annas, G. J. 1981. "Blue Jeans for You, Brown Lung for Us": OSHA's Cotton Dust Standard. *Hastings Center Report*, 11: 15–16.

Ashford, N. A., and Caldart, N. A. 1996. *Technology, Law, and the Working Environment* (rev. ed.). New York: Island Press.

Baker, E. L., Jr., et al. 1979. Occupational Lead Poisoning in the United States: Clinical and Biochemical Findings Related to Blood Lead Levels. *British Journal of Industrial Medicine*, 36(4): 314–322.

Baker, E. L., Jr., et al. 1985. The Neurotoxicity of Industrial Solvents: A Review of the Literature. *American Journal of Industrial Medicine*, 8(3): 207–217.

Barstow, D. 2003, December 22. U.S. Rarely Seeks Charges for Deaths in Workplace. *New York Times*, p. A1.

Baugh, C. M., et al. 2012. Chronic Traumatic Encephalopathy: Neurodegeneration following Repetitive Concussive and Subconcussive Brain Trauma. *Brain Imaging and Behavior*, 6: 244–254.

Bufton, M. W., and Melling, J. 2005. "A Mere Matter of Rock": Organized Labour, Scientific Evidence and British Government Schemes for Compensation of Silicosis and Pneumoconiosis Among Coalminers, 1926–1940. *Medical History*, 49(2): 155–178.

Bureau of Labor Statistics. 2004. *Census of Fatal Occupational Injuries, 1992–2004*. Washington, DC: U.S. Department of Labor.

Bureau of Labor Statistics. 2022, April 1. Economic News Release Employment Situation Tables A-1 and A-9. https://www.bls.gov/news.release/empsit.toc.htm. Accessed May 2, 2022.

Burmaster, D. 2000. Distributions of Total Job Tenure for Men and Women in Selected Industries and Occupations in the United States, February 1996. *Risk Analysis*, 20(2): 205–224.

Cordaro, T. L. 2015. Recent OSHA Inspection Statistics and Enforcement Initiatives. *JacksonLewis OSHA Law Blog*, https://www.oshalawblog.com/2015/03/articles/recent-osha-inspection-statistics-and-enforcement-initiatives/

Chemical Week. 1976, September 15. Polyvinyl Chloride Rolls out of Jeopardy, Into Jubilation, p. 34.

Cherniack, M. 1986. *The Hawk's Nest Incident: America's Worst Industrial Disaster*. New Haven, Conn.: Yale University Press.

Coglianese, C., Finkel, A., and Carrigan, C. 2015. *Does Regulation Kill Jobs?* University of Pennsylvania Press. https://www.law.upenn.edu/institutes/ppr/doesregulationkilljobs/

Corn, J. K. 1981. Byssinosis: An Historical Perspective. *American Journal of Industrial Medicine*, 2(4): 331–352.

Darby, S., Hill, D., and Doll, R. 2001. Radon: A Likely Carcinogen at All Exposures. *Annals of Oncology*, 12: 1341–1351.

Environmental Protection Agency. 1992. Draft Report: A Cross-Species Scaling Factor for Carcinogen Risk Assessment Based on Equivalence of $mg/kg^{3/4}/day$. *Federal Register*, 57(109): 24152–24173.

Environmental Protection Agency. 1999, June 17–18. Common-Sense Approaches to Protecting Workers and the Environment: Interagency Cooperation Towards Cooperative Solutions. *Conference Held in Washington, D.C.*

Environmental Protection Agency. 2000. EPA/OSHA Advisory on 2,4-Dichlorophenol. http://epa.gov/oppt/pubs/24dcp.htm.

Environmental Protection Agency. 2004. Toxic Substances Control Act, Section 8(e). http://www.epa.gov/opptintr/tsca8e/pubs/facts8e.htm.

Environmental Protection Agency. 2006a. Development of Acute Exposure Guideline Levels. http://www.epa.gov/oppt/aegl.

Environmental Protection Agency. 2006b. Region 8: Libby Asbestos. http://www.epa.gov/region8/superfund/libby/background.html.

Federal Advisory Committee Act Amendments. 2006. U.S.C. 5 App. (as amended). http://www.usdoj.gov/04foia/facastat.pdf.

Finkel, A. M. 2005, December. Kilo-Disparities? Prevailing Concentrations of Carcinogenic Air Pollutants in U.S. Workplaces and the Ambient Environment. *Paper Presented at the Annual Meeting of the Society for Risk Analysis*, Orlando, FL.

Finkel, A. M. 2008, September 16. There Is No "War" on Occupational Cancer. *Presentation before the President's Cancer Panel*, New Brunswick, NJ. https://healthandenvironment.net/uploads-old/No%20War%20on%20 Occupational%20Cancer-%20Finkel.doc

Finkel, A. M., Deubert, C. R., Lobel, O., Cohen, I. G., and Lynch, H. F. 2018. The NFL as a Workplace: The Prospect of Applying Occupational Health and Safety Law to Protect NFL Workers. *Arizona Law Review*, **60**: 291–368.

Fox, M. A., Spicer, K., Chosewood, L. C., Susi, P., Johns, D. O., and Dotson, G. S. 2018. Implications of Applying Cumulative Risk Assessment to the Workplace. *Environment International*, 115: 230–238.

Gochfeld, M. 2005. Chronologic History of Occupational Medicine. *Journal of Occupational and Environmental Medicine*, 47(2): 96–114.

Gomez, M. R. 1991. Validation of Sampling Data from the Occupational Safety and Health Administration (OSHA) Integrated Management Information System (IMIS). *American Industrial Hygiene Association Journal*, 52(9): A488.

Graham, J. D., and Wiener, J. B. 1995. *Risk Versus Risk: Tradeoffs in Protecting Health and the Environment*. Cambridge, MA: Harvard University Press.

Hattis, D., and Goble, R. L. 1991. Expected Values for Projected Cancer Risks from Putative Genetically Acting Agents. *Risk Analysis*, 11(3): 359–363.

The Histories of Herodotus, The Persian Wars, Book 7 Polymnia, c. 484–425 because n.d.

Hoang, A., Fagan, K., Cannon, D. L., et al. 2021. Assessment of Methylene Chloride-Related Fatalities in the United States, 1980–2018. *JAMA Internal Medicine*, 181(6): 797–805.

House Subcommittee on Workforce Protections. 2001, June 14. OSHA's Standard Setting Process. http://www.house.gov/ed_workforce/hearings/107th/wp/osha61401/seminario.htm.

Islam, K. M., and Anderson, H. A. 2006. Status of Work-Related Diseases in Wisconsin: Five Occupational Health Indicators. *Wisconsin Medical Journal*, 105(2): 26–31.

Johnson, J. M. 2001. A Review and Synthesis of the Costs of Workplace Regulations. (Working Paper) Arlington, VA: Regulatory Studies Program, Mercatus Center, George Mason University.

Johnson, M. S. 2020. Regulation by Shaming: Deterrence Effects of Publicizing Violations of Workplace Safety and Health Laws. *American Economic Review*, 110(6): 1866–1904.

Jones, J. H. 1981. Worker Exposure to Vinyl Chloride and Polyvinyl Chloride. *Environmental Health Perspectives*, 41: 129–136.

Kniesner, T. J., Leeth, J. D. 1995. Numerical simulation as a complement to econometric research on workplace safety. *J Risk Uncertainty* 10, 99–125. https://doi.org/10.1007/BF01083555

Kuempel, E. D., Sweeney, L. M., Morris, J. B., and Jarabek, A. M. 2015. Advances in Inhalation Dosimetry Models and Methods for Occupational Risk Assessment and Exposure Limit Derivation. *Journal of Occupational and Environmental Hygiene*, 12: S18–S40.

Landrigan, P. J. 1987. Benzene and Leukemia. *American Journal of Industrial Medicine*, 11(5): 605–606.

Landrigan, P. J., et al. 1980. Clinical Epidemiology of Occupational Neurotoxic Disease. *Neurobehavioral Toxicology*, 2(1): 43–48.

Lavoue, J., Friesen, M. C., and Burstyn, I. 2013. Workplace Measurements by the US Occupational Safety and Health Administration since 1979: Descriptive Analysis and Potential Uses for Exposure Assessment. *Annals of Occupational Hygiene*, 57(1): 77–97.

Leigh, P., et al. 1997. Occupational Injury and Illness in the United States: Estimated Costs, Morbidity, and Mortality. *Archives of Internal Medicine*, 157: 1557–1568.

Leigh, J. P., Waehrer, G., Miller, T. R., and Keenan, C. 2004. Costs of Occupational Injury and Illness Across Industries. *Scandinavian Journal of Work, Environment & Health*, 30: 199–205.

Lentz, T. J., Dotson, G. S., Williams, P. R. D., Maier, A., Gadgbui, B., Panadalai, S. P., et al. 2015. Aggregate Exposure and Cumulative Risk Assessment – Integrating Occupational and Non-Occupational Risk Factors. *Journal of Occupational and Environmental Hygiene*, 12:Suppl. 1: S112–S126.

Levine, D. I., Toffel, M. W., and Johnson, M. S. 2012. Randomized Government Safety Inspections Reduce Worker Injuries with no Detectable Job Loss. *Science*, 336: 907–911.

Lowell Center for Sustainable Production. 2006. *Integration of Occupational and Environmental Health*. Lowell, MA: University of Massachusetts. http://sustainableproduction.org/proj.inte.abou.shtml.

McMichael, A. J. 1976. Standardized Mortality Ratios and the "Healthy Worker Effect": Scratching Below the Surface. *Journal of Occupational Medicine*, 18: 165–168.

National Academy of Sciences. 1983. *Risk Assessment in the Federal Government: Managing the Process.* National Academy Press: Washington, DC, https://nap.nationalacademies.org/catalog/366/risk-assessment-in-the-federal-government-managing-the-process

National Institute for Occupational Safety and Health. 2020.*Current Intelligence Bulletin 69: NIOSH Practices in Occupational Risk Assessment.* By Daniels, R. D., Gilbert, S. J., Kuppusamy, S. P., Kuempel, E. D., Park, R. M., Pandalai, S. P., Smith, R. J., Wheeler, M. W., Whittaker, C., Schulte, P. A. Cincinnati, OH: U.S. Department of Health and Human Services, Centers for Disease Control and Prevention, National Institute for Occupational Safety and Health. DHHS (NIOSH) Publication No. 2020-106 (revised 03/2020). https://doi.org/10.26616/NIOSHPUB2020106revised032020.

NIOSH. 2016. *Criteria for a Recommended Standard: Occupational Exposure to Diacetyl and 2,3-Pentanedione.* By McKernan, L. T., Niemeier, R. T., Kreiss, K., Hubbs, A., Park, R., Dankovic, D., Dunn, K. H., Parker, J., Fedan, K., Streicher, R., Fedan, J., Garcia, A., Whittaker, C., Gilbert, S., Nourian, F., Galloway, E., Smith, R., Lentz, T. J., Hirst, D., Topmiller, J., Curwin, B. Cincinnati, OH: U.S. Department of Health and Human Services, Centers for Disease Control and Prevention, National Institute for Occupational Safety and Health, DHHS (NIOSH) Publication No. 2016-111.

NIOSH. 2016a. *Current Intelligence Bulletin 68: NIOSH Chemical Carcinogen Policy.* By Whittaker C, Rice F, McKernan L, Dankovic D, Lentz TJ, MacMahon K, Kuempel E, Zumwalde R, Schulte P, on behalf of the NIOSH Carcinogen and RELs Policy Update Committee. Cincinnati, OH: U.S. Department of Health and Human Services, Centers for Disease Control and Prevention, National Institute for Occupational Safety and Health, DHHS (NIOSH) Publication No. 2017-100.

National Toxicology Program. 2003. NTP-CERHR Monograph on the Potential Human Reproductive and Developmental Effects of 2-Bromopropane (2-BP). NTP-CERHR MON, 10, i–III11.

Recommend including the NIOSH Occupational Risk Assessment Document: n.d. https://www.cdc.gov/niosh/docs/2020-106/default.html

Occupational Safety and Health Administration. 1997, January 10. Occupational Exposure to Methylene Chloride. *Federal Register*, 62(7).

Occupational Safety and Health Administration. 2019. Chemical Exposure Health Data. Datafile "Inspection_NAICS_CY19b.csv," containing information on 41,850 samples taken during calendar year 2019. https://www.osha.gov/opengov/health-samples.

Office of Technology Assessment. 1995, September. Gauging Control Technology and Regulatory Impacts in Occupational Safety and Health: An Appraisal of OSHA's Analytic Approach (Report #OTA-ENV-635).

Pandanell, M. 2005. The Texas City Disaster: April 16, 1947. 2005. http://www.local1259iaff.org/disaster.html.

Piltingsrud, H. V., Zimmer, A. T., and Rourke, A. B. 2003. The Development of Substitute Inks and Controls for Reducing Workplace Concentrations of Organic Solvent Vapors in a Vinyl Shower Curtain Printing Plant. *Applied Occupational and Environmental Hygiene*, 18(8): 597–619.

Pratt, S. G., Kisner, S. M., and Helmkamp, J. C. 1996. Machinery-Related Occupational Fatalities in the United States, 1980 to 1989. *Journal of Occupational and Environmental Medicine*, 38(1): 70–76.

Rhomberg, L. R. 1997. A Survey of Methods for Chemical Health Risk Assessment Among Federal Regulatory Agencies. *Human and Ecological Risk Assessment*, 3(6): 1029–1196.

Robinson, R. 2004. Bromopropane: Ozone-Sparing Solvent Is Neurotoxic (News from the Annual Meeting). *Neurology Today*, 4: 15–16.

Rosenman, K. D., et al. 2006. How Much Work-Related Injury and Illness Is Missed by the Current National Surveillance System? *Journal of Occupational and Environmental Medicine*, 48(4): 357–365.

Rosner, D., and Markowitz, G. 2020. A Short History of Occupational Safety and Health in the United States. *American Journal of Public Health*, 110: 622–628.

Ruttenberg, R. 2004, February. *Not Too Costly After All: An Examination of the Inflated Cost-Estimates of Health, Safety, and Environmental Protections.* Report prepared for Public Citizen Foundation Inc. https://www.citizen.org/wp-content/uploads/migration/not_too_costly.pdf.

Schneider, A. 2006, August 3. House Members Fault Agency for Inaction on Flavoring Peril. *Baltimore Sun*.

Schulte, P. A. 2017. An Approach to Assess the Burden of Work-Related Injury, Disease, and Distress. *American Journal of Public Health*, 107(7): 1051–1057.

Schulte, P. A., Delclos, G., Felknor, S. A., & Chosewood, L. C. 2019. Toward an Expanded Focus for Occupational Safety and Health: A Commentary. *International Journal of Environmental Research and Public Health*, 16(24): 4946.

Selikoff, I. J., and Greenberg, M. 1991. A Landmark Case in Asbestosis. *Journal of the American Medical Association*, 265(7): 898–901.

Selikoff, I. J., et al. 1965. The Occurrence of Asbestosis Among Insulation Workers in the United States. *Annals of the New York Academy of Sciences*, 132(1): 139–155.

Selikoff, I. J., et al. 1967. Asbestosis and Neoplasia. *American Journal of Medicine*, 42(4): 487–496.

Service, R. F. 2005. Related Nanotechnology: Calls Rise for More Research on Toxicology of Nanomaterials." *Science*, 310, 1609.

Sinclair, U. 1985. *The Jungle*. New York: Penguin. (Originally published 1906.)

Smith, B. E. 1981. Black Lung: The Social Production of Disease. *International Journal of Health Services*, 11(3): 343–359.

Stout, N. A., and Linn, H. I. 2002. Occupational Injury Prevention Research: Progress and Priorities. *Injury Prevention*, 8(supp. 4): 9–14.

Sunstein, C. R. 1996. Health-Health Tradeoffs. Chicago Working Papers in Law and Economics, no. 42.

Takala, J., Hämäläinen, P., Saarela, K. L., et al. 2014. Global Estimates of the Burden of Injury and Illness at Work in 2012. *Journal of Occupational and Environmental Hygiene*, 11(5): 326–337.

Tamers, S. A., et al. 2020. Envisioning the Future of Work to Safeguard the Safety, Health, and Well-being of the Workforce: A Perspective from the CDC's National Institute for Occupational Safety and Health. *American Journal of Industrial Medicine*, 631: 1065–1084.

US Census Bureau. 2002, February. 2019 SUSB Annual Data Tables by Establishment Industry. https://www.census.gov/data/tables/2019/econ/susb/2019-susb-annual.html. Accessed May 2, 2022.

US District Court, District of New Jersey. *Adam M. Finkel v. U.S. Department of Labor, Civil Action No. 05-5525*, decided June 29, 2007. Opinion available at https://casetext.com/case/finkel-v-us-department-of-labor.

US EPA. 2017. Procedures for Chemical Risk Evaluation Under the Amended Toxic Substances Control Act, 82 FR 33726.

Upton, A. C. 1987. Prevention of Work-Related Injuries and Diseases: Lessons from Experience with Ionizing Radiation. *American Journal of Industrial Medicine*, 12(3): 291–309.

Urbina, I. 2013, March 30. As OSHA Emphasizes Safety, Long-Term Health Risks Fester." *New York Times*.

Vig, N., and Faure, M. G. (eds.). 2004. *Green Giants? Environmental Policies of the United States and the European Union*. Cambridge, MA: MIT Press.

Viscusi, W. K. 2013, October. Using Data from the Census of Fatal Occupational Injuries to Estimate the "Value of a Statistical Life". *Monthly Labor Review*, 1–16.

Von Drehle, D. 2003. *Triangle: The Fire That Changed America*. New York: Atlantic Monthly Press.

Winegar, D. A., et al. 1977. Chronic Occupational Exposure to Lead: An Evaluation of the Health of Smelter Workers. *Journal of Occupational Medicine*, 19(9): 603–606.

Yassin, A., Yebesi, F., and Tingle, R. 2005. Occupational Exposure to Crystalline Silica Dust in the United States, 1988–2003. *Environmental Health Perspectives*, 113(3): 255–260.

Young, R. C., Jr., and Rachal, R. E. 1996. Pulmonary Disability in Former Appalachian Coal Miners. *Journal National Medical Association*, 88: 517–522.

13 Children's Environmental Health Risk Assessment

Rebecca C. Dzubow
US Environmental Protection Agency, Office of Children's Health Protection

Ruth A. Etzel
Milken Institute School of Public Health, George Washington University, Washington, DC, United States

CONTENTS

Introduction 267
Children's Health in Risk Assessment 268
    Hazard Identification 268
    Toxicokinetics 269
    Toxicodynamics 270
    Dose Response 270
    Exposure Assessment 270
    Physiological Rates 271
    Activity Patterns 271
    Risk Characterization 273
    Thought Questions: Phthalates and Children 274
Web Resources 275
Literature Cited 275

LEARNING OBJECTIVES

Students who complete this chapter will be able to

1. Describe the history of children's environmental health;
2. Identify unique characteristics of children used in conducting children's risk assessments;
3. Determine how these characteristics influence exposure to environmental contaminants through the inhalation, dermal, dietary ingestion, and nondietary ingestion routes, as well as indirectly during fetal growth;
4. Identify relevant biomarkers of exposure to the fetus and child;
5. Describe current risk assessment methods and models used to assess children's risks to environmental contaminants; and
6. Identify deficiencies and uncertainties in available data and model defaults used to assess children's risks to environmental contaminants.

INTRODUCTION

Children are not just little adults. Nor is childhood a static point in time; it is a dynamic period full of changes across a series of life stages that extends from conception through in utero development, infancy, school age, and adolescence until adulthood is reached at 21 years of age (EPA 2005a). During childhood, there are observable changes in height, weight, behavior, language, cognition, and motor skills, as well as less observable structural and functional changes in the nervous, respiratory, endocrine, digestive, immune, circulatory, reproductive, digestive, renal and skeletal systems that mature in a sequential progression known as windows of development (Selevan, Kimmel, and Mendola 2000). Each of these changes influences how a child is exposed to, incorporates, and processes environmental contaminants and what organs or tissues will be affected by the contaminant to disrupt the normal progression of development.

Although not everyone is currently a child, everyone has been a child at some point in their lives, and exposures to environmental contaminants during early life can influence not only the health and well-being of the child but also the adult that this person becomes.

DOI: 10.1201/9780429291722-13

When conducting risk assessments, children should receive special consideration because children, or a particular subgroup of children (e.g., infants), may be at greater risk than the general population because of potential biological vulnerabilities or unique behaviors that may be occurring at certain developmental life stages. In some cases, children may be more sensitive to exposure to a contaminant but may have better repair mechanisms and greater potential for recovery. In other cases, children are less sensitive to the contaminant than adults.

The report *Pesticides in the Diets of Infants and Children* (NRC 1993) led to several laws and policies in the United States that require explicit consideration of children, including:

- The Food Quality Protection Act (FQPA) requires the assessment of *"whether infants and children have any special susceptibility to the residues (e.g., neurological differences or in utero exposure)"* and to apply *"an additional tenfold margin of safety to its assessments for infants and children, unless it has reliable data to show that a different margin of safety is appropriate to protect infants and children."*
- The Safe Drinking Water Act (SDWA) requires consideration of groups *"identified to be at greater risk of adverse health effects due to exposure to contaminants in drinking water than the general population"* (SDWA 1974).
- The Toxic Substances Control Act (TSCA) requires a determination of risk for *"potentially exposed or susceptible sub-populations"* defined as
  a group of individuals within the general population...who, due to either greater susceptibility or greater exposure, may be at greater risk than the general population of adverse health effects from exposure to a chemical substance or mixture, such as infants, children, pregnant women, workers, or the elderly. (TSCA 2016)
- The US Environmental Protection Agency (US EPA) Policy on Evaluating Risk to Children (EPA 1995), requires consideration of the
  risks to infants and children consistently and explicitly as a part of risk assessments generated during its decision making process, including the setting of standards to protect public health and the environment. To the degree permitted by available data in each case, the Agency will develop a separate assessment of risks to infants and children or state clearly why this is not done – for example, a demonstration that infants and children are not expected to be exposed to the stressor under examination.
- Executive Order 13045 (Clinton 1997) Protection of Children from Environmental Health Risks and Safety Risks requires each federal agency to *"make it a high priority to identify and assess environmental health risks and safety risks that may disproportionately affect children"* and *"ensure that its policies, programs, activities, and standards address disproportionate risks to children that result from environmental health risks or safety risks."*

CHILDREN'S HEALTH IN RISK ASSESSMENT

Steps required for conducting risk assessment include hazard identification; dose-response assessment; exposure assessment; and risk characterization (NRC 1983). Each of these risk assessment steps is described in this chapter with an emphasis on children's health. These topics are described in more depth elsewhere (e.g., EPA 2006; Felter et al. 2015; OECD 2019).

Hazard Identification

Hazard identification is the examination of data to determine whether a chemical or other environmental stressor has the potential to cause harm to humans and to characterize these health outcomes. In order to capture the health outcomes from early life exposures, studies need to be designed with consideration of whether the exposure occurred during critical windows of development, or whether there may be outcomes observed during development that are more frequent, more severe, or unique compared to adults.

Adverse effects can be identified early in life, such as at birth (e.g., low birth weight, reduced reflexes, cleft palate, hypospadias) or later during childhood (e.g., asthma, autism spectrum disorder, cancer). Some studies have explored the significance of early life exposure and outcomes that are not observed until later in life (e.g., cardiovascular disease, obesity, cancer) (De Long and Holloway 2017; Li et al. 2021; Mikeš et al. 2019; Yang et al. 2018).

Human evidence can come from epidemiology studies, such as the examination of a given population at a specific point in time or followed over time; incident or case reports; and human experimental data, typically conducted in adults only.

Animal toxicity studies are conducted using standardized methodologies, with some designed for observation of the impacts of early life exposure such as the two-generation reproduction toxicity study, the extended one-generation reproductive toxicity study, the prenatal developmental toxicity study, and the developmental neurotoxicity study.

In addition to the previously described in vivo studies, evidence for hazard can come from in vitro studies using cellular exposures or through predictive toxicity methods to quickly screen for possible adverse effects and prioritize further study. Although there is a movement to reduce the use of animals in toxicity studies, these new assessment methods may not capture the nuances that occur in a live animal, especially at different ages.

Toxicokinetics

Understanding what happens to the chemical after it enters the body, or *toxicokinetics*, consists of absorption, distribution, metabolism, and clearance, and can assist in determining whether an individual will likely have an adverse outcome. Much of what is known about toxicokinetic differences across life stages is from pharmaceutical research (Ginsberg et al. 2004; Ginsberg et al. 2002; Hattis et al. 2003), and much is applicable to environmental risk assessments (see Chapter 14).

Toxicokinetics starts with the **absorption** of the chemical into the body. Exposure routes common to all postnatal life stages are ingestion into the stomach, inhalation into the lung, or absorption through the skin (see Chapter 8 for an in-depth discussion). Prenatally, it is the mother's ingestion, inhalation, or dermal contact that exposes the fetus. These are typically referred to as transplacental exposures. Structural and functional differences during windows of development may be important contributors to the internal dose received. An infant's digestive tract is not fully developed and cannot absorb compounds to a similar degree to adults. An infant's lungs have fewer alveoli and bronchi) than adults which may alter the transfer of a chemical from the lung to the bloodstream. Infants, in particular for those born prematurely, have a higher skin permeability than adults (AAP 2019).

Once in the body, the contaminant is **distributed** through the body via the circulatory system to the brain, kidney, liver, fat, bone, etc. Where the contaminant is distributed depends on many factors including heart rate, blood pressure, and blood volume, which differ by age, as well as the chemical structure. Exposure to chemicals circulating through the body can be measured by taking blood samples. The National Health and Nutrition Examination Survey (NHANES), conducted by the US Centers for Disease Control and Prevention, collects nationally representative blood samples (CDC 2022) from various age groups. Blood samples are useful for a wide range of chemicals but have the limitation that it can be challenging to take blood from young children due to parental consent. The EPA's America's Children and the Environment (ACE) report displays trends of chemicals measured in the blood of children and females of reproductive age (16–49 years old), including for lead, mercury, per- and polyflouroalkyl substances (PFAS), polychlorinated biphenyls (PCBs), and polybrominated diphenyl ethers (PBDEs) (EPA 2019). Cord blood samples can be collected at birth and serve as indicators of contaminant exposure *in utero*.

When distributed to fat cells or bone, the chemicals can be stored, resulting in what is known as **body burden**. Importantly, these stored chemicals can be mobilized during pregnancy, lactation, and other periods of growth and weight loss. Therefore, the mother's behaviors, activities, and toxicokinetics are important considerations when addressing children's health in risk assessment (Kapraun et al. 2019).

Children may **metabolize** the chemical differently from the way adults do, or at a different rate. Depending upon whether the chemical or its metabolite is the more biologically active material, the rate and manner of metabolism may have a significant influence on how the chemical affects the individual. Enzyme ontogeny, or the development of the expression of enzymes, changes throughout growth. Some enzymes may be expressed at birth at levels equivalent to adults; however, many enzymes are not expressed until later in childhood (Ginsberg et al. 2017).

Eventually, the chemical or any metabolites formed will be **excreted** from the body in exhaled air, urine, feces, hair, nails, teeth, or breast milk. The measurement of chemicals in biological media, known as biomarkers, can be used to determine the amount of chemicals to which a person has been exposed. These samples can be used to indicate that exposure has occurred, or even back calculate to predict the amount of the chemical to which a person may have been exposed. Detailed information on similarities and differences in biomarkers of exposure for children of most age subsets is typically not well-characterized or difficult to interpret (Arbuckle 2010). Although urine collection is relatively easy, including from diapers, it usually can only serve as an indication of short-term exposure within 24–48 hours prior to the void. NHANES also collects nationally representative urine samples across the United States and age groups, and trends in the data for children and females of reproductive age (16–49 years old) are described in EPA's ACE report for phthalates, bisphenol A (BPA), and perchlorate measured in urine (EPA 2019). A few days after birth, measurements of chemicals in meconium, or an infant's first bowel movements, may represent cumulative prenatal exposures during the last two trimesters of pregnancy. Breast milk, as an excreted substance from the mother, becomes a source of exposure to the infant and is an important consideration in risk assessment (Lehmann et al. 2014).

Toxicodynamics

Whereas toxicokinetics is understanding what happens to the chemical after it enters the body, *toxicodynamics* data describe how the chemical impacts the various organ systems that can lead to observable adverse outcomes. The terms **mode of action (MOA)** and **adverse outcome pathway** are used to organize the series of biological events See Chapter 9 for more detail). However, the MOA that is applicable to an adult may not be the same as one for a child. Exposure during critical windows of development may result in MOAs leading to outcomes not observed in adults.

Dose Response

The dose-response step of risk assessment is the quantitative evaluation of how much exposure causes a given effect. This is typically calculated for the effects seen at the level of least exposure as doing so will protect against the effects seen in greater exposure.

Some chemicals such as lead have no known safe level of exposure. Others may not cause an adverse effect until a certain dose has been reached (known as a **threshold dose**); however, other chemicals, such as secondhand smoke, can have adverse effects at extremely small doses. A **point of departure** is the lowest dose at which an adverse response or at which no adverse response is observed (see Chapter 7).

Because of the uncertainties around the exact dose in a study that can actually cause harm, additional **uncertainties and variability factors** are applied to the point of departure, typically as a default tenfold factor:

- Variability in the human population (UF_H), including differences across life stages
- When using animal data, the differences between humans and animals (UF_A)
- Uncertainties related to identified database gaps (UF_{DB})
- Uncertainties based on the lack of a no adverse effect level (UF_L)
- Uncertainties due to extrapolating from a chronic study to a subchronic outcome (UF_S)

In certain circumstances, there are additional factors used. When calculating risk for pesticide exposure, the **FQPA Safety Factor** is used to account for any additional protection for infants and children (EPA 2002a; FQPA 1996). When calculating risk for a mutagenic carcinogen, EPA applies **Age Dependent Adjustment Factors** to account for early life sensitivity to these exposures (EPA 2005a).

Physiologically based pharmacokinetic (PBPK) models also can be used to convert the external dose into an internal target tissue dose using toxicokinetic data. When possible, these values can be preferred to the external dose and used for the point of departure in a risk assessment. Specific parameters for children and pregnant or lactating women must be used to account for the differences in toxicokinetics between children and adults (Dallmann et al. 2018; Yoon and Clewell 2016); however, many PBPK models lack a fetal or lactational compartment.

Exposure Assessment

Exposure assessment is the stage of risk assessment that examines the frequency, timing, and levels of exposure, which in turn are reflective of physiological rates and activity patterns and behaviors.

Population-based surveys have collected data about various factors that influence exposure across all ages. The US EPA's *Exposure Factors Handbook* (EPA 2011) summarizes the available data on a variety of topics such as body weight; dietary ingestion rates for drinking water, breast milk, and a variety of foods (fruits and vegetables; fish and seafood; meats, dairy products, and fats; grains); nondietary ingestion rates for incidental soil and dust; inhalation rates; dermal considerations; and a range of behaviors (e.g., mouthing), consumer product use, and activities to be considered when quantifying exposure at varying life stages, and provides a consistent set of default values for various life stages for use in US risk assessments.

One of the difficulties in creating exposure scenarios for risk assessments is that data for very young children are often lacking or are only from specific studies in which the children may not be representative of the larger population.

Physiological Rates

Water and food consumption rates differ across age groups; although the total amount consumed may be greater in adults than children, calculating exposure based on body weight demonstrates that children have higher intake rates per body weight than adults. When normalized for body weight, however, the amount of food or volume of water consumed by infants and toddlers is substantially greater than for older children. This is especially true for formula-fed infants because their diet for the first six months of life depends on the water used to reconstitute the infant formula. (Figure 13.1).

Inhalation exposure is influenced by both respiratory and inhalation rates. Respiratory rate is the number of breaths an individual takes per minute. Inhalation rate refers to the volume of air inhaled per day (m^3/day) and is a function of respiration rate and lung size. Although the respiratory rate of young children is more rapid than that of older children and adults, their lung capacity is smaller. When adjusted for body weight, children take in more air than do adults. This contributes to more frequent inhalation of airborne contaminants for children than for adults (Figure 13.2). For example, children may be more sensitive to the effects of secondhand tobacco smoke (Raghuveer et al. 2016) and wildfire smoke (EPA 2018)

Because adults are larger and have more skin surface area, dermal exposure may be assumed to be higher in adults. However, again considering the skin surface area along with body weight shows that children may have higher dermal exposures per body weight than adults (Figure 13.3).

Activity Patterns

Adults and children spend portions of their time in different locations, whether at home, in childcare or schools, at playgrounds, or at work. Also, contaminants can be brought home from the workplace. It is important to note that it is common for adolescents to have jobs, and therefore occupational exposures are to be considered for this life–stage.

While some behaviors are common to all life stages, unique behaviors typically observed at a specific life stage may significantly influence the exposure that an individual may experience. Young children display hand-to-mouth and object-to-mouth behaviors to a much greater degree than adults and are crawling, walking, and playing closer to the ground where some contaminants may concentrate (AAP 2019).

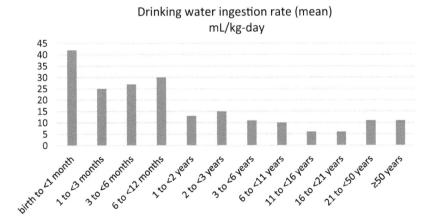

Figure 13.1 Mean drinking water ingestion rates for age groups when divided by mean body weight. *Source*: US EPA 2011, Table 3.1.

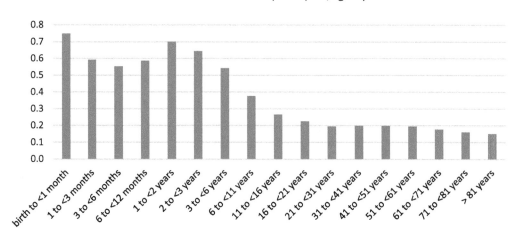

Figure 13.2 Mean inhalation rates for age groups when divided by mean body weight. *Source*: US EPA 2011, Tables 6.1 and 8.1.

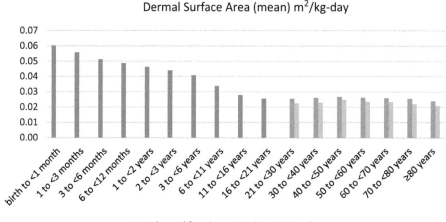

Figure 13.3 Mean dermal surface area for age groups when divided by mean body weight. *Source*: US EPA 2011, Tables 7.1 and 8.1.

For example, infants spend more time indoors each day than do older children, who in turn spend more time indoors than adults (Figure 13.4). Coupled with increased hand-to-mouth behaviors in infants and toddlers, time spent indoors can result in increased exposure to house dust. Because children at these ages also spend considerable time closer to the ground, they may also inhale increased levels of certain small particles or vapors that tend to be at higher doses closer to the ground (AAP 2019)

Soil and house dust can be important exposure pathways for all routes of exposure. Dermal exposure from soil may be higher in children than adults because of time spent outdoors, duration, and frequency of contact with soil. Dermal exposure from indoor dust is higher in children because of more time spent both indoors and on the floor than adults.

Outdoor activities are typically higher for older children, for instance spending more time each day playing in the grass (Figure 13.5) than do younger children and adults.

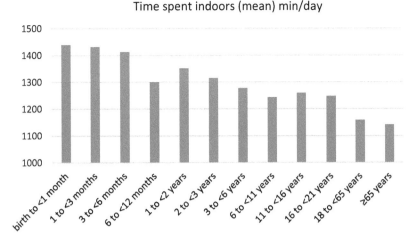

Figure 13.4 Mean time indoors for age groups. *Source*: US EPA 2011, Table 16.1

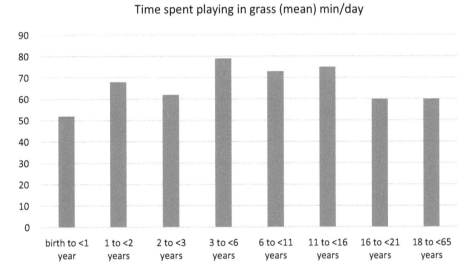

Figure 13.5 Mean time playing in grass for age groups. *Source*: US EPA 2011, Table 16.1.

Also, children as a whole spend more time doing certain activities than adults. For instance, children spend more time swimming in natural water bodies such as lakes and rivers as well as swimming pools each month than do adults (Figure 13.6). This may result in higher exposure to waterborne contaminants, which can occur through dermal exposure, inhalation exposure, and incidental ingestion. The US EPA's *Recommended Human Health Recreational Ambient Water Quality Criteria or Swimming Advisories for Microcystins and Cylindrospermopsin* (EPA 2019) is an example of a risk assessment that is based on increased childhood exposure.

Risk Characterization

Risk characterization is the summary of the data available to determine the nature and extent of risk from an exposure. It is the basis upon which the risk managers determine if interventions are needed and upon which regulatory decisions are made.

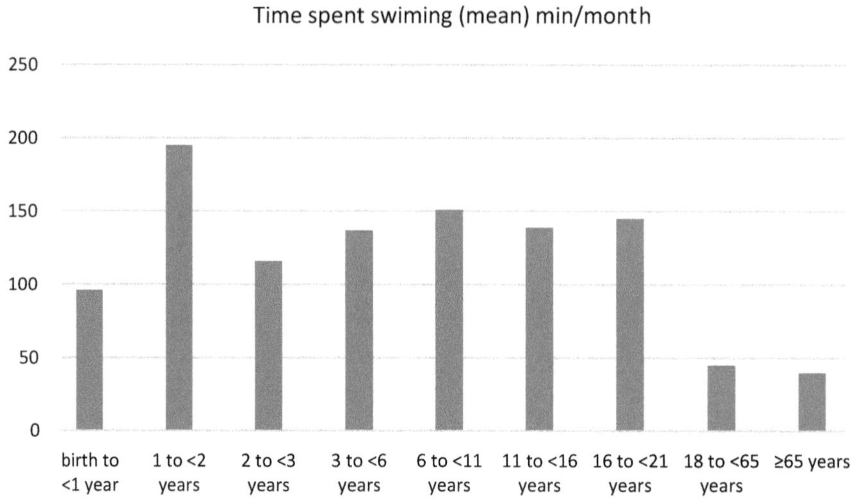

Time spent swiming (mean) min/month

Figure 13.6 Mean time swimming for age groups. *Source*: US EPA 2011, Table 16.1.

Typically, the risk characterization is for a single contaminant. However, in the real world, exposure is never in isolation and it is important to remember that there are other stressors that may be occurring in an individual's life. These include multiple sources of exposure to the same chemical, known as aggregate exposure, and exposure to multiple contaminants, known as cumulative exposure (Payne–Sturges et al. 2021), or nonchemical stressors such as poverty and racism (Trent, Dooley, and Dougé 2019), known as social determinants of health (WHO 2008). Issues of uncertainty and variability have made evaluating children's risks a challenge. Limited data or data generated for special populations that may not be representative of all children produce uncertainties in risk assessment when applied to other child populations. Data on the very young, that is, children under age 2 years, as well as data on adolescents tend to be lacking.

Without systematic exploration in population-based studies, we do not know if the variability is a result of the small sample size or is indicative of what can be expected with a larger population-based sample.

The US EPA has developed a number of risk assessment documents, which can be found at: www.epa.gov/risk. Of note, the following are of particular interest for children's risk assessment:

- *Guidelines for Developmental Toxicity Risk Assessment* (EPA 1991)
- *Guidelines for Reproductive Toxicity Risk Assessment* (EPA 1996)
- *A Review of the Reference Dose and Reference Concentration Processes* (EPA 2002b)
- *Supplemental Guidance for Assessing Susceptibility from Early-Life Exposure to Carcinogens* (EPA 2005a)
- *Guidance on Selecting Age Groups for Monitoring and Assessing Childhood Exposures to Environmental Contaminants* (EPA 2005b)
- *A Framework for Assessing Health Risk of Environmental Exposures to Children* (EPA 2006)

Thought Questions: Phthalates and Children

1. *Surveillance.* Use the US EPA's ACE (EPA 2019) to determine biological indicators (biomarkers) of exposure to phthalates.

2. *Hazard assessment.* Based on a review of available data, identify two phthalates that might be a concern for children, and determine what health outcomes are potential issues for children. Determine if data are available to address early life stage susceptibility.

3. *Exposure assessment.* Create an exposure scenario that takes into account the exposure factors, source of exposures, media, and routes of concern for children. Are some age groups of children more susceptible? What evidence is available to support your conclusion? What are the issues of uncertainty and variability that need to be addressed?

WEB RESOURCES

US EPA Risk Assessment https://www.epa.gov/risk

US EPA Risk Assessment Guidelines https://www.epa.gov/risk/risk-assessment-guidance

US EPA Superfund Risk Assessment https://www.epa.gov/risk/superfund-risk-assessment

US EPA Integrated Risk Information System https://www.epa.gov/iris

California EPA https://oehha.ca.gov/risk-assessment/childrens-health

ATSDR Minimum Risk Levels https://www.atsdr.cdc.gov/minimalrisklevels/index.html

Risk Evaluations for Existing Chemicals under TSCA https://www.epa.gov/assessing-and-managing-chemicals-under-tsca/risk-evaluations-existing-chemicals-under-tsca

LITERATURE CITED

AAP. 2019. Children's Unique Vulnerabilities to Environmental Hazards. In *Pediatric Environmental Health. 4th Edition*, edited by R. Etzel and S. Balk, pp. 17–31. Itasca, IL.: American Academy of Pediatrics.

Arbuckle, T. E. 2010. Maternal-Infant Biomonitoring of Environmental Chemicals: The Epidemiologic Challenges. *Rev. Birthdefects Res.: A Clin. Mol. Teratol.* 88 (10): 931–937.

CDC. 2022. National Report on Human Exposure to Environmental Chemicals: September 2022 Update. Available online at: https://www.cdc.gov/exposurereport/

Clinton, W. J. 1997. Executive Order 13045. Protection of Children from Environmental Health Risks and Safety Risks. *Fed. Reg.* 62: 19883–19888.

Dallmann, A., M. Pfister, J. van den Anker, and T. Eissing. 2018. Physiologically Based Pharmacokinetic Modeling in Pregnancy: A Systematic Review of Published Models. *Clin. Pharmacol. Ther.* 104 (6): 1110–1124. https://doi.org/10.1002/cpt.1084.

De Long, N. E., and A. C. Holloway. 2017. Early-Life Chemical Exposures and Risk of Metabolic Syndrome. *Diabetes Metab. Syndr. Obes* 10: 101–109. https://doi.org/10.2147/DMSO.S95296.

EPA, US. 1991. *Guidelines for Developmental Toxicity Risk Assessment.* 600-FR-91-001. Available online at: https://www.epa.gov/sites/default/files/2014-11/documents/dev_tox.pdf.

EPA, US. 1995. *Policy on Evaluating Risk to Children.* Available online at: https://www.epa.gov/children/epas-policy-evaluating-risk-children.

EPA, US. 1996. *Guidelines for Reproductive Toxicity Risk Assessment.* EPA/630/R-96/009. Available online at: https://www.epa.gov/sites/default/files/2014-11/documents/guidelines_repro_toxicity.pdf#:~:text=EPA%2F630%2FR-96%2F009%20October%201996%20Guidelines%20for%20Reproductive%20Toxicity%20Risk,Male%20Reproductive%20Risk%2C%20both%20dated%20June%2030%2C%201988.

EPA, US. 2002a. *Determination of the Appropriate FQPA Safety Factor(s) in Assessing Pesticide Tolerances.* Available online at: https://www.epa.gov/pesticide-science-and-assessing-pesticide-risks/determination-appropriate-fqpa-safety-factors

EPA, US. 2002b. *A Review of the Reference Dose and Reference Concentration Processes.* EPA/630/P-02/002F. Available online at: https://www.epa.gov/osa/review-reference-dose-and-reference-concentration-processes.

EPA, US. 2005a. *Supplemental Guidance for Assessing Susceptibility from Early-Life Exposure to Carcinogens.* EPA/630/R-03/003F. Available online at: https://www.epa.gov/risk/supplemental-guidance-assessing-susceptibility-early-life-exposure-carcinogens.

EPA, US. 2005b. *Guidance on Selecting Age Groups for Monitoring and Assessing Childhood Exposures to Environmental Contaminants.* (Washington, DC: Environmental Protection Agency).

EPA, US. 2006. *A Framework for Assessing Health Risk of Environmental Exposures to Children.* EPA/600/R-05/093F. Available online at: https://cfpub.epa.gov/ncea/risk/recordisplay.cfm?deid=158363.

EPA, US. 2011. *Exposure Factors Handbook: 2011 Edition*. EPA/600/R-09/052F. Available online at: https://www.epa.gov/expobox/about-exposure-factors-handbook.

EPA, US. 2018. *Protecting Children from Wildfire Smoke and Ash*. Available online at: https://www.airnow.gov/publications/wildfire-smoke-guide/protecting-children-from-wildfire-smoke-and-ash/.

EPA, US. 2019. *America's Children and the Environment*. Available online at: https://www.epa.gov/americaschildrenenvironment.

Felter, S. P., G. P. Daston, S.Y. Euling, H. Aldert, A.H. Piersma, and M.S. Tassinari 2015. Assessment of Health Risks Resulting from Early-Life Exposures: Are Current Chemical Toxicity Testing Protocols and Risk Assessment Methods Adequate? *Crit. Rev. Toxicol.* 45 (3): 219–244. https://doi.org/10.3109/10408444.2014.993919.

FQPA. 1996. *Food Quality Protection Act, Public Law 104–170, 1996*. Available online at: https://www.epa.gov/laws-regulations/summary-food-quality-protection-act. edited by FDA. Washington, DC: US Gov Printing Office.

Ginsberg, G., D. Hattis, R. Miller, and B. Sonawane. 2004. Pediatric Pharmacokinetic Data: Implications for Environmental Risk Assessment for Children. *Pediatrics* 113: 972–983. https://doi.org/10.1542/peds.113.4.S1.973. http://www.pediatrics.org/cgi/content/full/113/4/S1/973.

Ginsberg, G., D. Hattis, B. Sonawane, A. Russ, P. Banati, M. Kozlak, S. Smolenski, and R. Goble. 2002. Evaluation of Child/Adult Pharmacokinetic Differences from a Database Derived. *Toxicol. Sci.* 66: 185–200. https://doi.org/10.1093/toxsci/66.2.185.

Ginsberg, G., S. V. Vulimiri, Y. S. Lin, J. Kancherla, B. Foos, and B. A. Sonawane. 2017. Evaluation of Enzyme Ontogeny in Children's Health Risk Evaluation. *J. Toxicol. Environ. Health* 80 (10–12): 569–573. https://doi.org/10.1080/15287394.2017.1369915. https://www.ncbi.nlm.nih.gov/pmc/articles/PMC8018602/pdf/nihms-1675930.pdf

Hattis, D., G. Ginsberg, B. Sonawane, S. Smolenski, A. Russ, M. Kozlak, and R. Goble. 2003. Children's Variability in Drug Elimination Half-Lives and in Some Parameters Needed for Physiologically Based Pharmacokinetic Modeling. *Risk Anal.* 23 (1): 117–142. https://doi.org/0272-4332/03/1200-0117.

Kapraun, D. F., J. F. Wambaugh, R. W. Setzer, and R. S. Judson. 2019. Empirical Models for Anatomical and Physiological Changes in a Human Mother and Fetus During Pregnancy and Gestation. *PLoS One* 14 (5): e0215906. https://doi.org/10.1371/journal.pone.0215906.

Lehmann, G. M., M. A. Verner, B. Luukinen, C. Henning, S.A. Assimon, J. S. LaKind, E. D. McLanahan, L. J. Phillips, M. H. Davis, C. M. Powers, E. P. Hines, S. Haddad, M. P. Longnecker, M. T. Poulsen, D. G. Farrer, S. A. Marchitti, Y. M. Tan, J. C. Swartout, S. K. Sagiv, C. Welsh, J. L. Jr. Campbell, W. G. Foster, R. S. Yang, S. E. Fenton, R. Tornero-Velez, B. M. Francis, J. B. Barnett, H. A. El-Masri, and J. E. Simmons. 2014. Improving the Risk Assessment of Lipophilic Persistent Environmental Chemicals in Breast Milk. *Crit. Rev. Toxicol.* 44 (7): 600–617. https://doi.org/10.3109/10408444.2014.926306

Li, N., Y. Liu, G. D. Papandonatos, A. M. Calafat, C. B. Eaton, K. T. Kelsey, K. M. Cecil, H. J. Kalkwarf, K. Yolton, B. P. Lanphear, A. Chen, and J. M. Braun. 2021. Gestational and Childhood Exposure to Per- and Polyfluoroalkyl Substances and Cardiometabolic Risk at Age 12 Years. *Environ. Int.* 147: 106344. https://doi.org/10.1016/j.envint.2020.106344.

Mikeš, O., M. Vrbová, J. Klánová, P. Čupr, J. Švancara, and H Pikhart. 2019. Early-Life Exposure to Household Chemicals and Wheezing in Children. *Sci.Total Environ.* 663: 418–425. https://doi.org/10.1016/j.scitotenv.2019.01.254.

NRC. 1983. *Risk Assessment in the Federal Government: Managing the Process*. Washington, DC: National Academies Press.

NRC. 1993. *Pesticides in the Diets of Infants and Children*. Washington, DC: National Academies Press.

OECD. 2019. *Considerations When Assessing Children's Exposure to Chemicals from Products*. ENV/JM/MONO(2019)29. OECD (Stockholm). http://www.oecd.org/officialdocuments/publicdisplaydocumentpdf/?cote=ENV/JM/MONO(2019)29&docLanguage=en.

Payne–Sturges, D. C., D. Cory-Slechta, R. C. Puett, S. B. Thomas, R. Hammond, and P. S. Hovmand. 2021. Defining and Intervening on Cumulative Environmental Neurodevelopmental Risks: Introducing a Complex Systems Approach. *Environ. Health Persp.* 129. https://doi.org/10.1289/EHP7333.

Raghuveer, G., D. A. White, L. L. Hayman, J. G. Woo, J. Villafane, D. Celermajer, K. D. Ward, S. D. de Ferranti, J. Zachariah, American Heart Association Committee on Lifestyle and Cardiometabolic Health, and Council on Epidemiology and Prevention, and Stroke Council. 2016. Cardiovascular Consequences of Childhood Secondhand Tobacco Smoke Exposure: Prevailing Evidence, Burden, and Racial and

Socioeconomic Disparities: A Scientific Statement from the American Heart Association. *Circulation* 134(16): e336–e359. https://doi.org/10.1161/CIR.0000000000000443.

SDWA. 1974. *Summary of the Safe Drinking Water Act*. Available online at: https://www.epa.gov/laws-regulations/summary-safe-drinking-water-act. edited by Executive Branch. Washington, DC: US Government Printing Office.

Selevan, S., C. A. Kimmel, and P. Mendola. 2000. Identifying Critical Windows of Exposure for Children's Health. *Environ. Health Persp.* 108, no. 3: 451–456. https://doi.org/10.1289/ehp.00108s3451.

Trent, M., D. G. Dooley, and J. Dougé. 2019. American Academy of Pediatrics Section on Adolescent Health; Council on Community Pediatrics; Committee on Adolescence. The Impact of Racism on Child and Adolescent Health. *Pediatrics* 144 (2): e20191765. https://doi.org/10.1542/peds.2019-176.

US Congress. 2016a. *Frank R. Lautenberg Chemical Safety for the 21st Century Act*. Pub. L. No. 114-182, 130 Stat. 448 (114th Congress, 22 June 2016). https://www.congress.gov/114/plaws/publ182/PLAW-114publ182.pdf.

US Congress. 2016b. *Toxic Substances Control Act*. Available online at: https://www.epa.gov/laws-regulations/summary-toxic-substances-control-act. 15 U.S.C. §2601 et seq.

WHO. 2008. *Closing the Gap in a Generation: Health Equity Through Action on the Social Determinants of Health. Final Report of the Commission on Social Determinants of Health*. World Health Organization (Geneva: Commission on the Social Determinants of Health). Available online at: https://www.who.int/publications/i/item/WHO-IER-CSDH-08.1

Yang, C. L., H. K. Lee, A. P. S. Kong, L.L. Lim, Z. Cai, and A. C. K. Chung. 2018. Early-Life Exposure to Endocrine Disrupting Chemicals Associates with Childhood Obesity. *Ann. Pediatr. Endocrinol. Metab.* 23 (4): 182–195. https://doi.org/10.6065/apem.2018.23.4.182.

Yoon, M., and H. J. Clewell, 3rd. 2016. Addressing Early Life Sensitivity Using Physiologically Based Pharmacokinetic Modeling and In Vitro to In Vivo Extrapolation. *Toxicol. Res.* 32 (1): 15–20. https://doi.org/10.5487/TR.2016.32.1.015.

14 Addressing the Limits of Risk Assessment by Focusing on Safer Alternatives Risk Assessment for Environmental Health

Joel Tickner and Molly Jacobs
University of Massachusetts Lowell, Lowell, MA, United States

Margaret H. Whittaker
ToxServices LLC, Washington, DC United States

CONTENTS

Introduction 280
Limits of the Risk-Based Approach 280
    Overview 280
    Limits of Risk Assessment as a Tool 281
    Challenges When Integrated into Policy Decision-Making 283
    Addressing the Limits of Risk Assessment 286
From a Risk Focus to One Based on Safer Solutions 287
    Defining Alternatives Assessment 289
    History of Alternatives Assessment 291
Frameworks for Alternatives Assessment and Core Components 296
    Alternatives Assessment Frameworks 296
    Alternatives Assessment Components 296
Hazard Assessment 298
    Hazard Screening 298
    Full Hazard Assessment Methods and Tools 299
Comparative Exposure Assessment 301
Other Life Cycle Impact Considerations 304
Research Gaps in Alternatives Assessment – a Role for Risk Assessors 304
Data Gaps in Hazard Assessment 305
    NAMS in Alternatives Assessment 305
    Addressing Uncertainty in NAMs and IATAs 307
        Reducing Type I Uncertainties Related to the Input Data Used 307
        Reducing Type 2 Uncertainties Related to Extrapolations Made 307
        Example Uncertainty Analyses for Two Major Types of Uncertainties: Cyrene™
        (CAS#53716-82-8) 307
    Incorporating Toxicological Data and Exposure Information into the Design of
    Safer Alternatives 310
Conclusion 310
Additional Resources 312
References 312
Literature Cited 312

LEARNING OBJECTIVES

Students who complete this chapter will be able to

1. Understand some of the critiques and limitations of risk assessment and its application in chemicals decision-making,
2. Outline underlying rationale and history of alternatives assessment,
3. Understand the key steps of an alternatives assessment and research needs, and
4. Understand how the tools of alternatives assessment and risk assessment intersect through developments in toxicology.

DOI: 10.1201/9780429291722-14

INTRODUCTION

There are tens of thousands of chemicals in commerce today and an even greater number of chemical mixtures. While data on chemical hazards have increased significantly in the last decade, in part due to regulatory mandates and new tools like New Approach Methods (NAMs), information on chemical use and exposure across the life cycle of thousands of products is still limited. Since the 1980s, risk assessment has evolved as a science-policy tool for decision-making on chemical safety. Risk assessment is the standard tool for regulatory decision-making on chemicals in industrialized countries and is used by manufacturers to determine product safety. While risk assessment and its tool kit provide important input into decision-making, recent experience with Per- and Polyfluoroalkyl Substances (PFAS) provide clear evidence of the challenges of a risk-based approach to decision-making. More than 5,000 PFAS compounds have been identified in the literature, and while studies have been undertaken on uses, there is still limited knowledge as to all of the applications of this unique chemistry in practice. While significant research is increasing understanding of fate and transport, there are still important uncertainties with regard to this class of Persistent and Mobile Toxics (PMT). Tens of millions of dollars have been spent in recent years studying toxicity, exposures, and fate and transport, as well as on cleanup of contaminated water sources. A drinking water standard has yet to be established. Yet, PFAS have a unique chemistry that provide important functionality in a number of products, which, in many cases, is not equaled by alternatives. PFAS represent just a small portion of the universe of chemicals commonly used in manufacturing processes and products, which number in the tens of thousands, with hundreds of thousands of different mixtures. Assessing and then managing these in the current chemical-by-chemical, risk-by-risk decision-making process will take too long. Unfortunately, as risks are being studied, evaluated, debated, and actions proposed, the default is frequently no action, meaning exposure continues.

Nonetheless, there are increasing regulatory and market pressures to phase out chemicals of concern in products and production processes. But eliminating a chemical of concern without consideration of its replacements can lead to "regrettable substitutes" where risks of the alternative are greater or transferred to another population. The science-policy field of alternatives assessment evolved to provide a systematic and consistent approach to compare safer options to achieve the functionality of a chemical of concern in a particular application. Assessing potential chemical substitutes requires evaluation against a broad range of human, environmental, and physical hazard end points using established frameworks that allow for comparison between chemical alternatives. Such multiattribute assessments include evaluation of a broad array of health and environmental toxicity and fate end points. Over the past decade, the use of alternatives assessment in comparing chemicals for a particular application has grown significantly, and a new professional society for the field – the Association for the Advancement of Alternatives Assessment has been established.

Alternatives assessment utilizes many of the same toxicological and exposure-related tools as those in the risk assessment tool kit but applies these tools to understand the pros and cons of alternatives, supporting substitution decisions. Alternatives assessment provides a more proactive and expedited approach to addressing chemical risks through a focus on driving solutions. Increasingly, guidance pertaining to safer chemical selection and identification, such as the Organisation for Economic Co-operation and Development's (OECD) *Guidance on Key Considerations for the Identification and Selection of Safer Chemical Alternatives* published in 2021 (OECD 2021a), challenges risk assessors to actively participate in informed substitution activities and adhere to a consistent understanding of the minimum requirements to determine whether a chemical alternative is safer.

In this chapter, we present some of the limitations of risk assessment and the risk-based approach typically used to address the enormity of toxic chemical challenges. We introduce readers to the field of alternatives assessment, its history, and components, and then provide a detailed analysis of how alternatives assessment and the tools of risk assessment, including emerging directions in toxicology, intersect to support the development and substitution of safer chemicals and products.

LIMITS OF THE RISK-BASED APPROACH

Overview

There are tens of thousands of chemicals in commerce, many used in a multitude of applications with varying exposure profiles. The 2018 United Nations (UN) Global Chemicals Outlook II (identified the extent of global chemicals challenge). The authors stated, "The findings of the GCO-II indicate that the sound management of chemicals and waste and minimizing adverse impacts will not be achieved by 2020 (GCO 2019). Trends data suggest that the projected doubling of the global chemicals market between 2017 and 2030 will increase global chemical releases, exposures, concentrations and adverse health and environmental impacts unless the sound management of chemicals and waste is achieved worldwide. Business as usual is therefore not an option."

The authors spotlight the significant contributions of chemical exposures to the global burden of disease. The GCO identifies known or suspected health impacts from chemical exposures, such as cancer, nervous system damage, sensitization, and endocrine and reproductive system damage, that result in health costs upwards of 10% of global gross domestic product, while the US-based Collaborative on Health and Environment links chemical exposures to more than 180 different illnesses. The World Health Organization conservatively estimates that 1.6 million lives and 45 million disability-adjusted life years were lost in 2016 due to exposures to selected chemicals (not including many chemicals with known chronic impacts). The GCO II (GCO 2019) notes a number of challenges to better chemicals assessment and management globally, including the lack of data on toxicity and chemical uses and exposures for many chemicals and the fact that chemical exposures are ubiquitous in the environment. Importantly, chemical production and use are growing fastest in industrializing nations, which have the least scientific capacity to assess and evaluate chemicals.

These challenges limit our ability to evaluate chemical toxicity, use, and ultimately risks for tens of thousands of chemicals. There are simply insufficient resources to do that. However, over the past 40 years, the US regulatory and scientific response to chemical pollution has relied heavily on quantitative risk assessment. This response was heavily influenced by the US regulatory and political system, as well as the courts, where threats of judicial scrutiny force agencies to constantly construct formal, quantitative records (von Moltke 1987). Risk assessment methods presuppose the ability to objectively and adequately characterize and quantify complex hazards and their probability of occurrence. These predictions are then incorporated into decisions that are based on preestablished levels of "reasonable" or "acceptable" risks (for example, 1 in 1,000 excess cases of disease is considered acceptable for workplace exposures) and often economic and technical feasibility. Risk assessment was originally developed for mechanical problems such as bridge construction, where the technical process and parameters are well-defined and can be analyzed. Wynne (Wynne 1993) notes that by definition risk indicates that probabilities of occurrence are fairly well understood, whereas in most chemical risk decisions, available information and uncertainties do not allow for such precision.

While the techniques of risk assessment have evolved over the years to address different disease end points and to incorporate broader notions of exposure and greater analysis of uncertainty, the general framework for conducting risk assessments remains the same as when the National Research Council (NRC) *Red Book* was published in 1983: hazard identification, dose-response assessment, exposure assessment, and risk characterization research (NRC 1983). Risk assessment (science) is also generally separated from risk management (policy). The development of risk assessment has brought substantial advances in scientific understanding of exposure and disease and our ability to predict adverse outcomes from chemical exposures. Risk assessment is a useful tool for predicting outcomes in a data-rich environment when the nature of the harm is specific and well-characterized and probabilities are well established. It provides a useful tool to understand product safety and appropriate levels of clean up. And it provides a standardized, structured methodology for decision-making. Nearly all decisions involve some weighing of risks, either qualitatively or quantitatively.

Limits of Risk Assessment as a Tool

The reliance on risk assessment as the prominent analytical technique to address chemical exposures has significant disadvantages. Novel and complex risks – such as those associated with low-dose exposures to toxic chemicals during development and new materials, such as engineering nanomaterials – pose fundamental challenges to quantitative risk assessment. Specific criticisms of quantitative risk assessment and application regulatory decision-making include the following:

Limiting broader understanding of risks. Risk assessment can limit the breadth of information and disciplines used in examining chemical hazards. Numerical determinations can "crumple" into a single value, losing track of nuances and qualitative details about that information. This may inhibit a holistic understanding of complex systems and considerations such as multiple exposures, cumulative effects, sensitive populations, or less studied end points (such as

BOX 14.1   BISPHENOL A (BPA) – A CASE OF THE CHALLENGES OF A RISK-BASED
SYSTEM

Joel Tickner, Molly Jacobs and Margaret H. Whittaker

While research on the potential health impacts of BPA dates back some 60 years, it has grown significantly since 2000. During this period scientific understanding of BPA exposures and toxicity have grown significantly, though there have been some uncertainties about major sources of exposure, how the chemical is distributed and metabolized in the body, and the extent to which effects seen in animals are transferable to humans. For over a decade, these uncertainties led to vigorous debates over "how bad" BPA really is. Competing expert panels and agencies with different regulatory risk assessment approaches came to differing conclusions. In 2009, the US National Institutes of Environmental Health Sciences set aside more than 30 million dollars for research on the contribution of low-dose exposures of BPA to obesity, diabetes, and other chronic effects. However, no funds were provided for studying alternatives. Starting in 2009, government agencies in several states and countries moved to restrict BPA in baby bottles, thermal tape, and other children's articles. Well-organized advocacy efforts resulted in significant media attention and a very rapid marketplace substitution of BPA in specific high-profile applications, like baby bottles (Tickner, 2011). Given the short time frames for substitution, many manufacturers switched to similar bisphenol compounds, resulting in regrettable substitutes that were well documented. Finally, in 2021, the European Food Safety Authority, which for years had argued that BPA exposure from food contact uses was of low concern, lowered its recommended daily dose by fivefold, which will all but prohibit BPA use in food contact materials, though little mention is made of safer alternatives.

The BPA example highlights a large problem in our system: a narrow focus on characterizing problems in terms of causes and mechanisms as the basis for subsequent action. Such a reactive approach can lead to extended debates over mechanisms, dueling scientists and scientific panels, and ultimately inaction or, equally problematic, regrettable substitutes. While millions of dollars have been invested in studying detailed aspects of BPA exposure and toxicity, much less funding has been made available to evaluate alternatives to BPA. And given the wide range of uses of BPA – dental, food contact, solvents, safety items – and the range of agencies that regulate it in these different uses – there is no coordinated national approach to substituting uses of concern for BPA and implementing safer alternatives. Importantly, some manufacturers are taking an approach to developing and assessing BPA alternatives that meet functional requirements, while reducing risks. Valspar, in developing its valPure BPA-free can lining, used the tools of chemistry and toxicology to develop an alternative bisphenol-based lining that was evaluated by leading endocrine disruption scientists and found to be lacking endocrine activity (Tickner et al. 2021).

developmental toxicity) or potential alternatives to the chemical. O'Brien (2000) asks whether the "risk assessment frame is large enough" to address chemical challenges.

Limited interdisciplinary perspectives. In a risk assessment approach, scientists often study risks from a disciplinary perspective (for example, human toxicology), even though it might take an interdisciplinary approach to synthesize sufficient evidence to adequately characterize a problem or its solutions. Emerging risks, such as those of global change or endocrine-disrupting chemicals would never have been recognized without the combined effect of concerns raised by different disciplines (Colborn and Clement 1992; McMichael 1993). Multidisciplinary teams will be more likely to find new ways to frame hypotheses, evaluate qualitative and quantitative data, and examine options and trade-offs that lead to insights not possible from narrow disciplinary viewpoints. As Colborn and Clement noted when developing the endocrine disruption hypothesis, "[S]o shocking was this revelation (about the widespread observation of endocrine disruption in wildlife that no scientist could have expressed the idea using only the data from his or her discipline alone without losing the respect of his or her peers."

Limited consideration of uncertainties. Formal evaluation of uncertainty in risk assessment is generally limited to a narrow discussion of errors in main results or some type of sensitivity analysis. But these may leave out potentially more important sources of uncertainty such as errors in the model used to analyze and interpret data, variability and susceptibility of specific populations, systemic uncertainties such as the impacts of poverty on health, interactions of variables, and biases from limitations in the conduct of the study (see Bailar and Bailer 1999). Gaps in understanding about exposures, human behavior, chemical effects, and chemical fate are often addressed through assumptions or safety factors that may or may not be fully transparent in the assessment process. As a result, two risk assessments – even using the same data – may come up with fundamentally different answers depending on who conducts them. Further, current forms of uncertainty analysis leave out critical questions such as interpretations of what is known or not known or what is suspected.

Attempts to get overly precise estimates of risk. Because of the challenges that uncertainty poses in policy decision-making, scientists often focus efforts on assessing limited, quantifiable aspects of problems, like the relationship between a single chemical and a single disease, without examining the potentially important but more difficult to demonstrate aspects of disease such as exposure to multiple toxic substances, new end points, or the unique susceptibility of particular subpopulations like teenagers (see Kriebel et al. 2001). A related tendency is to refine understanding and increase detail about specific substances or hazards (for example, mechanisms of toxicity) rather than explore new questions. While such increased understanding is interesting from a scientific perspective, it often slows down preventive actions. In these cases, the search for more detailed understanding may be misinterpreted as insufficient knowledge to act and may mask what is already known about a hazard. Long debates on chemicals such as styrene and formaldehyde demonstrate this tendency. Legal scholar Carl Cranor notes that in these cases, "the attempt to have more fine-grained knowledge about the risks from a particular substance may actually increase the number of mistakes made" (Cranor 1993).

Failing to study cumulative exposures. Scientists generally study the direct effects of single exposures rather than exposures to multiple chemicals and other stressors – our everyday reality. For example, fence-line chemical manufacturing communities are exposed to air and water contaminants from the manufacturing process, in addition to chemicals in products they purchase and use in their homes, as well as workplace exposures. In part due to this complexity, the problem has received little attention to date but is gaining recognition with the growing importance of the environmental justice movement.

Failure to include affected communities in the assessment process. Risk assessments are often completed by experts far removed from the communities that they are assessing. This may lead to ignoring critical exposure or other information from workers, communities, or other "experts" potentially inhibiting the evaluation process. Further, affected communities may be more interested in specific preventive actions rather than a more nuanced understanding of the risks to which they are exposed.

Challenges When Integrated into Policy Decision-Making

Risk assessments are generally used for quantifying and analyzing problems rather than trying to solve or prevent them. Quantitative risk assessments are generally used to set "safe" levels of exposure rather than to identify and compare alternative actions that can prevent risk in the first place. This assumes that a "safe" or "acceptable" level of exposure can be established, particularly where there are gaps in knowledge about hazards, uses, or exposures. Evolving understanding of the toxicity of chemicals such as lead, mercury, bisphenol-a, phthalates, and now PFAS often reveal that "safe" exposures set by governments were vastly underestimated. Risk assessments also assume that particular chemicals and their applications and the risks they pose are inevitable. In essence, the necessity of risk is rarely considered. Risk assessments are generally expensive and time-consuming, tying up limited agency resources in developing detailed understandings of risk, while similar resource investments could be used to develop and implement safer processes, materials, and products. For example, while a typical two-year cancer bioassay for a single chemical may cost several million dollars, the US Environmental Protection Agency (US EPA) budget for safer chemicals and green chemistry – the design and application of chemicals – is less than that. The disproportional investment in risk assessment is not only costly and slows actions to protect health, but it is also inefficient and can be a hindrance to innovation in safer chemicals and products.

The regulatory system in the United States and in many other countries perpetuates the limits of risk assessment. To make decisions more defensible, decision-makers often prefer to release

BOX 14.2   A RISK ASSESSMENT CHALLENGE: HOW DO WE MANAGE THOUSANDS OF EXTREMELY PERSISTENT AND UBIQUITOUS CHEMICALS?

Simona Andreea Bălan

BACKGROUND

Per- and polyfluoroalkyl substances (PFASs) are a class of thousands of chemicals that contain at least one fully fluorinated carbon atom (OECD 2021). In recent years, PFASs have been recognized as a complex global problem due to their extreme environmental persistence combined with high mobility and potential toxicity. Nevertheless, due to their unique physico-chemical properties, PFASs continue to be used in over 200 applications, including textiles, food packaging, cosmetics, firefighting foam, cellphones, aircrafts, and alternative energy sources (Glüge et al. 2020). PFASs have improved the convenience of many consumer products but at the expense of widespread human and ecological exposures, with potential adverse impacts for generations to come. Depending on the chemical, adverse health outcomes may be observed at very low levels. For instance, some scientists recommend 1 part per trillion (ppt) in drinking water as the maximum safe level of exposure for perfluorooctanoic acid (PFOA) (Grandjean and Clapp 2015). The drinking water of more than 200 million Americans (Andrews and Naidenko 2020) and 450 million Chinese (Liu et al. 2021) may exceed that level.

So how can we deal with such a complex problem? The scientific community is making great progress at quantifying exposures and setting health benchmarks, but thus far only for a few members of the PFAS class. Faced with major data gaps, authorities around the world are employing a range of strategies for dealing with PFASs, including single chemical, mixture, arrowhead, and chemical class approaches.

As the name implies, the **single chemical approach** regulates individual chemicals based on available toxicity and exposure information through a formal risk assessment process. This approach has been used, for instance, by the Stockholm Convention (UNEP 2020), the European Chemicals Agency (ECHA 2020), the US EPA (US EPA 2020), and several US states seeking to regulate PFASs in drinking water (ASDWA 2021). However, fewer than a dozen PFASs have enough data for a standard risk assessment.

Unlike the single chemical approach, the **mixture approach** considers cumulative impacts and aggregate exposures, which is important since individual PFASs rarely occur in isolation. The US Food and Drug Administration (FDA) uses this approach, to some extent, when regulating PFASs in food packaging. Because the mixture approach requires detailed toxicity and exposure data for each mixture constituent, it allows for the continued use of chemicals in consumer products until sufficient toxicological evidence indicates concerns (FDA 2021).

The **arrowhead approach** sets standards for an arrowhead chemical that is well characterized and can be considered representative for a group of related chemicals. It assumes that by regulating the levels of the arrowhead chemical the levels of the other chemicals in the group will also be controlled. The arrowhead approach has been commonly applied to regulating PFASs in consumer products, typically targeting a perfluoroalkyl acid (PFAA) plus all its salts and precursors (Cousins et al. 2020). However, because of its focus on the toxicity of the PFAA arrowhead chemical, this risk management approach fails to consider the hazards of the PFAA salts and precursors, some of which can be more toxic (Rice et al. 2020).

The **chemical class approach** considers the aggregate exposures and cumulative impacts of a whole class of chemicals throughout their life cycle, including those of known and unknown environmental transformation products. Regulating PFASs as a class has been proposed as the most effective way to address the nonessential uses of PFASs (Cousins et al. 2019; Kwiatkowski et al. 2020) and drive the adoption of safer alternatives (Bălan et al. 2021).

The California Department of Toxic Substances Control (DTSC) is among the growing number of regulatory agencies approaching PFASs as a class. DTSC's Safer Consumer Products (SCP) program enacted regulations for carpets and rugs containing any member of the class of PFASs (DTSC 2021a) and is proposing similar regulations for treatments intended for use on converted textiles and leathers (DTSC 2021b). Several other US states and European Union countries are similarly taking a chemical class approach to regulating PFASs. Of note, as of July 2020, Denmark banned the intentional use of all PFASs in cardboard and paper used as food contact materials (Danish Ministry of Environment and Food 2019; Keller and Heckman LLP 2020). Furthermore, in December 2020, the European Parliament formally adopted a revised drinking water directive that includes the first limit for the sum of all PFASs in the world (European Commission 2020).

REFERENCES

Andrews, David Q., and Olga V. Naidenko. 2020. "Population-Wide Exposure to per- and Polyfluoroalkyl Substances from Drinking Water in the United States." *Environmental Science & Technology Letters*, October. https://doi.org/10.1021/acs.estlett.0c00713.

ASDWA. 2021. "Per- and Polyfluoroalkyl Substances (PFAS). Association of State Drinking Water Administrators (ASDWA)." https://www.asdwa.org/pfas/.

Bălan, Simona Andreea, Vivek Chander Mathrani, Dennis Fengmao Guo, and André Maurice Algazi. 2021. "Regulating PFAS as a Chemical Class under the California Safer Consumer Products Program." *Environmental Health Perspectives* 129 (2): 025001. https://doi.org/10.1289/EHP7431.

Cousins, Ian T., Jamie C. DeWitt, Juliane Glüge, Gretta Goldenman, Dorte Herzke, Rainer Lohmann, Mark Miller, et al. 2020. "Strategies for Grouping Per- and Polyfluoroalkyl Substances (PFAS) to Protect Human and Environmental Health." *Environmental Science: Processes & Impacts* 22 (7): 1444–1460. https://doi.org/10.1039/D0EM00147C.

Cousins, Ian T, Gretta Goldenman, Dorte Herzke, Rainer Lohmann, Mark Miller, Sharyle Patton, Martin Scheringer, et al. 2019. "The Concept of Essential Use for Determining When Uses of PFASs Can Be Phased Out." *Environmental Science: Processes & Impacts*, (11): 1803–1815. https://doi.org/10.1039/C9EM00163H.

Danish Ministry of Environment and Food. 2019. "The Minister of Food Is Ready to Ban Fluoride Substances." September 2, 2019. https://mfvm.dk/nyheder/nyhed/nyhed/foedevareministeren-er-klar-til-at-forbyde-fluorstoffer/.

DTSC. 2021a. "Effective July 1, 2021: Carpets and Rugs with Perfluoroalkyl or Polyfluoroalkyl Substances (PFASs). Department of Toxic Substances Control (DTSC)." Department of Toxic Substances Control. 2021. https://dtsc.ca.gov/scp/carpets-and-rugs-with-perfluoroalkyl-and-polyfluoroalkyl-substances-pfass/.

DTSC. 2021b. "Proposed Priority Product: Treatments Containing Perfluoroalkyl or Polyfluoroalkyl Substances for Use on Converted Textiles or Leathers. Department of Toxic Substances Control (DTSC)." Department of Toxic Substances Control. 2021. https://dtsc.ca.gov/scp/treatments-with-pfass/.

ECHA. 2020. "European Chemicals Agency (ECHA): Candidate List of Substances of Very High Concern for Authorisation." 2020. https://echa.europa.eu/web/guest/candidate-list-table.

European Commission. 2020. "The Revised Drinking Water Directive." 2020. https://ec.europa.eu/environment/water/water-drink/legislation_en.html.

FDA. 2021. "Food and Drug Administration (FDA): Packaging & Food Contact Substances (FCS)." *FDA*. September 1, 2021. http://www.fda.gov/food/food-ingredients-packaging/packaging-food-contact-substances-fcs.

Glüge, Juliane, Martin Scheringer, Ian T. Cousins, Jamie C. DeWitt, Gretta Goldenman, Dorte Herzke, Rainer Lohmann, Carla A. Ng, Xenia Trier, and Zhanyun Wang. 2020. "An Overview of the Uses of Per- and Polyfluoroalkyl Substances (PFAS)." *Environmental Science: Processes & Impacts* 22 (12): 2345–2373. https://doi.org/10.1039/D0EM00291G.

Grandjean, Philippe, and Richard Clapp. 2015. "Perfluorinated Alkyl Substances: Emerging Insights into Health Risks." *New Solutions* 25 (2): 147–163. https://doi.org/10.1177/1048291115590506.

Keller and Heckman LLP. 2020. "Denmark's PFAS Ban in Paper and Cardboard Effective in July 2020." *The National Law Review*. June 16, 2020. https://www.natlawreview.com/article/denmark-s-pfas-ban-paper-and-cardboard-effective-july-2020.

Kwiatkowski, Carol F., David Q. Andrews, Linda S. Birnbaum, Thomas A. Bruton, Jamie C. DeWitt, Detlef R. U. Knappe, Maricel V. Maffini, et al. 2020. "Scientific Basis for Managing PFAS as a Chemical Class." *Environmental Science & Technology Letters*, June. https://doi.org/10.1021/acs.estlett.0c00255.

Liu, Liquan, Yingxi Qu, Jun Huang, and Roland Weber. 2021. "Per- and Polyfluoroalkyl Substances (PFASs) in Chinese Drinking Water: Risk Assessment and Geographical Distribution." *Environmental Sciences Europe* 33 (1): 6. https://doi.org/10.1186/s12302-020-00425-3.

OECD. 2021. "Reconciling Terminology of the Universe of Per- and Polyfluoroalkyl Substances: Recommendations and Practical Guidance. Organisation for Economic Co-Operation and Development (OECD)." Series on Risk Management, No. 61. https://www.oecd.org/officialdocuments/publicdisplaydocumentpdf/?cote=ENV/CBC/MONO(2021)25&docLanguage=en.

Rice, Penelope A., Jason Aungst, Jessica Cooper, Omari Bandele, and Shruti V. Kabadi. 2020. "Comparative Analysis of the Toxicological Databases for 6:2 Fluorotelomer Alcohol (6:2 FTOH) and Perfluorohexanoic Acid (PFHxA)." *Food and Chemical Toxicology* 138 (April): 111210. https://doi.org/10.1016/j.fct.2020.111210.

UNEP. 2020. "United Nations Environment Programme (UNEP): All POPs Listed in the Stockholm Convention." 2020. http://chm.pops.int/TheConvention/ThePOPs/AllPOPs/tabid/2509/Default.aspx.

U.S. EPA. 2020. "U.S. Environmental Protection Agency (U.S. EPA): Risk Management for Per- and Polyfluoroalkyl Substances (PFASs) under TSCA." Overviews and Factsheets. 2020. https://www.epa.gov/assessing-and-managing-chemicals-under-tsca/risk-management-and-polyfluoroalkyl-substances-pfass.

seemingly precise estimates of risk and minimize the uncertainties underlying the numbers or fail to study specific problems – for example, cumulative effects of multiple exposures – if their tools or methods are not fully developed or might be challenged by regulated parties or others. Unfortunately, as the regulatory system generally assumes most chemical exposures are safe until demonstrated harmful by government agencies, it is often in the interest of those fighting regulation to convert political questions (should we act or not) into technical/scientific ones so as to delay regulation – also called manufactured or "smokescreen" uncertainty. Long debates over mechanisms of action (including whether animal models are relevant to humans) and exposure scenarios for halogenated solvents such as trichloroethylene and methylene chloride and other chemicals such as formaldehyde and styrene monomer have delayed regulatory actions for years while nuances in the science are debated. While these areas of research are interesting and important from a scientific knowledge perspective, they also have the potential to tie up research and regulatory policy in long debates over minute details of risk – all at the expense of primary prevention.

Unfortunately, limits in risk assessment to quantify risks or the decision to study a problem more are often misinterpreted as proof of safety. For example, when initially responding to concerns about the health impacts on children of phthalates used as plasticizers in polyvinyl chloride medical devices such as IV bags and tubing, the US Food and Drug Administration (FDA) and the medical device industry stated that these substances had been used safely for 40 years without any evidence of human impacts (Phthalate Information Center 2003). Biologist John Cairns has noted that scientists and policymakers often discount highly uncertain risks, concluding, "Unrecognized risks are still risks, uncertain risks are still risks, and denied risks are still risks" (Cairns 1999). For example, all chemicals on the market today that were on the market in 1980 were "grandfathered" under the Toxic Substances Control Act, meaning that to regulate them, the EPA must demonstrate a significant risk. While the Lautenberg Chemical Safety for the 21st Century Act reduced EPA's burdens significantly to act on chemical exposures, the agency is only required to assess and create risk management plans for 20 chemicals per year. Hence it will take decades until the agency adequately assesses risks and acts on most chemicals in commerce that are considered "approved" until then.

Addressing the Limits of Risk Assessment

Government agencies and the risk assessment community have made significant progress in recognizing and responding to criticisms about risk assessment and its use and developing recommendations to improve but still rely heavily on the process. Reports by the NRC (1994, 2007, 2008, 2009; Stern and Fineberg 1996) and the Presidential Commission on Risk Assessment and Risk Management (NRC 1997), among others, have recommended changes to the process of risk assessment that would

- better and more comprehensively examine uncertainty and variability,

- include affected publics throughout the risk assessment and management process (from problem definition through risk management),

- increase consideration of prevention and options in the risk assessment process,

- provide more holistic problem definition,

- include greater consideration of cumulative and interactive effects and sensitive subpopulations, and

- undertake a greater evaluation of actions taken.

While these recommendations point in the right direction, there is a need to expand the risk assessment toolbox to include consideration of safer alternatives that can avoid risks in the first place.

FROM A RISK FOCUS TO ONE BASED ON SAFER SOLUTIONS

"One of the most essential, and powerful steps to change is understanding that there are alternatives." – Mary O'Brien

In the previous section, we noted that analysts have criticized the current approach to chemicals assessment and management as resource intensive, slow, and reactionary. This has resulted in a relatively small number of chemicals being assessed or acted upon. High regulatory burdens are reinforced by a scientific research paradigm that focuses on securing detailed explanations of causality before issuing conclusions or recommendations – what might be called a "knowledge-first" approach. As the Leadership Council of the CDC/ATSDR-sponsored *National Conversation on Public Health and Chemical Exposures* noted,

Adequate protection of the public's health is hampered by deficient testing and information collection authority, fragmentation and segregation of critically related public health concerns into separate agency silos, lack of communication between agencies, limited transparency and accountability, inadequate funding, inappropriate placement of the burden to prove harm, and insufficient attention to the concerns of vulnerable communities.

A fundamental shift of emphasis is needed in our nation's approach to chemical exposures toward the development, adoption, and evaluation of safer alternatives. Preventing and eliminating problems at the source before harm occurs is a fundamental and proactive public health goal. Given that it is impossible to have full scientific certainty regarding public health risks, however, policymakers need decision-making tools that employ scientific rigor and encourage a common-sense, precautionary approach.

Developing a comprehensive understanding of human and ecosystem hazards and exposures is critical to prevention, but as the NRC noted in 2012, "The focus on problem identification sometimes occurs at the expense of efforts to use scientific tools to develop safer technologies and solutions. Defining problems without a comparable effort to find solutions can diminish the value of applied research efforts." If agency actions restrict the use of a specific chemical based on concerns over risks, there is a responsibility to understand alternatives and support a path forward that is environmentally sound, technically feasible, and economically viable.

An approach to chemicals assessment and management based on safer alternatives and substitution can help support responsible action and has several direct benefits to the environment and health, including the following:

1. *Focusing on solutions rather than problems.* Alternatives assessment reorients environmental protection discussions from problems to solutions – what might be termed a sustainable solutions agenda. Instead of examining the risks of one chemical of concern, alternatives assessment focuses on choices and opportunities. It draws attention to what a government agency or proponent of an activity could be doing to solve the problem at hand. Examining choices permits a broader range of questions and considerations about a chemical or product, including its need. Focusing on solutions provides hope rather than accepting the inevitability of impacts on human and ecosystem health.

2. *Stimulating innovation and prevention.* Alternatives assessment processes can lead to innovation and produce substantial cost-savings for firms as well as health and environmental benefits for society, including workers. Alternatives assessment calls attention to current and "on-the-horizon" alternatives and identifies gaps where further research to develop new solutions is needed. Resources that might otherwise be directed solely to resource-intensive processes of characterizing problems can focus on solutions.

3. *Multi-risk reduction.* Alternatives assessment can be an efficient means of reducing multiple risks. Problem-based approaches generally examine one risk or problem at a time and are met with one solution at a time. These solutions may be inflexible (e.g., pollution control equipment to reduce exposures to certain levels) and require successive investments of technology to meet each new problem or reduction in exposure limits. Or they may address only one particular problem or set of policy goals and ignore others. For example, efforts to enhance renewable energy technologies, such as solar energy, can involve the use of toxic materials that may adversely affect workers or communities.

4. *Avoiding regrettable substitutes.* Actions to address chemical risks without consideration of alternatives may fail to identify risk trade-offs that occur as a result of chemical or process changes. A regrettable substitution is one in which the alternative turns out either to have an unexpected hazard that results in similar or worse toxicity than the chemical of concern or involves shifting the burden of a hazard to another entity. An alternative may no longer be carcinogenic compared to the chemical of concern, but it may be toxic to aquatic organisms. For example, debates over the mechanism of action of methylene chloride delayed a regulatory process initiated by the US Occupational Safety and Health Administration (OSHA) for half a decade, prolonging worker exposure. When OSHA finally issued its exposure-based regulation, many small manufacturers substituted methylene chloride with n-propyl bromide, an equally problematic chemical. If OSHA had put even a small percentage of the resources spent debating the risk of methylene chloride into safer alternatives, costs in terms of worker health and safety and business substitution may have been reduced. Many other examples of regrettable substitutions exist in the literature (see Table 14.1). Another type of risk trade-off can occur when the assessment of the safety of a particular chemical or alternative in one agency may ignore risks that are not included in the "assessment lens" of that agency. For example, the FDA found the food additive diacetyl "generally recognized as safe" based on ingestion, despite it causing serious lung damage, bronchiolitis obliterans, in workers inhaling it when making microwave popcorn.

(Birnbaum 2010; CCOHS 2018; CDC 2008; ECHA 2013; Eladak et al. 2015; Harney et al. 2003; Ichihara et al. 2012; NTP 2011; Rochester and Bolden 2015; Siddiqi et al. 2003; Tomar et al. 2013; Velders et al. 2012)

Table 14.1: Notable Examples of Regrettable Substitutes

Chemical of Concern (Function)	Hazard	Substitute	Hazard
Bisphenol-A (plasticizer)	Endocrine disruption	Bisphenol-S, Bisphenol-F	Endocrine disruption
Bis(2-ethoxy phthalate (plasticizer; DEHP0	Endocrine disruption	Diisonyl phthalate (DiNP)	Carcinogenicity possible endocrine disruption
Lead, batteries, gasoline	Neurotoxicity	Methyl t-butyl ether (MBTE)	Aquatic toxicity
Methylene chloride (solvent (carrier in adhesives)	Acute toxicity, carcinogenicity	1–Bromopropane (nPB)	Carcinogenicity, neurotoxicity
Methylene chloride	Acute toxicity, carcinogenicity	n–Hexane	Neurotoxicity
Polybrominated diphenyl ethers (PBDEs) (flame retardant)	Persistence, neurotoxicity, reproductive, toxicity, carcinogen, penta, and deca	Tris (2,3–dibromopropyl) phosphate	Carcinogenicity, aquatic toxicity
Trichloroethylene (TCE) (metal decreasing)	Carcinogenicity	Bromopropane (nPB)	Neurotoxicity, carcinogenicity
Chlorofluorocarbons (CFCs) (Refrigerant)	Ozone depletion	Hydrofluorocarbons (HFCs)	Greenhouse gas

BOX 14.3 EXAMPLE: A SOLUTIONS-APPROACH TO TRICHLOROETHYLENE IN MASSACHUSETTS

Joel Tickner, Molly Jacobs and Margaret H. Whittaker

Trichlorethylene (TCE) is a commonly used chlorinated solvent that is a probable carcinogen and one of the most common contaminants found in hazardous waste sites in the United States. After almost 20 years, the US EPA completed a risk assessment for TCE in 2020 and as of 2021 has not issued any risk management actions for the substance. In the State of Massachusetts, under the 1989 Toxics Use Reduction Act, companies using listed toxic substances are required to annually quantify the use and emissions/waste of these chemicals and conduct an assessment of alternatives to reduce the use of the chemical every two years. With technical and research support from the Massachusetts Toxics Use Reduction Institute (TURI), funded by a small fee on chemicals, manufacturers using TCE in degreasing metal parts and other applications were able to evaluate and implement safer, water-based alternatives, reducing use of this chemical by some 95% in the state and saving companies millions of dollars. Even without definitive evidence on the mechanisms by which TCE causes cancer, there was enough evidence to indicate that the chemical should be avoided wherever possible.

The TCE case in Massachusetts demonstrates the critical importance of research and technical support in overcoming technical barriers to substitution. To avoid potential regrettable substitutes, TURI has been applying the successful approach taken to support companies in substituting TCE to other halogenated solvents as a class. While the European Commission took action on TCE under its Registration, Evaluation, and Authorization of Chemicals (REACH) regulations, little attention was paid to substitutes, and as a result, many metal finishers substituted to a less regulated drop-in solvent, perchloroethylene, a regrettable substitute.

1. *Better product design.* Ultimately the tools of alternatives assessment (and risk assessment can be used to design safer, more sustainable products. The cheapest and most advantageous point to address chemicals of concern is in the design phase, avoiding their use in the first place. By applying alternative assessment techniques in product design, chemicals can be reviewed for the potential hazard they pose to human health and the environment before they are used and safer alternatives can be designed and selected.

2. Used and safer alternatives can be designed and selected.

Defining Alternatives Assessment

Alternatives assessment is an iterative, step-defined, and solutions-oriented process *"for identifying and comparing potential chemical and non-chemical alternatives that could replace chemicals of concern on the basis of their hazards, comparative exposure, performance, and economic viability"* (Geiser et al. 2015; NRC 2014; Ziegler 1968). Alternatives assessment generally takes place after a determination to substitute a chemical of concern has taken place, but can be helpful in selecting safer options in product design or regular review of product chemistries, given the evolving nature of knowledge on chemicals. The US NRC notes that alternatives assessment is "a process for identifying, comparing, and selecting alternatives to chemicals of concern" that has a goal of "facilitating an informed consideration of the advantages and disadvantages of alternatives." The NRC further notes that alternatives assessment is not "a safety assessment, where the primary goal is to ensure that exposure is below a prescribed standard" or "a risk assessment where risk associated with a given level of exposure is calculated."

O'Brien (2000) notes that in its simplest form, alternatives assessment has three main components: (1) identification of a wide range of alternatives, (2) identification of the pros of alternatives, and (3) identification of the cons of alternatives. Alternatives assessment systematically provides critical information that is used to inform the transition to safer chemicals, materials, processes, or practices, reducing the potential for regrettable substitutions. The process may include modifications to how a product is engineered or used or may explore nonchemical alternatives, thereby shifting the focus from problem analysis to innovations and solutions (Geiser et al. 2015). This is similar to the planning approach that is central to pollution prevention. The ultimate goal of alternatives assessment is what the US EPA has termed "informed substitution," which is defined as "a considered transition from a chemical of particular concern to safer chemicals or non-chemical alternatives." Such a considered transition minimizes "the likelihood of unintended consequences, which can result from a precautionary switch away from a chemical of concern without fully understanding the profile of potential alternatives and enables "a course of action based on the best information – on the environment and human health – that is available or can be estimated." There are three general elements inherent in all alternative assessment processes.

1. *Alternatives assessments are action-oriented.* Alternatives assessments start with the goal of informed substitution. They ask a different set of questions than a traditional risk assessment. Rather than asking, "Is it safe?," or "Is the risk acceptable?" alternatives assessment asks, "Are there safer, feasible alternatives?" This action orientation helps to ensure that the analyses are sufficient to make decisions and avoid lengthy studies that lead to inaction. For example, Environmental Impact Assessment (EIS) regulations under the National Environmental Quality Act (NEPA) include a requirement for alternative assessment with regard to government proposals that might impact environmental quality. The regulations state that "NEPA's purpose is not to generate paperwork – even excellent paperwork – but to foster excellent action"; the EIS "should present the environmental impacts of the proposal and the alternatives in comparative form, thus sharply defining the issues and providing a clear basis for choice among options to the decision-maker and the public."

   • *Alternatives assessments reduce risks by identifying chemicals that are safer based on their inherent chemical and physical properties – what might be termed intrinsic impact reduction.* The objective of alternatives assessment is to reduce risk to humans and the environment by reducing intrinsic chemical hazards and exposure potential as a priority. For example, while perchloroethylene may be safely used in a closed loop dry cleaning system, it is an intrinsically dangerous chemical and at some point during production, use or disposal can lead to exposures. Aqueous solvents (including water) are intrinsically safer, and if released into the environment, they are unlikely to cause significant harm. Trevor Kletz, a corporate chemical engineer and originator of the concept of Inherent Safety in chemical process management, adeptly described the value of a focus on reducing intrinsic hazards, stating, "If the meat of lions were good to eat, then farmers would be asked to keep lions. But they would need cages and all sorts of safety systems. But why keep lions when lambs will do instead?" This is consistent with the principles of precaution and primary prevention in public health.

   • *The starting point of chemical alternatives assessment is the function or "service" of the chemical.* By focusing on function rather than the particular chemical of concern, the assessment of alternatives is able to move from "avoiding the chemical of concern" to considering a broader range of chemical and nonchemical alternatives, including whether the particular function is actually needed – termed "functional substitution" (see Table 14.2 for how this concept

Table 14.2: A Functional Substitution Approach for Chemicals in Products and Processes (J. A. Tickner et al. 2015)

Functional Substitution Level	Chemical Product Bisphenol-A in Thermal Paper	Chemical in Process Methylene Chloride in Degreasing Metal Parts
Chemical Function (Chemical Change)	Is there a functionally equivalent chemical substitute (i.e., chemical developer)? **Result: Drop-in chemical replacement.**	Is there a functionally equivalent chemical substitute (i.e., chlorinated solvent degreaser)? **Result: Drop-in chemical replacement.**
End Use Function Material, Product, Process Change	Is there another means to achieve the function of the chemical on the product (i.e., creation of printed image)? **Result: Redesign of thermal paper, material changes.**	Is there another means to achieve the function of the process (i.e., degreasing)? **Result: Redesign of the process (e.g., ultrasonic, aqueous).**
Function as Service (System Change)	Are cash register receipts necessary? Are there alternatives that could achieve the same purpose (i.e., providing a record of sale to a customer)? **Result: alternative printing systems (e.g., electronic receipts).**	Is degreasing metal parts necessary? Are there other alternatives that could achieve the same purpose (i.e., providing metal parts free of contaminants for other end uses? **Result: Alternative metal cutting methods.**

could be applied in practice). For example, the US FDA restricted the use of triclosan in hand soaps in the United States based on the fact that they provided no additional benefit over normal soap and water yet concerns over risks to humans and ecosystems existed. Chemical function can be narrowly defined at the chemical level or broadly defined at the product level.

The Commons Principles, developed by a collaboration of alternatives assessment researchers and practitioners, underscore the key elements of an alternatives assessment and guide the process of recognizing the need for transparency and openness about trade-offs.

History of Alternatives Assessment

The concept of chemical substitution has a long history internationally and in the United States. While there are many examples of policies to encourage or require substitution of chemicals of concern, there have traditionally been few that have included requirements or processes for alternatives assessment.

Internationally, the Swedish government instituted the "substitution principle" as a core principle of environmental policy in the 1970s. The 1985 Swedish Act on Chemical Products states,

> Anyone handling or importing a chemical product shall take such steps and otherwise observe such precautions as are necessary to prevent or minimize harm to human beings or to the environment. This includes avoiding chemical products for which less hazardous substitutes are available.

BOX 14.4   THE COMMONS PRINCIPLES FOR ALTERNATIVES ASSESSMENT

Joel Tickner, Molly Jacobs and Margaret H. Whittaker

REDUCE HAZARD. Reduce hazard by replacing a chemical of concern with a less hazardous alternative. This approach provides an effective means to reduce risk associated with a product or process if the potential for exposure remains the same or lower. Consider reformulation to avoid use of the chemical of concern altogether.

MINIMIZE EXPOSURE. Assess use patterns and exposure pathways to limit exposure to alternatives that may also present risks.

USE BEST AVAILABLE INFORMATION. Obtain access to and use information that assists in distinguishing between possible choices. Before selecting preferred options, characterize the product and process sufficiently to avoid choosing alternatives that may result in unintended adverse consequences.

REQUIRE DISCLOSURE AND TRANSPARENCY. Require disclosure across the supply chain regarding key chemical and technical information. Engage stakeholders throughout the assessment process to promote transparency in regard to alternatives assessment methodologies employed, data used to characterize alternatives, assumptions made and decision-making rules applied.

RESOLVE TRADE-OFFS. Use information about the product's life cycle to better understand potential benefits, impacts, and mitigation options associated with different alternatives. When substitution options do not provide a clearly preferable solution, consider organizational goals and values to determine appropriate weighting of decision criteria and identify acceptable trade-offs.

TAKE ACTION. Take action to eliminate or substitute potentially hazardous chemicals. Choose safer alternatives that are commercially available, technically and economically feasible, and satisfy the performance requirements of the process/product. Collaborate with supply chain partners to drive innovation in the development and adoption of safer substitutes. Review new information to ensure that the option selected remains a safer choice.

Denmark and Norway instituted similar provisions in national policies and used the precautionary principle (Raffensperger and Tickner 1999) and substitution principle as the foundation of several regional treaties addressing chemical contamination in the North Sea and Baltic regions.

The 1987 Montreal Protocol on Substances That Deplete the Ozone Layer represents the first global effort to identify substitutes for a group of chemicals of concern. The Chemical Technical Options Committees under the Montreal Protocol review "in-kind" and "not in kind" alternatives for ozone-depleting substances for specific applications and new replacements for ozone-depleting substances are reviewed under the US EPA Significant New Alternatives Policy (SNAP) before entering commerce. The 2001 Stockholm Convention establishes a legally binding means to address threats to health and the environment caused by persistent organic pollutants (POPs). Annex F of the Stockholm Convention requires the POPs Review Committee (POPRC) to complete an alternatives profile for all new candidate substances as part of its Risk Management Evaluation. In 2009, the POPRC adopted a new alternatives assessment policy, which states that having effective, available, and accessible alternatives are critical to any successful chemical phase-out strategy, particularly for developing and transition countries. The policy defines alternatives broadly as "a different chemical, material, product, product design system, production process or strategy that can replace a candidate substance while maintaining sufficient level of efficacy." In 2006, the UN Environment Programme established the Strategic Approach to International Chemicals Management (SAICM) to support the 2020 goal that chemicals are produced and used in ways that minimize significant adverse impacts on human health and the environment. The SAICM Overarching Policy Strategy includes the objective "[t]o promote and support the development and implementation of, and further innovation in, environmentally sound and safer alternatives, including cleaner production, informed substitution of chemicals of particular concern and non-chemical alternatives." The UN Global Chemicals Outlook II, a comprehensive review of chemicals management globally, outlines chemical substitution as a critical goal for chemicals management.

The European Union has issued policies since the 1990s calling for the substitution of chemicals of concern. A 2001 report commissioned by the European Commission evaluated substitution policies and opportunities in the region and defined the concept in the following manner:

> Substitution means the replacement or reduction of hazardous substances in products or processes by less hazardous or non-hazardous substances, or by achieving an equivalent functionality via technological or organizational measures.

Substitution is mandated in a number of European occupational health and safety regulations referring to carcinogens and hazardous substances in the workplace and in European cosmetics, toys, and formulated product regulations, which restrict the use of certain chemicals (primarily CMRs or carcinogens, mutagens, and reproductive toxicants). Substitution is a key goal of the European Union's REACH legislation. The European Chemicals Agency's (ECHA) Candidate List includes chemicals that will be subject to the REACH authorization procedures based on their intrinsic hazards (CMRs, Persistent Bioaccumulative, and Toxic Chemicals, and other chemicals of high concern), requiring firms to find substitutes for substances of concern unless they can provide clear justification for continued use through the completion of an alternatives assessment. The agency has developed a substitution strategy, authored reports, and developed training and guidance to support the process. The new European Chemicals Strategy for Sustainability extends the substitution focus of reach, with a stated goal of achieving chemicals that are "Safe and Sustainable by Design." The Chemicals Strategy extends the intrinsic hazards that require substitution processes (for example, endocrine-disrupting chemicals); institutes a "one chemical, one assessment" approach to chemical hazard evaluation, reducing the challenges posed by differing assessments from different agencies; and introduces the concept of "essential uses." This concept, inherent in the Montreal Protocol, restricts chemicals of concern for all uses, except those "necessary for health, safety or is critical for the functioning of society." How this concept will be integrated into a scientific assessment process is still under debate (Figure 14.1).

Several European countries have established alternatives assessment and substitution support centers, including Sweden, Denmark, and Germany, which hosts the SUBSPORT Plus database.

As noted, in the United States, perhaps the most comprehensive, institutionalized example of a requirement for alternatives assessment is the EIS process under the NEPA and similar state programs. NEPA regulations specify a process that the agency must follow before initiating an activity. Through an interdisciplinary approach, agencies must (1) comprehensively identify and examine environmental effects and values; (2) rigorously study, develop, and describe appropriate

	Protect Health and the environment	Encourage Innovation
Safe and sustainable chemicals	Use of safe chemicals while preventing harm to humans and the environment by avoiding substances of concern for non essential uses..	Promote the development of safe and sustainable chemicals and materials, clean production processes and technologies, innovative tools for testing and risk assessments.
Minimize and control	Minimize exposure of humans and environment to substances hazardous to health and environment, through risk management measures and full information to users of chemicals.	Promote modern and smart production processes, safe and sustainable uses and business models, chemicals as a service . IT solutions for tracking of chemicals.
Eliminate and remediate	Eliminate as far as possible, substances of concern in waste and secondary raw materials and restore human health and environment to a good quality. Status.	Promote safe and clean recycling solutions including chemical recycling waste management technologies, decontamination solutions.

Figure 14.1 Overview of the European chemicals strategy for sustainability.

(reasonable) alternatives in comparative form, including not moving ahead with an activity; and (3) recommended courses of action. Agencies are instructed to undergo a "scoping process" to broadly define potential impacts and to examine them in detail, including direct and indirect impacts, cumulative effects, effects on historical and cultural resources, impacts of alternatives, and options to mitigate potential impacts.

In the chemicals area, the earliest chemical substitution mandate is in the Delaney Clause of the Federal Food Drug and Cosmetics Act, which states, "the Secretary of the Food and Drug Administration shall not approve for use in food any chemical additive found to induce cancer in man, or, after tests, found to induce cancer in animals." Concerns about the impacts of problem pesticides, such as DDT, led to their early prohibition in the United States. The impacts of these pesticides and other chemicals, such as Polychlorinated Biphenyls (PCBs), on the fragile Great Lakes ecosystem led the United States and Canada to approve the 1978 Great Lakes Water Quality Agreement, which mandated that "the discharge of toxic substances in toxic amounts be prohibited and the discharge of any or all persistent toxic substances be virtually eliminated." The US-Canada International Joint Commission, the binational body that monitors boundary waters, noted in its Sixth Biennial report that to achieve the agreement's goals, "if a chemical or group of chemicals is persistent, toxic and bioaccumulative, we should immediately begin a process to eliminate it. Since it seems impossible to eliminate discharges of these chemicals through other means, a policy of banning or sunsetting their manufacture, distribution, storage, use and disposal appears to be the only alternative."

Substitution of hazards in the workplace has a long history. While substitution requirements are not explicitly built into the Occupational Safety and Health Act, the industrial hygiene hierarchy of controls identifies substitution as a priority for protecting workers from harmful exposures with personal protective equipment being the last resort. The hierarchy is mentioned in part of the first (1974) *NIOSH Pocket Guide* and Standards Completion Program and the *OSHA Respiratory Protection Standard*, and substitution was the basis of the never implemented 1979 *Generic Cancer Standard*, which stated that known and probable carcinogens should be substituted based on technical feasibility (Figure 14.2).

In 2014, OSHA published its *Transitioning to Safer Chemicals Toolkit*, designed to assist small and medium-sized employers and companies in undertaking a substitution process (Figure 14.3).

The Pollution Prevention Act of 1990 resulted in renewed attention to chemical reduction and substitution. The Act "declares it to be the national policy of the United States that pollution should be prevented or reduced at the source whenever feasible." The Act introduces the pollution prevention hierarchy – reduction of pollutants at source as the priority – as a compliment to its industrial hygiene counterpart. Pollution prevention, source reduction, and toxics use reduction planning – evaluating options to reduce emissions, waste, and chemical use are at the heart of pollution prevention (Figure 14.4).

Following the passage of the Act, the EPA established numerous programs to advance chemical substitution, including its Design for Environment Program. These efforts included projects to establish chemical hazard ranking and screening methods (a forerunner of the hazard assessment component of alternatives assessment), Cleaner Technology Substitutes Assessments, a methodology for evaluating alternatives for chemicals of concern in specific applications, and the Use Cluster Scoring System, designed to compare and rank chemicals for a specific functional

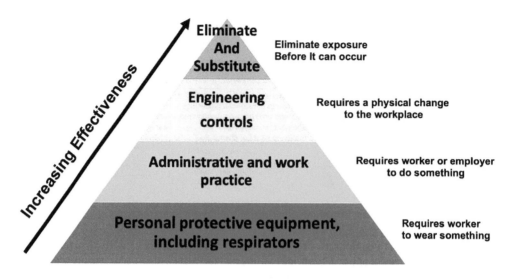

Figure 14.2 The industrial hygiene hierarchy of controls.

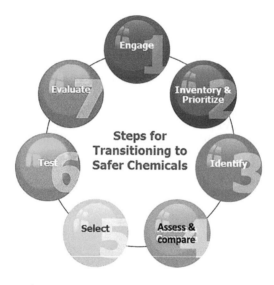

Figure 14.3 OSHA steps for transitioning to safer chemicals.

use, such as solvents. In 2008, EPA developed its Alternatives Assessment Criteria for Hazard Evaluation and initiated a series of alternatives assessment partnerships aimed at bringing together private sector and other stakeholders to identify and evaluate safer alternatives to specific chemicals of national concern, such as flame retardants. In 2010, the EPA launched its Safer Choice Program to stimulate market demand for safer chemicals by recognizing preferred products with its Safer Choice label and promoting the adoption of safer chemistries for specific functional uses through its Safer Chemical ingredients list (SCIL), which uses toxicological criteria for a range of hazard end points to identify safer options (US EPA 2018a). To achieve the label, ingredients are evaluated by a third-party certifier using stringent human health and environmental criteria.

Parallel to the growth of substitution efforts in the federal government, in the 1990s, EPA, along with the American Chemical Society, launched the concept of green chemistry and a recognition program that supports and rewards the design of inherently safer chemicals. In 2000, Paul Anastas and John Warner published the book *Green Chemistry: Theory and Practice*, which defined 12 principles of green chemistry (Anastas and Warner 1998). The 12 principles of green chemistry aim to alter the way products are manufactured in order to minimize their impact on human health and

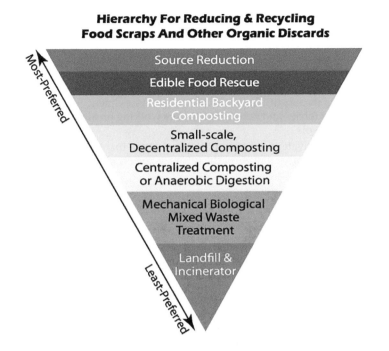

**Hierarchy For Reducing & Recycling
Food Scraps And Other Organic Discards**

Most-Preferred

Least-Preferred

Source Reduction

Edible Food Rescue

Residential Backyard Composting

Small-scale, Decentralized Composting

Centralized Composting or Anaerobic Digestion

Mechanical Biological Mixed Waste Treatment

Landfill & Incinerator

Figure 14.4 The pollution prevention hierarchy.

the environment throughout their life cycles. One principle specifically addresses the issue of safer alternatives:

Design safer chemicals and products: Design chemical products to be fully effective yet have little to no toxicity.

The field of green chemistry has grown significantly in academia and the private sector since Warner and Anastas' book.

Alternatives assessment requirements in policy have grown significantly in the past decade at the state level in the United States. The increased focus on alternatives assessment requirements comes as an outgrowth of state policies focused on restricting chemicals of concern where concerns had been raised about regrettable substitutes. The states have a long history of innovation in chemicals management and pollution prevention, dating back to the California Safe Drinking Water and Toxic Enforcement Act of 1986 (also known as Prop 65), which prohibits businesses from discharging chemicals that have carcinogenic or reproductive toxicity effects into sources of drinking water. In recent years states such as Washington, Maine, California, Oregon, Michigan, Minnesota, Connecticut, New York, Maryland, and Massachusetts have advanced policies requiring the substitution of problem chemicals with safer alternatives. These efforts have ranged from single chemical restrictions on mercury, phthalates, brominated flame retardants, and bisphenol-A, to procurement policies and broader chemical prioritization and substitution requirements for larger numbers of chemicals. For example, the California Safer Consumer Products Regulations require "responsible entities" to undertake alternatives assessments for chemical/product combinations of concern. The Safer Products for Washington policy, passed in 2019, requires the Washington Department of Ecology to identify high priority chemicals and product categories containing them and then to determine regulatory actions based on the results of alternatives assessments that outline availability of safer alternatives. Because of this evolution of state policies, and the frequent lack of resources for implementation, ten states have combined efforts to form the Interstate Chemicals Clearinghouse, which provides a mechanism to share data on chemical toxicity, uses, and alternatives.

Parallel to government efforts, retailers and manufacturers are beginning to work to avoid known chemicals of concern in products and identify safer alternatives as a result of increasing consumer pressure or regulations in some parts of the world. In some cases, large retailers and product purchasers, and brands have instituted chemicals policies, including restricted substances lists (RSL), with which their suppliers must comply. For example, Walmart has a sustainable chemistry program that requires information on chemical content in formulated products and safer alternatives to chemicals of concern. Other retailers and brands, such as Levi Strauss & Co., are screening their product chemistries to identify alternatives with lower hazard profiles.

The OECD established its Substitution and Alternatives Assessment Toolbox in 2013 (OECD 2013) to bring together countries and other stakeholders working on alternatives assessment and substitution policies and tools.

These government and private sector examples demonstrate that the need for alternatives assessment approaches will only increase in the future as governments, consumers, and large purchasers demand safer products.

FRAMEWORKS FOR ALTERNATIVES ASSESSMENT AND CORE COMPONENTS

Alternatives Assessment Frameworks

Over the past two decades, a variety of alternatives assessment frameworks, methods and tools have been developed to assist with the evaluation of potential substitutes in a particular process or product. A review by (M. M. Jacobs et al. 2016) documented nearly two dozen frameworks, the majority of which were published since 2006 by both institutions/organizations in Europe and in the United States (see Figure 14.3). This growth demonstrates an evolving trend in evaluating alternatives to inform a transition to safer options and to minimize regrettable substitutes as a key aspect of chemicals management science and policy. Many of the frameworks have been developed to support regulatory chemicals management programs. Others have been published as guidance documents, including those developed by the US NRC (2014), the US OSHA (2021), and the Interstate Chemical's Clearinghouse (IC2 2017). Although published as guidance, the IC2 framework as recently been incorporated into regulatory requirements for the evaluation of alternatives under the Safer Products for Washington law. In all cases, the level of detail needed for an assessment is context specific, as such alternatives assessment frameworks are generally flexible and adaptable to an individual company, sectoral, or policy decisions (Table 14.3).

Alternatives Assessment Components

Core components of an alternatives assessment are consistent across the majority of published frameworks and generally include a comparison to the incumbent chemical of concern. These

Table 14.3: **Examples of Alternatives Assessment Frameworks**

Framework	Organization	Purpose
Alternatives Analysis Guide, Version 1.0	CA Department of Toxic Substances and Control	Regulatory Guidance
Alternatives Assessment Guide V1.1	IC2	General Guidance
Massachusetts TURI 2006 and Eliason and Morose 2011	MA Toxics Use Reduction Institute	General Guidance
A Framework to Guide the Selection of Chemical Alternatives (guidance)	US National Research Council	General Guidance
Guidance on the Preparation for an Application for Authorization	ECHA	Regulatory Guidance
General Guidance on Considerations Related to Alternatives and Substitutes for Listed Persistent Organic Pollutants and Candidate Chemicals	UN Environment Program, Stockholm Convention	General Guidance
Technical Rules for Hazardous Substances (TRGS) 600 (regulatory)	German Institute for Occupational Safety and Health	Regulatory Guidance
Cleaner Technologies Substitute Assessment: A Methodology and Resource Guide	US EPA	General Guidance
Instructions for the SNAP Program Toxic Substances Control Act (TSCA)/SNAP Addendum (regulatory)	US EPA, SNAP Program	Regulatory Guidance
Transitioning to Safer Chemicals: A Toolkit for Employers and Workers	US OSHA	General Guidance

Table 14.4: What Does Alternative Assessment Involve? Overview of Key Components

Component/Step	What It Involves
1. Scoping and problem formulation	– Establishes the scope of and plan for assessment, including evaluation methods and criteria – Identifies decision rules that will guide the assessment (such as avoiding carcinogens) – Identifies stakeholders to engage – Gathers data on the chemical of concern, its function, and application and technical requirements – Identifies alternatives to be considered and potential concerns associated with them
Comparative Assessment Steps Comparing chemicals of concern and alternatives based on hazard, comparative exposure, technical feasibility, economic feasibility, and other life cycle considerations	
2. Hazard assessment	– Evaluates and compares human health and ecological hazards based on methods and criteria established in step 1
3. Comparative exposure assessment	– Evaluates and compares the intrinsic exposure potential of alternatives, based on methods and criteria established in step 1
3. Technical feasibility assessment	– Evaluates and compares performance of alternatives based on methods and criteria established in step 1
4. Economic feasibility assessment	– Evaluates and compares the costs of alternatives based on methods and criteria established in step 1
5. Other life cycle impacts	– Addresses additional potential upstream or downstream ecological and human health hazards, as well as other potential trade-offs such as energy, climate change impacts, and natural resource impacts
6. Decision-making	– Combines information from previous steps to evaluate trade-offs and preferences and identify acceptable alternatives – Addresses situations where no alternatives are currently viable by initiating Research and Development (R&D) to develop new alternatives or improve existing ones – Establishes an implementation and adoption plan to identify potential trade-offs during adoption

components are outlined in Table 14.4. While each component should be addressed in an alternatives assessment, as in risk assessment, the level of detail will vary based on the nature of the substitution process.

It is important to note that the assessment of alternatives is a series of steps to support the informed substitution decision. As described earlier, this action orientation ensures that data supporting the assessment are sufficient to make government and business decisions and to avoid lengthy analyses that lead to inaction. Making decisions about which alternative or alternatives to select requires considering data gaps, data uncertainties, and trade-offs. Decision-making is inherent to the process and made explicit in a few frameworks, including but not limited to, the US NRC (2014), IC2 (2017), and California Department of Toxic Substances Control (2017). frameworks.

The US NRC framework (2014) also recognizes the importance of implementation and further research and development. The fact that a safer alternative is identified through an alternatives assessment does not mean that it will work in practice; hence, consideration of and support for implementation of alternatives is essential and the US NRC framework (2014) provides important considerations for the adoption of alternatives, such as (a) implementing additional process design or formulation chemistry changes to achieve the necessary functionality that may not have been considered or identified during research and development stages or (b) changing environmental safety and health management practices to ensure that residual risks associated with the alternatives are sufficiently controlled across the life cycle, including controls for workers, the public and the environment during manufacturing, point of use, and disposal. There is a growing understanding that innovation in safer alternatives is needed. When safer, cost-effective, and high-performing alternatives do not exist, targeted research to develop those alternatives should be pursued. Alternatives assessment tools can inform those research and development efforts.

Hazard assessment and the assessment of technical and economic feasibility have been core to the alternatives assessment process since its inception (Geiser et al. 2015). Hazard assessment in the context of an alternatives assessment has historically focused on human toxicity and ecotoxicity (e.g., acute and chronic aquatic toxicity) end points. Stimulated in part by the publication of the US NRC framework (2014), there is a growing focus for alternatives assessments to also consider exposure and broader life cycle impacts. A brief overview of the assessment of hazard, exposure, and other life cycle impacts in an alternatives assessment is reviewed in the following sections. It is important to reiterate that the goal of alternatives assessment is to support thoughtful substitution decisions, and as the assessment process becomes more detailed, it is important to avoid "paralysis by analysis."

HAZARD ASSESSMENT

Hazard assessment is central to alternatives assessment since the goal is to identify safer substitutes. The purpose is to compare the hazards of alternatives to the chemical of concern for a given functional use. The evaluation of hazard in an alternatives assessment is similar to the hazard identification step in risk assessment in terms of the data sources used and health end points addressed. A key difference is the comparative nature of an alternative assessment – focused on evaluating a range of hazard end points to identify safer options. In contrast, a risk assessment focuses on formal dose-response or weight-of-evidence/mode-of-action evaluations to determine risk levels at specific exposure concentrations. Alternatives assessment seeks to answer a different question than that in a risk assessment: *Do specific alternatives present a high intrinsic hazard to human health and/or the environment considering an array of human and environmental health end points/assessment criteria in comparison to the chemical targeted for substitution?* The focus of hazard assessment in an alternatives assessment is to avoid regrettable substitutions, which can occur if an alternative with a similar or worse toxicity profile is adopted.

In a review of existing alternatives assessment frameworks and data/tools used to support hazard assessments, M. M. Jacobs et al. (2016) found that there is no standard set of hazard end points evaluated, and some frameworks are more general than others in terms of the end points that should be evaluated. The US NRC (2014) framework helped to better align which hazard end points should be considered in any alternatives assessment. These end points are noted in Table 14.5. In 2020, the OECD published a core set of hazard end points that must be evaluated to make a "safer" alternative determination. These end points are also noted in Table 14.5 (OECD 2020). Often, the specific hazard end points to be evaluated are determined during the scoping and problem formulation component of the alternatives assessment process based on an understanding of the chemical of concern and its application.

Jacobs et al. (2018) highlighted a range of data sources available to support hazard assessment including screening and hazard methods and assessment tools.

Hazard Screening

Authoritative lists are widely used in alternatives assessment to screen out problematic substances. Use of authoritative lists can help to focus on a smaller set of alternatives that should

Table 14.5: Hazard End Points to Consider in an Assessment of Alternatives as Outlined by the US NRC and OECD

Human Health Toxicity	Ecotoxicity	Environmental Fate/Transport	Physical/Safety Hazards
• Acute toxicity • Repeated dose/specific target organ toxicity • Eye/skin corrosion/irritation • Skin sensitization • Neurotoxicity • Chronic toxicity/repeated dose toxicity • Carcinogenicity^ • Mutagenicity/genotoxicity^ • Reproductive toxicity^ • Developmental toxicity^ • Endocrine activity • Respiratory sensitization	• Aquatic toxicity • Other ecotoxicity (avian, bees, terrestrial, air)	• Persistence*^ • Bioaccumulation*^	• Corrosivity • Flammability • Reactivity • Explosivity • Oxidizing properties • Pyrophoric properties

* US NRC considers these end points in the comparative exposure assessment component.
^ End points required to be evaluated to meet OECD's minimum requirements for making a safer alternative determination.

Table 14.6: **OECD Identified Authoritative Lists That Should Be Considered Determining a Safer Alternative (OECD 2020)**

List	Human Health and Environmental Health End Points Addressed – Reasons for Inclusion on the List
California Office of Environmental Health Hazard Assessment, Proposition 65	- Carcinogenic - Developmental Toxicant - Mutagenic - Reproductive Toxicant
Canadian Toxic Substances List and the Virtual Elimination List	- Persistent and Bioaccumulative Toxicant (PBT)
ECHA's Candidate List of Substances of Very High Concern for Authorization	- Carcinogenic - Mutagenic - Reproductive Toxicant - PBT Very Persistent and Very Bioaccumulative (vPvB) - Endocrine-disrupting properties – environmental - Endocrine-disrupting properties – human health - Respiratory sensitizer - Specific target organ toxicity after repeated exposure – human health - Equivalent level of concern having probable serious effects on human health (and/or) the environment
US EPA's Toxics Release Inventory's PBT Chemicals List and PBT Chemicals under the TSCA Section 6(h)	- PBT
US National Toxicology Program's Report on Carcinogens	- Known to be a human carcinogen - Reasonably anticipated to be a human carcinogen
World Health Organization's International Agency for Research on Cancer List of Agents Classified in the IARC Monographs	- Carcinogenic (including substances classified as Group 1, Group 2A, and Group 2B)
Montreal Protocol	- List of ozone-depleting substances
Stockholm Convention	- List of POPs

undergo a full hazard assessment. Authoritative lists are developed by governmental organizations or government-recognized expert institutions based on results from rigorous expert reviews of the scientific literature and stakeholder input. Some companies and sector-based organizations (such as the Zero Discharge of Hazardous Chemicals – ZDHC – for the footwear and appear industry) also use authoritative lists to create their own RSLs. Authoritative lists are not sufficient to indicate a chemical is safer, as most authoritative lists are not inclusive of all chemicals.

The OECD has identified a series of authoritative lists that should be reviewed when evaluating safer alternatives and are considered part of the minimum requirements for making a safer alternative determination (Table 14.6). These lists do not address all hazard end points that the US NRC framework suggests considering in an alternatives assessment but do address what are commonly considered hazards of high concern (e.g., carcinogenicity, mutagenicity, reproductive/ developmental toxicity, and persistent, bioaccumulative, and toxic substances among a few others). The GreenScreen® for Safer Chemicals (a hazard assessment method widely used by businesses and governments) includes a "List Translator" tool to help support the screening out of chemicals of concern, using 40 authoritative lists, including those that are in the OCED set of minimum requirements (CPA 2021). Each of the authoritative lists in the GreenScreen List Translator is then mapped to hazard end points and a hazard score based on GreenScreen Criteria. These criteria (and those included in many other hazard assessment processes are based on hazard classifications included in the UN Globally Harmonized System of Classification and Labelling of Chemicals (GHS). GHS is a globally established system of classification and labeling of hazardous chemicals.

Full Hazard Assessment Methods and Tools

A comprehensive hazard assessment resembles the hazard assessment component of a risk assessment, but it is more streamlined and summarized in a manner to support substitution decision-making. Most hazard assessment methods used in alternatives assessment are organized around the use of GHS criteria, which provides a standardized set of criteria for classifying hazards of chemicals. Using GHS criteria for human and environmental health end points as exampled in

Table 14.7: Generic Example of Hazard Assessment Results in an Alternative Assessment

	C	M	R	D	E	AT	ST Single	ST repeated	N Single	N repeated	SnS	SnR	IrS	IrE	AA	CA	P	B	RX	F
Chemical Targeted for Substitution	H	NE	DG	DG	M	*M*	*vH*	H	*vH*	*vH*	L	DG	H	H	M	*L*	*vH*	vL	L	L
Alternative A	L	L	*L*	M	DG	M	L	L	*M*	H	H	*L*	L	H	L	L	vL	vL	*L*	L
Alternative B	*L*	L	L	L	DG	L	L	H	DG	L	L	DG	*M*	H	L	L	vL	vL	*L*	M
Alternative C	*L*	L	L	L	DG	L	L	L	L	L	L	L	*M*	M	L	*L*	*L*	vL	*L*	M
Alternative D	L	L	L	*L*	DG	H	vH	*H*	vH	DG	L	DG	vH	vH	M	M	vL	vL	L	M

Abbreviations ([A] reflects OECD minimum requirements):

C = Carcinogenicity[A]
M = Mutagenicity[A]
R = Reproductive Toxicity[A]
D = Developmental Toxicity[A]
E = Endocrine Activity

AT = Acute Toxicity
ST = Systemic Organ Toxicity
N = Neurotoxicity
SnS = Skin Sensitization
SnR = Respiratory Sensitization
IrS = Skin Irritation
IrE = Eye Irritation

AA = Aquatic Toxicity
CA = Chronic Aquatic Toxicity
P = Persistence[A]
B = Bioaccumulation[A]
RX = Reactivity
F = Flammability

[Note how alternative C is the safer option compared to the compound that is targeted for substitution and compared To the other alternatives considered (alternatives A, B, and D). However, there are data gaps related to endocrine disruption that should be considered further in the substitution decision.]

Note: Hazard levels (Very High (vH), High (H), Moderate (M), Low (L), Very Low (vL) in italics reflect estimated (modeled values, authoritative lists, weak analogues, and lower confidence. **BOLD** are used with good quality data, authoritative A lists, or strong analogues. Group II human health end points have four hazard scores (vH, H, M, L) instead of three (H, M, L) and are based on single rather than repeated exposures. DG indicates insufficient data for assigning hazard level. NE indicates no determination was made.

Table 14.7 (note, there are no GHS criteria for endocrine activity, ecotoxicity other than aquatic, bioaccumulation, and persistence) allows assessors to review available hazard data and designate an alternative as **L**ow, **M**oderate, or **H**igh concern for a specific hazard (or some similar ranking scheme, such as green, yellow or red) and easily compare a chemical targeted for substitution with potential alternatives. Data sources used to establish the GHS classifications are often varied, depending on the expertise of the assessor. The most basic source of information is a Safety Data Sheet (SDS), which may report GHS hazard statements and/or actual toxicity or ecotoxicity data; however, SDSs often do not include full chemical ingredient information and/or hazard classification and may result in conflicting classifications depending on who conducts them. A more thoughtful approach involves reviewing the published literature as well as queries of hazard databases, such as eChemPortal curated by the OECD, or the CompTox Chemicals Dashboard curated by the US EPA, among others that compile hazard information on specific chemicals from a range of sources.

Some organizations have developed tools to support the comparison of alternatives based on their hazard profile, including Clean Production Action's GreenScreen for Safer Chemicals and US EPA Hazard Comparison Dashboard, among others, as summarized in Table 14.8.

The GreenScreen framework requires users to populate the comparison tables manually, while EPA's Hazard Comparison Dashboard automatically pulls hazard traits from its CompTox Chemicals Dashboard. Tools such as P2OASys and the Column Model are designed for use by workers and small businesses and use SDSs and other easily accessible data. The Healthy Building Network's Pharos Project and the GreenScreen Assessment Registry include published GreenScreen hazard assessments completed by expert toxicologists (some available for a fee). Other tools and databases, such as those by Chem*FORWARD*, utilize methods of both GreenScreen for Safer Chemicals Standard (CPA 2018) and the Cradle to Cradle Certified Product Standard (C2CPII 2021) to support a review of hazards by users.

Professional judgment is needed to evaluate the merits of specific toxicological and epidemiological studies when applying GHS criteria. Some hazard assessment methodologies pages, such as GreenScreen, use notations (such as italics or bolding) to discern whether there is uncertainty

Table 14.8: Hazard Assessment Tools to Support Alternatives Assessments

Tool	Developer
GreenScreen for Safer Chemicals	Clean Production Action
Quick Chemical Assessment Tool (QCAT)	Washington State Department of Ecology
P2OASys	Massachusetts TURI
Column Model	German Institute for Occupational Safety and Health
Chem*FORWARD* Platform or Intelligent Ingredient Report	ChemFORWARD
Hazard Comparison Dashboard	US EPA
Pharos	Healthy Building Network
GreenScreen Assessment Registry	Clean Production Action

in the quality of the evidence used in determining a hazard end point's classification and whether there are data gaps. Data gaps for specific hazard end points in the GreenScreen® method will often result in a lower, less desirable overall "benchmark" score for a chemical. In an alternatives assessment, it is crucial to evaluate data gaps, as there are many examples of regrettable substitutions because data were lacking key hazard end points for an alternative at the time of the replacement. For example, data were lacking on the endocrine-disrupting effects of bisphenol-S when it was used as a substitute for bisphenol-A in a number of applications, including as a resin in can linings (Rochester and Bolden 2015). Data were lacking on end points such as carcinogenicity for 1-bromo-propane when it was used as a substitute for methylene chloride. Its carcinogenicity has since been established (NTP 2013). Given the emergence of NAMs, the US NRC (NRC 2014)) and others have suggested increased use of these data streams to address data gaps in alternatives assessments.

COMPARATIVE EXPOSURE ASSESSMENT

Concerted consideration of exposure characteristics is relatively new in alternatives assessment practice. The goal has been to move to safer alternatives based on the inherent hazard profile of a substitute rather than limiting exposure. However, considering exposure can help to focus the relevance of the hazard assessment results, given the use conditions of the alternative, if more quantity or a higher concentration will be needed or if physicochemical properties of an alternative demonstrate a concern for increased exposure.

In an alternatives assessment, the purpose of assessing exposure is to answer the question, *Is the alternative preferable, equivalent to, or worse than the chemical being targeted for substitution for the specific function, given the potential for exposure?*

The goal of a comparative exposure assessment is to identify potential exposure for each alternative to assess whether each is

a. substantially equivalent,

b. inherently preferable, or

c. potentially worse than a chemical of concern.

If exposure is substantially equivalent between an alternative and the chemical of concern, then determination of "safer" can be limited to the relative hazard(s) of the chemicals.

In an alternatives assessment, exposure characterization is comparative and qualitative, as opposed to quantitative; it is not used to assess risk but to understand potential trade-offs for specific alternatives (NRC 2014). Considering exposure receptors, routes of exposure (dermal, oral, or inhalation), patterns of exposure (acute, chronic), and levels of exposure (irrespective of any exposure controls) when integrating hazard assessment evidence goes further in avoiding regrettable substitutes than just considering hazards alone. For example, one alternative paint stripper formulation to a methylene chloride-based paint stripper may contain dimethyl sulfoxide (DMSO), a less toxic solvent, although DMSO can increase skin uptake of other chemicals present in a mixture. As such, it is important to understand if DMSO's skin penetration enhancement would increase exposure to potentially problematic substances in an alternative paint stripper formulation during paint stripping operations.

As outlined by the OECD (2021b), the main components of a qualitative exposure assessment to support the identification and selection of a safer alternative includes (a) identifying exposure pathways and use scenarios and (b) comparing exposure potential. This simplification is a resulting synthesis of methods outlined in the NRC and IC2 frameworks.

Identifying exposure pathways and use scenarios that can reasonably be anticipated includes considering how a chemical is used across its life cycle. Identifying potential routes of exposure and relevant receptors is often supported by using conceptual exposure maps. In those circumstances where conceptual maps are not available, physicochemical properties are a valuable source of information that can be used to identify relevant routes of exposure for the alternatives and a method elevated in the US NRC and IC2 frameworks. The OECD (2021b) considers a review of physicochemical properties a minimum requirement for an assessment of exposure in order to determine that an alternative is indeed safer. Table 14.9 outlines those physicochemical properties and their influence on exposure parameters as outlined in the IC2 (2017) and NRC (2014) frameworks. Such properties are considered minimum requirements in the OECD guidance (2021b) for establishing that an alternative is safer. In cases where data on physicochemical properties are lacking, EPI (Estimation Programs Interface) Suite ™, a Windows®-based suite of physical/chemical property and environmental fate estimation programs developed by EPA and Syracuse Research Corp., is a useful tool to make such estimations (EPA 2021).

Physiochemical properties can be used to compare the exposure potential and environmental fate of the chemical of concern to alternatives under consideration. For example, an alternative in comparison to the chemical of concern may have a significantly lower log K_{ow} than the chemical of concern. A lower log K_{ow} is indicative of higher water solubility and, consequently, lower solubility in fatty tissues. This creates important differences in the potential for bioavailability and bioaccumulation among aquatic organisms that may be exposed following the release of the chemical in ambient waterways. If the alternative demonstrates even a moderate concern for aquatic toxicity (either acute or chronic) in the hazard assessment, this characterization of exposure potential may reveal an important trade-off worth highlighting as all information in the assessment (hazard, exposure, life cycle impacts cost, and performance) are considered.

As illustrated in Figure 14.5, the NRC framework states that if data on physicochemical properties are insufficient to identify a safer alternative, especially in situations where consideration of exposure is critical to interpreting the hazard assessment findings for specific end points of interest (i.e., Pathway B in Figure 14.5), then other tools can be used (i.e., Pathway A in Figure 14.5). These could include, for example, direct and indirect exposure measurements; use of exposure models, experimental values for transfer rates, dermal uptake, and bioavailability; questionnaires; and observational data to perform a more comprehensive qualitative exposure evaluation (NRC 2014; OECD 2021b).

Comparative exposure assessment is best suited for products with discrete end uses. Admittedly, it is challenging to assess exposure to chemicals that don't have clearly defined end

Table 14.9: Physicochemical Properties That Inform Exposure Potential in an Alternatives Assessment (IC2 2017)

Property	Reason
Physical state	Indicate which environmental compartments – air, water, sediment, biota, soil – into which the chemical will partition
Volatility/vapor pressure	Volatility/vapor pressure influences how likely the chemical is to be found in the air or how likely it is to enter the body
Molecular weight	Generally, as molecular weight and size increase, bioavailability decreases (leading to a lower toxicity potential)
Solubility in water	Generally, a chemical that is highly soluble in water will be more bioavailable and potentially toxic
Log K_{ow}	The log of the octanol-water coefficient is an indicator of potential for bioaccumulation, as well as bioavailability
Boiling point	The boiling point helps to determine if the chemical will be a liquid or gas at a certain temperature
Melting point	The melting point will determine if the chemical will be a solid or liquid at a certain temperature
Henry's law coefficient	Informs environmental partitioning and transport as well as human/mammalian alveolar absorption

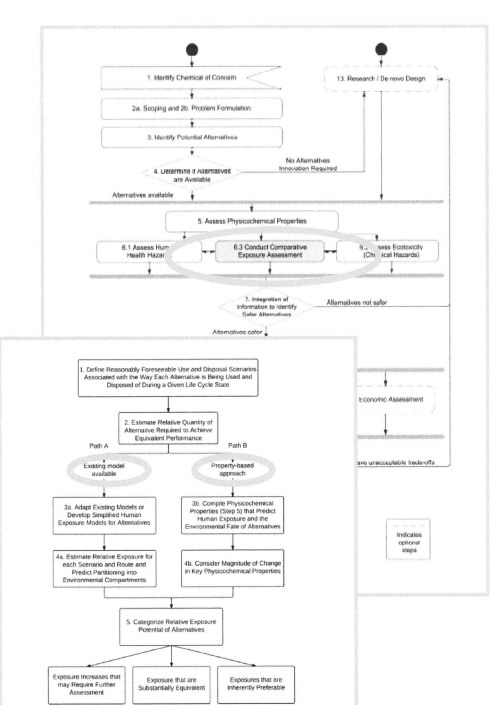

Figure 14.5 Comparative exposure assessment pathways (NRC 2014).

uses. Specific examples of ingredients that are good candidates for qualitative exposure assessments include the following:

- Injected vs. spray foam polyurethane insulation
- Methylene chloride-alternatives
- Fragrance raw materials (Greggs et al. 2018)

OTHER LIFE CYCLE IMPACT CONSIDERATIONS

Governments and companies are increasingly seeking to avoid a broader set of negative consequences of chemical substitutions, including "upstream" and "downstream" chemical or product impacts, resource depletion, energy use, and climate change potential. For example, a water bottle made from polyethylene terephthalate (PET) has a different life cycle impact profile than one produced from polylactic acid (PLA) due to the difference in the production of the two resins – which have very different feedstock and building-block chemicals – transportation of the resin to fabrication of bottles, and end of life.

Consideration of life cycle impacts in alternatives assessments is relatively new. It is required in alternatives assessment conducted under California's Safer Consumer Products regulation. Rather than use of life cycle assessment (LCA), which follows a well-defined quantitative methodology (e.g., ISO 14040), alternatives assessments typically use life cycle thinking or partial life cycle assessments. The purpose is to answer the question, *Is the alternative preferable in comparison to the chemical targeted for substitution given other relevant life cycle impacts?* The goal of considering life cycle impacts is to identify potential significant impacts across the life cycle but to do so using qualitatively versus the use of more time- and resource-intensive quantitative LCA processes. With its focus on averages and chemical emissions, LCA often does not thoroughly consider chemical hazards, a core component of alternatives assessment.

In an alternatives assessment, consideration of life cycle impacts includes first the mapping and identifying impact categories of potential concern during the scoping stage of the assessment. This scoping assessment of impacts is intended to help focus and streamline consideration of only those impacts of concern for the particular assessment. Subsequent analyses involve qualitatively evaluating the impacts (i.e., energy, and resource use), especially in relation to other attributes in the assessment (toxicity, performance, cost) in determining the best alternatives. Additional work is needed to adapt traditional LCA methods for the purpose and processes of alternatives assessment.

RESEARCH GAPS IN ALTERNATIVES ASSESSMENT – A ROLE FOR RISK ASSESSORS

Similar to risk assessment, research and discussions through the Association for the Advancement of Alternatives Assessment (A4) have identified a number of critical research and practice gaps for alternatives assessment (Tickner et al. 2019; Tickner and Jacobs 2016). Many of these overlap with gaps currently discussed in the field of risk assessment. Particular research needs identified, by the alternatives assessment component, include the following:

Hazard assessment

- Addressing *data gaps* through predictive toxicology and additional guidance, interpretation, and integration of predictive toxicology for chemical hazard assessment and best practice guidance for dealing with data gaps and associated uncertainties

- Developing methods to assess hazards of *chemical mixtures or specific forms*, including methods to assess hazards for formulated products and guidance for assessing nanomaterials in formulations

- Improving *ecological* hazard assessment, including consideration of applicable and sensitive species

Comparative exposure assessment

- Identifying needed intrinsic exposure information to understand comparative exposure trade-offs including, conceptual exposure models and critical exposure factors

- Identifying methods to integrate comparative exposure and hazard results without a full risk assessment to understand which option is safer and to understand potential exposure trade-offs between alternatives

Life cycle considerations

- Streamlining life cycle considerations in alternatives assessment by targeting relevant life cycle stages and impact categories that are comparatively different

- Developing guidance on integrating life cycle impact results into alternatives assessment processes to facilitate comparisons across components

Decision-making processes

- Developing tools or approaches to integrate and compare heterogeneous data across alternatives as well as address weighting of attributes for purposes of trade-off analysis

DATA GAPS IN HAZARD ASSESSMENT

It was all very well to say "Drink me," but the wise little Alice was not going to do that in a hurry. "No, I'll look first," she said, "and see whether it's marked 'poison' or not." — Chapter 1, Down the Rabbit-Hole, *Alice's Adventures in Wonderland* (Carroll 1946)

Major gaps in material health or performance attributes of a chemical, material, or product can result in harm to humans and/or environmental receptors or result in the commercialization of a product with a poor life cycle profile. Data are rarely available for all hazard end points in a chemical. A fundamental truth that should be remembered by all risk assessors is that the absence of declaration of hazard does not mean a chemical is safe. Unlike the *Alice in Wonderland* adage, most regrettable substitutions won't feature a discernable label that identifies a chemical as "poisonous."

It is critical for an assessor to know the identities of all chemicals used in a product and/or process and to characterize the human health and environmental hazard profiles of those chemicals, including those potentially formed upon release to the environment. Substituting a chemical of concern with a chemical that has similar or even dissimilar but undesirable hazard properties is a regrettable substitution. This section will explore how risk assessors can employ a variety of techniques and tools to address data gaps and minimize the likelihood that a regrettable substitution will occur.

NAMS in Alternatives Assessment

New Approach Methodologies (NAMs) are described as any nonanimal technology, methodology, approach, or combination thereof that can be used to provide information on chemical hazard and risk assessment (ICCVAM 2018)). More specifically, the term "NAM" applies to any nonanimal alternative that can be used alone or in combination to provide information for safety assessment (Madden et al. 2020)). NAMs hold the promise of faster and cheaper methods to evaluate chemical hazard and risk as compared to traditional methods for numerous end points (see Figure 14.6). Another advantage over conventional toxicology is that certain NAMs are designed to model human-specific physiology of tissues or organs (such as organ-on-a-chip assays),

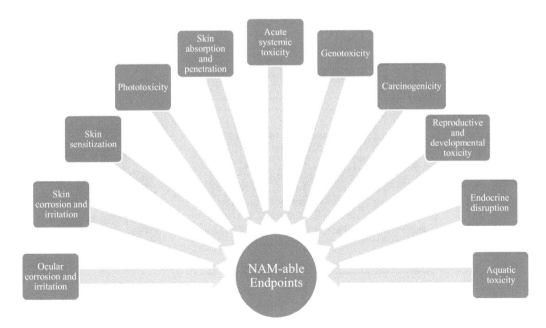

Figure 14.6 Example of NAM-Able endpoints (PISC 2021).

potentially reducing (or negating) the need for animal-to-human extrapolation, as well as significantly decreasing the use of animals (FDA 2021). One of the challenges of using NAMs lies in the interpretation of NAMs to derive equivalent estimates comparable with traditional toxicological methods (Parish et al. 2020).

A more expansive term "Integrated Approach to Testing and Assessment" (IATA) is often referenced in conjunction with NAMs, and like NAMs, IATAs are increasingly used to guide conclusions regarding potential hazards and/or risks of chemicals. An IATA can be defined (OECD 2016a) as an "approach based on multiple information sources used for the hazard identification, hazard characterization and/or safety assessment of chemicals." Within an IATA, relevant data including physicochemical properties, NAM predictions, Adverse Outcome Pathways, and human data are evaluated and integrated to draw conclusions on potential hazards and/or risks of an assessed chemical. Examples of published IATAs are indexed in the OECD IATA Case Studies Project and OECD Case Studies Reports (OECD 2016a, 2016b), which categorizes IATAs by type of assessment (e.g., safety assessment workflow, grouping (read across) for end points, including repeat dose toxicity, reproductive toxicity, developmental toxicity, endocrine disruption, and skin sensitization, among other end points).

Currently, there is not a uniformly accepted framework on how to report and apply individual NAMs or IATAs (EPA 2020; OECD 2020). A recent OECD (2020) report maps out 153 documents relating to various aspects of NAMs and IATAs, including guidance and publications relating to validation of test methods, *in vitro* approaches, *in silico* approaches, Quantitative Structure-Activity Relationships (Q)SARs, read-across approaches, -omics approaches, toxicokinetics, physiologically based pharmacokinetic (PBPK) modeling, uncertainty analyses, weight of evidence, and integration of data. This disarray and lack of uniformity of definitions, methods, and practices introduce significant uncertainty in NAMs and IATAs.

Figure 14.7 illustrates the building blocks of an IATA, including NAMs (OECD 2020). An IATA can be used to decide how and when to integrate information and data (including combinations of NAMs) to classify a chemical's specific hazard and potency. NAM-based and IATA-based assessments feed into many different types of work products, including chemical hazard assessments (such as GreenScreen for Safer Chemicals assessments), risk assessments, and chemical alternatives assessments for a myriad of product types (cosmetics, medical devices, pharmaceuticals, consumer products, cleaning products, home care products, and industrial use chemicals).

The expanded practice of NAM and IATA methods greatly amplifies the need to train practitioners in appropriate ways to select, conduct, and interpret NAMs and IATAs and, equally important, to recognize limitations and uncertainties in each type of assessment. As defined by the European Food Safety Agency (EEFSA 2018), uncertainty is "a general term referring to all types of limitations in available knowledge that affect the range and probability of possible answers to an assessment question."

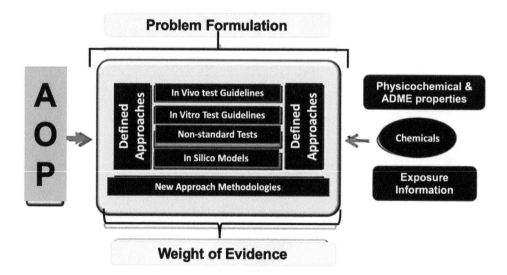

Figure 14.7 OECD building blocks of an IATA (OECD 2020).

Addressing Uncertainty in NAMs and IATAs

The quality, utility, and accuracy of the NAM and/or IATA predictions are greatly influenced by two primary types of uncertainties (OECD 2020):

- Type I: Uncertainties related to the input data used

- Type II: Uncertainties related to extrapolations made

Recognition of each type of uncertainty when conducting a NAM or IATA can greatly improve the quality and utility of the NAM and/or IATA assessment. As discussed in OECD (2020), most of the uncertainty analysis methods associated with NAMs and IATAs are qualitative in nature and are still undergoing development. Recommended approaches to reduce each type of uncertainty are discussed below.

The expanded practice of NAM and IATA methods greatly amplifies the need to train practitioners in appropriate ways to select, conduct, and interpret NAMs and IATAs, and equally important, to recognize limitations in each type of assessment.

Reducing Type I Uncertainties Related to the Input Data Used

Uncertainties related to the input data used in a NAM or IATA relate to the relevance, reliability, and completeness of the data. The universe of NAMs includes many methodological approaches, including (Q)SARs (i.e., read-across approaches, and *in chemico*, *in vitro*, and -omics (such as toxicogenomics) technologies). No single NAM serves as a one-to-one replacement for more complex assays based on whole animal or clinical (human) tests.

To ensure that input data are relevant, reliable, and complete, it is critical to follow a framework when applying NAMs or IATAs to ensure that they are appropriate for the end point of interest, able to accomplish the job at hand (e.g., chemical prioritization, hazard screening, or assessing risk), and transparent, accurate, and clearly disclose limitations and assumptions. There are two guidelines that most NAM practitioners reference:

- OECD Guideline 34 (2005)

- OECD Guideline 211 (2014)

A NAM-related workgroup sponsored by Health and Environmental Sciences Institute (HESI) published a useful three-step NAM framework (Parish et al. 2020) that is built upon OECD Guidelines 34 and 211. The HESI three-step framework reminds the practitioner to specify the intended use of the NAM, adhere to core principles relating to accuracy and transparency (among other principles), and tailor criteria based on the intended use of the NAM.

Reducing Type 2 Uncertainties Related to Extrapolations Made

Uncertainties related to extrapolations made refer to the interpretation, extrapolation, and integration of data (OECD 2020). Ideally, an assessor needs to have a strong understanding of the end point being assessed by the NAM or IATA, recognize the limitations of the test method(s) being used, and take care not to extend the reach of the test data. If specific NAMs are not used to assess a chemical (for example, if a chemical is outside of a (Q)SAR model's applicability domain), the assessment report should clearly state this so the entire assessment process is transparent. If NAM and conventional data sets have conflicting results, it is usually a good idea to default to a more conservative hazard classification until an additional assessment is possible.

Publications that include NAMs and/or IATAs should include access to complete copies of the NAM and IATA predictions to facilitate transparency and widespread dissemination of best practices. If precluded by page limitations, supplementary appendices should accompany a published article.

Table 14.10 summarizes ways to reduce uncertainties related to input data used.

Example Uncertainty Analyses for Two Major Types of Uncertainties: Cyrene™ (CAS#53716-82-8)

Cyrene (also known as Dihydrolevoglucosenone) is a bio-based heterocyclic cycloalkanone solvent derived from cellulose. Cyrene is a potential alternate to N,N-dimethylformamide, which is classified as a GHS Category 2 eye irritant (H319) and a GHS Category 1B reprotoxicant (H360D) (ECHA 2021). As explained previously, IATAs provide guidance on how and when to integrate

Table 14.10: Steps to Reduce Uncertainties Related to the Input Data Used and Extrapolations Made

Appropriate Selection of Alternative Test Method for Specific End Points	Methods accepted in the United States: >114 separate alternative methods	Indexed end points: acute oral, dermal, and inhalation toxicity; dermal irritation, phototoxicity, sensitization, and corrosion; developmental and reproductive toxicity; endocrine disruption; genotoxicity; carcinogenicity; ocular corrosion and irritation; pyrogenicity; ecotoxicity (NTP 2022)
	Methods accepted in Europe: European Union Tracking System for Alternative Methods for Regulatory Acceptance (TSAR)	Indexed end points: acute oral toxicity; dermal irritation, phototoxicity, sensitization, and corrosion; ocular irritation; genotoxicity; carcinogenicity (EC 2022)
	Methods accepted in Japan: The Japanese Center for the Validation of Alternative Methods (JaCVAM): > 22 separate alternative methods	Indexed end points: acute oral toxicity; dermal irritation, phototoxicity, sensitization; ocular corrosion and irritation (JaCVAM 2022)
(Q)SAR Resources	ECHA (2016) tabulates freeware and commercial ware (Q)SARs by hazard end point	
	European Joint Research Commission database indexes 154 (Q)SAR models searchable by hazard end point (EC 2021)	
Read-Across and Grouping Guidance	ECHA Read-Across Assessment Framework	ECHA 2017
	OECD Guidance on Grouping	OECD 2007, 2014b
	Examples of automated tools to perform read across and grouping: (Q)SAR Toolbox, ToxMatch, US EPA Analog Identification Methodology (AIM) tool, US EPA CompTox dashboard	
IATA Frameworks and Case Studies	OECD *Guidance Document on the Reporting of Defined Approaches (Das) to Be Used within IATA. Series on Testing and Assessment: No. 255* (OECD 2016a)	
	OECD *Guidance Document on the Reporting of Defined Approaches and Individual Information Sources to be Used within Integrated Approaches to Testing and Assessment (IATA) for Skin Sensitization: No. 256* (OECD 2016b)	
	OECD *Guidance Document for the Use of AOPs to Develop IATAs* (OECD 2017)	
	OECD *Guidance Document on Integrated Approaches to Testing and Assessment (IATA) for Serious Eye Damage and Irritation. No. 263* (OECD 2019a)	
	OECD *Overview of Concepts and Available Guidance Related to Integrated Approaches to Testing and Assessment (IATA)* (OECD 2020)	
	OECD's IATA Case Studies Project 2015–Present: Online compilation of more than one dozen case studies applying different approaches (Grouping, (Q)SAR, Adverse Outcome Pathways) to assess hazards of chemicals as part of an IATA (OECD 2022)	

information sources and minimize use of animals to the extent possible while ensuring human safety. The OECD (2019a) recommends two IATA testing approaches for the assessment of serious eye damage and eye irritation:

- Bottom-Up Approach: Starting with *in vitro* test methods that can accurately identify non-eye irritants (not GHS classified)

- Top-Down Approach: Starting with *in vitro* test methods that can accurately identify severe eye irritants (GHS Category 1)

OECD's Top-Down Approach IATA was used to assess the eye irritancy potential of Cyrene. As shown in Figure 14.3, the IATA Top-Down Approach specifies starting with an *in vitro* test that can identify chemicals that are either seriously damaging to the eye (GHS Category 1) or GHS not classified. An *in vitro* assay that can assess serious eye damage is the Bovine Corneal Opacity and Permeability Assay (BCOP) following OECD Test Guideline 437 (OECD 2020). BCOP test data are used to calculate an *In Vitro* Irritancy Score (IVIS), which is then used to classify eye damage following the Globally Harmonized System of Classification and Labeling (GHS) (Figure 14.8).

As shown in Table 14.11, when a chemical produces an IVIS between 3 and 55 in a BCOP assay, OECD's Top-Down IATA recommends conducting a second *in vitro* test to classify chemicals irritating to the eye. Cyrene's ECHA dossier describes an *in vitro* ocular irritation (OI) assay

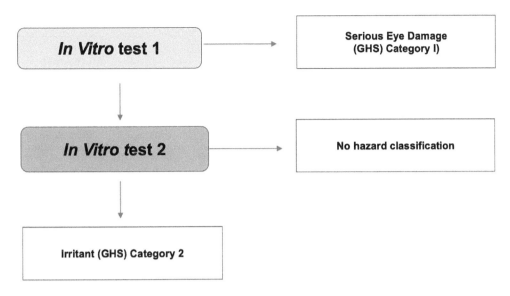

Figure 14.8

Table 14.11: **Cyrene Classified According to the Serious Eye Damage and Irritation Studies IATA (OECD 2019a)**

BCOP *IVIS*	Irritation Draize Equivalent (IDE) MQS	GHS Eye Damage Classification
< 3	0–12.5	No Category
>3–< 55	> 12.5–30	No prediction can be made
> 55	> 30	Category 1 ("Irreversible Effects on the Eye")
Eye Damage/Eye Irritation Hazard Classification following OECD Top-Down IATA		
Cyrene IVIS Score from BCOP	36.37 IVIS (ECHA 2021)	No prediction can be made based on IVIS reported in ECHA dossier (ECHA 2021)
Cyrene IVIS Score from OI Assay	13.5 MQS (ECHA 2021)	OECD Test Guideline 496 (OECD 2019) notes that No Prediction Can be Made (NPCM) based on OI^{O} MQS of >12.5 – 30 Despite Test Guideline 496, ECHA dossier (ECHA 2021) uses OI^{O} MQS to classify Cyrene as Category 2B ("Reversible effects to the eye")(H320) ECHA dossier (ECHA 2021) then reports overall conclusion that Cyrene is a GHS Category 2 eye irritant (H319)

with a Maximal Qualified Score (MQS) of 13.5. Although the OECD Test Guideline 496 for the *In Vitro* Macromolecular Test Method for Identifying Chemicals Inducing Serious Eye Damage and Chemicals Not Requiring Classification or Eye Irritation or Serious Eye Damage (OECD 2019b) states that MQS results > 12.5 – 30 should not be used in isolation for GHS classification, Cyrene's ECHA dossier uses the OI MQS score to classify Cyrene as a GHS Category 2B eye irritant, which corresponds to mildly irritating to the eyes (H320). Cyrene's ECHA dossier subsequently reports an overall eye irritation classification as Category 2 (H319), which corresponds to irritating to the eyes.

Table 14.12 provides examples of Type I and Type II uncertainties associated with Cyrene's eye damage and irritation data set. This analysis indicates that there are uncertainties associated with the completeness and relevance of the input data (i.e., BCOP and OI test protocols) used to classify Cyrene's eye irritation potential (a Type I Uncertainty), as well as the extrapolation of the BCOP and OI test data to support a Category 2 eye irritation classification (Type 2 Uncertainty). This example demonstrates the utility of considering both types of uncertainty when applying and

Table 14.12: Type I and II Uncertainty Analysis of Cyrene's Eye Damage and Irritation Potential

Chemical	IATA	Uncertainty Type I: Input Data Uncertainties	Uncertainty Type II: Extrapolation of Data Uncertainties
Cyrene™ (CAS #53716-82-8)	IATA Top-Down Approach (OECD 2019a) for Serious Eye Damage and Irritation	Limited data set: Only two *in vitro* studies (BCOP and Ocular Irritection (OI^O) Assay System) No other NAM used to classify eye damage end point Questionable relevance of Top-Down strategy compared to Bottom-Down Strategy: Top-Down Strategy is for highly irritating substances (OECD 2019a)	BCOP and OI are not recommended for identifying Category 2 eye irritants (OECD 2019a, 2019b, 2020) Cyrene's BCOP IVIS test results in ECHA (2021) can't be used on its own for classifying eye damage, per the IATA (OECD 2019a) Cyrene's OI MQS test results in ECHA (2021) can't be used on its own for classifying either Category 1 or 2 eye damage, per the IATA (OECD 2019a, 2019b)

interpreting an IATA so that inherent weaknesses in the assessment are clearly and prominently communicated.

Incorporating Toxicological Data and Exposure Information into the Design of Safer Alternatives

There is increasing interest in incorporating the tools of toxicology commonly used for risk assessment – and now increasingly used in alternatives assessment – into the design of new chemicals. Because safer alternatives do not always exist, developing new safer options, while controlling exposure to incumbent chemicals, may be the best option. For example, Vlisco, a Dutch company that makes batik printed formal African textiles evaluated alternatives to trichloroethylene in its printing processes in order to continue using trichloroethylene as required to under the European Union's REACH Authorization process. The company found no alternative, except other problematic drop-in halogenated solvents, that would maintain the quality of the printing. The company chose instead to invest in application of switchable solvents, a green chemistry innovation. However, chemists are not generally trained in toxicology and hence in most cases do not consider toxicity when designing new molecules.

One promising approach, that of rational design, has emerged from medicinal chemistry, where human safety is paramount (Joudan 2016)). It uses toxicological knowledge to inform the design of safe medicines rather than screening them after development (DeVito 2018). During the design phase of pharmaceutical molecules, high throughput chemical screening and *in vitro* data are used to ensure that the active ingredient has the desired effect on the target without adverse side effects. Development of new in silico and high throughput tools to better understand chemical toxicity and potential exposures, including property-toxicity relationships and toxicological mechanisms of action at the molecular level, has been identified as an important priority for green chemistry. A number of research efforts have been undertaken to develop high throughput models to predict chemical toxicity and exposure based on molecular structure and NAMS to develop tiered assays to assess specific end points, such as endocrine disruption, in the design stage of molecules and to design molecules based on an understanding of interrelationships between physical-chemical properties, structure, mechanisms, and modes of action. Filling such data gaps to inform chemical design and selection of safer alternatives requires greater collaboration between the chemistry and toxicology communities to develop a robust tool kit to aid both chemical design and selection. The development of Valspar's valPure is an example of this type of collaboration.

CONCLUSION

Alternatives assessment is an action and solutions-oriented approach to managing chemical risks. It is grounded in primary prevention, the industrial hygiene hierarchy of controls, and the pollution prevention hierarchy. Alternatives utilize the same toxicological tool kit as risk assessment but apply it in a different way aimed at comparative assessment of options to replace a particular chemical function/application. The level of detail needed to compare options should

Table 14.13: **Examples of Alternatives Assessment Frameworks**

- California Department of Toxic Substances Control. 2017. *Alternatives Analysis Guide, Version 1.0.* June.
- Interstate Chemicals Clearinghouse. 2017. *Alternatives Assessment Guide Version 1.1.* January.
- Massachusetts Toxics Use Reduction Institute. 2006. *Five Chemicals Alternatives Assessment Study.*
- Eliason, P. and G. Morose. (2011) Safer Alternatives Assessment: The Massachusetts Process as a Model for State Governments. *Journal of Cleaner Production* 19: 517–526.
- US NRC (US National Research Council). 2014. Committee on the Design and Evaluation of Safer Chemical Substitutions: A Framework to Inform Government and Industry Decision, Board on Chemical Sciences and Technology, Board on Environmental Studies and Toxicology, Division on Earth and Life Studies, & National Research Council. *A Framework to Guide Selection of Chemical Alternatives.* National Academies Press.
- European Chemicals Agency. 2011. *Guidance on the Preparation of an Application for Authorisation.* ECHA-11-G-01-EN. Helsinki, Finland.
- United Nations Environment Program. 2009. *Report of the Persistent Organic Pollutants Review Committee on the Work of Its Fifth Meeting. Addendum General Guidance on Considerations Related to Alternatives and Substitutes for Listed Persistent Organic Pollutants and Candidate Chemicals.*
- German Federal Institute for Occupational Safety and Health. 2008. Committee on Hazardous Substances (AGS). *Technical Rules for Hazardous Substances, Substitution, TRGS 600.*
- US Environmental Protection Agency. 1996. *Cleaner Technologies Substitute Assessment: A Methodology and Resource Guide.* Office of Pollution Prevention. EPA744-R-95-002. December.
- US Environmental Protection Agency. 2011. *Instructions for the Significant New Alternatives Policy (SNAP) Program Information Notice and TSCA/SNAP Addendum.* EPA-1265-07. Washington, DC. US EPA, Office of Atmospheric Programs.
- US Occupational Health & Safety Administration. 2021. *Transitioning to Safer Chemicals: A Toolkit for Employers and Workers (online).*
- California Department of Toxic Substances Control. 2017. *Alternatives Analysis Guide, Version 1.0.* June.
- Interstate Chemicals Clearinghouse. 2017. *Alternatives Assessment Guide Version 1.1.* January.

Table 14.14: **The OECD's Set of Authoritative Lists That Should Be Considered in a Hazard Assessment to Support Identifying and Selecting a Safer Alternative (OECD 2020)**

- California Office of Environmental Health Hazard Assessment. *The Proposition 65 List.* https://oehha.ca.gov/proposition-65/proposition-65-list
- Government of Canada. *Toxic Substances List and the Virtual Elimination List.*
- ECHA. *Candidate List of Substances of Very High Concern for Authorization.* https://echa.europa.eu/candidate-list-table
- ECHA. *Substances Classified as Substances with Carcinogenic, Mutagenic or Reproductive Toxicity Properties (CMR) 1a or 1b under Annex VI of CLP.* https://echa.europa.eu/information-on-chemicals/annex-vi-to-clp
- US Environmental Protection Agency. *Toxics Release Inventory's Persistent, Bioaccumulative and Toxic (PBT) Chemicals List and PBT Chemicals under the Toxic Substances Control Act (TSCA) Section 6(h)*
- US National Toxicology Program. *Report on Carcinogens.* https://ntp.niehs.nih.gov/whatwestudy/assessments/cancer/completed/index.html?utm_source=direct&utm_medium=prod&utm_campaign=ntpgolinks&utm_term=rocevals
- World Health Organization's International Agency for Research on Cancer. *Agents Classified by the IARC Monographs.* https://monographs.iarc.who.int/agents-classified-by-the-iarc/
- Montreal Protocol. *List of Ozone Depleting Substances.* https://ozone.unep.org/treaties/montreal-protocol/summary-control-measures-under-montreal-protocol
- Stockholm Convention. *List of Persistent Organic Pollutants.* http://chm.pops.int/TheConvention/ThePOPs/ListingofPOPs/tabid/2509/Default.aspx

Table 14.15: **Hazard Assessment Tools to Support Alternatives Assessments**

- Clean Production Action. *GreenScreen® for Safer Chemicals. https://www.greenscreenchemicals.org/learn/full-greenscreen-method*
- Washington State Department of Ecology. QCAT. https://ecology.wa.gov/Regulations-Permits/Guidance-technical-assistance/Safer-alternatives/Quick-tool-for-assessing-chemicals
- Massachusetts TURI. P2OASys. https://www.turi.org/Our_Work/Alternatives_Assessment/Alternatives_Assessment/Tools_and_Methods/P2OASys_Tool_to_Compare_Materials
- German Institute for Occupational Safety and Health, Column Model. https://www.dguv.de/ifa/praxishilfen/hazardous-substances/ghs-spaltenmodell-zur-substitutionspruefung/index.jsp
- ChemFORWARD. ChemFORWARDPlatform or Intelligent Ingredient Report. https://www.chemforward.org/safer-alternatives
- US EPA. Hazard Comparison Dashboard forthcoming.
- Healthy Building Network. Pharos Project. https://pharosproject.net/
- Clean Production Action. GreenScreen® Assessment Registry. https://registry.greenscreenchemicals.org/about/registry

be significantly less than that to determine a "safe" level of exposure. Given the thousands of chemicals in commerce, it would be impossible to assess each and hence an approach focused on identifying and evaluating the best option(s) will permit a broader evaluation of chemical non-chemical options for specific functional uses, including considering whether the chemical use is even needed.

Alternatives assessment suffers from the same concerns over data gaps as risk assessment and hence NAMs will play an increasingly important role in developing a more thoughtful understanding of chemical hazards, safer options, and how to apply these results in designing safer chemicals in the future. For alternatives assessment to be supportive of the transition to safer chemicals, the approaches will need to be flexible and applicable to a variety of business and government contexts. Marketplace decisions are being made to phase out certain chemicals in products and manufacturing processes, even before government regulations. As such, alternatives assessment cannot become bogged down in paralysis by analysis as has been the case in many risk assessment processes. This will require that governments design regulatory processes for chemical substitution that facilitate thoughtful but expeditious assessment and that the alternatives assessment community design tools and approaches that support thoughtful but not overburdensome assessments.

Alternatives assessment is an interdisciplinary approach, requiring the input of toxicologists, exposure scientists, environmental health professionals, engineers, chemists, and others. To drive safer chemistry, it is essential to break down the silos that have divided the health sciences and chemistry/engineering to develop thoughtful approaches to safer chemical assessment and design, as well as to train next-generation practitioners to focus on safer chemistry from the design stage of chemicals and products, where the greatest possibilities for primary prevention of impacts lie. It is critical that the risk assessment community utilize its skills and knowledge in driving safer alternatives that result in both benefits for health and safety but also for the economy.

ADDITIONAL RESOURCES

OECD Substitution and Alternatives Assessment Toolkit and Guidance on Key Considerations of the Identification and Selection of Safer Chemical Alternatives

https://www.oecd.org/chemicalsafety/substitution-of-hazardous-chemicals.htm

Massachusetts TURI – www.turi.org

SUSBPORT Plus Database – https://www.subsportplus.eu/subsportplus/EN/Home/Home_node.html

OSHA Transitioning to Safer Chemicals Toolkit – https://www.osha.gov/safer-chemicals

Interstate Chemicals Clearinghouse – https://theic2.org/#gsc.tab=0

Association for the Advancement of Alternatives Assessment – www.saferalternatives.org

NRC – Framework to Guide Selection of Chemical Alternatives – https://www.nap.edu/catalog/18872/a-framework-to-guide-selection-of-chemical-alternatives

EPA Safer Choice and related programs – https://www.epa.gov/saferchoice/safer-choice-related-programs

REFERENCES

Resources Referenced in Tables and Figures

LITERATURE CITED

Anastas, P. T., and J. C. Warner. 1998. *Green Chemistry: Theory and Practice*. New York: Oxford University Press.

Bailar, J. C., and A. J. Bailer. 1999. Risk Assessment – the Mother of All Uncertainties: Disciplinary Perspectives on Uncertainty in Risk Assessment. *Annals N.Y. Acad. Sci* 895: 273–285.

Birnbaum, L. S. 2010. Brominated and Chlorinated Fame Retardants: The San Antonio Statement. *Environ. Health Persp.* 118: A-514–A515. http://doi.org/10.1289/ehp.1003088.

C2CPII. 2021. *Cradle to Cradle Certified*. London: Cradle to Cradle Products Innovation Institute. https://www.c2ccertified.org/get-certified/product-certification.

Cairns, J. J. 1999. Absence of Certainty Is Not Synonymous with Absence of Risk. *Environ. Health Persp.* 107 (2): A56–A57.

Carroll, L. 1946. *Alice's Adventures in Wonderland. Special Edition.* Special ed. Fantasy. New York: Random House.

CCOHS. 2018. *OHS Answers Fact Sheets: Trichloroethylene.* Canadian Centre for Occupational Health and Safety. Ottowa, CA: Canadian Centre for Occupational Health and Safet.

CDC. 2008. Neurologic Illness Associated with Occupational Exposure to the Solvent 1-Bromopropane – New Jersey and Pennsylvania, 2007–2008. *M. M. W. R.* 57 (48): 1300–1302.

Colborn, T., and C. A. Clement. 1992. *Chemically-Induced Alterations in Sexual and Functional Development: The Wildlife/Human Connection.* Vol. Xxi. Princeton, NJ: Princeton Scientific Publishing.

Control, CA DTSC [California Department of Toxic Substances]. 2017. *Alternatives Analysis Guide.* Sacramento, CA: California Department of Toxic Substances Control.

CPA. 2018. *GreenScreen® for Safer Chemicals: Hazard Assessment Guidance.* Clean Production Action (Clean Production Action). http://www.greenscreenchemicals.org.

CPA. 2021. *Tools for Safer Chemicals – from Chemicals to Products to Organizations.* Brussels.

Cranor, C. 1993. *Regulating Toxic Substances.* New York: Oxford University Press.

DeVito, S. C. 2018. The Need for, and the Role of the Toxicological Chemist in the Design of Safer Chemicals. *Toxicol. Sci.* 161 (2): 225–240. https://doi.org/10.1093/toxsci/kfx197.

European Commission (EC). 2022. Tracking System for Regulatory Acceptance, Joint Research Centre. https://tsar.jrc.ec.europa.eu/

ECHA. 2013. *Evaluation of New Scientific Evidence Concerning DINP and DIDP in Relation to Entry 52 of Annex XVII to REACH Regulation (EC) No 1907/2006.* Helsinki: European Chemicals Agency.

ECHA. 2022. Summary of Classification and Labeling: N,N-Dimethylformamide (CAS#68-12-2). https://echa.europa.eu/information-on-chemicals/cl-inventory-database/-/discli/details/2384

EEFSA. 2018. Guidance on Uncertainty Analysis in Scientific Assessments. *EFSA J.* 16: 5123 (1): 39. https://doi.org/10.2903/j.efsa.2018.5123. https://www.efsa.europa.eu/en/topics/topic/uncertainty-scientific-assessments.

Eladak, S., T. Grisin, D. Moison, G. Livera, V. Rouiller-Fabra, and R. Habert. 2015. A New Chapter in the Bisphenol A Story: Bisphenol S and Bisphenol F Are Not Safe Alternatives To This Compound. *Fert. Steril.* 103 (1): 11–21. DOI:https://doi.org/10.1016/j.fertnstert.2014.11.005.

EPA. 2020. *EPA Innovative Approaches for DART Related Toxicities.* (EPA). Estimation Programs Interface Suite™ for Microsoft® Windows, v 4.11. EPA, online.

European Chemicals Agency (ECHA). 2016. Practical Guide: How to Use and Report (Q) SARs. Version 3.1. July 2016. https://echa.europa.eu/documents/10162/13655/pg_report_qsars_en.pdf/407dff11-aa4a-4eef-a1ce-9300f8460099.

European Chemicals Agency (ECHA). 2017. Read-Across Assessment Framework (RAAF). ECHA-17-R-01-EN. https://echa.europa.eu/documents/10162/13628/raaf_en.pdf

FDA. 2021. *FDA in Brief: FDA Publishes Report on Advancing Alternative Methods.* US HHS. Washington, DC: FDA.

GCO. 2019. The Full Global Chemicals Outlook II. https://www.unep.org/explore-topics/chemicals-waste/what-we-do/policy-and-governance/global-chemicals-outlook.

Geiser, K., J. Tickner, S. W. Edwards, and M. Rossi. 2015. The Architecture of Chemical Alternatives Assessment. *Risk Anal.* 15 (12): 2152–2161. https://doi.org/10.1111/risa.12507.

Greggs, W., T. Burns, P. Ereghy, M.R. Embry, P. Fantke, B. Gaborek, L. Heine, O. Jolliet, C. Lee, D. Muir, K. Plotzke, J. Rinkevich, N. Sunger, J.Y. Tanir, and M. Whittaker. 2018. Qualitative Approach to Comparative Exposure in Alternatives Assessment. *Int. Environ. Assess. Mgt. J.* 15 (6): 880–894. https://doi.org/10.1002/ieam.4070.

Harney, J. M., J. B. Nemhauser, C.M. Reh, D. Trout, and S. Schrader. 2003. *NIOSH Health Hazard Evaluation Report: HETA #99-0260-2906. Marx Industries, Inc. Sawmills.* NIOSH, CDC. Washington, DC: OSHA. https://www.cdc.gov/niosh/hhe/reports/pdfs/1999-0260-2906.pdf.

IC2. 2017. *Alternatives Assessment Guide Version 1.1.* Washington, DC: Interstate Chemicals Clearinghouse (United States). http://theic2.org/article/download-pdf/file_name/IC2_AA_Guide_Version_1.1.pdf.

ICCVAM. 2018. *Biennial Progress Report.* NIEHS (RTP: NTP). https://ntp.niehs.nih.gov/go/2019iccvamreport.

Ichihara, G., J. Kitoh, W. Li, X. Ding, S. Ichihara, and Y. Takeuchi. 2012. Neurotoxicity of 1-Bromopropane: Evidence from Animal Experiments and Human Studies. *J. Adv. Res.* 3: 98–98. https://doi.org/10.1016/j.jare.2011.04.005.

Jacobs, E. T., J. L. Burgess, and M. B. Abbott. 2018. The Donora Smog Revisited: 70 Years After the Event That Inspired the Clean Air Act. *Am. J. Public Health* 108: S85–S88.

Jacobs, M. M., T. F. Malloy, J. A. Tickner, and S. W. Edwards. 2016. Alternatives Assessment Frameworks: Research Needs for the Informed Substitution of Hazardous Chemicals. *Environ. Health Persp.* 124: 265–280. http://dx.doi.org/10.1289/ehp.1409581.

JaCVAM. 2022. The Japanese Center for the Validation of Alternative Methods (JaCVAM). http://www.jacvam.jp/en/international-acceptance-test-methods.html.

Joudan, S. 2016. Challenges in Designing Non-Toxic Molecules: Using Medicinal Chemistry Frameworks to Help Design Non-Toxic Commercial Chemicals. *Green Chemistry Blog.* February 22. https://greenchemuoft.wordpress.com/2016/12/20/challenges-in-designing-non-toxic-molecules-using-medicinal-chemistry-frameworks-to-help-design-non-toxic-commercial-chemicals/

Kriebel, D., J. Tickner, P. Epstein, J. Lamons, R. Levins, E. L. Loecher, M. Quinn, R. A. Rudel, T. Schetter, and M. Stoto. 2001. The Precautionary Principle in Environmental Science. *Environ. Health Persp.* 109: 871–876. http://ehpnet1.niehs.nih.gov/docs/2001/109p871-876kriebel/abstract.html.

Madden, J. C., S. J. Enoch, A. Paini, and M. T. D. Cronin. 2020. A Review of In Silico Tools as Alternatives to Animal Testing: Principles, Resources and Applications. *Alt. to Lab. Animals* 48 (4): 146–172. https://doi.org/10.1177/0261192920965977journals.sagepub.com/home/atl.

McMichael, T. 1993. *Planetary Overload: Global Environmental Change and the Health of the Human Species.* Cambridge University Press.

NRC. 1983. *Risk Assessment in the Federal Government: Managing the Process.* Washington, DC: National Academies Press.

NRC. 1994. *Science and Judgment in Risk Assessment.* Washington, DC: National Academy Press.

NRC. 1997. *Risk Assessment and Management at Deseret Chemical Depot and the Tooele Chemical Agent Disposal Facility. In Risk Assessment and Management at Deseret Chemical Depot and the Tooele Chemical Agent Disposal Facility.* Washington, DC: National Academies Press.

NRC. 2007. *Models in Environmental Regulatory Decision Making.* Washington, DC: National Academies Press.

NRC. 2008. *2008 Amendments to the National Academies Guidelines for Human Embryonic Stem Cell Research.* Washington, DC: National Academies Press.

NRC. 2009. *Science And Decisions: Advancing Risk Assessment.* Washington, DC: National Academies Press.

NRC. 2014. *A Framework to Guide Selection of Chemical Alternatives.* National Academies Press.

NTP. 2011. *Toxicology and Carcinogenesis Studies of 1- Bromopropane in F344/N Rats and B6C3F1 Mice (Inhalation Studies).* NIEHS (RTP, NC: NIEHS/NTP).

NTP. 2013. *Report on Carcinogens Monograph on 1-Bromopropane: RoC Monograph 01.* NIEHS/NIH. Research Triangle Park, NC: NIEHS/NTP. https://ntp.niehs.nih.gov/ntp/roc/thirteenth/monographs_final/1bromopropane_508.pdf.

NTP. 2022. NTP Interagency Center for the Evaluation of Alternative Toxicological Methods (NICEATM). Alternative Methods Accepted by U.S. Agencies, https://ntp.niehs.nih.gov/whatwestudy/niceatm/accept-methods/index.html

O'Brien, M. K. 2000. *Making Better Environmental Decisions: An Alternative to Risk Assessment.* Cambridge, MA: MIT Press.

O'Brien, M. K. 2000. *Making Better Environmental Decisions: An Alternative to Risk Assessment.* Cambridge, MA: MIT Press.

OECD. 2005. Series on Testing and Assessment: Publications by Number. OECD. Accessed February 28. https://www.oecd.org/chemicalsafety/testing/series-testing-assessment-publications-number.htm.

OECD. 2007. Guidance Document on Grouping of Chemicals. Series on Testing and Assessment. No. 80. ENV/JM/MONO(2007)28, (2007). http://www.oecd.org/officialdocuments/publicdisplaydocumentpdf/?cote=env/jm/mono(2007)28&doclanguage=en

OECD. 2013, November 28. *Current Landscape of Alternatives Assessment Practice: A Meta-Review. Series on Risk Management.* Organisation for Economic Co-operation and Development. https://www.oecd.org/officialdocuments/publicdisplaydocumentpdf/?cote=env/jm/mono%282013%2924&doclanguage=en.

OECD. 2014a. *Series on Testing and Assessment: Publications by Number.* OECD. Accessed February 28. https://www.oecd.org/chemicalsafety/testing/series-testing-assessment-publications-number.htm.

OECD. 2014b. Guidance on Grouping of Chemicals. Second Edition. ENV/JM/MONO(2014)4, 2014. http://www.oecd.org/officialdocuments/publicdisplaydocumentpdf/?cote=env/jm/mono(2014)4&doclanguage=en

OECD. 2016a. *Series on Testing and Assessment No. 255: Guidance Document on the Reporting of Defined Approaches (Das) to Be Used within IATA.* OECD. https://www.oecd.org/officialdocuments/publicdisplaydocumentpdf/?cote=env/jm/mono(2016)28&doclanguage=en.

OECD. 2016b. *Guidance Document for the Use of Adverse Outcome Pathways in Developing Integrated Approaches to Testing and Assessment (IATA).* Organisation for Economic Co-operation and Development. Ttp://www.oecd.org/officialdocuments/publicdisplaydocumentpdf/?cote=ENV/JM/MONO(2016)67/&doclanguage=en.

OECD. 2017. *Guidance Document for the Use of Adverse Outcome Pathways in Developing Integrated Approaches to Testing and Assessment (IATA),* OECD Series on Testing and Assessment, No. 260, OECD Publishing, Paris, https://doi.org/10.1787/44bb06c1-en.

OECD. 2019a. *Streamlined Summary Document Supporting OECD Test Guideline 438 on the Isolated Chicken Eye for Eye Irritation/Corrosion.* Brussels.

OECD. 2019b. *In vitro Macromolecular Test Method for Identifying Chemicals Inducing Serious Eye Damage and Chemicals not Requiring Classification for Eye Irritation or Serious Eye Damage.* Test Guideline 496. 24 October 2019. https://www.oecd-ilibrary.org/docserver/970e5cd9-en.pdf?expires=1613921672&id=id&accname=guest&checksum=7E526AB84E74E916E8405C45D6943464

OECD. 2020. *Overview of Concepts and Available Guidance related to Integrated Approaches to Testing and Assessment (IATA).* Stockholm: OECD.

OECD. 2021a. *Guidance on Key Considerations for the Identification and Selection of Safer Chemical Alternatives.* OECD (Environmental Directorate OECD).

OECD. 2021b. *Reconciling Terminology of the Universe of Per- and Polyfluoroalkyl Substances: Recommendations and Practical Guidance.* Environment Directorate, Organisation for Economic Co-Operation and Development (OECD). Stockholm: OECD. https://www.oecd.org/officialdocuments/publicdisplaydocumentpdf/?cote=ENV/CBC/MONO(2021)25&docLanguage=en.

OECD. 2022. Case Studies Project. Integrated Approaches to Testing and Assessment (IATA). http://www.oecd.org/chemicalsafety/risk-assessment/iata-integrated-approaches-to-testing-and-assessment.htm.

OSHA. 2021. *Transitioning to Safer Chemicals: A Toolkit for Employers and Workers.* US Occupational Health & Safety Administration. https://www.osha.gov/safer-chemicals.

Parish, S.T.M., M. Aschner, W. Casey, M. Corvaro, M. R. Embry, S. Fitzpatrick, D Kidd, Kleinstreuer. N.C., B. S. Lima, R.S. Settivari, D. C. Wolf, D. Yamazaki, and A. Boobis. 2020. An Evaluation Framework for New Approach Methodologies (NAMS) for Human Health Safety Assessment. *Reg. Toxicol. Pharmacol.* 112: 104592. https://doi.org/10.1016/j.yrtph.2020.104592.

Phthalate Information Center. 2003. *Phthalates.* Phthalate information Center.

Raffensperger, C. A., and J. A. Tickner. 1999. *Protecting Public Health and the Environment: Implementing the Precautionary Principle.* Washington, DC: Island Press.

Rochester, J. R., and A. L. Bolden. 2015. Bisphenol S and F: A Systematic Review and Comparison of the Hormonal Activity of Bisphenol A Substitutes. *Environ. Health Persp.* 123 (7): 643–650. https://doi.org/10.1289/ehp.1408989.

Siddiqi, M. A., R. M. Laessig, and K. D. Reed 2003. Polybrominated Diphenyl Ethers (PBDEs): New Pollutants-Old Diseases. *Clin. Med. Res.* 1 (4): 281–290. http://www.mfldclin.edu/clinmedres.

Stern, P. C., and H.V. Fineberg. 1996. *Understanding Risk: Informing Decision in a Democratic Society.* National Academies Press.

Tickner, J. A. 2011. Science of Problems, Science of Solutions, or Both: A Case Example of Bisphenol A. *Journal of Epidemiology and Community Health* 65: 649–650.

Tickner, J. A., J.N. Schifano, A. Blake, C. Rudisill, and M.J. Mulvihill. 2015. Advancing Safer Alternatives Through Functional Substitution. *Environ. Sci. & Technol.* 49 (2): 742–749. http://doi.org/10.1021/es503328m

Tickner, J. A., and M. Jacobs. 2016. *Improving the Identification, Evaluation, Adoption and Development of Safer Alternatives: Needs and Opportunities to Enhance Substitution Efforts within the Context of REACH.* Lowell: U. Mass (European Chemical Agency). https://substitution.ineris.fr/sites/substitution-portail/files/documents/substitution_capacity_lcsp_en_0.pdf.

Tickner, J. A., M. M. Jacobs, and N. B. Mack. 2019. Alternatives Assessment and Informed Substitution: A Global Landscape Assessment of Drivers, Methods, Policies and Reeds. *Sust. Chem. Pharm.* 13:100161. https://doi.org/10.1016/j.scp.2019.100161.

Tickner, J. A., Rachel V. Simon, Molly Jacobs, Lindsey D. Pollard & Saskia K. van Bergen. 2021. The Nexus between Alternatives Assessment and Green Chemistry: Supporting the Development and Adoption of Safer Chemicals, *Green Chemistry Letters and Reviews* 14(1): 21–42. https://doi.org/10.1080/17518253.2020.1856427

Tomar, R.S., J.D. Budroe, and R. Cendak. 2013, October. *Evidence on the Carcinogenicity of Diisonoyl Phthalate (DINP).* California Environmental Protection Agency. CALOEHHA: Sacramento, CA.

Velders, G. J. M., A. R. Ravishankara, M. K. Miller, M. J. Molina, J. Alcamo, J. S. Daniel, D. W. Fahey, S. J. Montzka, and S. Reimann. 2012. Preserving Montreal Protocole Climate Benefits by Limiting HFCs. *Science (Washington)* 335: 922–923. https://doi.org/10.1126/science.1216414.

von Moltke, K. 1987. *The Vorsorgeprinzep in West German Environmental Policy in Royal Commission on Environmental Pollution.* Institute for European Environmental: London.

Wynne, B. 1993. Public Uptake of Science: A Case for Institutional Reflexivity. *Public Understand. Sci.* 2 (4): 321–337. https://doi.org/10.1088/0963-6625/2/4/003.

Ziegler, E. 1968. Zur Prophylexe der Zivilisationskrqnkheiten [On the Prevention of Civilization Dseases]. *Praxis* 23: 1032–1035.

15 How European Countries Approach Regulatory Risk Assessment

Helmut Greim
Technical University of Munich, München, Germany

CONTENTS

Introduction 317
Regulation of Hazardous Chemicals...317
The Elements of the Registration, Evaluation, Authorisation, and Restriction of
    Chemicals (REACH) Regulation 318
    Registration 318
        Occupational Safety Rules..318
        Joint Registration of Same Substances...319
        Testing and Assessment Requirements 319
    Evaluation...319
        Examination of the Testing Proposals 319
        The Compliance Check...319
        Substance Evaluation 320
    Authorization...320
    Restriction..320
    Allocation of Responsibilities and Administration of REACH 320
        Status and Function of ECHA...320
        Role of the European Commission 321
        Role of Member States 321
    Downstream Users..321
        Submission of the Notification Documents and Decisions 321
    Cosmetics..321
    Medicinal Products for Human and Veterinary Use...322
    Medical Devices..323
    General Requirements for Risk Assessment..323
        Selection of a Point of Departure..324
        Extrapolation to Lower Risk Levels..324
Note..325
Further Reading 325

INTRODUCTION

Until the 50th of the last century, each European country regulated technical dangers and chemical substances differently. The increased trade between the European countries and worldwide required harmonization, especially within the increasing common market in Europe. As a first step, the European Coal and Steel Community (ECSC) was established in 1952, followed by the Treaty of Rome in 1958, which established the *European Economic Community (EEC)* and the *European Atomic Energy Community (Euratom)*. In 1993, the Treaty of Maastricht established at first the *European Community (EC)*, and the Treaty of Lisbon of 2009 defined the function of the European Union (EU). These treaties entered into force in December 2009 and were amended later. In the meantime, the number of Member States of the Community increased from 6 to 28. In the Member States, EU legislation has replaced national law for the purpose of harmonization, and the national authorities are responsible for implementing EU legislation in national law. The *Court of Justice of the European Union* interprets EU legislation.

REGULATION OF HAZARDOUS CHEMICALS

To regulate trade of dangerous substances within the EC, directives for the harmonization of national law have been established. The Council Directive 67/548/EEC on the approximation of laws, regulations, and administrative provisions relating to the classification, packaging, and labeling of dangerous substances requests that Member States take measures to ensure that dangerous substances can only be placed on the market after classification, packaging, and labeling. Accordingly, the 6th Amendment of Directive 67/548/EEC introduced a uniform notification and test procedure throughout the Community, which has replaced or modified national laws in many areas to harmonize and achieve common regulations among the Member States. The authorities in each Member State are responsible for implementing EU legislation in national law.

Accordingly, the Chemicals Act requests to notify, test, and, if necessary, label new substances. New substances are all substances not listed in the European Inventory of Existing Commercial Chemical Substances (EINECS). Substances, preparations, or products that are regulated by special laws are generally exempted. The notifier must reside or have his business premises in a Member State. After notification, producers or importers may freely market the substance throughout the entire EU area, as well as in states within the European Economic Area.

The Chemicals Act provides for the tonnage-related notification of each new substance placed on the market in quantities of ≥ 10 kg per year. Once the next tonnage threshold has been reached, further documents have to be submitted. The decisive factor regarding import notifications is the total quantity of the substance which is imported into the EU and the European Economic Area (EEA) states per producer.

THE ELEMENTS OF THE REGISTRATION, EVALUATION, AUTHORISATION, AND RESTRICTION OF CHEMICALS (REACH) REGULATION

Evaluation, authorization, and restriction of substances are tools of the authorities to address potential deficiencies or risks. If the available information is insufficient for risk assessment, authorities may ask registrants to generate the necessary information and present it to the authorities. If there is a suspicion that certain uses of a substance cause relevant health or environmental risks, such uses may be banned by means of 'restriction,' which must be justified by the authorities. Substances with properties of very high concern may be subjected to authorization, which implies that applicants must provide evidence that the intended use is safe.

Registration

Manufacturers and importers register their substances with the European Chemicals Agency (ECHA) by submitting a registration dossier. The notifier, who intends to place chemical substances and preparations on the market, is requested to label them and provide relevant information based on the criteria defined in Annex V to Directive 67/548/EEC or Directive 1999/45/EC. Classification is the substance-related assignment of danger categories (such as flammable, toxic, carcinogenic, dangerous for the environment). The regularly updated Annex I of Directive 67/548/EEC contains a list of the dangerous substances for which an EU-harmonized, binding classification already exists ("legal classification"). The data, which lead to a specific labeling, have to be described in the safety data sheet according to Directive 88/379/EEC, which describes the requirements for the establishment of the safety data sheet. Directive 91/155/EEC ensures that the safety data sheet is accepted within Europe. This documentation provides the information which supports classification and labeling and the principal risks of the substance or preparation.

The registration dossiers contain information about the identity of the substance, and its physical, chemical, toxic, and eco-toxic properties. Part of the registration dossier is the chemical safety report, which describes the use conditions, an assessment of exposure and risk, and information on the risk management measures applied or recommended by the registrant.

For existing substances, registration is applied to quantities of one ton or more per year. To enable registrants and ECHA to handle the expected vast number of substances, deadlines for the registration have been defined depending on the annual tonnage. For substances produced or imported at a volume of more than 1,000 tons per year, the deadline for registration was November 30, 2010. Substances with an annual tonnage between 100 and 1,000 tons had to be registered by May 31, 2013, and for substances between 1 and 100 tons, the deadline for registration was May 31, 2018. New, so-called non-phase-in substances, have to be registered before the annual volume exceeds one ton.

Occupational Safety Rules

In accordance with Article 138 of the European Treaty, Directive 98/24/EC and the other EU safety directives relating to the handling of chemicals (production and use) contain requirements for the protective measures in the individual Member States. The national requirements can exceed those of the European legislation. The safety data sheet should consider specific national rules and the resulting protective measures.

After examination of their completeness, the manufacturer or importer is allowed to produce or import the substance. In case of changes of uses or if new data about hazardous properties become available, the registration dossiers need to be adopted by the registrant.

Joint Registration of Same Substances

Since many substances are produced by more than one manufacturer, REACH requests that the registrants submit a joint registration dossier of the specific substance. This only applies to the parts of the registration dossier which are related to the hazard assessment, whereas the chemical safety report which describes use-specific exposure and risk assessments are submitted separately. Originally the aim of joint registration was to avoid non-necessary repetition of tests using vertebrate animals. Because the registration dossier may contain confidential business information, it has been agreed that they must not be presented in the joint registration dossier.

Testing and Assessment Requirements

The required physical, chemical, toxicological, and eco-toxicological studies depend on the annual tonnage of a substance and are defined in the annexes of the REACH regulation.

For the tonnage range between 1–10 tons per year, information on acute toxicity, skin and eye irritation/corrosion, and mutagenicity is requested. Substances used between 10–100 tons need data on mutagenicity and a 28-day repeated dose study, whereas substances used by more than 100 tons require a sub-chronic toxicity study (90 days) and a developmental toxicity study. For substances above 1,000 tons, an additional reproductive toxicity study is required. However, according to Annex XI of the REACH Regulation, standard tests may be waived if the existing data provide equivalent information as compared to the standard test (weight of evidence approach). Testing may also be replaced by a prediction of toxicity by qualitative or quantitative structure-activity relationship (QSAR) models or read across. However, since registrants extensively propose to waive testing, especially of the expensive toxicological tests, it often leads to discussions about whether an adequate prediction of toxicity is possible without testing and usually delays the administrative procedure: To reduce the likelihood that relevant toxic effects of a substance remain undetected, the regulatory site usually insists on providing the tests.

Based on the toxicological (and environmental) data, the registration dossier needs to provide a risk assessment for the use-specific exposure of consumers and workers. Since use of the specific substance is considered safe if exposure during its life circle is below the derived no-effect level (DNEL), the assessment of the use-specific exposure is essential, including the use of a substance as a component of a mixture.

DNELs are derived from the available human or animal studies by applying assessment factors to account for differences of sensitivity between the tested animal species and humans (interspecies variability) and within the same species (intraspecies variability). The assessment of exposure is based on exposure scenarios which are representative of the use of the specific compound. For many professional and industrial standard processes, exposure scenarios have been developed and algorithms derived to facilitate the estimation of the level of exposure.

ECHA has published comprehensive and detailed guidance documents on the methodology for risk assessment.

Evaluation

The evaluation process evaluates whether the registration dossiers meet the REACH information requirements and decides whether the submitted information is sufficient for risk assessment. It includes three evaluation processes: Examination of the testing proposals, the compliance check, and substance evaluation.

Examination of the Testing Proposals

ECHA examines the submitted studies as well as proposals for additional studies, including the study designs, animal species, route of application, etc., to decide on the testing proposals or the argumentation for waiving. To avoid unnecessary animal tests and costs, in particular, of the long-term animal studies, registrants need to obtain ECHA's permission if additional studies are considered necessary. However, in practice, the agency frequently concludes that the data on reprotoxicity are insufficient and requests additional studies.

The Compliance Check

ECHA evaluates the information submitted by registrants regarding the quality and adequacy of the data. Due to the enormous resources required to meet the high standards for comprehensiveness and depth of the assessment, REACH requests that a minimum of 5% of the registration dossiers are checked for compliance by ECHA. It is at the agency's discretion to decide which dossiers are selected preferentially when there is a concern that the use of a substance presents a risk to human health or the environment.

Substance Evaluation

If there is a concern that the use of a substance presents a relevant risk to human health or the environment, competent authorities of EU Member States carry out the technical examination of the dossiers, and registrants may be required to generate and submit additional information, which may not be part of the REACH standard information requirements. After ECHA or a Member State authority has prepared a draft decision specifying the required information, registrants and, subsequently, Member State authorities may provide comments on the draft. If no Member State objects, the decision is accepted by ECHA. If not, ECHA submits the draft decision to the Member State Committee which is composed of representatives of EU Member States. In case no unanimous agreement is reached, the draft decision is forwarded to the European Commission for final decision.

Authorization

Authorization is applied to substances of very high concern (SVHC), which include carcinogenic, mutagenic, and reprotoxic substances (CMR); persistent, bioaccumulative, and toxic (PBT); and very persistent and very bioaccumulative (vPvB) substances. More recently, compounds with endocrine disrupting (ED) potential are also considered SVHC. Substances that require authorization are listed in Annex XIV of the REACH regulation. In case Member States provide evidence that substances with hazardous properties other than CMR, PBT, or vPvB properties, they may also be included in this annex.

The authorization process usually is initiated by a Member State which proposes to include a substance of at least one of the SVHC criteria into the ECHA inventory candidate list. Inclusion into this list does not (already) entail that use of the substances requires authorization. ECHA selects a substance from the candidate list and proposes its inclusion into Annex XIV, which needs approvement by the European Commission. After a sunset date, further use of the substance is prohibited unless users have obtained an authorization. This is granted by the European Commission after the user has submitted an application for specific uses, which has been evaluated by the scientific committees of ECHA, which forward the conclusion to the Commission.

Restriction

The restriction process may be initiated by EU Member States to prohibit production, marketing, or use of substances and to define risk management measures by submitting a dossier to ECHA. In this dossier, an assessment of the risks to human health or the environment must be presented to justify the proposed restrictions and risk management measures. ECHA evaluates the scientific and technical validity, including the socio-economic consequences of the restriction, and presents its conclusion to the European Commission for final decision.

Allocation of Responsibilities and Administration of REACH

The rather complex REACH concept is designed to ensure that decisions are based on high scientific/technical quality, to make the administrative procedures robust toward corruption and manipulation, and to ensure that all steps of the process and their outcome can be followed by the public.

Status and Function of ECHA

The independent agency ECHA examines the submitted dossiers for restriction and authorization and publishes the conclusions in opinions. The process includes public consultations on submitted dossiers to allow submission of additional information and comments.

ECHA is comprised of several committees and a secretariat managed by an executive director, which carries out the administrative tasks for registration and evaluation. The scientific-technical evaluation of the submitted dossier's assessment is carried out by the Committee for Risk Assessment (RAC) and the Committee for Socio-economic Assessment (SEAC). These committees are composed of independent experts proposed by the EU Member States. RAC examines the submitted risk assessment, and SEAC analyses the socio-economic impact of restrictions or uses applied for under authorization. The opinions are published on ECHA's website. The publication includes the opinion and the names of committee members, which intends to provide an incentive for the members to conduct a thorough analysis.

The ECHA secretariat s responsible for the administrative part of the REACH process evaluating the completeness of registration dossiers, the testing proposals, and the compliance with the regulations. During the evaluation processes, Member States retain considerable influence, and the ECHA secretariat must obtain approval from all Member States for all evaluation decisions.

Role of the European Commission

To guaranty that the final decisions on restrictions and authorizations under REACH are taken by institutions having sufficient democratic legitimacy, the decision-making power remains with the European Commission. However, in practice, the decision of the European Commission relies on the scientific opinions of RAC and SEAC as reference points regarding the nature and level of risk and benefit, which are legitimized by unanimous approval of the Member States. In case Member States cannot reach a unanimous agreement, the Commission may request additional information from the registrants for compliance or to clarify a concern.

Role of Member States

If a competent authority (or ECHA) identifies a substance which raises concern that its use presents a risk to human health or the environment substance, it carries out the technical examination of the dossier. In consequence of this evaluation, registrants may be asked to generate and submit additional information to verify or dismiss the concern.

After the Member State authority (or ECHA) has prepared a draft decision specifying the required information, registrants and, subsequently, Member State authorities may provide comments on the draft. If no Member State objects, the procedure is finalized, and the decision is taken by ECHA. Otherwise, ECHA submits the draft decision to the Member State Committee, which is composed of representatives of EU Member States. If the Committee fails to reach a unanimous agreement, the draft decision is forwarded to the European Commission for decision-making.

Based on their evaluation, EU Member States may propose a restriction on the production or use of a hazardous substance. The proposal is submitted to ECHA, which forwards it to RAC and SEAC for evaluation. The scientific committees evaluate the proposal and submit their conclusion to ECHA.

Downstream Users

Downstream users are natural or legal persons who use a substance either on its own or in a mixture. They are obliged to assess whether their uses are covered by the exposure scenarios defined by registrants. Since a substance may be used in several products and may have changed owners several times, the registrant may not be aware of the final use of his product, so the use conditions described in the chemical safety report may be different. For this reason, the downstream user has to check whether its use condition is covered by the original registration dossier. If not, the downstream user needs to perform an additional safety assessment and submit it to ECHA.

Submission of the Notification Documents and Decisions

The notification procedure requires the completion of a form (in English or the national language) which the notifier, usual industry, submits to ECHA. About 5% of the dossiers, or if the substance may raise concern, are checked for completeness. In case the documents meet the notification requirements, the notifier is informed. If the documents and test reports do not allow adequate assessment, the notifier is asked to supplement additional information or correct the notification document. After the notification has been accepted, producers or importers may market the substance throughout the entire EU. In case of specific concerns, which require classification and labeling, the documents are evaluated by the scientific committees RAC and SEAC. After public consultation and adoption by the scientific committees, ECHA forwards the final document to the European Commission. In addition to ECHA, competent authorities of the Member States may also evaluate the submitted dossiers and may request additional information – e.g., additional studies – and propose classification and labeling, restrictions on use, or authorization for specific use. This needs to be justified and submitted to ECHA for further evaluation.

Cosmetics

Legislation on cosmetics is part of the special legislation of products. Regulation 1223/2009/EC on cosmetic products is the main regulatory framework for finished cosmetic products. Cosmetic products include substances or mixtures, which are applied to skin, hair, lips, nails, teeth, and the mucous membranes of the oral cavity formulated as rinse-off and leave-on products.

According to Annex I of the regulation, a *product information file* (PIF) should be sent to the competent authority in the Member State, which documents normal and reasonable and foreseeable use; composition, including impurities, properties, and manufacture; and microbiological quality and that a safety assessment has been performed.

For information of the consumers, the ingredients in a cosmetic product should be indicated on its packaging, in case of nanomaterials, the word 'nano' should be added in brackets to the specific ingredient. To allow appropriate medical treatment appropriate information should be provided to an internet portal at the European Commission so that confidential information about the formulation can be made available in particular to poison control centers and assimilated entities.

The Cosmetic Regulation contains various annexes for prohibited or restricted substances. Prohibited substances are listed in Annex II (around 1,400 entries); Annex III contains substances with use and concentration restrictions or warning labels (around 300 entries). In addition to the manufacturer's safety assessment, the Scientific Committee on Consumer Safety (SCCS) provides a safety evaluation and, finally, authorization is required. These include Annex III substances, skin and hair colorants (Annex IV), preservatives (Annex V), active UV-filter substances for sunscreens (Annex VI), manufactured nanomaterials, and category 2 carcinogens, mutagens or toxic for reproduction (CMR substances according to Regulation 1272/2008/EC). The use of CMR substances classified as category 1A or 1B in cosmetics is generally prohibited unless they comply with food safety requirements because they are naturally occurring in food or if no suitable alternative substances exist, and the SCCS considers the use of the substance as safe.

Since 2013 all animal studies for testing of cosmetic ingredients are forbidden, which implies development of alternative methods according to the "reduce, reuse, and recycle" (RRR) principles.

Medicinal Products for Human and Veterinary Use

'Medicinal product' (drugs or pharmaceuticals) includes substances that can act within or on the body. The regulation is based on Directive 2001/83/EC and Regulation 726/2004/EC and consists of a network between the regulatory authorities for medicines in the EU Member States (in addition, Iceland, Liechtenstein, and Norway), the European Commission and the *European Medicines Agency (EMA)*. All medicines must be authorized before they can be placed on the market in the EU. Different routes for *authorization* are possible.

For the *centralized procedure*, which is valid for all EU Member States, pharmaceutical companies submit a single authorization application to EMA. The agency's Committee for Medicinal Products for Human Use (CHMP) or Committee for Medicinal Products for Veterinary Use (CVMP) evaluates the application and recommends whether the European Commission authorizes marketing in all EU Member States. This authorizing procedure applies to most innovative medicines, including medicines for rare diseases (orphan drugs).

However, most of the medicines are authorized by National competent authorities (NCAs) in the Member States if authorization is requested for several Member States only. This *decentralized procedure* grants authorization of a medicine in more than one EU Member State if it has not yet been authorized in any EU country. The *mutual recognition* procedure applies when authorization has been granted in one EU Member State, and the industry applies for authorization in other EU countries. In this case, Member States may rely on the scientific assessment by the first Member State.

All decisions are documented in a European Public Assessment Report (EPAR), which is available in the Public Assessment Report.

Specific regulations apply for the authorization of innovative medicinal products developed from certain biotechnological processes, medicines for rare (orphan) diseases, advanced therapy medicinal products, and new active substances for the treatment of most immunological diseases, cancer, neurodegenerative disorders, diabetes, and viral diseases. Traditional herbal medicines may be authorized through a simplified registration procedure.

In the work of EMA, external experts participate as members of its scientific committees, working parties, etc., or as members of the national assessment teams that evaluate medicines. EMA also prepares scientific guidelines in cooperation with experts of its scientific committees and working groups.

Manufacturers, importers, and distributors of medicines in the EU must be licensed by the regulatory authorities of the Member States. All manufacturing and importing licenses are entered into EudraGMDP, the publicly available European database operated by EMA. The network between the national regulatory, the Commission, and EMA enables the exchange of information in the regulation of medicine, the clinical trials, and the inspections of manufacturers and compliance with good clinical practice (GCP), good manufacturing practice (GMP), good distribution practice (GDP), and good pharmacovigilance practice (GVP). Manufacturers listed in the application of a medicine are inspected by a national competent authority. The outcome is made publicly available across the EU through EudraGMDP. This also applies to inspections of manufacturers located outside the EU unless a mutual recognition agreement (MRA) is in place between the EU and the country of manufacture.

The European Commission and EMA work in close cooperation with partner organizations around the world such as the WHO, with one of the main forums being the International Council for Harmonization of Technical Requirements for Pharmaceuticals for Human Use (ICH), which brings together medicines regulatory authorities and pharmaceutical industry from around the world. The Veterinary International Conference on Harmonization (VICH) is the equivalent platform for veterinary medicines.

Medical Devices

Medical devices are technical or physical products and comprise plasters, pregnancy tests, hip implants, state-of-the-art pacemakers, X-ray machines, or genetic tests. Placed in or outside of the human body, they may cause skin sensitization or other types of allergies or may release toxic substances such as metal ions.

They are regulated similar to consumer products and are not subject to pre-market authorization. Instead, they require a *conformity assessment* to establish whether they meet existing standards, which is performed by '*notified body*,' such as a laboratory or a national authority. The recent *scandals* related to metal-on-metal artificial hips or faulty silicone breast implants have strengthened the case for modernizing the current directives for medical devices.

For these and other reasons, the current medical device directives were revised and replaced by two regulations, the Medical Device Regulation 2017/745/EU (MDR) and the In Vitro Diagnostic Medical Device Regulation 2017/746/EU (IVDR). These new regulations place a special focus on *pre-market conformity* with requirements on safety and quality standards and contain a series of important improvements. These include a risk classification system for in vitro diagnostic medical devices, stricter ex-ante control for high-risk devices, reinforcement of the criteria for designation and processes for oversight of *notified bodies*, reinforcement of the rules on clinical evidence, *post-market oversight* by manufacturers, and *traceability* of all medical devices throughout the supply chain. The latter shall be achieved *inter alia* by the establishment of a Unique Device Identification system (UDI system) and the creation of a European database on medical devices (Eudamed). Both regulations will apply with transitional periods of several years, the MDR in 2020 and the IVDR in 2022.

General Requirements for Risk Assessment

Humans may be exposed to chemicals in the air, water, food, or on skin. The external dose at which a chemical exerts its toxic effects is a measure of its potency, i.e., a highly potent chemical produces its effects at low doses. Ultimately, the response to the chemical depends upon duration and route of exposure, the toxicokinetics of the chemical, the dose-response relationship, and the susceptibility of the individual. To characterize the risk of a given or potential exposure, the adverse effects of chemicals have to be identified, the dose-response relationship must be characterized, and the exposure at which the chemical which is associated with adverse effects must be identified.

It is obvious from this that risk characterization comprises three elements:

- Hazard identification, i.e., a description of the agent's toxic potential.

- Evaluation of the dose response, including information on the concentration above which the agent induces toxic effects to identify the no observable adverse effect level (NOAEL).

- Exposure assessment to understand the concentration of the agent in the relevant medium, time, and routes of human exposure.

The hazard identification requests information on toxicokinetics/pharmacokinetics (intake, distribution, metabolism, excretion), infection-related effects (e.g., pathogenicity, infectivity) toxic effects, e.g., acute toxicity, sub-chronic/chronic toxicity, mutagenicity, carcinogenicity, reproductive toxicity, neurotoxicity, and their dose responses to derive the NOAEL, Lowest Observable (Adverse) Effects Level (LO(A)EL), incidence figures and other information on frequency. If applicable, health-relevant dosage limits are derived and stated, such as the Acceptable Daily Intake (ADI), Acute Reference Dose (ARfD), or Acceptable Operator Exposure Level (AOEL).

Exposure assessment requests information on exposed population groups, different exposure situations for consumers, users, sick persons, pregnant women, taking into account age and body weight, in case of microbial agents, the contaminated products. In addition, information on consumption data and other information on the frequency of exposure, and the qualitative and quantitative presence of a microbial agent and/or the residue levels in and on foods or other products is documented.

The risk characterization comprises a comparison between the potential damage caused by the product, substance, or microbial agent and the calculated or estimated exposure, considering the dose-effect relationships and the exposure limit values. Description of incidence data should be as accurate as possible. This approach applies to compounds for which a NOAEL can be identified. In such cases, an ADI can be derived, usually using a factor of 100 taking into account intraspecies and interspecies differences in sensitivity. To identify a DNEL, ECHA may use additional assessment factors to cover remaining interspecies differences or severity of effects. More recently, an additional factor to cover potential effects of mixtures is discussed.

In the case of genotoxic compounds, which do not allow identification of a NOAEL, the risk at certain exposures is identified to set a risk-based standard. Extrapolation (including quantitative extrapolation) is generally assumed when the substance is genotoxic, and a genotoxic mode of action is assessed as relevant for carcinogenicity. In the case of animal studies, these are based either on the identification of a benchmark dose (BMD) or of the TD_{25} (a dose or concentration at which cancer occurs in an additional 25% of the animals). In case appropriate epidemiologic studies are available, in general, analytical study designs with an individual exposure estimate are to be selected for risk assessment. Both cohort and case control studies can be used for risk assessment.

Where the genotoxicity is not relevant or is of limited relevance, mechanistic findings and mode of action (e.g. cytotoxicity, endocrine activity) can be used for the extrapolation.

The tumor incidences in the various organs are quantified separately and compared with each other. In the standard case, risk quantification is based on the tumor site with the lowest TD_{25} (a dose or concentration at which cancer occurs in an additional 25% of the animals) taking into account the different background rates. In specific cases such as mesotheliomas and lung tumors induced by asbestos, the different tumor sites are combined.

Selection of a Point of Departure

The point of departure (POD), usually the TD_{25} is the starting point for extrapolation. The TD_{25} value is calculated according to Sanner et al. (2001) and Dybing et al. (1997) and is determined by linear interpolation. This procedure is used if a qualified benchmark calculation cannot be made.

If data of sufficient quality are available, the benchmark concentration or BMD is determined. Usually, the central estimated value (BMD) rather than the 95-percent confidence interval (BMDL) is used, and, depending on sufficient information on species-species differences the human equivalent (hBMD) is determined.

Extrapolation to Lower Risk Levels

For extrapolation to lower concentrations, the models selected for curve fitting should be consistent with the mechanistic considerations about carcinogenicity. In general, the multistage model (or function) or gamma function, which both correspond to the multistage model of carcinogenicity, are used. Other models should be considered if the data can be better adjusted.

In cases when genotoxicity is of no predominant importance but no threshold for carcinogenicity is determined, a sublinear dose response into the low-risk range is generally assumed. However, linear extrapolation is applied if sublinearity cannot be justified – i.e., when the concentration range in which the slope becomes steeper for the risk of developing cancer is not clear.

If a carcinogenic substance has acute or chronic, non-carcinogenic effects, these effects are taken into account. If the limit concentration for a non-carcinogenic effect lies in the medium-risk area, this value is adopted as a tolerable concentration.

Finally, the following points are essential for risk characterization:

- Characterization of a hazard/risk for the population or individual subgroups

- Evaluation of the probability of the occurrence of impairment of, or damage to, health

- Evaluation of the extent of health impairment or damage

- If relevant, an assessment of user and consumer safety

In addition, the presumed effectiveness of governmental monitoring measures may be considered as well as methods of detection and monitoring.

NOTE

This chapter is partially based on the contributions by J. Lebsanft ("The Concept of REACH") and W. Lilienblum and K. M. Wollin ("Regulations on Chemical Substances in the European Union") both published in *Toxicology and Risk Assessment: A Comprehensive Introduction*, H. Greim and R. Snyder eds., John Wiley & Sons Ltd, 2019.

FURTHER READING

Dybing, E., Sanner, T., Roelfzema, H., Kroese, D., Tennant, R.W. 1997. T25: A Simplified Carcinogenic Potency Index: Description of the System and Study of Correlations between Carcinogenic Potency and Species/Site Specificity and Mutagenicity. *Pharmacol Toxicol* 80: 272–279

ECHA. 2017a. *Guidance on Information Requirements and Chemical Safety Assessment*. European Chemicals Agency. http://ECHA.europa.eu/

ECHA. 2017b. Guidance on the Application of the CLP Criteria, Version 5.0, January 2017 http://echa.europa.eu/

EU SCCS (EU Scientific Committee on Consumer Safety). n.d. https://ec.europa.eu/health/scientific_committees/consumer_safety_de

EU SCHEER (EU Scientific Committee on Health, Environmental and Emerging Risks). n.d. https://ec.europa.eu/health/scientific_committees/consumer_safety_de

Greim, H. and Snyder, R. 2019. *Toxicology and Risk Assessment. A Comprehensive Introduction*. Second Edition, John Wiley & Sons.

IARC (International Agency for the Research of Cancer). *Monographs on the Evaluation of Carcinogenic Risks to Humans*. Geneva.

Sanner, T., Dybing, E., Willems, M.I., Kroese, E.D. 2001. A Simple Method for Quantitative Risk Assessment of Non-threshold Carcinogens Based on the Dose Descriptor T25. *Pharmacol Toxicol* 88: 331–341.

The Globally Harmonized System for Hazard Communication. 2009. *Hazard Communication. Occupational Safety & Health Administration*, United States Department of Labor, 10. June 2009.

Website of the European Commission. n.d. https://europa.eu/european-union/index_en

16 Envirome Disorganization and Ecological Riskscapes

The Algal Bloom Epitome

Matteo Convertino

Institute of Environment and Ecology, Tsinghua Shenzhen International Graduate School, Tsinghua University, Shenzhen, China

Nexus Group, Laboratory of Information Communication Networks, Graduate School of Information Science and Technology, Hokkaido University, Sapporo, Japan

Haojiong Wang

Nexus Group, Laboratory of Information Communication Networks, Graduate School of Information Science and Technology, Hokkaido University, Sapporo, Japan

CONTENTS

Ecosystem Risk: Ecology-Environment Nexus..327
    Ocean Health: Algal Bloom as Epitome of Ecosystem Health................................327
    On Phytoplankton and Algal Blooms: A Two-Faced Coin....................................330
    Ocean Viruses, Algal Blooms, Carbon Cycling, and Climate Risk 331
    Land-Ocean Interface, Carbon Dynamic Transition, and Eco-hydrologic Restoration 333
Systemic Risk Quantification: Complex Networks and Predictions 334
    Geospatial Probabilistic Risk Assessment 334
        Optimal Information Flow 334
        Florida Bay Case Study...335
Planetary Health via Ecosystem Science and Engineering.......................................338
    Ecosystem Portfolio Risk Management 338
Synopsis and Perspectives...340
Acknowledgments 343
Literature Cited 343

> *"Everything flows nothing stands still."*
>
> –Heraclitus of Ephesus – 501 BC

LEARNING OBJECTIVES

Students who complete this chapter will be able to

1. Summarize the feedback between ocean microbiome, environmental pressure and climate change risk;
2. Analyze the envirome and phytoplankton co-organization and quantify the resulting impacts as algal bloom magnitude, distribution and persistence; and
   Define optimal network-based algal bloom controls to minimize ecosystem risks.

ECOSYSTEM RISK: ECOLOGY-ENVIRONMENT NEXUS

Ocean Health: Algal Bloom as Epitome of Ecosystem Health

Oceans are the basis of life in an ecological and evolutionary perspective from the origin of Earth (Bonan and Doney 2018). It is fundamental to base any conversation about ecosystem health and risk on oceans, which are the starting and end points of any Earth transformation at multiple levels (Scheffers et al. 2016). Oceans are also particularly important considering the very large anthropogenic pressure they are experiencing (with impacts evident over the last 20–30 years), their role in climate regulation, and the rise of threatening pathogens emerging from oceanic alteration. Coastal ecosystems especially, are crucial for land-ocean feedback (positive and negative), considering both social and ecological actors, i.e., humans and other species. These ecosystems have the highest biodiversity, the largest Blue Carbon (carbon sequestration), and the fastest temporal changes among all ecosystems worldwide. Oceans serve as eco-indicators of terrestrial and global anthropogenic pressure and provide countless ecosystem services such as food provision, flood protection, recreation, and local-global climate regulation. These features are invariant across epochs; therefore, oceans are at the center stage of local ecosystem and planetary health. The aquatic microbiome is the biotic core underpinning all ocean functions. The microbiome is composed of a multiphylotype community of microbes, ranging from the numerically dominant viroplankton (viruses and phages), the bacterioplankton (prokaryotes and archaea), the phylogenetically diverse unicellular phytoplankton (mostly eukaryotes), to the zooplankton in order of abundance. Interestingly, fish and mammals (i.e., "nekton" that swims actively in the water in contrast to plankton) are lower in abundance than plankton; all of these life-forms are distributed along a power-law abundance spectrum (Hatton et al. 2021) that is an ecological pattern revealing an optimal organized distribution of biota. Deviation from this pattern has relevance for measuring ecosystem dysbiosis (J. Li and Convertino 2019) (Figure 16.1), yet for ecosystem risk assessment based on deviations from desired ecosystem functions manifested by phytoplankton probabilistic distribution (Figure 16.2).

Information is about ecosystem states (state uncertainty and uncertainty reduction between communities and populations). Predictive causality is based on uncertainty reduction of abundance underpinning biological interactions (Li and Convertino 2021a). Persistently disorganized or highly organized envirome around one strong environmental factor can cause systemic impacts

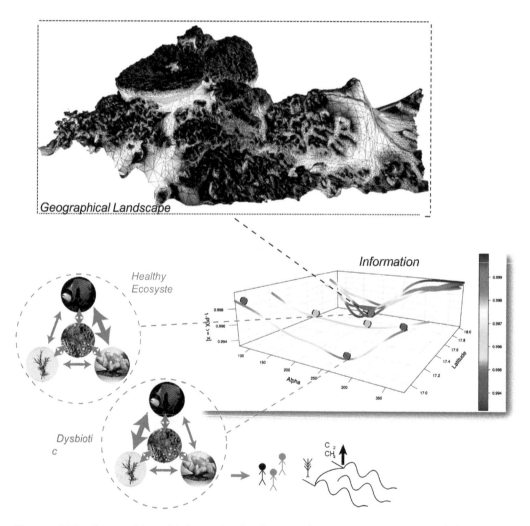

Figure 16.1 Geographic and information landscapes of ocean ecosystems across habitats.

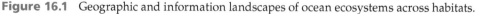

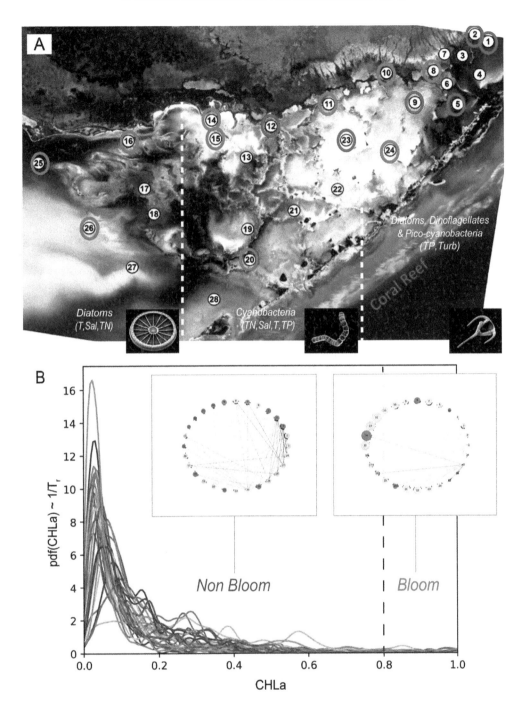

Figure 16.2 Map. Probability distribution function of normalized CHL-a. Blue-green-red color gradient for nodes is proportional to the Shannon Entropy of each station reflecting the disorganization of CHL-a. Small-world and scale-free organization of non-bloom and bloom CHL-a networks underpinning habitat networks: both environmental and ecogeomorphological gradients (water flow and quality as well as vegetation-habitat configuration) determine distribution and intensity of CHL-a over space and time. NB and B networks are determined via time-delayed CHL-a probabilistic changes (values, probability, and their divergence). The salient connections are between salient source and sink areas for blooms. (Source areas are "endemic" blooming areas contributing to export of CHL-a (or nutrients) to other "epidemic" areas. Images of diatoms, Cyanobacteria, and dinoflagellates are used under license from Shutterstock.com.)

on ecosystem function (the former and the latter determining critical slowing down and sudden critical transitions), particularly for disorganized microbiomes. Images in the network are used under license from Shutterstock.com.

On Phytoplankton and Algal Blooms: A Two-Faced Coin

Blue Carbon ecosystems (marine, estuarine, and freshwater) are important primarily for survival of all life on Earth, including that of humans. Occasionally, these ecosystems experience phytoplankton or algal blooms, compromising short and potentially long-term ecosystem function. Blooms are sudden population explosions of phytoplankton, mostly in the form of microalgae (eukaryotes) or blue-green bacteria causing green blooms (e.g., the most common are Cyanobacteria, that are prokaryotes) living in the water. More generally, some phytoplankton are bacteria, protists, but most are single-celled plants. Other common kinds of phytoplankton are silica-encased diatoms, dinoflagellates, green algae, and chalk-coated coccolithophores. Phytoplankton "plants," underpinning photosynthesis that transform carbon dioxide and release oxygen, are the base of aquatic food webs, including zooplankton, bacterioplankton, and nekton. In balanced ecosystems, phytoplankton provides food for a wide range of sea creatures. Phytoplankton growth depends on water temperature and salinity, water depth, wind, availability of carbon dioxide, sunlight, and inorganic nutrients (nitrate, phosphate, silicate, calcium, and sulfur at various levels depending on the species) and predators, which graze on them. A balance of these factors is critical for ecosystem health, which may be defined by outcomes of ecosystem functional organization such as algal blooms (Figure 16.3). Phytoplankton biomass is often estimated by the concentration of chlorophyll-a concentration, which provides a useful bioindicator or index of potential primary production. Primary productivity is defined as the amount of organic material produced per unit area and time or simply as the product of phytoplankton biomass times phytoplankton growth rate. This marine primary production plays an important role in food-web dynamics, in biogeochemical cycles (converting inorganic to organic carbon), and in marine fisheries, yet any imbalance causes undesired ecosystem effects such as algal blooms. Of particular note are the relatively rare harmful algal blooms (HABs), which are algal bloom events involving toxic or otherwise harmful phytoplankton. Cyanobacterial HABs produce multiple toxins, including liver, nerve, and skin toxins, which can affect human and animal health. Cyanobacteria are not the only species producing HABs; e.g., marine dinoflagellates produce red tides and ichthyotoxins, and *Karenia brevis* is an algal species found in South Florida coastal ecosystems (Milbrandt et al. 2021). Other microalgae, such as *Chattonella* and *Heterosigma akashiwo*, which cause red tides, determine a variety of multitrophic impacts such as large-scale fish deaths and unprecedented die-off of seagrass (e.g., *Thalassia testudinum*) that is a Blue Carbon keystone species and constituting a critical habitat for many species (e.g., turtle and sponges). Note that all red tides are not strictly categorized as "HABs" (in terms of toxin release), but all algal bloom tides are harmful because their ecosystem impacts are linked to poor environmental quality. The blooms that are highly visible are widely publicized events, drawing concerns from fishermen, citizens, resource managers, and scientists alike. However, not all blooms are clearly visible, and this complicates the assessment of their risks.

However, ephemeral "boom and bust" blooms are also extremely important because they regulate carbon flux across marine food webs, vertically for the same habitat and horizontally across habitats. Independently of blooms' visibility, most of the processed carbon is returned to near-surface waters when phytoplankton are eaten or decomposed, but some fall into the ocean depths. This "biological carbon pump" (strictly speaking related to phytoplankton only, but interacting also with the microbial and viral carbon pumps) transfers about 10 Gigatonnes of carbon from the atmosphere to the deep ocean each year. Even small changes in the growth of phytoplankton may affect atmospheric carbon dioxide concentrations, which creates feedback to global surface temperatures. Algal blooms affect biota, humans, and climate via local-global teleconnections that have been poorly quantified so far. The key is in the balance of bloom frequency, magnitude, and duration that has been compromised.

There is a lack of understanding about the biocomplexity of algal blooms considering their biodiversity and environmental determinants (envirome) considering both global climate change factors (e.g., ocean temperature and hydroclimatological extremes) and local stressors (e.g., biogeochemical loads from rivers and coastal development). All of this is important both in terms of basic research and ecosystem risk assessment, protection, and restoration.

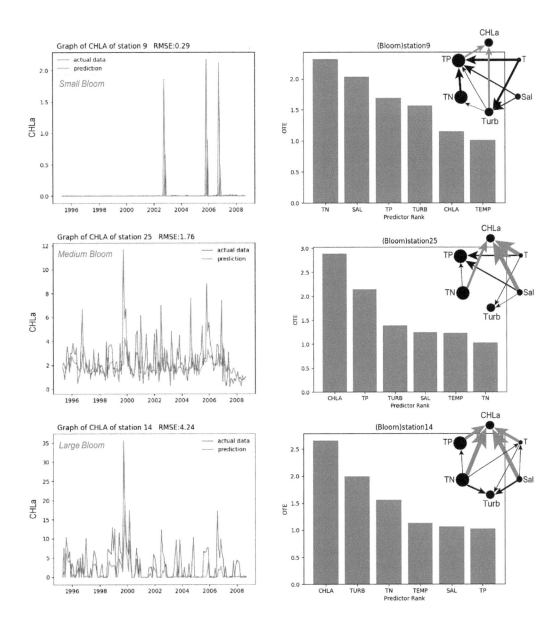

Figure 16.3 Bloom dynamics characterization and top environmental determinants. Discuss the relationship between complexity, predictability, and sensitivity (biocomplexity) of these three dynamics, also considering biodiversity of blooming species, and the hydro ecogeomorphological drivers (considering also how they changed over time).

Ocean Viruses, Algal Blooms, Carbon Cycling, and Climate Risk

A quarter teaspoon of seawater contains on the order of a million cells and ten million viruses. Despite their microscopic size, marine microbes catalyze chemical reactions that are critical for maintaining Earth's habitability. Virus infections of marine microbes can transform the fate of individual cells and also cascade up to influence population dynamics, community diversity, and even carbon and other essential nutrient cycling. Yet, the understanding of how virus-microbe interactions are organized, and their environmental-triggered disorganization, is fundamental for quantifying biogeochemical cycles and alterations of Earth, as well as for designing climate solutions. Host-virus interaction during algal blooms can span more than ten orders of magnitude, from the individual cell (~10^{-6} m, detectable *via* microbiological sampling) to mesoscale oceanic patches (~10^5 m, detectable *via* Unmanned Aerial Vehicle and satellites); therefore, the lack of large-scale quantifications of host-virus dynamics hinders our understanding of the ecological and biogeochemical role of viruses and related processes in oceans.

This quantification will improve our ability to incorporate these dynamics into large-scale ecological and biogeochemical models that assess local ecosystem trajectories of habitat and biodiversity and global trajectories of climate. In terms of data, time series of species abundance, chlorophyll-a (CHL-a), particulate inorganic carbon, particulate organic carbon (POC), and other water chemistry features were documented by many studies, including satellite images. These efforts are increasingly using large-scale oceanographic campaigns that are targeting the microbiological world, e.g., TARA (Sunagawa et al. 2020; Vernette et al. 2021). It is relevant to say that POC was found to closely follow the CHL-a trend, serving as a proxy for organic carbon from phytoplankton. These studies further corroborate the pattern of bloom demise exerted by viruses and their impact on carbon sequestration.

Algal viruses are the most abundant life-form in oceans and seem to have a profound impact on global ecosystems by regulating carbon cycling in oceans. In particular, the term 'girus' (for giant virus) was coined to refer to a new group of viruses with extremely large genome size and complex viral infections that had never been observed previously. Additionally, more than 80% of their genes are of unknown function and those genes have few database matches. These giant viruses are for instance: Cafeteriavirus (544 genes), Pithovirus (467 genes), Sambavirus (938 genes), Megavirus (1,120 genes), and the recent Pandoravirus (2,556 genes). With the presence of all those viruses in the oceans, even with a highly heterogenous host population dominating one region, viral infection becomes almost inevitable. Interestingly, these giant viruses have been found to be one of the major causes of bloom demise (decay) and yet blooms offer an excellent opportunity to isolate viruses and study the fundamental ecosystem dynamics underpinning ecosystem function and environmental quality.

Large DNA viruses infecting unicellular marine and freshwater eukaryotes are thus likely an important component of the aquatic ecosystem as part of the "viral shunt" (Wilhelm and Suttle 1999), i.e., carbon sequestration in oceans and Blue Carbon ecosystems within the larger microbial and biological carbon pump (Guidi et al. 2016; Jover et al. 2014). As a special case of viral shunt, giant viruses were found to induce episodic mass-scale mortality of algal blooms: the virus-induced demise of large-scale blooms was reported for the coccolithophore, *Emiliania huxleyi* (Lehahn et al. 2014); the *Heterosigma akashiwo* virus that affects eukaryotes by forming seasonal harmful blooms (Tomaru et al. 2004); and the *Emilian huxleyi* viruses that form vast oceanic blooms at temperate latitudes (Pagarete et al. 2009; Pagarete et al. 2011).

Interestingly, Brum and colleagues (Brum et al. 2016) reported a lytic-lysogenic infection switch during Antarctic phytoplankton blooms where CHL-a was highly proportional to Megaviruses and bacteria in predicting the onset of blooms, and lysogeny/lysis are predominant in pre-bloom spring and bloom summer periods, respectively. These results also suggested that virus-host interactions were critical to predicting carbon-driven changes in microbial dynamics brought on by warming. If eukaryotes contribute significantly to ocean biomass and net production (>40%), then their viruses play a large role in the biological carbon pump. The oceanic biological pump accounts for up to 90% of the annual export of POC that occurs during the few episodic pulses throughout the year, following strong seasonal phytoplankton blooms. This implies that extreme blooms are necessary to cycle the Earth's carbon and are part of the self-organizing climate system. However, if these blooms become more erratic in terms of frequency and size, by overload of nitrogen and phosphorus, then there is an imbalance and both biodiversity and carbon can be affected via species loss and carbon pump inversion. Deep-sequencing molecular data generated by TARA Oceans (Sunagawa et al. 2020), found that the abundance of giant viruses explained ~49% of the variation in carbon export (compared with ~89% by bacterial viruses). The data also substantially explained the variation in net primary production (~76%) and carbon export efficiency (~50%) (Blanc-Mathieu et al. 2019). The amount of organic carbon produced during the bloom was estimated ~24,000 tons every 30 km^2 (Lehahn et al. 2014). Thus, viruses of the eukaryotic plankton are predicted to increase carbon export efficiency in the global sunlit ocean (Blanc-Mathieu et al. 2019).

Considering this positive viral effect, researchers are also attempting to isolate virus strains capable of killing *Cyanobacteria* sp. and related blooms. Nonetheless, other giant viruses cause diseases in fish and can lead to economic damage in aquacultural industries (Kurita and Nakajima. 2012); thus, not all of their effects are ecologically positive.

Land-Ocean Interface, Carbon Dynamic Transition, and Eco-hydrologic Restoration

Wetlands have a major influence on the global carbon cycle, with capacity to act as both carbon 'sinks' or 'sources.' The source-sink capacity of wetlands is governed by microbially mediated biogeochemical processes, which are modulated by abiotic environmental conditions. In particular, the breaking down of bacteria by viruses (lysis) has been shown to enhance nitrogen cycling and stimulate phytoplankton growth.

The viral shunt pathway facilitates the flow of dissolved organic matter and particulate organic matter through the food web. In hydrology-controlled ecosystems such as coastal wetlands, viruses seem to infect prokaryotes. However, this finding may be related to disturbed conditions or biased data and further research is needed to understand whether coastal habitats are characterized by a reverse viral shunt (with respect to oceans) and prokaryote-infected carbon release.

Studies found that in response to watering related to wetland hydrologic restoration, viral-induced prokaryotic mortality declined by 77%, resulting in limited carbon released by viral shunt that was significantly correlated with the 2.8-fold reduction in wetland carbon emissions (Bonetti et al. 2021). Thus, these findings substantiate the hypothesis of beneficial eukaryote-virus interactions in healthy ecosystems, mimicking the oceanic virus shunt and their role as a major controller of bacterial mortality and algal blooms. The shift toward prokaryote-virus interactions when hydrology or hydrodynamics is compromised results in an unhealthy ecosystem.

Likely, hydrologic restoration also affects soil oxidation and subsidence where the latter may decrease with optimal hydrologic restoration, yet contributing to the minimization of Sea Level Rise effects (Convertino et al. 2013; see Figure 16.4). Other positive effects of virus-controlled eukaryote-prokaryote balanced feedback are about the diversion of nutrient flows, the promotion of genetic exchange across distantly related species, and their roles as components of sinking particles (Bonetti et al. 2019). Freshwater and transition fresh/saltwater wetlands, characterized by erratic flooding events and frequent dry/wet cycles with extreme salinity gradients have higher metabolic (bacterial) and viral (lysogeny-dominated) activity in the dry phase (with aerobic processes), and low prokaryotic diversity and carbon sequestration implicating high greenhouse gas (GHG) emissions (Bonetti et al. 2019). This strong lysogenic infection and "reversed" viral shunt might increase the rates of microbial-mediated recycling of the sedimentary organic matter, thus resulting in CO_2 and CH_4 production and emission, because soils are exposed and microbial growth efficiency (MGE) is lower. Alternatively, the transition to restored wetlands or stable flooded phases determines a shift from soil- to water-dominated viruses, which may trigger beneficial viral (lytic) infections of prokaryotes involved in carbon metabolism that lead to higher carbon stock and lower GHG emissions. The Dissolved Organic Carbon released by the viral shunt is typically consumed by prokaryotes; however, if infections of prokaryotes are too high this does not happen and DOC becomes labile. All of the previous reasoning, of course, assumes the same vegetation type since vegetation is a primary driver in carbon cycling. In the dry phase, focus is on infection of prokaryotes because eukaryotes come into play mainly in the flooded phase. Physical disturbance of sediments, e.g., from dredging and certain aquaculture may expose previously anoxic sediment layers to oxygen (O_2), which could turn them into carbon sources instead of carbon sinks.

The aforementioned dynamics consider interfacial habitats vs. marine/oceanic ones; however, similar gradients in lysogenic-lytic infections were reported across an estuarine-deep water transect where lysis was observed in marine systems rather than riverine (Chen et al. 2019), although in deep oligotrophic waters, lysogeny becomes predominant due to nutrient limitation. Overall, lysogeny is associated with harsh environmental conditions, either coastal or oceanic, and may be the most favorable strategy for viruses to survive until environmental conditions improve. The amount of organic carbon that prokaryotes uptake into their biomass or synthesis versus what is respired as CO_2, CH_4, or N_2O depends on MGE that is likely higher in the lytic cycle (Bonetti et al. 2019).

Strong lysogenic infection might decrease the MGE and the associated substrate usage, resulting in the increase of the carbon not consumed, i.e., remineralized by the prokaryotic members of the microbial loop that is then emitted. Faster microbial growth, microbial biomass, production, and diversity promotes soil carbon accumulation, yet lower MGE has an impact on climate change.

In conclusion, it seems mandatory to consider land-ocean connections for any biodiversity-carbon security plans since these fundamental ecosystem services are anchored on structural and functional ecosystem connections.

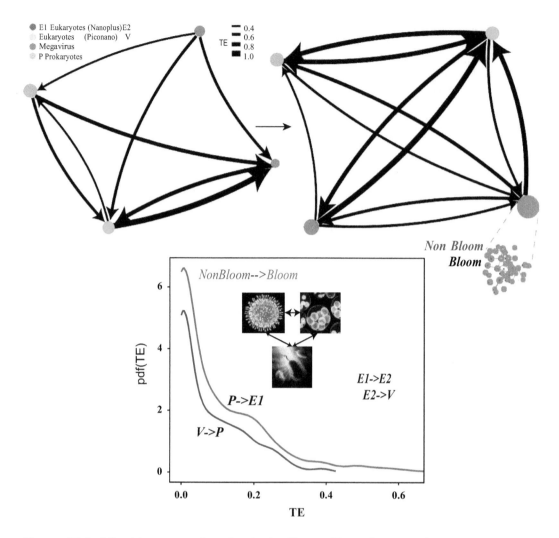

Figure 16.4 Microbiome network underpinning blooms. Networks are predictions representing the ensemble dynamics of seawater E-P-V seen in a set of databases mined in literature (see Section "Geospatial Probabilistic Risk Assessment"). These databases cover spatial and/or temporal dynamics of communities related to blooms or habitat gradients with E-P-V changes attributable to biotic and abiotic factors. The 0.8–3 μm and ¿3 μm fractions are typically referred to as the (Eukaryote) PicoNano and NanoPlus fractions, respectively. E-P make "the ocean microbiome dance" that is modulated by viruses (V). Eukaryotes are altered in abundance by environmental alterations (e.g. systemic ocean temperature change and/or local nutrients loads, in particular, nitrogen). Images in the inset network are used under license from Shutterstock.com.

SYSTEMIC RISK QUANTIFICATION: COMPLEX NETWORKS AND PREDICTIONS
Geospatial Probabilistic Risk Assessment
Optimal Information Flow

In the following, we discuss methodological advances, concepts, and issues in assessing ecosystem risk for the case of blooms in Florida Bay, an estuarine bay south of the Everglades National Park (Figure. 16.2). For this case study, we show preliminary results of a pattern-oriented model (see recently developed to infer ecosystem information flows to predict critical ecosystem patterns) (J. Li and Convertino 2021a).

This "Optimal Information Flow" model is coupled to a deep-learning model (Xu et al. 2020) that extracts features (sets of variables that are dynamically changing over time) for each node in order to maximize predictions. Predictions are focused on chlorophyll-a (CHL-a); that is, the ecosystem pattern that better represents the systemic variability of ecosystem flows from microbiological ones (such as viruses and eukaryotes to higher trophic levels) to environmental ones, such as water and nutrient flows. Additionally, CHL-a variability in magnitude, frequency, and spatial distribution is a leading indicator of algal blooms emergence: is then intuitive to use this bioindicator for assessing short- and long-term bloom risks (i.e., occurrence and magnitude of blooms) and risk of cascading effects on species and ecosystem functions (e.g., carbon sequestration).

Florida Bay is a 2,200 km^2 shelf lagoon located at the intersection of the Everglades, Florida Keys, Gulf of Mexico, and Atlantic Ocean at the tip of the Florida peninsula. A mixture of mud banks, seagrass beds, and hard-/soft-bottom habitats compose this ecosystem, that is yet largely composed by Blue Carbon habitats. Land development (the city of Miami and agricultural fields) and associated water management practices in Central and South Florida have starved the Everglades of freshwater over the past century and, as a result, reduced Florida Bay's freshwater (and its quality) to only a fraction of the historical flow. For some of the preliminary analyses presented about algal blooms in Florida Bay (USA), monthly water quality data from the Florida International University Water Quality Monitoring Program (http://serc.fiu.edu/wqmnetwork/SFWMD-CD/index.htm) were used. The most complete data span roughly 16 years, from August 1992 through September 2008 (194 time steps per station). The vast majority of these data were used in a multiple regression model to extract quantiles revealing spatiotemporal shifts in phytoplankton biomass between bloom and non-bloom conditions (Nelson, Munoz-Carpena, and Philips 2017). The model is mildly discussed in a comparative way (Nelson, Munoz-Carpena, and Philips 2017). The information-theoretic framework (Figure 16.1) permits analysis and predictions that are faster and completely probabilistic than acting on the geographical space, e.g., *via* regression modes assuming linearity. The characterization of ecosystem components (structure as habitats, biota, and services) is done by characterizing them in terms of probability distribution functions, assessing their stability, and mutual interdependencies. In this way, it is possible to identify ecosystem states, i.e., how ecosystem components are organized in networks for all geographical areas of interest. In the *long-term* or stationary state, considering *the whole probability distribution*, the higher the average probability of being in a certain state or exceedance probability of being in that state or another with a larger magnitude of the tracked ecosystem indicator, e.g., higher microbial diversity to explore its use as an environmental quality indicator the more stable that state and the lower its energy dissipation with respect to other states. Energy dissipation is about the ecosystem functioning in a particular state that is the lowest for the healthy state; conversely, the free energy, that is the energy available (~1-entropy, where the entropy is roughly proportional to the energy dissipation), is the highest. States are represented by different organizations of species underpinning ecosystem structure and function. It should be noted that the exceedance probability can be linked to climate or other extremes' return periods to establish the predictive link between causes and outcomes. Note that using the probability exceedance distribution or the probability distribution function would provide the same results for the energy landscape where each depression corresponds to an attractor. In *short-term* (or transitory states, considering single events and their probability value vs. their distribution, the extreme events with a lower probability of exceedance have higher energy dissipation, e.g., algal blooms or extreme nutrient loading associated with climate extremes. The question is how these disturbances can tip the ecosystem from one stable state to another over a long time; thus, it is of paramount importance to assess the transition probability among states and their causes. Long-term distributions reflect processes underpinning self-organized criticality (SOC) of natural systems (Bak, Tang, and Wiesenfeld 1987). While short-term dynamics reflect time-point events with critical slowing down (CSD) that may alter long-term trends in case of persistency of unbalanced or extreme environmental pressures (Scheffer et al. 2009). It should be noted that normal environmental pressure is precisely responsible for sculpting ecosystem patterns and species fitness in a punctuated evolutionary process; however, problems arise when environmental pressure is altered in magnitude and distribution such as climate change pressure.

Florida Bay Case Study

Figure 16.1 shows two ideal functional species networks connecting different trophic groups for reef/ocean habitats to estuarine Blue Carbon habitats (blue and red networks, respectively) in Florida Bay depicted in Figure 16.2. Healthy ecosystems correspond to more balanced fish-coral-seagrass species networks, while dysbiotic ecosystems are characterized by shifts in fish populations (herbivore-dominated) that lead to seagrass decay and increase in algal blooms, and decays in coralline species and sponges. All these networks are modulated by the ocean microbiome at the center of functional networks in Figure 16.1 that regulate food-web dynamics and carbon sequestration *via* microbial and biological pumps.

In the Florida Bay case, the latitudinal gradient coincides with the gradient in systemic environmental pressure (or envirome), but these two do not necessarily coincide. Systemic pressure is typically power-law distributed (considering the predominance of one extreme affecting biota), but it can also be organized according to other distributions. More generally, systemic pressure causes systemic impacts that can be caused by more disorganized or complex environmental factors, e.g., distributed exponentially or multimodally, such as a combination of global ocean extremes and local nutrient loading.

Figure 16.4 shows *in silico* simulations of the interaction dynamics of Eukaryotes (E), Prokaryotes (P), and Viruses (V) of the ocean microbiome observed in several databases from around the world to capture universal dynamical patterns. Namely, these are the Shenzhen (Yantian) E-P-V dynamics (Du et al. 2020) during blooms of *Gymnodinium catenatum* (a dinoflagellate causing blooms and paralytic shellfish poisoning); E-P-V in Shenzhen (Pearl River Delta sampled via the QingYan No. 1 boat of Tsinghua SIGS in a July 2019 cruise) along a salinity gradient without reported blooms; E-P-V in the Quantuck Bay (Zhang et al. 2021) and Weesuck Creek (Shinnecock Bay along the southern shore of Long Island, New York) (Moniruzzaman et al. 2016) also during harmful brown tides caused by the pelagophyte *Aureococcus anophagefferens* (affected by Megaviridae); E-P-V in the San Pedro Channel (Southern California, USA) (Needham, Sachdeva, and Fuhrman 2017; Sieradzki et al. 2020) (The Port of Los Angeles data set), Santa Catalina Island Two Harbors (CAT dataset), and the San Pedro Ocean Time series (data set) without declared blooms (Sieradzki et al. 2020; Giovannoni 2017) are emphasizing SAR11 as the most abundant bacteria in the ocean, in oceans' plankton leading to salient virus interactions; E-P-V in a large Arctic marine ecosystem gradient (Sandaa et al. 2018) during diverse blooms; E-P-V in the Kerguelen Island in the Southern Ocean during spring phytoplankton blooms (KEOPS2 dataset) (Christaki et al. 2014); E-P-V along a Pacific Ocean gradient also during blooms (Needham et al. 2019); E-P-V across the North Atlantic Ocean (Mojica et al. 2016) during blooms; E-P-V in the Antarctic Peninsula, one of the most rapidly warming regions on the planet (Brum et al. 2016) during blooms and Megaviruses; and (Prodinger et al. 2022) in the Uranouchi Inlet, Kochi (JP), during diverse species blooms and Megaviruses.

Other studies reporting only one or two microbiome group interactions (predominantly EP or P) can also be considered; for instance, the E-P dynamics in the Florida Reef Tract (Laaset et al. 2021), also considering blooms of Scrippsiella (a nontoxic dinoflagellate causing red blooms with oxygen depletion resulting in fish kills); E-P dynamics associated with blooms the ichthyotoxic dinoflagellate Cochlodinium (Margalefidinium) causality (linked to any model) vs. true causality, where the latter requires a detailed investigation of processes beyond the sole use of models. Diverse morphology of species causing blooms can be related to different environmental niches whose alteration may also lead to morphological changes and new species emergence.

An interesting research question is whether species morphological complexity is associated with bloom complexity (in terms of microbiological network and biodiversity at higher trophic levels), habitat complexity (related to hydrodynamical and biogeochemical features), environmental pressure diversity and complexity. This seems most likely the case as highlighted by preliminary findings shown in Figure 16.2A where the number of eukaryote species (and their morphological asymmetry) is higher for more complex habitats that are sensitive to fewer environmental factors. This is also aligned with principles of optimal Pareto evolution under environmental pressure that forces species to differentiate themselves from the rest and become more resilient to change (Convertino and Valverde 2019; Shoval et al. 2012); polykrikoides in New Yorkestuaries (USA) (Hatterath–Lehmann et al. 2019); E-P dynamics in a Salt Pond in the Nauset Marsh System (Cape Cod, Massachusetts, USA) (L. Liu et al. 2019) during a marine dinoflagellate bloom; E-P dynamics in Xiamen, southeast China (L. Liu et al. 2019) during cyanobacterial blooms over six years in two subtropical reservoirs; E-P dynamics (microeukaryotes and bacterioplankton) (Tan et al. 2015) during algal Scrippsiella trochoidea blooms; E-P dynamics (Zhao et al. 2016) during Cyanobacteria blooms; E-P in two subtropical Florida estuaries (Philips et al. 2020) during diverse algal blooms; E-V (rather rare coupling being investigated) in Hiroshima Bay (Tomaru et al. 2004) also during blooms of Heterosigma akashiwo (that is very famous for causing extensive red blooms); P-V dynamics (rare to investigate) in the water column along a large North Atlantic latitudinal transect (De Corte et al. 2012) (where V-P direct scaling was found); P dynamics in indoor marine microcosms (S.W. Jung et al. 2021) during Akashiwo sanguinea (Dinophyceae) blooms; P dynamics only in regions of Taihu Lake with different nutrient loadings (Cao et al. 2018); and E dynamics only in the eastern Gulf of Mexico (Milbrandt et al. 2021) during dinoflagellate Karenia brevis red tide/

blooms. It should be noted that by considering one or two microbiome pairs, interactions certainly vary from those inferred by considering viruses due to both virus-induced change in information dynamics and the model-related structure that selects information with the highest predictability (J. Li and Convertino 2021a). The same argument is true when considering any other group that can be added, such as zooplankton, which was not accounted for in our review. In this perspective, one should always be careful in distinguishing predictive causality.

Figure 16.5A shows predictive causality networks where the non-bloom dynamics also appear as long-range connections driven by probabilistic dependence (similarity of endemic bloom dynamics) rather than physical dependence. North East areas are much more similar in terms of dynamics than others. *Vice versa* bloom dynamic networks likely reflect physical connections of endemic and epidemic areas (in terms of blooms) driven by abiotic (water, nutrient, and particulate matter) and biotic fluxes (eukaryotes and viruses dispersal). Figure 16.5 emphasizes the CSD of blooms that are getting smaller but more erratic and widely distributed in space. This is evident from 2005 after a hiatus between 2000 and 2005 approximately, which is a classical signature of critical transition from one dynamic to another: variance and average diminishing before a change in regime (Scheffer et al. 2009). It is also interesting to observe that after 2005, blooms started to expand to NE areas of Florida Bay closer to South Florida agricultural and urban areas, yet manifesting an increasing pressure from these areas. Unfortunately, that sector of Florida Bay hosts many unique

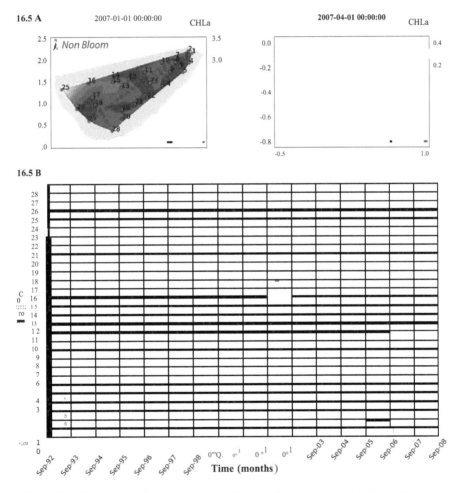

Figure 16.5 Non-bloom and bloom average pattern and persistency of extreme blooms. Environmental data are for the period 1992–2008 with a monthly resolution. The data used are the same as in Nelson, Munoz-Carpena, and Philips (2017) obtained from the FIU Water Quality Monitoring Program (http://serc.fiu.edu/wqmnetwork/SFWMD-CD/index.ht) based on 28 spatially distributed stations maintained in Florida Bay from 1989 to 2008.

species, such as marine sponges, and due to the shallow-water habitats, ecological communities are very sensitive to environmental change, which poses a greater risk.

PLANETARY HEALTH VIA ECOSYSTEM SCIENCE AND ENGINEERING
Ecosystem Portfolio Risk Management

Ecosystems are shaped according to structural and functional networks that are portfolios of "assets" (such as areas, species, and interactions) where the collective organization is critical for optimal function. Natural systems have a tendency toward optimality and equilibrium *via* Pareto evolutionary strategies that increase fitness for survival against the majority of environmental shocks at the population scale. Evolution of populations over time, and communities, in turn, is observable *via* information evolution of features (such as abundance and other traits) characterized probabilistically where the optimal state is often a critical state with power-law distributed features, reflecting the envisioned SOC of Bak (Bak, Tang, and Wiesenfeld 1987). Then, divergence from the optimal portfolio is a signature of ecosystem dysbiosis (J. Li and Convertino 2019) and engineering portfolio approaches, considering collective dynamics of ecosystems and interventions, are suitable to minimize divergence from the naturally optimal, desired, or trade-off state. A clear example of ecosystem engineering where both ecological interventions (species-specific interventions such as vegetation protection and planting) and environmental restoration (e.g., habitat restoration via re-nourishment) are implemented by taking into account nonlinear temporal trajectories related to climate and development, spatial dependencies, and ecosystem-intervention portfolio feedback (Convertino and Valverde 2013).

In the Florida Bay case, information like that shown in Figures 16.3 and 16.6 can be highly useful to target key environmental factors associated with persistent and large blooming areas, e.g.,

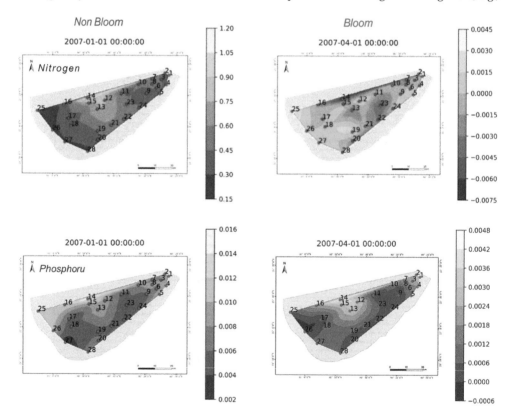

Figure 16.6 A, B, C Average environmental determinants associated with non-bloom and bloom dynamics. The value of environmental determinants is different for each station in the NB and B but their network interdependence is fairly robust for these two regimes. Chlorophyll-a (µg/L), total nitrogen and phosphorus (mg/L), surface salinity (practical salinity units, psu), surface water temperature (Celsius), surface turbidity (Nephelometric turbidity units).

critically nitrogen-affected areas that are high-risk, considering either hazard or vulnerability as opposite functions for ecological communities of which humans are a part.

Not all environmental determinants are controllable because of their natural variability. Detecting critical drivers of anomalous blooms can lead to the detection of coastal sites responsible for the overload of nutrients and particularly sensitive areas prone to change. Note the centrality of the environment, its equilibrium, and its optimality. It is a common misconception to consider the environment in equilibrium as the "pristine" or "healthy" state of nature. This could be false because (i) the current equilibrium state may be completely unhealthy or different from the original "pristine" condition as is the case for deforested ecosystems or natural ecosystems converted to agriculture. (ii) Evolution implies punctuated disequilibrium, and transitory states may lead to more optimal states and instability, which could be the desired state of an ecosystem; this is the case for the Venice "natural" environment for instance. (iii) Healthy states may occur in disequilibrium conditions; e.g., in constructed bays, the ocean microbiome may be optimally

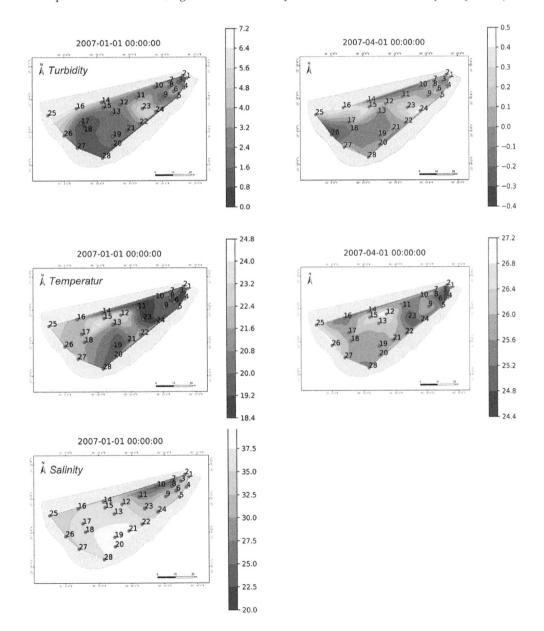

Figure 16.6 (Continued)

organized with balanced positive and negative feedbacks with higher trophic scales. Pristineness does not exist because nature always evolves (leaving aside the invariance of optimal configurations that are inevitable canonical forms of nature) and any natural ecosystem has been somewhat impacted at a certain level either by local conditions or global forcing. Yet, the target should not be about restoring ecosystems as they were originally, which is an unsolvable question, but how we can preserve, enhance, or design new ecosystems as Venetians did and are currently doing in maintaining its lagoon and islands by optimizing their functions such as biodiversity dynamics and carbon cycling.

We are transforming Earth, so we cannot get back to how it was because that would imply deleting history that is a utopian vision. Creating the best future should be our effort, as well as optimizing ecosystem monitoring. The questions are what, where, and how many features to monitor to anticipate critical short- and long-term changes; an example is water microbiological monitoring since the microbiome is the first life fingerprint of environmental change.

SYNOPSIS AND PERSPECTIVES

The ocean contains 97% of all water on our planet and is thus a fundamental biodiversity reservoir and driver of global ecosystems. Marine plankton form the base of ocean food webs and play a major role in the planet's global biogeochemistry by accounting for half of the net primary production (Falkowski, Fenchel, and Delong 2008), and thus drive ocean oxygen production and the biological carbon pump (Bauer et al. 2013). Alteration of these processes leads to deoxygenation (Breitburg et al. 2018), acidification, tropicalization, which includes impacts on deep-sea biodiversity (Yasuhara and Danovaro 2016) and human health (Baker-Austin et al. 2013; Fleming et al. 1999; Harvell et al. 1999). Within marine systems, microalgal blooms are natural phenomena related to the seasonality of photosynthetic organisms, from coastal areas to deep oceans. They are key components of the architecture and dynamics of these ecosystems and sustain a variety of ecosystem services, including climate regulation of Earth. Particularly, abundant microeukaryotes and Cyanobacteria (phytoplankton) contribute to half of the total primary production of microflora on Earth and are the basis of the marine food web. However, some microalgal blooms can cause harm to humans and other species. These HABs, which are rapid expansions of phytoplankton populations, and other noncarrying toxin blooms have direct impacts on human health and potential long-term influence on human well-being. Consequences to coastal ecosystem services, e.g., fisheries, tourism and recreation, and other marine organisms and environments show evident negative outcomes of blooms, mostly because of their erratic cycle with increased frequency, magnitude, and/or duration. Thus, in order to assess ecosystem health from land to ocean and to better quantify the impact of one or multiple species or on one or multiple ecosystem services, we recommend considering the collective dysbiosis of ecosystem function (multitrophic network) mapped as a complex network. For both research and application, it is important to map the functional symbiosis between hosts and associated prokaryotes, eukaryotes, and viruses in an ecosystem context that is often called the "holobiont." Unraveling holobiont associations has proven to be both difficult and controversial, but the convergence of studies demonstrating this biocomplexity is starting to reveal important and surprising linkages between biota and climate with local-global and micro-macro feedback. For instance, it is interesting to note that phytoplankton blooms can undergo a synchronized demise following infection by viruses, which can reach $\sim 10^8$ virions per liter of seawater and therefore are thought to control the fate of phytoplankton blooms, including the subsequent release of organic matter fueling microbial life and the viral shunt enhancing carbon sequestration.

Considering preliminary estimates, viruses are roughly responsible for half of the global annual carbon dioxide fixation and sustain higher trophic levels in marine ecosystems, yet they influence global-scale processes. It is important for the public and ecosystem manager to understand the impact of environmental quality on invisible microbiological processes, which have tangible and long-lasting macroscale impacts. Other things that are important to investigate are how the disappearance of large marine (and iconic) mammals will impact microbiology and climate considering the proven dependence on the food web and biogeochemical dynamics. Also, microorganisms in the environment have a tendency to react with pharmaceutical pollutants by developing resistance to drugs. These microorganisms could develop into superbugs, which implies that when humans get infected, available medication will no longer work. This issue is related to antimicrobial resistance genes spreading in the water, which is a largely unexplored research topic in ecology. Other largely unexplored topics include how metals, compounds of emerging concerns, and microplastics interact with microorganisms to affect human health.

In conclusion, synthesizing our preliminary analyses, we highlight the following:

- Environment-modulated viruses in marine ecosystems control the eukaryote-prokaryote balance whose alteration affects biodiversity and biogeochemistry via the food web across trophic scales. These ecosystem functions underpin ecosystem metabolism that is regulating the energy expenditure of processes involving species (biota) and abiotic transformations. Yet ocean viruses have an incredibly important ecological role because they control blooms and enhance the biological and microbial carbon pump, provided the environment is not altered dramatically. Viruses can also grow faster (exponentially) than eucaryotes therefore, virus concentrations can be early warning signals (EWS) of blooms, leaving aside the complication of measuring viruses (see Figure 16.4). That is why it is fundamental to map the "envirome" (or key species/bioindicators; Whitfield et al. 2016) to determine microbiological dynamics that can serve both to understand environment-driven changes and as an EWS of biota. Capturing the holobiont dynamics is reflecting the zoonoses framework in epidemiology where environment-biota transmission chains are investigated, and epigenetics where the effect of the environment on human biology is assessed. It is crucial to integrate abiotic and biotic dynamics because the variation of the latter cannot be explained without the former. Biotic variations are habitat specific, but for the same habitat, biotic dynamics can be different because of local biogeochemical stress. Overall, optimal balance, captured by network topology and likely habitat-specific due to niche attraction, is key for optimal ecosystem function. In time, the natural bloom cycle may experience long-term changes, e.g., because of temperature trends and nitrogen increases that lead to permanent ecosystem changes from oligotrophic to eutrophic, although blooms are quite rapid with respect to these states. Eutrophic ecosystems are in fact experiencing more persistent or erratic blooms manifested by disorganized network topologies. Small and repeated stress should not be overlooked because they can have large effects in the long run via CSD (Batt, Eason, and Garmestani 2019; J. Li and Convertino 2021b)

- Ecosystem structure, function, and services (ecosystem connectome) are tightly and nonlinearly connected. It is compelling to protect the natural ecosystem structure and function (e.g., water flow and quality, or more generally environmental flows that avoid undesired blooms or support needed functions and services) that define habitat structure and suitability leading to multiple ecosystem services. Everything starts from the ocean, including pathogens emerging from ocean dysbiosis, and impacts on human populations arise when there is a tension and physical proximity between the natural and built environment: this is for instance the case of the Everglades and nearby marine ecosystems whose alteration is leading to ecological collapse and emergence of toxins and viruses. The health of humans hugely depends on ecological health, yet the importance of organized biota feedback on habitat/environment and climate is crucial. Thus, the centrality of oceans and climate connections is related to the centrality of ecohydrology and land-water connections in an ecosystem perspective that goes beyond single species populations and microbiology. Preserved ecosystem structure is the key to adsorbing environmental shocks (until a certain level) and guaranteeing proper function. Global forcing has much higher systemic impacts if local conditions are largely altered due to the higher sensitivity of biota and habitats that have a lower degree of freedom to bounce back.

- Nature-based solutions with an ecosystem portfolio approach (considering interdependencies of areas, species, and ecosystem functions) should be adopted for ecosystem health at the local and planetary scale. Efforts in this direction are addressing fundamental ecosystem services such as carbon sequestration and biodiversity accounting for past changes (Dinerstein et al. 2020; Dinerstein et al. 2019; M. Jung et al. 2020; Sala et al. 2021). Saving biodiversity is typically oriented toward protecting one species (e.g., iconic species that can be a major anchor); however, that may certainly miss habitat protection and keystone species that are actually accounted for via carbon-centered solutions. For instance, protecting the Sundarbans tiger or the mangroves in isolation is not enough; we need both to sustain carbon sequestration and biodiversity because both mangroves and the tiger are interconnected via a tangled and important food web whose fluxes establish species and biogeochemical interactions. To do so, water quantity and quality that largely define habitat and habitat suitability must be considered. For the aforementioned reasons, several recent plans have identified biodiversity-carbon ecosystem protection areas (Dinerstein et al. 2020; Dinerstein et al. 2019). In terms of ecosystem engineering, approaches should also aim to restore compromised hydrologic flows (Convertino and Valverde 2019; Macreadie et al. 2017) and keystone vegetation with "umbrella" positive effects on other species, e.g., macroalgae (S. Liu et al. 2020b) (that can also generate biofuel for food and feed production), regulation of biogeochemical loads from rivers into oceans (S. Liu et al. 2020a) and in the potential enhancement of carbon drawdown via artificial upwelling or downwelling i.e., "climate engineering" also combined with selected aquaculture (Fan et al. 2020; Fan et al. 2019; Oschlies et al. 2010). Portfolio approaches selecting the Pareto optimal set of all these actions (Convertino and Valverde 2013) are useful especially in the presence of resource constraints and the spatial dependence of land-ocean ecosystems. In general, we believe it is important to shift the discussion from risk to ecosystem performance and put environmental quality at center stage; it is not just the local "health" of humans; it is also about global survivability. The previous collapse of civilizations (Egyptian, Rapa Nui, Angkor, and Maya civilizations are epitomic cases) should have taught us about the centrality of environmental degradation in determining the fate of humanity, caused by co-occurring and linked climate-driven alterations of environmental flows, spread of emerging pathogens, and overexploitation of resources – i.e., the systemic risk by definition. To restore human health, we must restore our relationship with the natural environment, with a greater sense of unity, place, and purpose within nature. Our planet is losing biodiversity at an unprecedented rate, and it is urgent to preserve Earth's biodiversity locally in order to counter global climate change.

- Predictive pattern-oriented computational models serve the triple purpose of (i) data selection in terms of biota and envirome, including the detection of critical stations to monitor that leads to the creation of salient ecosystem monitoring networks informing about critical spatiotemporal changes; (ii) investigate potential causality of envirome-biota processes by quantifying nonlinearity and extending discrete space-time point predictive causality (fundamental mechanisms vs. the whole "tangled web" of reality) to the continuum; and (iii) define precise ecosystem engineering actions (e.g. to restore habitat, protect species, and enhance carbon drawdown) based on (i) and (ii) and short-/long-term trajectory of climate and anthropogenic change, as well as deep uncertainty (the latter considering the whole stochastic variability of biota and envirome). Information- and network-theoretic models are quite suitable for uncertainty reduction that is about magnitude, probability, and delay in the occurrence of events considering the whole collective dynamics as an information portfolio (J. Li and Convertino 2021a). As for predictability, it should be recognized the unpredictability of the unpredictable ("Dragon King" events (Sornette 2009): spillover of viruses from the environment to humans with staggering impacts, are largely unpredictable phenomena since these are one-time fortuitous events related to unstable and anti-persistent (or stuttering vs. sustained) transmission chains in the food web (Llyod–Smith et al. 2009) For many pathogens, e.g., Megaviruses in the oceans, the food-web distance is rather long (considering as well the phylogenetic distance) but cascading events can occur along the trophic chain through causal mechanisms that are unknown or extremely unlikely, yet unpredictable. In a terrestrial context, for instance, for COVID-19, the food web between bats and humans was fairly long; therefore, the spillover probability between these two hosts was quite small; nonetheless, this caused the largest pandemic in human history. Of course, this makes risk assessment quite of no practical value, but in a systemic risk purview, the need would be to build up a system of EWSs and response that efficiently counteract these unpredictable "Dragon Kings." As for causality, we showed how predictive causality may arise for non-bloom dynamics, but these spatial long-range connections are driven by probabilistic dependence rather than physical connections; vice versa the bloom dynamic networks reflect much more physical connections of endemic and epidemic areas (in terms of blooms) with abiotic (nutrient and particulates) and biotic fluxes (eukaryotes and viruses). Further studies need to unveil the Virus-Prokaryote relationships, particularly before and after blooms with more clarity. This causality investigation should keep in mind the limitation exerted by discrete sampling over space-time and care must be placed when the sampling scale is larger than the event scale (e.g., monthly microbiome sampling vs. weekly blooming cycles); a factor may not be relevant just because there is a mismatch between its scale of variability and one of predicted patterns (e.g., virus and carbon cycling scales). Additionally, integrating different data, from microbiological, environmental quality, satellite, and human health impacts is novel and useful but scale issues and scale dependence on what is relevant at what scale must be considered numerically. research and climate actions should move beyond predictions especially in a constantly changing and yet unpredictable future in the long term (Dawson et al. 2011).

ACKNOWLEDGMENTS

M. C. acknowledges the High Talent Scheme ("A" Talents) of the Shenzhen Government and the Talents Hiring Funding of Tsinghua University, Shenzhen International Graduate School. M.C. also acknowledges funding of the project " Climate and Anthropogenic Impacts on Coastal Ecosystems: Key Species-Habitat and Blue Carbon Feedbacks" from the Ministry of Science and Technology, China. M. C. acknowledges extensive discussions with H. Ogata and F. Prodinger at the Institute for Chemical Research, Kyoto University.

LITERATURE CITED

Bak, P., C Tang, and K. Wiesenfeld. 1987. Self-organized Criticality: An Explanation of the 1/f Noise. *Phys. Rev. Lett* 59 (4): 381–384.

Baker-Austin, C., J. A. Trinanes, N. G. H. Taylor, R. Hartnell, A. Siitonen, and J. Martinez-Urtaza. 2013. Emerging Vibrio Risk at High Latitudes in Response to Ocean Warming. *Nat Clim Chang* 3 (1): 73–77. https://doi. org/10.1038/nclimate1628.

Batt, R. D., T. Eason, and A. Garmestani. 2019. Time Scale of Resilience Loss: Implications for Managing Critical Transitions in Water Quality. *PLoS One* 14 (10): e022336. https://doi.org/10.1371/journal.pone.0223366.

Bauer, J. E., W.-J. Cai, P. A. Raymond, T. S. Bianchi, C. S. Hhopkinson, and P. A. G. Regnier. 2013. The Changing Carbon Cycle of the Coastal Ocean. *Nature (London)* 504 (478)): 61–70. https://doi.org/10.1038/nature12857

Blanc-Mathieu, R., H. Endo, S. Chaffron, R. Hern'andez-Vel'azquez, C. H. Nguyen, H Mamitsuka, N. Henry, C. de Vargas, and M. B. Sullivan. 2019. Viruses of the Eukaryotic Plankton Are Predicted to Increase Carbon Export Efficiency in the Global Sunlit Ocean. *bioRxiv*, 710228. https://doi.org/10.1101/710228

Bonan, G. B., and S. Doney. 2018. Ecosystems, and Planetary Futures: The Challenge to Predict Life in Earth System Models. *Science (Washington)* 359: 6375. https://doi.org/10.1126/science.aam8328.

Bonetti, G., S. M. Trevathan-Tackett, P. E. Carnel, and P. I. Macreadie. 2019. Implication of Viral Infections for Greenhouse Gas Dynamics in Feshwater Wetlands: Challenges and Perspectives. *Front. Microbiol.* 10:1962. https://doi.org/10.3389/fmicb.2019.01962.

Bonetti, G.. 2021. The Potential of Viruses to Influence the Magnitude of Greenhouse Gas Emissions in an Inland Wetland. *Water Res.* 193 (2021): 116875. https://doi.org/10.1016/j.watres.2021.116875.

Breitburg, D., L. A. Levin, A. Oschlies, M. Grégoire, F. P. Chavez, D. J. Conley, V. Garçon, D. Gilbert, D. Gutiérrez, K. Isensee, G. S. Jacinto, K. E. Limburg, I. Montes, S. W. A. Naqvi, G. C. Pitcher, N. N. Rabalais, M. R. Roman, K. A. Rose, B. A. Seibel, M. Telszewski, M. Yasuhara, and J. Zhang. 2018. Declining Oxygen in the Global Ocean and Coastal Waters. *Science (Washington)* 359: 11. https://doi.org/10.1126/science.aam724.

Brum, J. R., B. L. Hurwitz, O. Schofiel, H. W. Ducklow, and M. B. Sullivan. 2016. Seasonal Time Bombs: Dominant Temperate Viruses Affect outhern Ocean Microbial Dynamics. *ISME J.* 10 (2): 437–449. https://doi.org/10.1038/ismej.2015.125.

Cao, X., D. Zhao, H. Xu, R. Huang, J. Zeng, and Z. Yu. 2018. Heterogeneity of Interactions of Microbial Communities in Regions of Taihu Lake with Different Nutrient Loadings: A Network Analysis. *Sci. Rep.* 8 (1 e8890): 1–11. https://doi.org/10.1038/s41598-018-27172-z.

Chen, X., W. Wei, J. Wang, H. Li, J. Sun, R. Ma, N. Jiao, and R. Zhang. 2019. Tide Driven Microbial Dynamics Through Virus-Host Interactions in the Estuarine Ecosystem. *Water Res.* 160 (1): 118–129. https://doi.org/10.1016/j.watres.2019.05.051.

Christaki, U., D. Lef'evre, C. Georges, J. Colombet, P. Catala, C. Courties, T. Sime-Ngando, S. BlaIN, and I. Obernosterer. 2014. Microbial Food Web Dynamics During Spring Phytoplankton Blooms in the Naturally Iron-Fertilized Kerguelen Area (Southern Ocean). *Biogeosciences* 11 (23): 6739–6753. https://doi.org/10.5194/bg-11-6739-2014.

Convertino, M., C. M. Foran, J. M. Keisler, L. Scarlett, A. LoSchiavo, G. A. Kiker, and I. Linkov. 2013. Enhanced Adaptive Management: Integrating Decision Analysis, Scenario Analysis and Environmental Modeling for the Everglades. *Sci. Rep.* 3 (1): 1–10. https://doi.org/10.1038/srep02922.

Convertino, M., and J. Valverde, Jr. 2013. Portfolio Decision Analysis Framework for Value–Focused Ecosystem Management. *PLoS One* 8 (6) (2013): e65056. https://doi.org/10.1371/journal.pone.0065056.

Convertino, M.. 2019. Toward a Pluralistic Conception of Resilience. *Ecol. Ind.* 107 (2019): 105510. https://doi.org/10.1016/j.ecolind.2019.105510.

Dawson, T. P., S. T. Jackson, J. House, I. C. Prentice, and G. M. Mace. 2011. Beyond Predictions: Biodiversity Conservation in a Changing Climate. *Science (Washington)* 332 (6025): 53–58. https://doi.org/10.1126/science.1200303.

De Corte, D., E. Sintes, T. Yokokawa, T. Reinthaler, and G. J. Herndl. 2012. Links Between Viruses and Prokaryotes Throughout the Water Column Along a North Atlantic Latitudinal Transect. *ISME J.* 6 (8): 1566–1577. https://doi.org/10.1038/ismej.2011.214.

Dinerstein, E., A. R. Joshi, C. Vynne, A. T. L. Lee, F. Pharand-Deschenes, M Franca, S. Fernando, T. Birch, K. Burkhart, P. Asner, and D. Olson. 2020. A Global Safety Net to Reverse Biodiversity Loss and Stabilize Earth's Climate. *Sci. Adv.* 6 (36:eabb2824). https://doi.org/10.1126/sciadv.abb2824.

Dinerstein, E., C. Vynne, E. Sala, A. R. Joshi, S. Fernando, T. E. Lovejoy, J. Mayorga, D. Olson, G. P. Asner, J. E. M. Baille, N. D. Burgess,.K. Burkart, R. F. Noss, Y. P. Zhang, A. Baccini, T. Birch, N. Hahn, L. N. Joppa, and E. Wikramanayake. 2019. A Global Deal for Nature: Guiding Principles, Milestones, and Targets. *Sci. Adv.* 5: 17. https://doi.org/10.1126/sciadv.aaw2869.

Du, X.-P., Z.-H. Cai, P. Zuo, F. Xu, F-X. Meng, and J. Zhou. 2020. Temporal Variability of Virioplankton During a Gymnodinium Catenatum Algal Bloom. *Microorganisms* 8 (107): 15. https://doi.org/10.3390/microorganisms8010107.

Falkowski, P. G., T. Fenchel, and E. F. Delong. 2008. The Microbial Engines That Drive Earth's Biogeochemical Cycles. *Science (Washington)* 320 (5879): 1034–1039. https://doi.org/10.1126/science.1153213.

Fan, W., C. Xiao, P. Li, Z. Zhang, T. Lin, Y. Pan, Y. Di, and Y. Chen. 2020. Intelligent Control System of an Ecological Engineering Project for Carbon Sequestration in Coastal Mariculture Environments in China. *Sustainability* 12 (13): 5227. https://doi.org/10.3390/su12135227.

Fan, W., R. Zhao, Z. Yaoi, C. Xiao, Y. Pan, Y. Chen, N. Jiao, and Y. Zhang. 2019. Nutrient Removal from Chinese Coastal Waters by Large-scale Seaweed Aquaculture Using Artificial Upwelling. *Water* 11 (9): 1754. doi:10.3390/w11091754.

Fleming, T. P., A. J. Watkins, M. A. Velazquez, J. C. Mathers, A. M. Prentice, J. Stephenson, M. Barker, R. Saffery, C. Yajnik, and J. J. Eck. 1999. Origins of Lifetime Health around the Time of Conception: Causes and Consequences. *Lancet* 391: 1842–1852.

Giovannoni, S. J. 2017. Sar11 Bacteria: The Most Abundant Plankton in the Oceans. *Annu. Rev. Marine Sci.* 9: 231–255. https://doi.org/10.1146/annurev-marine-010814-015934.

Guidi, L., S. Chaffron, L. Bittner, D. Eveillard, A. Larhlim, Roux S., Y. Darzi, S. Audic, L. Berline, J. R. Brum, L. P. Coehlo, J. C. I. Espinoza, and M. Malviya. 2016. Plankton Networks Driving Carbon Export in the Oligotrophic Ocean. *Nature (London)* 532 (7600): 465–470. https://doi.org/10.1038/nature16942.

Harvell, C. D., K. Kim, J. M. Burkholder, R. R. Colwell, P. R. Epstein, D. J. Grimes, E. E. Hofmann, E. K. Lipp, A. D. D. M. E. Osterhaus, R. M. Overstreet, J. W. Porter, G. W. Smith, and G. R. Vasta. 1999. Emerging Marine Diseases–Climate Lnks and Anthropogenic Factor. *Science (Washington)* 285 (5433): 1505–1510. https://doi.org/10.1126/science.285.5433.1505.

Hatterath-Lehmann, T. K., J. Jankowiak, F. Koch, and C. J. Gobler. 2019. Prokaryotic and Eukaryotic Microbiomes Associated with Blooms of the Ichthyotoxic Dinoflagellate Cochlodinium (Margalefidinium Polykrikoides in New York, USA, Estuaries). *PLoS One* 14 (11): e0223067. https://doi.org/10.1371/journal.pone.0223067.

Hatton, I. R., R. F. Heneghan, Y. M. Bar-On, and E. O. Galbraith. 2021. The Global Ocean Size-Spectrum From Bacteria to Whales. *Sci. Adv.* 7: eabh3732. https://doi.org/10.1126/sciadv.abh3732.

Jover, L. F., T. C. Effler, A. Buchan, S. W. Wilhelm, and J. S. Weitz. 2014. The Elemental Composition of Virus Particles: Implications for Marine Biogeochemical Cycles. *Nat Rev. Microbiol.* 12 (7): 519–528. https://doi.org/10.1038/nrmicro3289.

Jung, M., A. Arnell, X. de Lamo, S. García-Rangel, M. Lewis, J. Mark, C. Merow, and L. Miles. 2020. Areas of Global Importance for Terrestrial Biodiversity, Carbon, and Water. bioRxiv. *Nat. Ecol. Evol.* 5 (11): 1499–1509. https://doi.org/10.1038/s41559-021-01528-7.

Jung, S. W., J. Kang, J. S. Park, H. M. Joo, S.-S. Suh, D. Kang, T-K. Lee, and H-J. Kim. 2021. Dynamic Bacterial Community Response to Akashiwo Sanguinea (Dinophyceae) Bloom in Indoor Marine Microcosms. *Sci. Rep.* 11 (6983): 1–11. https://doi.org/10.1038/s41598-021-86590-8.

Kurita, J., and K. Nakajima. 2012. Megalocytiviruses. *Viruses* 4 (4): 521–538. https://doi.org/10.3390/v4040521.

Laaset, P., K. Ugarelli, M. Absten, B. Boyer, H. Bricen⁻o, and U. Stingl. 2021. Composition of Prokaryotic and Eukaryotic Microbial Communities in Waters Around the Florida Reef Tract. *Microorganisms* 9 (6): 1120. https://doi.org/10.3390/microorganisms9061120.

Lehahn, Y., I. Koren, M. Frada, U. Sheyn, E. Boss, D. Schatz, M. Trainic, S. Sharoni, C. Laber, C. R. DiTullio, M. J. L. Coolen, A. M. Martins, B. A. S. Van Mooy, K. D. Bidle, and A. Vardi. 2014. Decoupling Physical From Biological Processes to Assess the Impact of Viruses on a Mesoscale Algal Bloom. *Curr. Biol.* 24 (17): 2041–2046. http://dx.doi.org/10.1016/j.cub.2014.07.046

Li, J., and M. Convertino. 2019. Optimal Microbiome Networks: Macroecology and Criticality. *Entropy* 21 (5). https://doi.org/10.3390/e21050506.

Li, J., and M. Convertino. 2021a. Inferring Ecosystem Networks as Information Flows." *Sci. Rep.* 11 (1): 11:7094. https://doi.org/10.1038/s41598-021-86476-9.

Li, J.. 2021b. "Temperature Increase Drives Critical Slowing Down of Fish Ecosystems." *PloS One* 16 (10): e0246222. https://doi.org/10.1371/journal.pone.0246222.

Liu, L., H. Chen, M. Liu, Yang, J. R., P. Xiao, D. M. Wilkinson, and J. Yang 2019. "Eukaryotic Plankton Community to the Cyanobacterial Biomass Cycle Over Six Years in Two Subtropical Reservoirs." *ISME J.* 13 (9): 2196–2208. https://doi.org/10.1038/s41396-019-0417-9.

Liu, S., Y. Deng, Z. Jiang, Y. Wu, X. Huang, and P. I. Macreadie. 2020a. "Nutrient Loading Diminishes the Dissolved Organic Carbon Drawdown Capacity of Seagrass Ecosystems." *Sci Total Environ.* 740. https://doi.org/10.1016/j.scitotenv.2020.140185.

Liu, S., S. M. Trevathan-Tackett, C. J. Ewers-Lewis, X. Huang, and P. I. Macreadie. 2020b. Macroalgal Blooms Trigger the Breakdown of Seagrass Blue Carbon. *Environ. Sci. & Technol.* 54: 14750–14760. https://dx.doi.org/10.1021/acs.est.0c03720.

Llyod-Smith, J. L., D. George, K. M. Pepin, J. R. C. Pulliam, A. P. Dobson, P. J. Hudson, and B. T. Grenfell. 2009. Epidemic Dynamics at the Human-Animal Interface. *Science (Washington)* 326 (5958): 1362–1367. https://doi.org/10.1126/science.1177345.

Macreadie, P. I., D. A. Nelsen, J. J. Kelleway, Y. B. Atwood, J. R. Seymore, K. Petrou, and P. J. Ralph. 2017. Can We Manage Coastal Ecosystems to Sequester More Blue Carbon? *Front. Ecol. Environ* 15 (4): 206–217. https://doi.org/10.1002/fee.1484.

Milbrandt, E. C., A. J. Martignette, M. A. Thompson, R. D. Bartleson, E. J. Philips, S. Badylak, and N. G. Nelson. 2021. Geospatial Distribution of Hypoxia Associated with a Karenia Brevis Bloom. *Estuar. Coast. Shelf. Sci.* 259: 107446. https://doi.org/10.1016/j.ecss.2021.107446.

Mojica, K. D. A., J. Huisman, S. W. Wilhelm, and P. D. Brussaard. 2016. Latitudinal Variation in Virus-Induced Mortality of Phytoplankton Across the North Atlantic Ocean. *ISME J.* 10 (2): 500–513. https://doi.org/10.1038/ismej.2015.130.

Moniruzzaman, M., E. R. Gann, LeCleir, G. R., C. J. Kang, C. J. Gobler, and S. Wilhelm. 2016. Diversity and Dynamics of Algal Megaviridae Members During a Harmful Brown Tide Caused by the Pelagophyte, Aureococcus Anophagefferens. *FEMS Microbiol. Ecol.* 92 (5): fiw058. https://doi.org/10.1093/femsec/fiw058.

Needham, D. M., Sachdeva, R., and J. A. Fuhrman. 2017. Ecological Dynamics and Cooccurrence Among Marine Phytoplankton, Bacteria and Myoviruses Show Microdiversity Matters. *ISME J.* 11 (7): 1614–1629. https://doi.org/10.1038/ismej.2017.29.

Needham, D. M., S. Yoshizawa, T. Hosaka, L. A. Poirier, C. J. Choi, E. Hehenberger, N. A. Irwin, S. Wilken, C-M. Yung, C. Bachy, R. Kurihara, Y. Nakajima, K. Kojima, T. Kimura-Someyac, G. Leonard, R. R. Malmstrom, D. R. Mende, D. K. Olsoni, S. Yudof, S. Sudeka, T. A. Richards, E. F. De Long, P. J. Keeling, A. E. Santoro, M. Shirouzu, W. Iwasaki, and A. Z. Wordena. 2019. A Distinct Lineage of Giant Viruses Brings a Rhodopsin Photosystem to Unicellular Marine Predators. *Proc. Natl. Acad. Sci. (USA)* 116 (41): 20574–20583. https://doi.org/www.pnas.org/cgi/doi/10.1073/pnas.1907517116.

Nelson, N. G., R. Munoz-Carpena, and E. J. Philips. 2017. A Novel Quantile Method Reveals Spatiotemporal Shifts in Phytoplankton Biomass Descriptors Between Bloom and Non-Bloom Conditions in a Subtropical Estuary. *Marine Ecol.Prog. Ser.* 567: 57–78. https://doi.org/10.3354/meps12054.

Oschlies, A., M. Pahlow, A. Yool, and M. J. Matea. 2010. Climate Engineering by Artificial Ocean Upwelling: Channelling the Sorcerer's Apprentice. *Geophys. Res. Lett.* 37 (4): L04701. https://doi.org/10.1029/2009GL041961.

Pagarete, A., M. J. Allen, W. H. Wilson, S. A. Kimmance, and C. de Vargas. 2009. Host–Virus Shift of the Sphingolipid Pathway Along an Emiliania Huxleyi Bloom Survival of the Fattest. *Environ. Microbiol.* 11 (11): 2840–2848. https://doi.org/10.1111/j.1462-2920.2009.02006.x.

Pagarete, A., G. Le Corguille, B. Tiwari, H. Ogata, C. de Vargas, W. H. Wilson, and M. J. Allen. 2011. Unveiling the Transcriptional Features Associated with Coccolithovirus Infection of Natural E Miliania Huxleyi Blooms. *FEMS Microbiol. Ecol.* 78 (3): 555–564. https://doi.org/10.1111/j.1574-6941.2011.01191.x.

Philips, E. J., S. Badylak, N. G. Nelson, and K. E. Havens. 2020. Hurricanes, el Niño And Harmful Algal Blooms in Two Sub-Tropical Florida Estuaries: Direct And Indirect Impacts. *Sci. Rep.* 10 (1): 1910. https://doi.org/10.1038/s41598-020-58771-4.

Prodinger, F., H. Endo, Y. Takano, Y. Li, K. Tominaga, T. Isozak, R. Blanc-Mathieu, Y. Gotoh, H. Tetsuya, E. Taniguchi, K. Nagasaki, T. Yoshida, and H. Ogata. 2022. Dynamics of Amplicon Sequence Variant

Communities Differ Among Eukaryotes, Mimiviridae, and Prokaryotes in a Coastal Ecosystem. *FEMS Microbiol. Ecol.* 97 (12): fiab167. https://doi.org/10.1093/femsec/fiab167.

Sala, E., J. Mayorga, D. Bradey, R. B. Cabral, T. B. Atwood, A. Auher, W. Cheung, C. Costello, F. Feretti, A. M. Friedlande, S. D. Gaines, C. Garilao, W. Goodell, B. S. Halpern, A. Hinson, K. Kaschner, K. Kesner-Reyes, F. Leprieur, J. McGowan, L. E. Morgan, D. Mouillot, J. Palacios-Abrantes, H. P. Possingham, K. D. Rechberger, B. Worm, and J. Lubchenco. 2021. Protecting the Global Ocean for Biodiversity, Food and Climate. *Nature (London)* 592 (7854): 397–402. https://doi.org/10.1038/s41586-021-03371-z.

Sandaa, R-A., J. E. Storesund, E. Olesin, M. L. Paulsen, A. Aud Larsen, G. Gunnar Bratbak, and J. Louise Ray. 2018. Microbial Community Structure, Shaping Both Eukaryotic and Prokaryotic Host-viral Relationships in an Arctic Marine Ecosystem. *Viruses* 10 (12): 715. https://doi.org/:10.3390/v10120715.

Scheffer, M., J. Bascommpte, W. A. Brock, V. Brovkin, Carpenter, S. R., V. Dakos, H. Held, E. H. Van Nes, M. Rietkerk, and G. Sugihara. 2009. Early-Warning Signals for Critical Transitions. *Nature (London)* 461 (7260): 53–59. https://doi.org/10.1038/nature08227.

Scheffers, B. R., L. De Meester, T. C. L. Bridge, A. A. Hoffmann, J. M. Pandolfi, Corlett, R. T., H. M. Butchart, P. Pearce-Kelly, K. M. Kovacs, D. Dudgeon, M. Pacifici, C. Rondinin, W. B. Foden, T. G. Martin, C. Mora, D. Rickford, and J. E. M. Watson. 2016. The Broad Footprint of Climate Change from Genes to Biomes to People. *Science (Washington)* 354 (6313): aaf7671–11.

Shoval, O., H. Sheftel, G. Shinar, Y. Hart, O. Ramote, A. Mayo, E. Dekel, K. Kavanagh, and U. Alon. 2012. Evolutionary Trade-Offs, Pareto Optimality, and the Geometry of Phenotype Space. *Science (Washington)* 336 (6085): 1157–1160. https://doi.org/10.1126/science.1217405.

Sieradzki, E. T., C. I. Ignacio-Espinoza, D. M. Needham, E. B. Fichot, and J. A. Fuhrman. 2020. Dynamic Marine Vral Infections and Major Contribution to Photosynthetic Processes Shown by Spatiotemporal Picoplankton Metatranscriptomes. *Nature Communic.* 10 (1): 1–9. https://doi.org/10.1038/s41467-019-09106-z.

Sornette, D. 2009. Dragon-Kings, Black Swans and the Prediction of Crises. *Int. J. Terraspace Sci. Eng.* 2 (1), 1–18.

Sunagawa, S., S. G. Acinas, P. Bork, C. Bowler, D. Eveillard, G. Gorsky, L. Guidi, D. Iudicone, E. Karsenti, and F. Lombard. 2020. Tara Oceans: Towards Global Ocean Ecosystems Biology. *Nat. Rev. Microbiol.* 18 (8): 428–445. https://doi.org/10.1038/s41579-020-0364-5.

Tan, S., J. Zhou, X. Zhu, S. Wu, W. Zhan, B. Wang, and Z. Cai. 2015. An Association Network Analysis Among Microeukaryotes and bacterioplankton Reveals Algal Bloom Dynamics. *J. Phycol.* 51 (1): 120–132. https://doi.org/10.1111/jpy.12259.

Tomaru, Y., Tarutani, K., M. Tarutani, and K. Nagasaki. 2004. Quantitative and Qualitative Impacts of Viral Infection on a Heterosigma Akashiwo (Raphidophyceae) Bloom in Hiroshima Bay, Japan. *Aquat. Microb. Ecol.* 14 (3): 227–238. https://doi.org/10.1128/AEM.66.11.4916-4920.2000.

Vernette, C., N. Henry, J. Lecubin, C. de Vargas, P Hingamp, and M. Lescot. 2021. A Web Service to Explore the Biodiversity and Biogeography of Marine Organisms. *Mol. Ecol. Resour.* 21 (4): 1347–1358. https://doi.org/10.1111/1755-0998.13322.

Whitfield, A. K., N. C. James, S. J. Lamberth, J. B. Adams, R. Perissinotto, A. Rajkaran, and T. G. Bornman. 2016. The Role of Pioneers as Indicators of Biogeographic Range Expansion Caused by Global Change in Southern African Coastal Waters. *Estuar. Coast. Shelf. Sci.* 172: 138–153. https://doi.org/10.1016/j.ecss.2016.02.008.

Wilhelm, S. W., and C. A. Suttle. 1999. Viruses and Nutrient Cycles in the Sea: Viruses Play Critical Roles in the Structure and Function of Aquatic Food Webs. *BioScience* 49 (10): 781–788.

Xu, H., Y. Huang, Z. Duan, X. Wang, J. Feng, and P. Song. 2020. Multivariate Time Series Forecasting With Transfer Entropy Graph. *Tsingua Sci. Technol.* (or arXiv:2005.01185v4 (Xu et al.) for this version). https://doi.org/10.48550/arXiv.2005.01185.

Yasuhara, M., and R. Danovaro. 2016. Temperature Impacts on Deep-Sea Biodiversity. *Biol. Rev.* 91 (2): 275–287. https://doi.org/10.1111/brv.12169.

Zhang, C., X-P. Du, Y-H Zeng, J-M. Zhu, S-J. Zhang, and Z-H. Cai. 2021. The Communities and Functional Profiles of Virioplankton along a Salinity Gradient in a Subtropical Estuary. *Sci. Total Environ* 759: 143499. https://doi.org/10.1016/j.scitotenv.2020.143499.

Zhao, D., F. Shen, J. Zeng, R. Huang, Z. Yu, and Q. L. Wu. 2016. Network Analysis Reveals Seasonal Variation of Co-Occurrence Correlations Between Cyanobacteria and Other Bacterioplankton. *Sci. Total Environ.* 573: 817–825. https://doi.org/10.1016/j.scitotenv.2016.08.150.

17 Risk Communication

Elaine M. Faustman and Jill C. Falman
Institute for Risk Analysis and Risk Communication, School of Public Health, University of Washington, Seattle, WA, USA

Susan L. Santos
FOCUS GROUP, New Orleans, LA, USA

CONTENTS

The Relationship between Risk Communication, Risk Assessment, and Risk-Management
  Decision-Making 347
Current and Evolving Risk Communication Approaches 348
Legal and Regulatory Considerations...349
What Is Risk Communication?..350
Typology of Risk Communication..350
The Purpose(s) of Risk Communication 353
Risk Communication and Stakeholder Involvement...354
Audience and Stakeholder Considerations..356
Distinctions between Lay and Expert Opinions..357
NRC's Committee on Risk Characterization 357
Principles of Effective Risk Communication...358
Goals and Objectives 358
Audiences and Concerns 359
Understanding Risk Perception and the Importance of Establishing Trust and Credibility 360
Issues in Explaining Risk and Designing Messages 362
Dealing with Uncertainty 362
Risk Comparisons 363
Thought Questions 364
References...364

LEARNING OBJECTIVES

Students who complete this chapter will be able to

1. Understand what risk communication is and how it fits in the risk assessment and risk-management decision-making process;
2. Understand context for risk communication;
3. Using lessons learned, identify key principles for effective risk communication;
4. Recognize the importance of risk perception;
5. Understand best practices in how to explain/present risk information;
6. Discuss types of risk communication messages; and
7. Recognize the importance of two-way, iterative approaches for effective risk communication.

THE RELATIONSHIP BETWEEN RISK COMMUNICATION, RISK ASSESSMENT, AND RISK-MANAGEMENT DECISION-MAKING

As our society has become more technology-based, public awareness and concern over the effects of technology on human health and the environment have heightened. Risk assessment has been used as a tool to estimate the risks to human health and the environment posed by various agents, products, technologies, and activities. Legislation in the early 1970s and creation of several regulatory agencies, such as the US Environmental Protection Agency (US EPA), elevated the role of risk assessment in the regulatory process. In 1983, the National Academy of Science (NRC 1983) developed *The Red Book*, formally titled *Risk Assessment in the Federal Government: Managing the Process*

DOI: 10.1201/9780429291722-17

to lay out and frame essential elements of risk assessment and clearly distinguish risk assessment from risk management.

To address the risks that were identified as part of this process, increased interest by the public about regulatory and other risk-management actions resulted in several regulatory actions to address how we communicated and to whom about risks. Discovery of abandoned hazardous waste sites such as Love Canal prompted Congress to pass the landmark Superfund legislation in 1980. Concerns over the potential for a major chemical incident such as that which occurred in Bhopal, India, in 1984 resulted in passage of the Emergency Planning and Community Right-to-Know (RTK) Act (SARA Title III) in late 1986. With these new pieces of legislation also came the call by local citizens and citizen groups for both access to information and more involvement in decision-making. In 1986, former EPA administrator William Ruckelshaus noted that the question facing government agencies and industry was not whether to involve the public in decisions about risk, but how (Davies, Covello, and Allen 1987). For the first time, an agency head noted that the responsibility for communicating with stakeholders, including the public, rested upon those making the decisions.

While risk assessment is intended to be an objective process, social scientists, among others, point out that the definition and assessment of risk are, in fact, a social process that goes far beyond the empirical process of risk envisioned by the 1983 NRC Committee. Professional affiliation instead of scientific training and expertise affects toxicologists' views of whether the risk assessment process is overly conservative or needs more conservatism to account for uncertainties (Johnson and Slovic 1995; Slovic and Johnson 1995). The recognition that scientific and other forms of expert knowledge are socially constructed has set the stage for acceptance among scientists of a broader analytic-deliberative process as necessary to fully define and characterize risks (NRC 1994). Analysis involves the use of rigorous and replicable scientific methods to address factual questions, and deliberation involves processes such as discussion, reflection, and often recognition of risk perception to raise issues, increase understanding, and ultimately collectively arrive at decisions using a multidirectional dialogue (NRC 1994). Similarly, the Presidential/Congressional Commission on Risk Assessment and Risk Management (Moore et al. 1997) stated,

> Results of a risk assessment are not scientific estimates of risk; they are conditional estimates of the risk that could exist under specified sets of assumptions and – with political, engineering, social, and economic information – are useful for guiding decisions about risk reduction.

As the boundaries and context of risk assessment have changed, so has the importance of the third part of the original National Academy of Sciences paradigm: risk communication. As we will explore in this chapter, the practice and theoretical underpinnings of this field have greatly changed over the last 40 years, and risk communication has become a formal recognized part of the risk assessment and risk-management decision-making process. It was fortuitous that the Society of Risk Analysis on its 40th Anniversary completed a review of the evolving field of risk communication (Balog-Way, McComas, and Besley 2020) the findings of which we will share in this chapter.

CURRENT AND EVOLVING RISK COMMUNICATION APPROACHES

In 2020, the Society for Risk Analysis (SRA) undertook a review of risk communication. The resulting paper, entitled "The Evolving Field of Risk Communication," came at a critical time as WHO had just acknowledged the importance of noncommunicable diseases and climate change disasters, which was published just at the start of the COVID-19 pandemic (following on the emergence of MERS and SARS coronaviruses). This review provides an excellent background for contextual and methodological changes that we are experiencing across hazards in the multidisciplinary field of risk communication (Balog-Way, McComas, and Besley 2020). Important lessons that have been noted in the 21st century include (1) trust remains a key focus of risk communication and methods to enhance transparency and have been critical for the evolution of this field, and (2) the public seeks to understand their personal risk in the context of public health recommendations or measures. Confidence in who communicates and understanding the reasons for health advice are key elements for public acceptance. Thus, a broader frame for risk communication that considers personal factors such as gender, race, age, and social and political values is necessary to consider personalized health approaches, as well as population- and citizen-based inclusion to frame each risk problem.

LEGAL AND REGULATORY CONSIDERATIONS

As public awareness and concern about environmental issues have increased, federal legislation aimed at protecting public health and the environment has included more extensive communication and public participation requirements. For example, under the Comprehensive Environmental Response, Compensation, and Liability Act (CERCLA), commonly referred to as *Superfund*, public involvement provisions have become a central and also controversial part of the site investigation and cleanup process, and the use of risk assessment as a tool for making site cleanup decisions has corresponding communication challenges. The Superfund Amendments and Reauthorization Act of 1986 (SARA) broadened the public's role in the decision-making process and refer to the importance of stakeholder involvement. The Community RTK Act of 1986 (SARA TITLE III) requires corporations to annually provide state and local communities and the EPA with information about the chemicals they release to the land, air, and water. Corporations must also provide information on spills and unintentional releases. EPA maintains all of this information in a variety of formats and makes it available to the public. SARA Title III was grounded in the belief that industrial disclosure of risk-related information, and its potential effects on public attitudes, would serve as a powerful tool for motivating company behavior.

The implementation of TITLE III has resulted in a significant reduction in facility emissions and releases; also, companies report that they pay more attention to their pollution-prevention activities and have increased their communication with the public (Santos, Covello, and McCallum 1996). Subsequent expansion of the RTK provisions in the late 1990s requiring utilities to report their emissions has resulted in similar pressure for industry actions to restrict emissions. Section 112-r of the Clean Air Act Amendments of 1990 requires companies meeting certain criteria to prepare facility risk-management plans for unintentional or catastrophic accidents that could occur for specific hazardous substances, and it requires corporations to anticipate worst-case scenarios. Communicating the results of these complex risk analyses and their inherent uncertainties and assumptions has resulted in risk communication efforts by industry and activist groups alike. The events of 9/11 called into question, at least on the part of some industry and agency officials, how much of this potentially sensitive information should be made public. Amendments to the Safe Drinking Water Act of 1996 (42 U.S.C. 3009-3 (c)(4) require water suppliers to provide annual "consumer confidence reports" on the quality and source of their drinking water. The Food Quality Protection Act of 1996 provides for a comprehensive set of pesticide food safety initiatives covered by the EPA, Food and Drug Administration (FDA), and US Department of Agriculture (USDA). That landmark legislation also included a series of RTK provisions on the health effects of pesticides, including recommendations for how to avoid risks by reducing exposure to pesticides and maintaining an adequate diet, and noting which foods have tolerances for pesticide residues based on benefits considerations. The law requires that EPA publish this information annually in pamphlets to large retail grocers for public display. The law also allows states to require provisions for labeling or requiring warnings. In addition, for the first time, industry petitions for tolerances must include informative summaries that can be made publicly available. Similarly, agencies such as the USDA and FDA have conducted quantitative microbiological risk assessments for purposes of making food safety decisions and also recognizing that communication of such assessments must be a structured part of the process (Wu and Rodricks 2020).

The requirements for risk communication have also been extended to the private sector. Passage of laws such as the Occupational Safety and Health Administration's (OSHA) Hazard Communication or worker RTK standards requires firms producing or using certain substances to provide workers with risk information on workplace hazards so that they might understand the hazards, determine personal risks, and take appropriate action to reduce their risks. The law requires chemical manufacturers and importers to assess the hazards of chemicals that they produce or import.

Employers must provide training and education on hazardous substances including their effects, emergency procedures, and proper handling. These examples illustrate the shift over the last 40 years in the focus and scope of communication and public participation/involvement provisions contained in various agency regulations. Access to information by the public, activist groups, and the media has become a regulatory and policy tool for a wide variety of environmental and health-related issues. The majority of environmental laws and regulations have focused on performance-based standards or provided technology-based specifications. In contrast to these traditional command-and-control approaches, requirements that focus on the provision of information often provide indirect pressure through market dynamics, private litigation, and moral pressure by nongovernmental entities. Risk communication is thus a major thrust of such legislation. Further, movement on the part of some toward a *precautionary principle* in which safety must be established prior to allowing for the introduction of new products, technologies, and certain facilities will also likely require a focus on risk communication.

WHAT IS RISK COMMUNICATION?

In its simplest form, *risk communication* is communication about some risk. In this book, it is used to refer to communicating about a health, safety, or environmental risk. Risk communication was defined as "any purposeful exchange of information about health or environmental risks between interested parties" (Covello, von Winterfeldt, and Slovic 1987). This definition assumes that communication is essentially unilateral, where communication flows from the transmitter or source, the "experts," *via* some transmission channel to a receiver or target audience (Fisher 1991). In a *one-way model of communication*, scientists and health officials have historically assumed that rejection of the message was due to a lack of understanding on the part of the recipient rather than to the public's disagreement with either risk messages or, more often, risk-management decisions. The term *two-way communication* is used to describe a communication process whereby an exchange of information occurs between source and receiver in a process of reciprocal disclosure (Gurabardhi, Gutteling, and Kuttschreuter 2005). Both of these descriptions of risk communication fail, however, to account for the social and cultural context in which the communication exchange takes place. In reality, risk communication takes place in a multilayered and complicated environment involving a variety of stakeholders, communicators, and a spectrum of risk definitions and messages. Participants in the communication process play very different roles. Source and receiver are continually interchanged, requiring an appreciation for the multidirectional nature of communication and the need for feedback mechanisms (Santos and McCallum 1997).

Efforts to broaden the understanding of risk communication as a socially constructed process have come from the work of a number of social scientists (see, for example, Douglas and Wildavsky 1982; Krimsky and Plough 1988; Renn 1992) who have shown that communication occurs and is interpreted within a cultural frame and sociopolitical context. This *social constructionist model* suggests that policy or risk-management decisions "should not be made in private by some arhetorical means and then, through rhetoric, attempt to impose that policy on our fellows" (Waddell 1995). Such an approach would have technical experts providing the technical knowledge to conduct a risk assessment while allowing for the input of the stakeholders' values, beliefs, and perceptions in the risk-management process. It is also possible to have nonexperts provide input into the technical decisions to be made in a risk assessment, for example, determining what exposure pathways are of most importance or adjusting the parameters used for exposure as opposed to relying on default assumptions. In 1989, the NRC conducted an extensive study of the communication of risk information and defined risk communication as

> (an) interactive process of exchange of information and opinions among individuals, groups, and institutions, concerning a risk or potential risk to human health or the environment. It involves multiple messages about the nature of risk and other messages not strictly about risk, that express concerns, opinions or reactions to risk messages or to legal and institutional arrangements for risk management.
>
> (NRC 1989)

This definition of risk communication goes beyond the one-way unilateral model and allows for the social construction of risk. It is offered here as a more useful means of integrating risk communication within the context of the risk assessment and risk-management process.

TYPOLOGY OF RISK COMMUNICATION

There are many types of risk communication objectives. Box 17.1 shows "A Typology of Risk Communication Objectives" as described in 1986 (Covello, Slovic, and von Winterfeldt 1986). This typology continues to be important, as it summarizes the purpose and identifies both a temporal context (urgent messaging during emergencies) from a more deliberative dialog where the public can be involved in joint decision-making and conflict resolution. The typology describes four types of objectives. Type 1 discusses the importance of increasing public knowledge about risks and ensuring an "educational" construct to support the process of public health education and understanding about various risks. For this chapter, our application of Type 1 risk communication

BOX 17.1   TYPOLOGY OF RISK COMMUNICATION OBJECTIVES

Elaine Faustman, Jill Falman and Susan Santos

- *Type 1: Information and Education*
- *Type 2: Behavior Change and Protective Action*
- *Type 3: Disaster Warnings and Emergency Information*
- *Type 4: Joint Problem-Solving and Conflict Resolution*

(Covello, Slovic, and von Winterfeldt 1986)

messages is interpreted to educate and ensure a risk-informed platform to support understanding of risks and the process of risk assessment.

The objective of Type 2 risk communication is to describe messages that are designed to support risk-based interventions and risk reduction behaviors. These are usually directed to specific audiences for whom their risky behaviors are of concern and involve context relevancy for individuals as well as at-risk populations such as seen with cigarette cessation and recent COVID-19 messaging. To change a behavior, such as smoking cessation, a holistic understanding of what drives that behavior including barriers to change, is needed to develop an effective communication message. In this smoking example, a social marketing campaign should consider social behavior (who, when, where, and how smoking activities take place), as well as the biophysical additive properties of cigarettes due to the presence of nicotine. Many of the successful Type 2 risk communication objectives must both understand the target risks (e.g., lung cancer) and also understand the broad interrelated "risks and benefits.". Such messages for smoking cessation must address broader issues such as perceived weight loss benefits from smoking, as well as chronic and delayed aspects of the risks of lung cancer. All of this must then be placed within an understanding of habits (associated with common cigarette use triggers), as well as physical addition to cigarette nicotine contents.

Urgent emergency warnings are considered Type 3 messages, and these are designed to be specific and provide time-sensitive messages for which both quick understanding of the risk and rapid actions are required. This type of risk communication usually combines risk information with the change action required to reduce the identified risk. This is an essential component in public health for responding to natural disasters, disease outbreaks, and chemical and hazardous waste spills. Risk communication includes using risk indices with which the public may be most familiar, such as hurricane-force winds and earthquake disaster scales. This does not mean that these indices are as informative as our usage would suggest. In fact, several of these frequently used risk index approaches appear to be confusing and can make the message more complex. For storm surge hazards, the Saffir-Simpson Hurricane Wind Scale has been an effective storm surge risk communication tool to improve risk perception, but the index alone is not sufficient in providing the resources needed for every person to respond to risk via evacuation or other behaviors (Camelo and Mayo 2021) Similarly, the widely used Richter scale uses log scaling to communicate an earthquake's magnitude, which is done by comparing the earthquake severity to a standard (Boore 1989). The Richter scale measures the largest amplitude of an earthquake recording, which is especially important for identifying the maximum potential for structural damage (USGS 2022a). However, Richter scale information can be misinterpreted by the public, both because it uses a log scale, with which the general public is often not familiar, and this scale does not capture the public health impact that people are interested in knowing for individual and community effects. This has led to the development of other risk scales, such as the Modified Mercalli Intensity Scale where the intensity of the earthquake is ranked based on observed effects (i.e., degree of shaking experienced by an individual and type of damage observed such as dishes, windows, and doors moving and walls making cracking sounds) (USGS 2022b). This example using a linear scale is conceptually easier for nonscientists to understand and provides a framework in which individuals experiencing the earthquake can place their observations on the scale. It also presents an opportunity to interpret how earthquakes affect public health by matching a similar linear scale for potential human health hazards.

Such revised risk indices are examples of how crafting risk messages for the public requires consideration of what risk questions the public is asking and what factors will drive behaviors. Both considerations contribute important information but are not necessarily emphasizing the urgent information needed for appropriate health responses by the general public via risk communication. Although we frequently look at such emergency communications as generally coming from experts in a "top-down" messaging approach, recent events in the COVID-19 pandemic have shown that Type 3 messages benefit from regular public feedback to improve familiarity and acceptance of recommendations and mandates (Varghese et al. 2021). Acknowledging and incorporating the public perspective into the development and revision of communication plans is essential in delivering clear communication messages during emergencies.

Type 4 risk communication messages are those that arise from joint public health decision-making. Examples of Type 4 messages include those released from agencies with advisory groups where stakeholders, scientists, the public, nongovernmental organizations, and specific governmental and regulatory entities can be represented and their voices contribute to the final message and decision. In order to issue risk communication messages, such groups frequently use an analytical deliberative dialogue to resolve conflict, prioritize key messages, and format and issue joint communication on public safety and environmental concerns. Examples of such groups can include those federally assembled groups that advise the Centers for Disease Control and Prevention (CDC), FDA, OSHA, and EPA, as well as international advisory groups to the Environmental Food Safety Authority (EFSA) and World Health Organization (WHO). Crafting tailored messages can take time and require agency-wide approaches that are consistent with this broader context. Several examples of these are highlighted in Box 17.2. Depending upon the agency or organization, specific types of risk communication messages may be mandated, and many of these legal and regulatory considerations were presented earlier in this chapter.

BOX 17.2   EXAMPLES OF TAILORING MESSAGES/TOOLS FOR SPECIFIC AUDIENCES

Elaine Faustman, Jill Falman and Susan Santos

- The CDC has developed two parallel risk information sheets for Vitamin A. One is for consumers and the other is for health professionals. These examples illustrate the difference in context and operation of specific risk messages related to Vitamin A intakes for two user groups (National Institutes of Health 2022a, 2022b).
- The FDA prescription drug package inserts have been complex to produce and even more confusing to interpret by the user community. The Epilepsy Foundation provides an excellent example of a specific group packaging information to guide the public on how to read prescription inserts and inform them on what to expect, what is there and how can they use this information to make informed decisions about their health (Epilepsy Foundation 2014).
- OSHA produces fact sheets in an effort to communicate health and safety conditions for workers. The fact sheet for working safely with ethylene oxide provides long-term as well as short-term considerations and also presents this information in a straightforward manner for a professional audience (Occupational Safety and Health Administration 2002).
- EFSA's annual report on pesticide residues (European Food Safety Authority 2022b) and informational video on pesticides (European Food Safety Authority 2022a) provide a more user-friendly platform for the public to understand their risk-based activities. These materials are the result of the EFSA's implementation of new risk communication guidance on how to share information with both the public and professional audiences. This EFSA annual report shares example fact sheets on surveillance for 12 food products and statistics on how many of these products contain pesticide residues exceeding the legal maximum value of pesticides each year. These reports are supported with browsable charts, graphs, and a model program to determine personalized dietary intake (DietEx tool) (European Food Safety Authority 2022b).

- The EPA CompTox Chemicals Dashboard has been an important communication tool for professionals to access data for more than 900,000 chemicals (US Environmental Protection Agency 2022). Providing a "one-stop" location for the types of data needed for risk analysis, this communication tool has been a phenomenal success. Besides accessing specific data and data sets across the toxicological domains, this site also provides links to specific regulatory contexts and action levels by regulation. Launched in 2016 and now through multiple versions, the site now provides access to data on physiochemical properties and fate and transport data, as well as both *in vivo* and *in vitro* test data on an increasingly user-friendly, web-based interface (Williams et al. 2017).
- The WHO's web page on the *infodemic* provides a portfolio of risk communication fact sheets, tools, and interactive dialogue options for managing excessive information during health emergencies that often include false and misleading content (World Health Organization 2022b). One example is the Early AI-supported Response with Social Listening platform to share how people are talking about COVID-19 online (World Health Organization 2022a). The tool is creative and dynamic with applications for global audiences.

THE PURPOSE(S) OF RISK COMMUNICATION

Historically, many scientists and health officials in government agencies viewed communication as a way to guide recipients on how to take appropriate measures to reduce risks. Whether it was explicitly stated or not, communication was viewed as a way of getting people to calm down or to somehow simplify risk-related information so that results would be accepted. For public health professionals and those who conduct risk assessments and then must explain their results, a more useful focus is to view risk communication as a reciprocal process whereby health officials and risk assessors may obtain valuable information that can be used in conducting the risk assessment. Ideally, effective risk communication can be used as a means of empowering the public in decision-making.

Covello, von Winterfeldt, and Slovic (1987) described four broad classes of risk communication based on their primary objective or intended effect: (1) information and education, (2) encouraging behavior change and protective action, (3) disaster warnings and emergency information, and (4) joint problem-solving and conflict resolution.

In all but the last category, communication tends to be one-way, where the goal ranges from telling people what has been done or what decision has been made to telling them what specific actions to take. A different perspective on the purposes of risk communication, which include (1) to make sure that all receivers of the message are able and capable of understanding and decoding the meaning of the messages sent to them, (2) to persuade the receivers of the message to change their attitude or their behavior with respect to a specific cause or class of risk, and (3) to provide the conditions necessary "for a rational discourse on risk issues so that all affected parties can take part in an effective and democratic conflict–resolution process has been proposed" (Renn 1992). This categorization broadens the notion that risk communication should simply be message-driven and focus on the processes to obtain understanding and reach consensus on risk-management decisions. Lundgren describes a topology of risk communication along functional and subject-related lines that embraces the three goals outlined by Renn; it is useful for the purposes of identifying the various and often conflicting goals and purposes of risk communication from a practitioner's perspective (Lundgren and McMakin 2018). Lundgren differentiates *care communication* from *consensus* or *crisis* communication. *Care communication* is risk communication about health and safety risks "for which the danger and the way to manage it have already been well determined by scientific research that is accepted by most of the audience" (Lundgren and McMakin 2018). Included in this category are health care or medical communications seeking to inform or advise the audience about health risks such as smoking and AIDS and industrial health and safety risk communications to impart workplace health and safety information or the safe application of pesticides.

Crisis communication is communication in the face of extreme or sudden danger (or perceived danger). Situations for which crisis communications are appropriate range from an accident at a nuclear power plant or industrial complex to the outbreak of a disease (*E. coli*, mad cow disease, COVID-19, Ebola, or monkeypox) to a natural disaster to more recent concerns about a terrorist event, such as bioterrorism or a dirty bomb. In crisis communication, getting the attention of the target audience(s) is extremely important. A third form of communication is *consensus communication*, which is most appropriate for informing and encouraging groups to work together to reach a decision about how risks should be managed, that is, prevented or mitigated. Included in this form of communication are public participation-related communications and *stakeholder involvement processes*. Examples include reaching decisions on the cleanup of a hazardous waste site, siting of a facility, or establishing regulations such as the appropriate drinking water standard. Consensus communication implies that the decision about how to manage the risks results from the participation of all those with an interest in how the risk is to be managed in the decision-making process (Lundgren and McMakin 2018). The concept of consensus communication thus broadens the definition of risk communication beyond that of information disclosure or even exchange. For purposes of this text, consensus communication includes the full range of public participation and stakeholder involvement activities whereby the goal is to enable a mutual discourse and empower all parties to participate in democratic decision-making.

The "Ladder of Citizen Participation" (Arnstein 1969) provides a framework for critically examining citizen participation and communication activities to uncover both explicit and implicit goals on the part of agencies and those making risk-management decisions. This ladder has been adapted to illustrate the distinctions among various forms of citizen participation (Chess, Hance, and Sandman 1988). One's position on the ladder can be viewed as a function of the goals of the communication and further used to examine the degree of control or power citizens are given in decision-making and the corresponding form of communication. Arnstein's ladder consists of eight rungs, each corresponding to the extent of citizen power in determining the end product. The bottom rungs of the ladder are forms of nonparticipation. The objective is not participation but to enable power holders to educate or "cure" the participants. Hance and colleagues refer to this as government power. In both of these schemes, communication is one-way. The next several rungs represent degrees of tokenism ranging from informing to consultation to placation (Chess, Hance, and Sandman 1988). Here too communication is one-way. Many public meetings and opportunities for public comment fall into this range. One problem with activities falling into this range is that they may simply be an attempt to make the information more palatable to the recipient and thus obscure issues surrounding the transfer of knowledge or power. Further, simplistic representations can misinform as many people as they inform. It is unlikely that a one-way model would ever be appropriate or useful for consensus-type communications. Even in care and consensus communications, reciprocal disclosure and feedback from the recipients may be needed to ensure that the goals of increased attention, comprehension, or behavioral change can be achieved.

At the top of Arnstein's ladder are forms of participation that allow for various degrees of citizen power, where communication is used as a means of enabling people. Here communication must be multidirectional, allowing for the full expression and inclusion of multiple sources and receivers who may have conflicting messages and information needs (Merkelson 2011). In this model, risk communication would be used to enable people to make their own decisions about risks under their control. In the context of risk assessment and risk management, communication that is higher up the ladder would be structured to enable stakeholders to have input in the selection and framing of the problems to be studied as well as the processes used for assessing risks (e.g., data and assumptions used) and decision-making.

Risk communication does not occur in a vacuum. In order to both fully understand the risk communication process and evaluate its effect, the impact of multiple communicators with their various perspectives and goals must be considered.

RISK COMMUNICATION AND STAKEHOLDER INVOLVEMENT

Historically, the process of risk communication has been embedded in the democratic process. It has been argued that agency officials and policymakers are responsible for more than the programs they administer; they have a responsibility to go beyond outcomes to preserve and promote the constitutional democracy of which they are the agents (Landy, Roberts, and Thomas 1990). A similar challenge might be posed to scientists and those conducting risk and health assessments: Is there an obligation in communicating risk-related information to go beyond mere informing or transferring information to the public? In this context, the purpose of risk communication is not to tell citizens what to think (Needlemen 1987). Rather, experts, officials, and decision-makers use their stature and expertise to frame questions so that the debate can be made understandable (Plough and Krimsky 1987).

A 1994 symposium on the role of public involvement in environmental decision-making entitled "Addressing Agencies Risk Communication Needs" helped illuminate the evolution of risk communication in government deliberation and decision-making. Baruch Fischoff, in his keynote address, suggested that risk communication has evolved in seven stages. While each stage is characterized by a focal communication strategy (Fischoff 1995), the evolutionary process is not linear. Different organizations have been at different stages at the same time, and even within the same organization, it is possible for different stages to be present. The stage of evolution may depend on a number of internal and external organizational factors. According to Fischoff, the earliest stage of risk communication involves experts perfecting their profession or "getting the numbers right." These experts see no need to communicate because they view the risks as reasonably small or controlled.

By relying solely on the results of risk analysis or assessment, these professionals often ignore the fact that the public wants to be part of the discussion about risk and, in particular, how the problem gets defined and which questions are to be answered. By institutionalizing the methods used to assess risk, experts may become too comfortable with their discipline and assume it represents some objective truth. Further, their status as experts corresponds to a judgment that they hold valued knowledge that is expressed in a language that is usually scientific and statistical.

In the second stage, risk assessors and managers discover that they are not trusted to do their work in private, so they "hand over the numbers" to the public. Often, such communications only serve to reflect the distance between the technical analysts and the recipients. For example, attempts to clarify the uncertainty surrounding risk estimates may only serve to admit the subjectivity that exists, which extends beyond issues of technical merit and also reflects ethical values.

The third stage of risk communication focuses on the goal of trying to explain risk information more clearly by "explaining the numbers." To be meaningful, this requires understanding people's decision processes so that communications can fill in their knowledge gaps, reinforce correct beliefs, and correct misunderstandings (Fischoff 1995).

The danger at this stage is that professionals may rely solely on their limited technical framework to determine what information is relevant. The results at this stage of communication are evident in the growing number of public debates over government and industry decision-making. Because public values are not a legitimate part of the process, the public enters into a debate about the merits of the science or methods used to determine risk. It is only by challenging the technical basis of decisions that the public can influence the decision-making process. Government agencies' tendency to "decide, announce and defend" has led to citizen challenges and the recognition that scientific explanations alone do not lead to improved risk communication or decision-making.

The fourth developmental stage, and the one that is frequently used by technical professionals, including risk assessors, focuses on providing some reference risk or comparisons among risks to convince the public about which risks to take seriously. Experts use comparisons to downplay or highlight the magnitude or probability of a risk. Fischoff refers to this stage as "all we have to do is show them that they've accepted similar risks in the past." This form of communication is fraught with peril and subject to manipulations by those who claim expert status and have access to information.

The fifth stage of risk communication involves giving people information on both the risks and benefits of a particular action or activity. Providing information on benefits, especially if done as a means of suggesting compensation for the risk, raises a number of ethical issues: "Analyses can be specified in different ways, with alternative specifications representing different ethical positions— belying their ostensible objectivity" (Fischoff 1995). Research regarding the communication of both benefits and trade-offs suggests that framing effects may occur whereby equivalent representations of the same trade-offs evoke inconsistent evaluations. The presence of framing effects suggests that how we balance risks and benefits may depend on how the information is presented. The result may lead to instability in preferences over time and distrust in how information is framed (Santos and McCallum 1997).

The sixth stage, "all we have to do is treat them nice," focuses on the communicators, their demeanor, and perceived trustworthiness. The focus of this stage is to train the communicator and allow for more one-on-one exchanges. Unfortunately, the focus often becomes one of packaging versus substance.

The last and the most highly evolved stage of risk communication involves building partnerships with the public. Partnering is needed to reduce the social amplification of technically small risks, as well as generate concern when it is warranted. The public has demonstrated their ability to understand complex scientific information when sufficiently motivated. In this context, risk communication ensures that all sides have relevant information to learn and to share. According to Fischoff, effective risk communication can fulfill part of the social contract between those who create risks (as a by-product of other activities) and those who bear them (perhaps along with the benefits of those activities).

> Ideally, risk management should be guided by the facts. Those facts concern not just the sizes of the risks and benefits involved, but also the changes in political and social status that arise from the risk–management process.
>
> (Fischoff 1995)

In spite of the growing recognition that risk communication must be linked with meaningful public involvement and partnering, much of the practice of risk communication remains focused at the third and fourth evolutionary stages of explaining and putting risks into perspective for the public. Such attempts at risk communication focus on getting the public to accept risks that officials or experts believe are necessary for our technological society to function. In this next section entitled "Audience and Stakeholder Considerations," examples are given to address these issues.

AUDIENCE AND STAKEHOLDER CONSIDERATIONS

Essential to effective risk communication is the recognition of the audience or stakeholders for the risk communication messages. Stakeholders are at the heart of the risk assessment process and not only are necessary for the risk formulation step of risk assessment but are also essential in how we identify and communicate our risks during the risk assessment process. There are many suggestions on how and who should be involved as stakeholders, and these include agency-specified representatives. An example of this is the Federal Advisory Committee Act (FACA), which governs the establishment and activities of federal advisory committees in the United States. FACA has requirements on how to establish committees to ensure open and transparent procedures and includes an emphasis on representation, reporting, and public involvement (USGSA 2022). Stakeholders can also be self-identified through community meetings and via a process entitled "snowballing," where key informants, community leaders, or influencers are identified and included in the development of risk communication processes (Leighton et al. 2021). The focus of this chapter is not to review all of these aspects but to emphasize that having inclusive representation and transparent processes has consistently proven to improve risk communications activities. Case studies can illustrate the importance of these practices and how they are applied at various venues. Boiko and her colleagues illustrate the process for identifying Advisory Board members for two former nuclear waste facilities under a FACA process (Boiko et al. 1996). One of the earliest public dialogues with a risk communication context was during the early 1980s when the US EPA, then led by William Ruckleshaus, ensured public involvement in the risk assessment process at the Asarco Tacoma Smelter Superfund site (Heifetz 1994). In the 1980s, such engagement was rare, but this early case helped inform key lessons on the capacity of the public to participate and learn, which supported approaches for future risk communication strategies. In this case, there was enthusiasm by the public and affected families to become involved in deciding the future of the smelter that polluted surrounding communities with arsenic, lead, and other contaminants. However, there was a failure to communicate technical information in a manner that the general public would understand to actively make decisions. Complex statistical graphs of cancer risk estimates were presented that did not make it easy for the public to participate in decision-making. The public in attendance wanted to know whether it was safe to eat from their gardens rather than the details about complex statistics on future cancer risks for former workers.

Another illustrative early event in risk communication includes the Alar case in 1989. Initially, the EPA announced in a press release they would begin to cancel food uses of Alar, a growth regulator absorbed into fruit, given "interim analyses of new data" on the chemical and a metabolite (US EPA 1989). The Natural Resources Defense Council wanted to accelerate the process and released a report finding that the diets of American children faced "intolerable risks" as a result of apples sprayed with Alar (Friedman et al. 1996; Hathaway 1993; Sugarman 1989). This report was amplified by the "60 Minutes" coverage that sparked media outlets to emphasize the risk story, and the repetition and long news coverage subsequently elevated public fears (Friedman et al. 1996). The Alar issue was sensationalized by the mass media, and experts disagreed on the risk information, which had consequences for a number of groups, including the apple industry (revenue loss), supermarkets (demand for organic produce), and the public (food safety concerns)

(Friedman et al. 1996). This case emphasized the importance of presenting and explaining data and being responsive to audiences to help them understand the information to make informed decisions.

Sensitivity to what matters to the public is paramount and needs to be considered in developing risk messaging. For example, the evacuation processes during Hurricane Katrina showed that for the public to hear the evacuation messages and to act on those messages, they needed to know how to save what mattered to them (i.e., could they evacuate with their pets? what might be the length of time they would be gone? how could they get pocket money for buses or transportation beyond the immediate events?). There were long lists of these issues which illustrated the much broader context with the affected public that was needed for effective and actionable behavior change as a response to this disaster risk communication. Additionally, the complex factors that influenced evacuation behaviors of minority and vulnerable communities were not factored into communication strategies. The strong social ties of these groups influenced factors such as access to shelter, transportation, and perception of evacuation messages, meaning that community-based communication is essential to tailor preparation strategies and communication (Eisenman et al. 2007; Lachlan et al. 2009). The analytic-deliberative dialogue, which involves an iterative and engaging process among affected actors, was envisioned by the National Research Council (NRC) and underscores the importance of two-way communication between decision-makers and those who are being informed (Stern and Fineberg 1996).

Judd and her colleagues present case studies of three groups – one Asian and Pacific Islander community coalition and two Native American Tribes – who are actively involved in framing scientific analyses of health risks related to contaminated seafood (Judd et al. 2005). Each study demonstrated different approaches, but all were successful in engaging the community/tribal partners and researchers in framing activities and outcomes (Judd et al. 2005).

Indigenous tribes in the United States provide a broader context for conversations on risk. One of the important lessons learned from tribal communities is the "social and cultural" context that they bring to understanding concepts of health and well-being. These contexts are necessary for communicating, especially for risk communication considerations. Such an approach is seen in a paper from the Swinomish Community (Donatuto, Campbell, and Gregory 2016), which describes some of the values-based approaches specific to their tribal populations. In this paper, six specific Swinomish Indigenous Health Indicators are identified that provide a values-based context for tribal activities: *cultural use, community connection, self-determination, resilience, education* (i.e., intergenerational knowledge transfer), and *natural resources security* (Donatuto, Campbell, and Gregory 2016).

DISTINCTIONS BETWEEN LAY AND EXPERT OPINIONS

The illustrative examples of early risk communication efforts given in the previous section show that the initial foundation of risk communication was structured around an "objective, expert" risk assessment process versus one inclusive of "lay" perspectives that had been qualified as "subjective and irrational" (Balog-Way, McComas, and Besley 2020). This dichotomy has now been recognized as a basis for futile disconnections. Fortunately, a more inclusive and adaptive mechanism has been embraced, especially since reports from the National Academies of Sciences, Engineering, and Medicine emphasize that effective risk communication requires interactive, deliberative, and joint problem formulation (NRC 1994, 1996, 2009). Consequently, this has sparked the need for understanding the social and mental constructs for understanding risks (Slovic et al. 2005). This has also supported the need for community-based participatory research within the context of risk communication (Thompson et al. 2017).

NRC'S COMMITTEE ON RISK CHARACTERIZATION

In 1996, the NRC published a report by a group of experts on how the process of risk assessment, risk management, and risk communication could be improved (NRC 1996). This group advocated a strong stakeholder participation process. They stated that risk assessments should be directed toward informing decisions and that this process should start at the very beginning of the risk assessment process and continue throughout the course of risk management and communication. "Many decisions can be better informed and their information base can be more credible if the interested and affected parties are appropriately and effectively involved" (NRC 1996). The Committee offers a rich view of the interconnectedness of risk assessment to risk communication and risk-management risk assessment process and continues throughout the course of risk management and communication. "Many decisions can be better informed and their information base can be more credible if the interested and affected parties are appropriately and effectively involved" (NRC 1996. The Committee offers a rich view of the interconnectedness of risk assessment to risk communication and risk management: A risk characterization must address the interests of affected and other interested parties *believe to be the risk* in the particular situation, and it must incorporate their perspectives and specialized knowledge. It may need to consider alternative sets of assumptions that may lead to divergent estimates of risk and to address social, economic, ecological, and ethical outcomes as well as consequences to human health and safety. Adequate risk analysis and characterization thus depend on incorporating the perspectives and knowledge of the interested and affected parties from the earliest phases of the efforts to understand the risks (NRC 1996), emphasis added].

The Committee spent a great deal of effort criticizing the current process of risk characterization. The problem, according to the Committee, is that the current process of risk characterization fails to pay adequate attention to questions of central concern to affected stakeholders. The failure is not with the scientific analysis, but with the integration of the analysis with a broad-based process of deliberation. The Committee called for risk characterization to be an analytic-deliberative process. A series of criteria are identified for judging the success of any such process; they must have sufficiently broad participation, and the information, viewpoints, and concerns of those involved must be adequately reflected, including the fact that "their participation has been able to affect the way risk problems are defined and understood" (NRC 1996).

PRINCIPLES OF EFFECTIVE RISK COMMUNICATION

Risk communication is a process rather than a set of specific gimmicks or techniques. It requires awareness of the factors that affect the communication process and how individuals perceive risk and risk information. Focusing on the communication process rather than just the risk may be one of the most important considerations for successful risk communication.

Effective risk communication recognizes that the public has a right to receive information and to be actively involved in both the dialogue regarding the nature of the risk and the decisions about ways to minimize or control identified risks. This dialogue often blurs the distinction between risk assessment – Is there a risk?

What is it? How bad is it? – and risk management – What should we do about the risk? Another important principle of risk communication is that those communicating risk information be perceived as credible. If not, the message will not be believed, especially if it involves risk information. It has been suggested that several factors influence source credibility including the degree of empathy and caring conveyed, the degree of openness and honesty, the extent to which the source is considered competent, and, finally, the extent to which a communicator shows commitment and dedication to health and safety and resolving the risk (Peters, Covello, and McCallum 1997). No single approach or method to communicating risk or risk assessment information can be universally applied to all purposes or audiences, but certain steps can be followed to foster more effective communication.

Developing an effective risk communication program involves the following:

1. Determining communication goals and objectives

2. Identifying the audience and its concerns

3. Understanding issues of risk perception that will influence the audience

4. Designing risk communication messages and testing those messages

5. Selecting the proper communication channels

6. Implementing the plan

7. Evaluating the risk communication program

Some of these steps are discussed in the following sections.

GOALS AND OBJECTIVES

Risk communication can have several goals and objectives. Sometimes the goal is to alert people to a particular risk and move them to action. At other times, the goal is to tell them not to worry, to calm down. In the latter instances, the communicator wants to inform individuals that a particular situation does not pose a health risk. Because the public has different concerns and information needs when being alerted or being calmed down, strategies for communicating also need to vary. As discussed earlier in this chapter, purposes of risk communication include

- education and information,
- improving public understanding,
- behavior change and protective action,
- organizationally mandated goals,
- legally mandated or process goals, and
- **joint problem-solving and conflict resolution.**

BOX 17.3   QUESTIONS TO CONSIDER

Elaine Faustman, Jill Falman and Susan Santos

A federal agency conducts a so-called baseline risk assessment of a hazardous waste site and determines that the risk from drinking water contaminated with volatile organic compounds and perchlorate exceeds EPA's "acceptable risk levels of 1×10^{-5}" and also exceeds safe drinking water standards for two compounds. No federal or state drinking water standard exists for perchlorate, but levels are shown to exceed the state's "action limit" and public water supply wells have been closed. The risk assessment shows that in the absence of consuming water from potable wells, there is no exposure but clearly cleanup is required. How do you communicate the risk to area residents who also wonder about their personal risks given possible historic consumption of water for a short period of time prior to perchlorate being detected? What would your goal be for holding a meeting to discuss resident health concerns?

Each event prompting the need for risk communication will have its own objectives. In designing a risk communication program, the particular risk-communication needs and corresponding objectives lay the framework for the design of specific messages and activities. This framework establishes what needs to be communicated and why.

AUDIENCES AND CONCERNS

Often those responsible for communicating risk-related information and risk assessment results inadvertently place too much emphasis on designing a particular message or ways of simplifying the technical information. To ensure that communication is two-way, more attention should be focused on the receivers of the information. This means first identifying the various audiences or stakeholders.

Although it may not be possible to reach everybody, it is important to try to identify individuals and groups who have an interest or stake in the issue and to provide an opportunity for those people to be involved. Within a particular geographical area, several tiers of stakeholders will exist that may include individuals or groups with a particular interest in the issue. Your audience, however, should not be limited to just geographical neighbors. Other audiences may exist based on common demographic, educational, or other interests (see Box 17.4).

Identifying stakeholders goes beyond just determining who needs to be informed; it includes understanding the concerns and information needs of the various interested parties. Characterizing target audiences is similar to a data collection effort for conducting a risk assessment: without knowing what chemicals are present in what quantities and in what forms, it is impossible to characterize risk. Characterizing target audiences involves looking at such areas as demographics, psychographics, and information and source-utilization characteristics. For effective communication to occur, public concerns must be known prior to conducting the risk assessment or relaying risk information. Only then can the message be presented and disseminated in a manner that acknowledges and addresses the apprehensions and needs of the receivers.

BOX 17.4   CHECKLIST TO AID IN AUDIENCE IDENTIFICATION

Elaine Faustman, Jill Falman and Susan Santos

Local government agencies, education groups, academic institutions
Local, state, and federal officials; chambers of commerce
Unions
Professional organizations
Local, regional, and national environmental groups; local businesses
Civic associations, property owners, religious organizations
Senior-citizen associations, public interest groups
Sporting and recreational clubs, media
Other interest groups

Although audience concerns vary from situation to situation, it is possible to categorize them. Four general categories of concerns are (1) health and lifestyle concerns, (2) data and information concerns, (3) process concerns, and (4) risk-management concerns (Chess, Hance, and Sandman 1988). Health and lifestyle concerns are often the most important because in any risk situation people inevitably want to know what the implications are for themselves and their families. These what-does-it-mean-to-me series of questions are often the most difficult for risk assessors to respond to; instead, they often rely on default assumptions used to characterize risk. However, such questions may also be thought of as a sensitivity analysis of sorts to better bound the risk estimates provided.

Data and information concerns are usually associated with the technical basis for – and uncertainties involved in – any estimation of risk. For example, the target audience may ask, "Are your studies correct? Did you sample for the right parameters? Have you considered the interaction of exposures to multiple toxicants?" Process concerns relate to how decisions are made by the entity responding to a risk and to how communication occurs. They may ask, "Who decides? How are we informed?" Obviously, trust and credibility are important in these issues, as is the control the public feels they have in the decision-making process. Finally, risk-management concerns relate to how and when the risk will be handled: Will it be effectively mitigated, avoided, or reduced?

A variety of techniques are available for documenting audience information needs and concerns, including interviews, written or telephone surveys, the use of existing public poll information, review of news coverage and letters to the editor, small informal community group meetings, and focus groups that are structured group interviews with participants from specific target groups or from the general population.

Internationally, such techniques include the collaborative maps of OpenStreetMap, where in collaboration with local communities, maps are developed to reflect how the communities view their local context and where resources are available for addressing local problems (Herfort et al. 2021). Another example is participatory epidemiology where engagement with community leaders and key stakeholders to promote a participatory process in understanding their risk perception, health risks, and options for surveillance, control, and health evaluation in populations provides an informed local context for real social behavior changes (Alders et al. 2020). By involving the community in the approach and instilling a sense of ownership, the community is subsequently more likely to embrace ideas for change.

UNDERSTANDING RISK PERCEPTION AND THE IMPORTANCE OF ESTABLISHING TRUST AND CREDIBILITY

Those who conduct health risk assessments and other technical experts often discuss frustration in that the public often makes erroneous judgments as to the nature or magnitude of a particular risk. Another principle of effective risk communication is to recognize that the public's often differing perception of risk is not misperception and that perception equals reality. The field of risk communication has a rich literature examining the gap between "expert" and "lay" perception of risk. For example, studies have illustrated the effect that gender, professional affiliation, and race have on perception of risk (Flynn, Slovic, and Mertz 1994; Slovic, Fischhoff, and Lichtenstein 1981). Researchers have identified and classified a number of dimensions or attributes of a risk that affect perception of riskiness. Risk is seen as multidimensional and represents the confluence of a variety of public

BOX 17.5 PRIMARY RISK PERCEPTION FACTORS

Elaine Faustman, Jill Falman and Susan Santos

Primary risk perception factors include whether the risk is perceived as

Voluntary or involuntary
Controlled by the system, or controlled by the individual
Fair or unfair
Having trustworthy or untrustworthy sources
Morally relevant or morally neutral
Natural or artificial
Exotic or familiar
Memorable or not memorable
Certain or uncertain
Detectable or undetectable
Dreaded or not dreaded

Based on (Slovic, Fischhoff, and Lichtenstein 1981)

values and attitudes (Slovic 1987, 2000). The difference in definition affects the likelihood that risk messages will be "received" (Santos and McCallum 1997). For example, a risk assessor might define risks narrowly in terms of the likelihood of developing cancer, whereas some concerned citizens might include a wider range of harms such as that the risk is involuntary, outside their control, or artificial. Sandman popularized the risk perception work of Baruch Fischhoff and Paul Slovic among others by stating that the public's perception of risk is a function of the hazard plus outrage, whereby *outrage* is everything about a risk except its actual magnitude, or how likely it is to actually produce harm (Sandman 1987). A quantitative risk assessment may arrive at estimates of excess incremental cancer risks that experts or regulatory agencies deem insignificant. However, the public may respond as if severe harm was evident and be angered at the lack of concern on the part of experts. Several of the major characteristics affecting perception of risk are described in Box 17.5.

Voluntary or involuntary. Risks that are voluntary are usually perceived by the public as less serious or dangerous than those that seem to be involuntary, regardless of the actual hazard. A voluntary risk (such as smoking or sunbathing) should never be compared to a perceived involuntary risk (such as exposure to contaminated air or water).

Controlled by the system or by the individual. People tend to view risks that they cannot control as more threatening than those that they can control, regardless of the actual hazard. Pesticide residues on food products (whether regulations deem them allowable or not) or emissions from a facility that are permitted are perceived to be beyond the control of the individual.

Trustworthy or untrustworthy sources. How individuals view a risk is often a function of how much they trust the organization that seems to be imposing or allowing the risk and of how credible they believe the source of risk information to be. Trustworthiness and credibility can be increased by the source's collaboration with credible sources outside the organization who can help to communicate the message to the public.

Exotic or familiar. Exotic risks appear riskier than familiar risks. Toxic pollutants, with their long names, can certainly seem exotic. Further, the use of units of measurement that are also unfamiliar such as parts per billion or μg/L add to the exotic nature of the risk.

Dreaded or not dreaded. Risks that are dreaded seem more serious than those that carry less dread. For example, nuclear radiation or chemicals that are carcinogens may seem riskier and less acceptable than common household cleaners or COVID-19 versus a common illness such as a cold. It is important that communication efforts recognize and acknowledge this dread.

Certainty or uncertainty. Risks that are thought to be more certain or known are often perceived by the public to be less serious (and more acceptable) than those that are not. Conversely, risks that scientists are uncertain about are considered far more serious. In these cases, the public tends to want to err on the side of caution. Risk communication efforts must acknowledge points of uncertainty, but it is important to be careful not to overwhelm people by pointing out all the uncertainty associated with risk estimates.

In summary, risk-perception considerations cannot be ignored or minimized as emotional, not factual, or irrelevant. Emotions, feeling, values, and attitudes carry as much – if not more – importance for the public than the technical magnitude of the risk situation.

ISSUES IN EXPLAINING RISK AND DESIGNING MESSAGES

The potential for distorted communication is not solely based on the public's lack of a technical background or the relevance of the information provided. Those assessing risk need to be aware that the varying and often conflicting interpretations of risk results that get communicated are a function of several factors. In part, the problems may stem from the lack of a clear message as to what the results are or the limitations of scientists and risk assessors to place results in context for various stakeholders. Messages about risk are further obscured by technical jargon. For example, simply listing tables of carcinogenic risk estimates or hazard indices for noncarcinogens will not answer concerns about safety and possible health consequences. In addition, results are interpreted not only by the scientists themselves but also by other parties and institutions, including government agencies, activists or interest groups, and the media.

The two-way nature of risk communication requires that messages contain the information the audience wants and the information the communicator wishes to convey. Effective messages should also clarify points that might be difficult to understand. For example: Are the risks to children, to fetuses, or to adults? Was exposure assumed over a lifetime or of a shorter duration? As stated earlier in this chapter, the goal of risk communication should be to make the differences in language (and rationalities) between experts and others more transparent. Strong differences between the two languages serve as barriers to dialogue and deliberation, and impede the possibility of developing a shared understanding. For example, experts may not be aware of or value information that the various stakeholders have including pertinent value issues and beliefs that influence their decisions of perceived riskiness. In general, the public receivers of the information have limited access to the information used in decision-making. Even when the information is available, it may not be fully understood or accepted due to a lack of trust.

Written messages and oral presentations must transmit the information to the public in an understandable form. Many risk analysts tend to use overly technical or bureaucratic language, which may be appropriate for the risk assessment document and for discussions with other experts but not for communicating with the general public. Similarly, experts, in seeking to simplify risk messages, may leave out important content that provides context. The challenge is to provide sufficient detail and content – while taking time to explain concepts that are key to understanding. Take care in using words such as *insignificant* or *significant* risk. At a minimum, explain what you mean by the term. Is it based on a regulation? Expert judgment? And risk to whom? Health effects associated with acute exposure must be differentiated from those associated with chronic exposure, and carcinogenic effects must be differentiated from noncarcinogenic effects. Risk messages need to place health effect information into the proper perspective so that people can comprehend the difference between significant and less significant risks. Messages should explain, as simply and directly as possible, such things as risk estimates, exposure considerations, and what uncertainties drive the risk estimate.

Because different audiences have different concerns and levels of understanding, one risk message may not be appropriate for all interested parties. It may be necessary to develop a series of messages on the same topic. Finally, a critical part of successful message design is testing or trying out the message. This can be done formally, for example, by the use of focus groups or citizen advisory committees, or informally, for example, by testing the material on uninformed third parties.

DEALING WITH UNCERTAINTY

Scientists by nature are precise and, as such, tend to describe all the uncertainties and limitations associated with a risk assessment. This may be overwhelming for the public, who is trying to figure out what the risk means and wants certainty, not caveats. It is important to discuss the major sources of uncertainty. When interpreting the results of health risk assessments for the public, explaining how health standards were developed and their applicability to the population at risk may be very important. In other instances, limited sampling data may be the most important uncertainty to explain. While the public may press for assurances of whether it is safe or unsafe, experts need to take care to be neither overly reassuring nor overwhelming with uncertainties. Explaining what you will do to reduce uncertainty may be especially important to communicate.

RISK COMPARISONS

In an attempt to make risk information understandable to the public, experts often focus on providing comparison as a means of placing risks in context. Care must be taken in attempting to make such comparisons. Research on risk comparisons is limited and contradictory (Lundgren and McMakin 2018). Comparisons can be useful, but only when they are part of an overall communication strategy that requires the communicator to understand the nature of the risk, both the hazard that it presents and the qualitative attributes that influence perception by the target audience; understand the audiences that are being addressed and their relationship to the hazard; understand how the risk comparison interacts with other components of the message; and have a way to evaluate the audience's response (Santos and McCallum 1997).

A hierarchy for risk comparisons is given in Box 17.6 (Covello, Sandman, and Slovic 1988). Comparisons based on quantity are considered the most intelligible and accessible. Comparisons of the probability of an event, such as the probably of being struck by lightning versus the probability of getting cancer from exposure to a particular substance, are considered much less useful. It is also important that risk comparisons take into account the variables that determine risk acceptability, which includes issues of fairness, benefits, alternatives, control, and voluntariness (Slovic 1987, 2000).

The complex nature of risk communication calls into question the value of requiring simple comparisons of risk end points with either common risks of daily life or other risks posed by chemical or physical agents or bright-line risk values. Without context, this information might provide inaccurate or confusing messages for the public. For most individuals, these types of comparisons ask the primary question: What does the information mean to me? And, more specifically, What does the risk mean to me? To address such broad issues, risk communication efforts should seek to inform and enhance a recipient's understanding by providing information within a context. To be complete, risk messages should also provide information that can help facilitate individual decision-making.

BOX 17.6   ACCEPTABILITY OF RISK COMPARISON

Elaine Faustman, Jill Falman and Susan Santos

MOST ACCEPTABLE

- Same risk at different times
- Risk vs. standard
- Different estimates of the same risk

LESS DESIRABLE

- Doing something vs. not doing it
- Alternative ways of lessening risk
- Risk in one place vs. risks in another place

EVEN LESS DESIRABLE

- Average risk vs. peak risk at a particular time or location
- Risk from one source of harm vs. risk from all sources of that harm
- Occupational risk vs. environmental risk

RARELY ACCEPTABLE

- Risk vs. cost
- Risk vs. benefit
- Risk vs. other specific causes of same harm

Adapted from Covello, Sandman, and Slovic (1988).

Experience in risk communication suggests that risk comparisons should be presented in ways that provide cues to action and respect the values of participants in the process. Failure to consider social and political issues and values will increase the likelihood that a comparison will not be meaningful (Santos and McCallum 1997).

THOUGHT QUESTIONS

1. How would you develop a risk communication plan for addressing environmental health concerns in an urban community? What message considerations are important given the variety of audiences, for example, government workers, local politicians, community residents with multiple racial and ethnic backgrounds? What tools would you use to determine these different audience concerns and information needs?
2. How do you explain the concept of a one in one million cancer risk to a nontechnical audience?
3. How would you explain exposure to a nontechnical audience concerned about their possible health risk to contamination in air and water from a hazardous waste site?
4. How would you describe the risk for several chemicals of concern to a nontechnical audience where the hazard indices are all less than one? How would you address their concern about possible cumulative risk or the possible interactions?
5. Describe how a maximum contaminant level is set for a drinking water contaminant. Consider how to explain building in uncertainty factors and accounting for the most sensitive receptor from a risk communication perspective.
6. Cite an example of an effective risk message, either from a government agency or a corporation.
7. Describe how you would address people's concerns about health effects from historical exposures in a risk assessment.
8. Describe options for engaging specific groups to develop effective risk messages and management.
9. How would you go about evaluating the effectiveness of your risk communication program?

REFERENCES

Alders, R. G., S. N. Ali, A. A. Ameri, B. Bagnol, T. L. Cooper, A. Gozali, M. M. Hidayat, E. Rukambile, J. T. Wong, and A. Catley. 2020. Participatory Epidemiology: Principles, Practice, Utility, and Lessons Learnt. *Front. Vet. Sci.* 7: 532763. https://doi.org/10.3389/fvets.2020.532763.

Arnstein, S. 1969. A Ladder of Citizen Participation.
J. Amer Inst. Planners 35 (16): 216–224. https://doi.org/org/10.1080/01944366908977225.

Balog-Way, D., K. McComas, and J. Besley. 2020. The Evolving Field of Risk Communication. *Risk Anal.* 40 (S1): 2240–2262. https://doi.org/10.1111/risa.13615.

Boiko, P. E., R. L. Morrill, J. Flynn, E. M. Faustman, G. van Belle, and G. S. Omenn. 1996. Who Holds the Stakes? A Case Study of Stakeholder Identification at Two Nuclear Weapons Production Sites. *Risk Anal.* 16 (2): 237–249. https://doi.org/10.1111/j.1539-6924.1996.tb01454.x

Boore, D. M. 1989. The Richter Scale: Its Development and use for Determining Earthquake Source Parameters. *Tectonophysics* 166 (1): 1–14. https://doi.org/10.1016/0040-1951(89)90200-X.

Camelo, J., and T. Mayo. 2021. The Lasting Impacts of the Saffir-Simpson Hurricane Wind Scale on Storm surge risk Communication: The need for multidisciplinary Research in Addressing a Multidisciplinary Challenge. *Weather Clim. Extrem.* 33: 100335. https://doi.org/10.1016/j.wace.2021.100335.

Chess, C., B. J. Hance, and P. M. Sandman. 1988. *Improving Dialog With Communities: A Risk Communication Manual for Government.* Trenton, NJ: Environ. Commun. Res. Prog.NJ Agr. Exper. Sta.. doi:https://doi.org/10.7282/T3CV4HBB

Covello, V. T., P. M. Sandman, and P. Slovic. 1988. *Risk Communication, Risk Statistics, and Risk Comparisons: A Manual for Plant Managers.* Chemical Manufacturers Association.

Covello, V. T., P. Slovic, and D. von Winterfeldt. 1986. Risk Communication: A Review of the Literature. In *Carcinogen Risk Assessment*, edited by T. C. Travis, In Contemporary Issues in Risk Analysis, 193–207. New York: Springer.

Covello, V. T., D. von Winterfeldt, and P. Slovic. 1987. *Risk Communication: An Assessment of the Literature on Communicating Information About Health, Safety, and Environmental Risks.* EPA: Washington, DC.

Davies, J., V. T. Covello, and F. W. Allen. 1987. Risk Communication. *Proceedings of the National Conference on Risk Communication*, January 29–31, 1986, Washington, DC.

Donatuto, J. L., L. Campbell, and R. Gregory. 2016. Developing Responsive Indicators of Indigenous Community Health. *Int. J. Environ. Res. Publ. Health* 13 (9): 16. https://doi.org/10.3390/ijerph13090899.

Douglas, M., and A. Wildavsky. 1982. *Risk and Culture: An Essay on the Selection of Technological and Environmental Dangers*. Berkeley, CA: University of California Press.

Eisenman, D. P., K. M. Cordasco, S. Asch, J. F. Golden, and D. Glik. 2007. Disaster Planning and Risk Communication With Vulnerable Communities: Lessons From Hurricane Katrina. *Amer. J. Public Health* 97 (Suppl.1): S109–S115. https://doi.org/10.2105/AJPH.2005.084335.

Fischoff, B. 1995. Risk Perception and Communication Unplugged: Twenty Years of Process. *Risk Anal.* 15 (2): 137–145. https://doi.org/10.1111/j.1539-6924.1995.tb00308.x.

Fisher, A. 1991. Risk Communication Challenges. *Risk Anal.* 11 (2): 173–179. https://doi.org/10.1111/j.1539-6924.1991.tb00590.x.

Flynn, J., P. Slovic, and C. K. Mertz. 1994. Gender, Race, and Perception of Environmental Health Risks. *Risk Anal.* 14 (6): 1101–1108. https://doi.org/10.1111/j.1539-6924.1994.tb00082.x.

Friedman, S. M., K. Villamil, R. A. Suriano, and B. P. Egolf. 1996. Alar and Apples: Newspapers, Risk and Media Responsibility. *Publ. Underst. Sci.* 5 (1): 1–20. https://doi.org/10.1088/0963-6625/5/1/001.

Gurabardhi, Z., J. M. Gutteling, and M. Kuttschreuter. 2005. An Empirical Analysis of Communication Flow, Strategy and Stakeholders' Participation in the Risk Communication Literature 1988–2000. *J. Risk. Res.* 8 (6): 499–511. https://doi.org/10.1080/13669870500064192.

Hathaway, J. S. 1993. Alar: The EPA's Mismanagement of an Agricultural Chemical. In *The Pesticide Question: Environment, Economics, and Ethics*, edited by D. Pimentel and H. Lehman, 337–343. Boston, MA: Springer US.

Heifetz, R. A. 1994. *Leadership Without Easy Answers*. Cambridge, MA: Belknap Press of Harvard University Press.

Herfort, B., S. Lautenbach, J. Porto de Albuquerque, J. Anderson, and A. Zipf. 2021. The Evolution of Humanitarian Mapping Within the OpenStreetMap Community. *Sci. Reports* 11 (1): 3037. https://doi.org/10.1038/s41598-021-82404-z.

Johnson, B. B., and P. Slovic. 1995. Presenting Uncertainty in Health Risk Assessment: Initial Studies of Its Effects on Risk Perception and Trust. *Risk Anal.* 15 (4): 485–494 https://doi.org/10.1111/j.1539-6924.1995.tb00341.x.

Judd, N. L., C. H. Drew, C. Acharya, T. A. Mitchell, J. L. Donatuto, G. W. Burns, T. M. Burbacher, and E. M. Faustman. 2005. Framing Scientific Analyses for Risk Management of Environmental Hazards by Communities: Case Studies with Seafood Safety Issues. *Environ Health Perspect.* 113 (11): 1502–1508. https://doi.org/10.1289/ehp.7655.

Krimsky, S., and A Plough. 1988. *Environmental Hazards: Communicating Risks as a Social Process*. Dover, MA: Auburn House.

Lachlan, K. A., J. M. Burke, P. R. Spence, and D. Griffin. 2009. Risk Perceptions, Race, and Hurricane Katrina. *Howard J. Commun.* 20 (3): 295–309. https://doi.org/10.1080/10646170903070035.

Landy, M. K., M. J. Roberts, and S. R. Thomas. 1990. *The Environmental Protection Agency – Asking the Wrong Questions*. New York: Oxford University Press.

Leighton, K., S. Kardong-Edgren, T. Schneidereith, and C. Foisy-Doll. 2021. Using Social Media and Snowball Sampling as an Alternative Recruitment Strategy for Research. *Clin. Simul. Nurs.* 55: 37–42. https://doi.org/10.1016/j.ecns.2021.03.006.

Lundgren, R. E., and A. H. McMakin. 2018. *Risk Communication: A Handbook for Communicating Environmental, Safety, and Health Risks*, 6th ed. New York: John Wiley.

Merkelson, H. 2011. Risk Communication and Citizen Engagement: What to Expect from Dialogue. *J. Risk. Res.* 14 (5): 631–645. https://doi.org/10.1080/13669877.2011.553731.

Moore, J. A., J. R. III Fowle, G. S. Omenn, S. C. Lewis, G. M. Gray, and D. W. North. 1997. Risk Characterization: A Bridge to Informed Decision Making. *Fundam. Appl. Toxicol.* 39: 81–88.

Needlemen, C. 1987. Ritualism in Communicating Risk Information. *Sci. Technol. & Human Values* 12 (3/4): 20–25. https://www.jstor.org/stable/689378.

NRC. 1983. *Risk Assessment in the Federal Government: Managing the Process*. Washington, DC: National Academies Press.

NRC. 1989. *Improving Risk Communication*. Washington, DC: National Academies Press.

NRC. 1994. *Science and Judgment in Risk Assessment*. Washington, DC: National Academy Press.

NRC. 1996. *Understanding Risk: Informing Decisions in a Democratic Society*. Washington, DC: National Acadamies Press.

NRC. 2009. *Science and Decisions: Advancing Risk Assessment*. Washington, DC: National Academies Press.

Peters, R. G., V. T. Covello, and D. B. McCallum. 1997. The Determinants of Trust and Credibility in Environmental Risk Communication: An Empirical Study. *Risk Anal.* 17 (1): 43–54.

Plough, A., and S. Krimsky. 1987. The Emergence of Risk Communication Studies: Social and Political Context. *Sci. Technol.& Human Values* 12 (3/4): 4–10.

Renn, O. 1992. Risk Communication: Towards a Rational Discourse with the Public. *J. Hazard. Mater.* 29: 465–519.

Sandman, P. M. 1987. Risk Communication: Facing Public Outrage. *EPA J*: 21–22. http://www.psandman.com/articles/facing.htm#.

Santos, S. L., V. T. Covello, and D. B. McCallum. 1996. Industry Response to SARA Title III: Pollution Prevention, Risk Reduction and Risk Communication. *Risk Anal.* 16 (1): 57–66. https://doi.org/10.1111/j.1539-6924.1996.tb01436.x.

Santos, S. L., and D. B. McCallum. 1997. Communicating to the Public: Using Risk Comparisons. *Human and Ecol. Risk Ass.: An Intl. J.*, 3 (6): 1197–1214 https://doi.org/org/10.1080/10807039709383747.

Slovic, P. 1987. Perception of Risk. *Science (Washington)* 236: 280–285.

Slovic, P. 2000. *Perception of Risk*. Edited by R. E. Löfstedt. *Risk, Society and Policy Series*. London: Earthscan, Routledge.

Slovic, P., B. Fischhoff, and S. Lichtenstein. 1981. Perceived Risk: Psychological Factors and Social Implications. *Proc. Royal Soc. Series A* 376 (1764): 17–34. https://doi.org/10.1098/rspa.1981.0073.

Slovic, P., and B. Johnson. 1995. Explaining Uncertainty in Health Risk Assessment: Initial Studies of Its Effects on Risk Perception and Trust. *Risk Anal.* 15 (4): 485–494. https://doi.org/10.1111/j.1539-6924.1995.tb00341. xCitations:213.

Slovic, P., E. Peters, M. L. Finucane, and D. G. Macgregor. 2005. Affect, Risk, and Decision Making. *Health Psychol.* 24 (4S): S35–S40. https://doi.org/10.1037/0278-6133.24.4.S35.

Stern, P. C., and H.V. Fineberg. 1996. *Understanding Risk: Informing Decision in a Democratic Society*. National Academies Press.

Sugarman, C. 1989. The Alarm Over Alar. *Washington Post*, 1989/03/08/T12:00-500, 1989. Accessed 2022/05/18/23:04:05. https://www.washingtonpost.com/archive/lifestyle/food/1989/03/08/the-alarm-over-alar/23e6fde1-61ea-4f56-ab87-17f362915755/.

Thompson, B., E. Carosso, W. Griffith, T. Workman, S. Hohl, and E. M. Faustman. 2017. Disseminating Pesticide Exposure Results to Farmworker and Nonfarmworker Families in an Agricultural Community: A Community-Based Participatory Research Approach. *Journal of Occl. Environ. Med.* 59 (10): 982–987. https://doi.org/10.1097/JOM.0000000000001107.

US EPA. 1989/02 /01/, 1989, Daminozide, press release.

USGS. 2022a. *How Are Earthquakes Recorded? How Are Earthquakes Measured? How Is the Magnitude of an Earthquake Determined?* https://www.usgs.gov/faqs/how-are-earthquakes-recorded-how-are-earthquakes-measured-how-magnitude-earthquake-determined.

USGS. 2022b. *The Modified Mercalli Intensity Scale*. https://www.usgs.gov/programs/earthquake-hazards/modified-mercalli-intensity-scale.

USGSA. 2022. *Federal Advisory Committee Act (FACA) Management Overview*. https://www.gsa.gov/policy-regulations/policy/federal-advisory-committee-act-faca-management-overview.

Varghese, N. E., I. Sabat, Neumann-B. S., J. Schreyögg, T. Stargardt, A. Torbica, J. Exel, P. P. Barros, and W. Brouwer. 2021. Risk Communication during COVID-19: A Descriptive Study on Familiarity with, Adherence to and Trust in the WHO Preventive Measures. *PLOS ONE* 16 (4): e0250872. https://doi.org/10.1371/journal.pone.0250872.

Waddell, C. 1995. Defining Sustainable Development: A Case Study in Environmental Communication. *Tech. Commun. Qtely* 4 (2): 201–216. https://doi.org/10.1080/10572259509364597.

Wu, F., and J. V. Rodricks. 2020. Forty Years of Food Safety Risk Assessment: A History and Analysis. *Risk Anal.* 40 (S1): 2218–2230. https://doi.org/10.1111/risa.13624.

Index

Page numbers in **bold** refer to tables/exhibits and page numbers in *italics* refer to figures

1-bromopropane, 252–253, 301, 313–314
    example, 248
    presumed human carcinogen, 241
2-bromopropane, 252, 264
2-ethoxy phthalate, 288
2-ethylhexyl, 93
3-phenoxybenzoic acid, 94
8-tetrachlorodibenzo, 156
9H-fluoren-2-yl, 141
1,1,1-trichloroethane, 159–160, 168, 173–175
1,3-butadiene, 237, 240
1,4-dioxane, 199, 223
2,3,7,8-tetrachlorodibenzofuran, 32
2,3,7,8-tetrachlorodibenzo-p-dioxin (TCDD), 5, 74, 88, 91, 97, 171, 174–175, 191
2,3-dimercaptopropanol, 136
2,4,5-trichlorophenoxyacetic acid, *see* Agent Orange
2,4- dichlorophenoxyacetic acid, 2

A

absorption, 81, 116
    distribution, metabolism, and excretion (ADME), 80–81, 154
absorption barrier, 60, 62
absorption simulation, 155
acceptable daily intake (ADI), 41–42, 118
    NNS, **44**
acceptable risk levels, 69
acesulfame potassium, 43
acetylcholinesterase, 180
acrylamide, 45
acslX, 159–160
active sampling, 78
active transport, 116
activity patterns, and children's health, 271–272, *273*
Acute Exposure Guideline Levels (AEGSs), 238–239
additives, 19
adhesives, 11
adipose tissue, in exposure assessment, 85
administrative controls, 225, 253, 255–256, 259
Advanced Continuous Simulation Language (ACSL), 158
adverse outcome pathways (AOPs), 180
    AOP-Wiki, 181
    application to environmental health risk assessment, 182–184
    approach, 32
    and children's health, 270
    basic principles, 180–181
    components, *179*
    development and assessment, 27, 180–182
    Development Program, 181
    and epigenetics, 194
    framework, *27*, 28, 145, 183
    future directions and challenges, 184
    overarching concept of, 181
    overview, 179–180

affected communities, failure to include, 283
aflatoxins, 19, 48–49
age dependent adjustment factors, 270
Agency for Toxic Substances and Disease Registry (ATSDR), 139
Agent Orange, *3*, 5, 46, 91, 171
aggregate and cumulative risks, characterizing, 205–209
aggregate assessments, 203
aggregate exposure, 200, 202–203
agricultural biotechnology, 49–50
agricultural chemicals, regulations, 239
AhR action, *137*
AhR-activating HAHRLs, 5
air pollution, 3, 16, 97, 106
    air quality index (AQI), 259
    exposure assessment, 70–71
    invisible, 17
ALARA, 34
albumin, 82
alcohol, drinking by pregnant women, 133
alcohol metabolism, *132*
alcohols, 133
    metabolic pathways, *134*
alcohols and aldehyde metabolites, relative toxicities, **132**
alcohol use disorder (AUD), 133
aldrin, 2
algal blooms, 332
    dynamics characterization and top environmental determinants, *331*
    microbiome network underpinning, 334
algal viruses, 332
allergies, wheat gluten, 48
alternatives assessment, 280, 290
    conclusions, 310, 312
    core components, 296, **297**
    focusing on solutions, 287
    frameworks, **296**, **311**
    history of, 292, 294–295
    research gaps in, 305
American Community Survey (ACS), 109
American Conference of Governmental Industrial Hygienists (ACGIH), 236
American Homebuilders, 4
American Housing Survey (AHS), 109
American National Standards Institute (ANSI), 236
American Society for Testing and Materials, 236
amines, primary, conjugation of, *140*
amniotic fluid, 85
analytical chemistry, 9
analytic-deliberative dialogue, 357
anaphylactic shock, 48
Anastas, Paul, 294–295
animal bioassays, in occupational risk assessment, 248
animal testing, seeking alternatives to, 180–181, 183
animal to human extrapolation, 26
AOPs, *see* adverse outcomes pathways

Applications of Toxicogenomics Technologies to Predictive Toxicology and Risk Assessment, 18
ArcGIS, 145
Area Deprivation Index (ADI), 108
Aristotle, on alcohol, 133
Arnstein, S., 354
arrowhead approach, 284
arsenic, 46–47, 83
    in drinking water, 135
    health effects of, 135–136
arsenicosis, indicators of, 135
artificial intelligence (AI), 29
    potential applications to PBPK modeling, 170–171
asbestos, 79, 101, **227**, 237, 258, 324
    carcinogenicity of, 99
    in the workplace, 234, 236
    removal, 17
Asian flush syndrome, 48
aspartame, 43
assay for transposase accessible chromatin using sequencing (ATAC-seq), 192
assays, local lymph node, 182
Association for the Advancement of Alternatives Assessment, 280
asthma, 3, 48
atomic absorption spectrometry (AAS), 88
authoritative lists, 298, **299**
    in alternatives assessment, **311**
auxins, 2
average global temperatures, increases in, 4

B

baby foods, 47
Bayesian framework, 222–223
Bayesian population approach, 169
Bazelon, David, 16
behavioral sciences, 26
benchmark dose (BMD) approach, in occupational risk assessment, 248–249
benefits and trade-offs, communication of, 355
benzene, 100, 139
    metabolism, *140*
    worker exposure to, 242–243
benzo(α)pyrene, metabolism of, *138*
Berkeley Madonna, 158–162
best available technology, use of, 34
beta distribution, 215
bias, recall, 79
big data, 9
binomial distribution, 215
bioaccumulative metals, 83
bioallergens, 83
bioassays, 88
bioavailability, 61
    independent variable in risk assessment, 90–91, 171–172
biodiversity
    accounting, 341
    dynamics, 340
    loss of, 342
biodiversity-carbon ecosystem protection areas, 341
biodiversity-carbon security plans, 333

bioinformatics, 26, 31
biological agents, exposure to, 9
biological end points, **19**
biologically effective dose, 78
biological markers of exposure, in occupational risk assessment, 247
biological pathways, 184
biological plausibility, 182
biomarkers, 26, 103–104
    and 9/11 terrorist attacks, 101, 103–104
    continuum of, *102*
    definition, 101
biomolecular adducts, in exposure assessment, 86
biomonitoring, 68, 78–79, 82
    of children and adolescents, 83
    of exposure, 81
    of fetuses and infants, 83–84
biostatistics, 26
biphenyls, 5
Birth Defects Monitoring Program, 3
birth weight, reduced, 10
bisphenol A (BPA), and challenges of risk-based system, 282
bisulfite modification, 192
blood, 79, 82
    in exposure assessment, 84
Blue Carbon, 327
body burden, 269
Body Chip, 118
Box, George E. P., 80
Bradford-Hill criteria, 182
breast milk, in exposure assessment, 85
breathing zone, 78
bromine, 5
Bt corn, 50
Buehler Test, 182
built environment, 3
    as influencer of health, 4

C

cadmium, 47
Cafeteriavirus, 332
caffeine consumption, 111–112
Cairns, John, 286
California Safe Drinking Water and Toxic Enforcement Act, 295
California Safer Consumer Products Regulations, 295
Campylobacter, 49
cancer risk, estimating, 200–201
carbon cycling, 340
carbon drawdown, 342
carbon monoxide, 19, 70
    exposure to, 83
carbon sequestration, 332, 340–341
carcinogenic contaminants, 42
carcinogenicity to humans, **25**
carcinogens, 6, 10, 47
    classification of, 244
    known, 11
cardiac diseases, 4
care communication, 353
career decisions, 4

Carson, Rachel, *Silent Spring*, 1, 16, 51
cell fate decisions, example, *188*
cell phone data, 105
cellular membrane, structure of, *117*
censored data, 220
Centers for Disease Control and Prevention (CDC), 3, 109, 199
chemical analysis methods, organic chemicals, 87–88
chemical class approaches, 284
chemical classes, behavior in the body, 81–83
chemical mixtures, 280
chemical risk assessment, emerging areas, 26–29, 31–32
chemicals
    common, toxic and lethal doses, **125**
    extremely persistent and ubiquitous, risk assessment of, 284–285
    general behavior in the body, 81
    natural and man-made, *113*
    risk assessment of, challenges, 23–24
Child Health Data, 107
childhood lead exposure, reducing, 127–128
childhood lead poisoning, 3
Child Lead Data, 107
children, 7, 83, 116, 123, 267–268
Children's Health Exposure Analysis Resource (CHEAR), 106
Chi-Square test, 215
chloracne, 5–6, 10, 91
chlorinated naphthalenes, 5
chlorination of water, 19
chlorine, 5
chlorpyrifos, 205
chlorpyrifos aggregate exposure assessment, **206**
cholangiocarcinoma, study in vinyl-chloride workers, 99
cholera, 9
Cholera Map, 143
chromatin immunoprecipitation, 192
chronic traumatic encephalopathy (CTE), 259
chrysotile, 234
circadian disruption, 260
classical pharmacokinetic models and PBPK models, differences between, 155–156
classical pharmacokinetics, 155
Clean Air Act, 19, 26
    Amendments, 21, 34, 349
Cleaner Technology Substitutes Assessments, 293
climate change, and occupational risk, 258–259
climate engineering, 342
cluster analysis, 100
CO_2, increases in, 4
Collaborative on Health and Environment, 281
color additives, 44
Column Model, 300
communication, 16, 31, 70, 253, 287
    two-way model, 350
, *see* risk communication
communities, 141–142
    fishing, 10
    tribal, 357
communities of color, 142
Community Health Survey (CHS), 107

Community RTK Act, 349
comparative exposure assessment pathways, *303*
Comparative Toxicogenomics Database (CTD), 122–123
compliance safety and health officers (CSHOs), 235–236
compounds
    halogenated, 5
    polychlorinated, 2, *3*, 5
Comprehensive Environmental Response, Compensation, and Liability Act (CERCLA), 349; *see also* Superfund
CompTox Chemicals Dashboard, 300, 353
computational models, predictive pattern-oriented, 342
computational toxicology, 28–31, 173–174, 176, 181
concentration levels, 69
concentrations, in occupational risk assessment, 245
consensus communication, 354
conservative assumptions, 115
Consumer Financial Protection Bureau, 239
consumption, accidental, 10
contaminants and additives to food, 39
contaminants in food and water, 19
contamination, microbial pathogen, 42
controls
    NIOSH hierarchy of, *253*
    profit, employment, and health, 256
correlated input parameters, 220
cosmetics, EU legislation, 322
cotinine, 88
cotton dust, in US workplaces, 243
Court decisions affecting occupational risk assessment, 242–244
Court of Justice of the European Union, 317
COVID-19 pandemic, 1, 9
    impacts of, 105–106
    testing data, 109
CpG islands, 188
Cranor, Carl, 283
criteria air pollutants (CAPS), 70, 83
crop protection chemicals, 45
crops, glyphosate-tolerant, 50
cumulative exposures, 200, 204
cumulative risk, 204
cumulative risk assessment, 205
    equations for calculating, 204
Cuyahoga River, 1
Cyanobacteria, 330, 332
CYP1 enzymes, 5
CYP1A1, 136, 137, 142
cyrene classified according to serious eye damage and irritation studies IATA, **309**
cytochrome P450, 136, 141; *see also* CYP1A1

D

Dannenberg, Andrew, 4
data, ecologic, 77
databases, *30*
data sets, useful for environmental epidemiology, 107–109
DDT, *see* dichlorodiphenyltrichloroethane

Delaney Clause, 16, 41–42
deoxynivalenol (DON), 48
Departments of Health Surveys, 107
depression, 4
derived no-effect levels (DNELs), 319
dermal absorption, 1
    exposure by, 58
dermal surface area for age groups, 272
dermatitis, 48
Design for Environment Program, 293
deterministic models, 209
deterrence, power of, 257
developmental delays, 10
Developmental Origins of Health and Disease
        (DOHaD) hypothesis, 135, 190–191
diacetyl, NIOSH risk assessment for, 247–248
diarrhea, 48
dibenzofurans, 5, 28
dichlorodiphenyltrichloroethane (DDT), 1, 2, 6, **7**, 45,
        51, 130, 293
dichloromethane (DCM), 169
diethylstilbesterol (DES), 45
    maternal exposure to, 116
diffusion, 116
dioxins, *3*, 5, 91
diphenyl ethers, 5
direct environmental measurements, 77
direct measurements, 67
Dirty Dozen, **7**
disasters, environmental health effects of, 105–106
disclosure, 291
diseases
    cardiac, 4
    congenital Minamata, 130
    ecogenomic, 120
    first noted in occupational settings, **227**
    infectious, 3, 9
    ischemic, 47
    occupational, 232, 235
    peripheral vascular, 47
    respiratory, 47
disinfectants, humidifier, exposure to, 183
distribution, 81
D-limonene, 25
DNA,
    accessibility and function, regulation of, 188
    adducts, 82
    bisulfite modification, *193*
    cytosine methylation, 188
    double helix, 187
    methylation, 191–192, 194
    overview, *189*
    quantitative assessment of, *194*
Donora Pennsylvania, 1
dose, 61–63
    in occupational risk assessment, 245
dose response, 112
    analysis, in occupational risk assessment, 247
    assessment, 2, 21, 182
    and children's health, 270
    concept of, 111
    curve, *114, 115*
    inverted U-shaped, *125*

experiments, 115
    relationship, extrapolation of, 24–25
    study, complete, range-finding for, *114*
dread, 361
drinking water,
    contaminants, 11
    directive, revised, 285
    ingestion rates for age groups, *271*
drowsiness, 11
duration of exposure, 58, 125
    in occupational risk assessment, 246
Dutch Famine, World War II, 191

E

eating fish, 130
Ebola, 9
eChemPortal, 300
ecohydrology, 341
E. coli, 49
ecologic measures, 76
economic health, as determinant of physical and
        mental health, 142
ecosystem,
    connectome, 341
    dysbiosis, 338
    metabolism, 341
    portfolio approach, 341
    risk management, 339–340
ecosystems, eutrophic, 341
electron capture, 87
elimination of hazards, 253
Emergency Planning and Community Right-to-Know
        (RTK) Act, 348
emergency procedures, 349
empirical support, 182
endocrine disruption, 189–190
engagement, of stakeholders, 33
engineering controls, 254–255
envirome, 341
envirome-biota processes, 342
environmental contaminants, 40
    and human health, 6
environmental degradation, centrality of, 342
environmental epidemiology
    biomarkers in, 101, 103, 105
    definition, 99
    future goals, 107
    spatial analysis in, 100–101
environmental health research, role of geography in,
        100
environmental health risk assessment, definition, 15
environmental health risk management, framework,
        23
environmental justice, 23, 105, 107, 141–142, 200, 210,
        222
environmental lead (Pb) exposure, 203
Environmental Protection Agency (EPA), 1, 16
    Policy on Evaluating Risk to Children, 268
    role in occupational risk management, 236,
        237–239
    Toxic Substances inventory, 24
environmental public health, careers in, 3

environmental regulations, 16
environmental risk assessment, 7
environmental stress, 70
environmental xenobiotics, hazard of, 90
environment-biota transmission chains, 341
enzyme systems, xenobiotic-metabolizing, *131*
EPA, *see* Environmental Protection Agency
epidemiology, 3, 25
    definition, 99
    and environmental health problems, 99–100
    zoonoses framework in, 341
epigenetic changes, observed, 191
epigenetic landscape model, 187
epigenetic programming, 189
epigenetic regulation, 187–188
epigenetic reprogramming of gametes by HAHRLs, 6
epigenetic variation, 192
epigenetics, 9, 116, 341
    applying in risk assessment, 194
    limitations, 196
    assessing, 192
    definition, 187
equipment, electrical, 10
essentiality, 182
estimated daily intake (EDIs), 43
ethanol, 41, **125**, 131, *132*, 133
ethical perspectives, 141
ethylene glycol, 131
EudraGMDP, 322
eukaryote-prokaryote balance, 341
eukaryotes, 334, 336
European Atomic Energy Community (Euratom), 317
European Chemicals Strategy for Sustainability, 292
    overview, *293*
European Coal and Steel Community (ECSC), 317
European Commission (EC), 30
European Economic Area (EEA), 318
European Economic Community (EEC), 317
European Inventory of Existing Commercial Chemical
    Substances (EINECS), 318
European Parliament, 285
European Public Assessment Report (EPAR), 322
European Union Cosmetics Directive, 183
evaluation of individual hazards and risks, 20
excessive information, managing, 353
excess lifetime cancer risk, 201
    cumulative distribution calculated through one-
        dimensional Monte Carlo simulation, *218*
    cumulative distribution calculated through two-
        dimensional Monte Carlo simulation, *219*
excretion, 82
exhaled breath, 85
expert elicitation, 222
expert judgment, 222–223
exponential distribution, 214
exposome, 32, 106, 116, 121, 143
    concept of, 31, *107*, *108*
    interacting with human genomes, 120
exposome analyses, 31
exposome-genome approach, 145
exposome-genome interaction, 116
exposome-informed epidemiologic research, *109*
EXPOsOMICS Project, 121

exposure
    community-based, 80
    definition, 58, 74
    in occupational risk assessment, 245
    unintentional, 118
    xenobiotic, 118
exposure and dose in source-to-outcome framework,
    63
exposure and dose terms by routes of exposure, *62*
exposure and risk modeling, tiered approach, *210*
exposure assessment, 2, 21, 31–32, 74, 112
    applying to estimate risk, 68–69
    basic concepts and key components, 58–60
    biological matrices for, 84–85
    and children's health, 270–271
    definition, 58
    methods and approaches, 67–68, 73–75, *76*, 77–80,
        246
    in occupational risk assessment, 246
    overview, 57
    process, overview, 64, 66–67
    retrospective, 80
    role in risk assessment, 63–64
    throughout life cycle, 83–84
exposure concentrations, 58
    and occupational risk assessment, 241
exposure factors, 59
Exposure Factors Handbook, 125
exposure medium, 59
exposure minimization, 291
exposure misclassification, 77
    biases, 78
exposure modeling, 73, 79–80
exposure pathways, 1, 59
    identification, 66
    relative importance of, *208*
exposure patterns, and occupational risk assessment,
    241
exposure period, 58, 74
exposure points, 66
exposure profile, in occupational risk assessment, 246
exposure quantification, 66
exposure reconstruction, 68
exposure routes, 66
exposure scenarios, 69
exposure science, 9
Exposure Science in the 21st Century, 9
exposure setting characterization, 65
exposure surface, 74
exposures to multiple chemicals, risk assessment for,
    32
extrapolation models, 115

F

fatal and non-fatal workplace injuries by race, **231**
fate and transport, 59, 66
fatigue, 10
fatty acids, polyunsaturated, 130
fatty foods, 10
Federal Advisory Committee Act (FACA), 356
Federal Insecticide, Fungicide, and Rodenticide Act
    (FIFRA), 7, 239

federal legislation, 16, **17**, 349
feedback mechanisms, need for, 350
fetal alcohol spectrum disorder (FASD), 133, 135
fetal alcohol syndrome (FAS), 133
filtration, 116
Fischoff, Baruch, 355, 356
fish, 10, 48
    eating, 130
fish oil capsules, 130
five-step process of risk assessment, and GIS, **145**
fixed-site monitoring, 71
flame photometric, 87
Flint, lead exposure in, 127–128
Florida International University Water Quality
        Monitoring Program, 335
fluidics, 118
fluids, cleaning, 11
fluorene metabolism, *141*
fluorescence, 87
fluorescent lights, 10
food additive petition (FAPs), 43–44
food additives and contaminants, 40, 42, 43–44
    classes of, **41**
    deaths, 49
    of industrial origin, organics, 45–47
food allergies, 48
Food and Drug Administration (FDA), 16
food fraud, 39
food integrity, 39
food intolerances, 48
food processing, 40, 43
food production, 42
Food Quality Protection Act (FQPA), 32, 200, 349
    in relation to children, 268
    Safety Factor, 270
food safety,
    history of, 40–42
    regulation, 41
    risk analysis, 39
    risk assessment, summary, 42
Food Safety Modernization Act (FSMA), 43
food safety science, 40
food spoilage, 42
food supply chains, 42, 43
foodborne pathogens, 49
formaldehyde, 17
Frank R. Lautenberg Chemical Safety for the 21st
        Century Act, 17, 18, 200, 237
frequency of exposure, 58
    in occupational risk assessment, 246
Frumkin, Howard, 4
fumonisins, 48
functional substitution approach for chemicals in
        products, **290**

G

gamma distribution, 215
gas chromatography (GC), 87
gene-environment interactions, 26
gene polymorphisms, 139
genetically modified organisms (GMOs), 49–50
genome wide association studies (GWAS), 121

genomics, 9, 121
geographic information systems (GIS), 77, 143–144
    data layers visualization, *143*
    in Five-Step Risk Assessment, **145**
girus (giant virus), 332
global carbon cycle, 333
Global Chemicals Outlook II, 280–281, 292
global pandemic, 9
global survivability, 342
glucuronidation, 137, *138*, 139
glyphosate, 50, 52
glyphosate-containing products (GCPs), 52
Golden Rice, 50
goodness-of-fit tests, 215
GRAS, 50
    substances, 44–45
Great Lakes Water Quality Agreement, 293
GreenScreen® Assessment Registry, 300
Guinea Pig Maximization Test, 182

H

half-life, 59
Halifax Project, 168
halogenated aryl hydrocarbon receptor ligands
        (HAHRLs), 5
    exposure to, 6
halogens, 5
Halowax, 5
Hanna-Attisha, Mona, 128
harmonization, 317
Harvard Football Players Health Study, 259
Hazard Communication Standard (HazCom), 257
hazard identification, 2, 20, 112, 182, 190
    and children's health, 268
    in occupational risk assessment, 244
hazard quotient (HQ), 201
hazardous air pollutants (HAPs), 71
hazards
    control strategies, 253, 255–258
    emerging, 258–259
    occupational, 226
    workplace, 5
headaches, 10–11
head trauma, repeated, 259
health, adolescent, 83
Health and Environmental Sciences Institute (HESI),
        32, 307
Health and Exposome Research Center:
        Understanding Lifetime Exposures
        (HERCULES), 106
health benchmarks, 201–203
health disparities, 143
Healthy Building Network, Pharos Project, 300
heat exchangers, 10
heat islands, 4
heavy metals, 46–47
heavy metals and metalloids (HMMs), sample
        preparation process for, 88
hemoglobin, 82–83
herbicides, 2, *3*
Herodotus, 226
high-performance liquid chromatography (HPLC), 87

high-priority designation, 17
high production volume (HPVs), 9
    industrial chemicals, 23–24
high-resolution mass spectrometry (HRMS), 32
high-risk groups, 7
Hippocratic concept of health and disease, 143
histamine content, 48
histone proteins, 187–188
historical perspectives, 15
HIV/AIDs, 9
hives, 48
holobiont dynamics, 341
hormesis, 123
human cell culture, 118
human exposure assessment, 78
human genome, 187
    sequencing, 26, 120
Human Health Exposure Analysis Resource
    (HHEAR), 106
human health risk assessment, definition, 2
human on a chip, *120*
Hurricane Harvey, 105
Hurricane Katrina, 105, 357
Hurricane Sandy, 101
hybrid measurement-modeling approach, 79
hydraulic fluids, 10
    water pump, 10
hydrocarbons, 19
hydrologic restoration, 333
hyperkeratosis, 6, 47
hypertension, 47
hypospadias, 3

I

immune response, 10
immune system, 11
immunoassays, 88
immunoglobins, 48
inactivity, 4
inclusion, population- and citizen-based, 348
Indigenous tribes, 357
indole-3-acetic, 2
inductively coupled plasma-mass spectrometry
    (ICP-MS), 88
industrial hygiene, 245
    evolution of, 258
Industrial Revolution, 226
industry, metal machining, 11
inequitable mindset/philosophy, 142
infodemic, 353
information
    disclosure, 257
    overload, 35
    using best available, 291
ingestion, 1, 123
    exposure by, 58
inhalation, 1, 123
    exposure by, 58
input parameters for calculating cancer risk, example,
    216
in silico toxicology (IST), 29–30
insecticides, 6, 51

organochlorine, 81
Institute of Medicine (IOM), 18
intake, 61
Integrated Approaches to Testing and Assessment
    (IATAs), 306, 308, 310
interdisciplinary perspectives, limited in risk
    assessment approach, 282
International Agency for Research on Cancer (IARC),
    25
Interstate Chemicals Clearinghouse, 295
intolerances, lactose, 48
intuitive approaches, 34
isolation, in hazard control, 254–255
isopropanol, 131

J

job-exposure matrix approach, 80
Joint Expert Committee on Food Additives (JECFA), 43

K

key events (KEs), 180–182
key event relationships (KERS), 180–181
Key National Academies Reports, **18**
key species/bioindicators, 341
kidneys, 11
    tumors, in male rats, 25
kinetics of transport, *119*
Kolmogorov-Smirnov test, 215
Krishnan, Kannan, 168

L

labeling, drug, 48
lactase, 48
"Ladder of Citizen Participation", 354
Lake Cuyahoga, 16
Land and Copper Rule (LCR), 126–127
land-ocean,
    feedback, 327
    interface, 333
land-water connections, 341
lead, 19, 47, 70
    in drinking water, 126–127
    toxicity of, 127
learning deficits, 10
legislation, federal, 16, **17**, 349
lesions, 10
Lethal Dose 50, 115
leukemia, chronic B-cell, 6
Levi Strauss & Co., 296
life cycle assessment (LCA), 304
lifetime excess cancer risks associated with OSHA
    substance-specific PELs, **240**
light-headedness, 11
limits of detection (LODs), 88
linearized multistage model (LMS), in occupational
    risk assessment, 248
liver cancer, 11
local health departments, 109
lockdowns, 105
lognormal distribution, 214

lowest observed adverse effect level (LOAEL), 115, 116
low-priority designation, 17
lung-on-a-chip, *119*
lungs, 116
lysis, 333
lysogeny, 333

M

machine learning, 9
    application to PBPK modeling and analysis, 171
magnitude of exposure, 58
    in occupational risk assessment, 246
Magnolia, 158
manganese, 78
margin of exposure (MOE), 202
margins of safety (MOS), 115
Markers of Autism Risk in Babies – Learning Early
        Signs (MARBLES), 86
mass spectrometry, 87–88
maternal-fetal biological matrix selection and
        considerations for exposure assessment, *90*
maternal-fetal exposure diagram, *75*
maternal smoking, sustained, 191
MATLAB, 158
measurement studies, 199, 205–208, 210–211
Meat Inspection Act (1906), 41
meconium, 85
Megaviruses, 332
mercury, 47, 128–129
    average concentration in selected fish species, *129*
mercury poisoning, 129
    fetal, 130
MERS, 9
message tailoring for specific audiences, 352
metabolism, 81–82
metabolome, 31
metabolomics, 121
methanol, 131, 133
    metabolism, *133*
methanol poisoning, 133
methods, point-of-contact, 67
methylene chloride (MC), industrial use of, 249–252
methylmercury, 47, 83
    exposure from fish consumption, 128–129
methylmercury poisoning, symptoms, 129
Michaelis-Menten kinetic parameters, 163
microbial growth efficiency (MGE), 333
microbial pathogens, 49
microbiological dynamics, 341
microbiome, 340
microbiome network underpinning algal blooms, 334
microplastics, 183, 340
Minnesota Children's Pesticide Exposure Study
        (MNCPES), 205
mixture approach, 284
mixtures, 25
    exposure to, and occupational health risk, 261
mobility, sociodemographic component of, 105–106
mobility analysis, 106
modeling studies, 209
model uncertainty, 221

mode of action (MOA),
    and children's health, 270
    concept, 181
    data, 26
    in cancer risk assessment, 27
modern food supply, 42–43
Modified Mercalli Intensity Scale, 351
molecular biology, 9
    methods used in toxicology, *124*
    tools applied to toxicology, *122*
molecular initiating events (MIEs), 27–28, 180–182
molecular signatures, 26
monitoring, personal exposure, 78
monoculture, 43
monooxygenases, 131, 132, 136
Monte Carlo simulation, 216, 218–219, 222
    fundamental concept of, *217*
Montreal Protocol on Substances That Deplete the
        Ozone Layer, 292
Muller, Paul, 51
multidisciplinary teams, 282
multimedia exposure, 203
multipathway exposure, 203
multiple myeloma, 6
multi-risk reduction, 288
mycotoxins, 48, **49**
myelodysplastic syndromes (MDS) cases, spatial
        analysis, *101*
myocardial infarction, 47

N

NAMs, *see* new approach methodologies
nanomaterials (NMs), risk assessment of, 12
nanotechnology, and occupational risk, 258
National Academies of Sciences, Engineering and
        Medicine (NASEM), 18, 239
National Ambient Air Quality Standards (NAAQS),
        19, 70–71, 234
National Cancer Institute, 100
National Center for Environmental Health (NCEH), 3
National Center for Health Statistics (NCHS), 107
*National Conversation on Public Health and Chemical
        Exposures*, 287
National Environmental Protection Act (NEPA), 1
National Fire Protection Association, 236
National Health and Nutrition Examination Surveys
        (NHANES), 3, 31, 107, 199, 233
National Institute for Environmental Health Sciences
        (NIEHS), 106
National Institute for Occupational Safety and Health
        (NIOSH), 226–227, 235
    Chemical Carcinogen Policy, 235, 238
    Health Hazard Evaluations, 233
    Practices in Occupational Risk Assessment, 235
National Research Council (NRC), 1–2, 9, 180
    framework, 297
Natural Resources Defense Council, 356
nausea, 48
Neighborhood Atlas, 123
neotame, 43
neurotoxicants, 51
new approach methodologies (NAMs), 9, 280, 306

NAM-able endpoints, *305*
three-step framework, 307
night shift work, and breast cancer risk, 260
nitrogen, 338–339
nitrogen dioxide, 70
nitrogen oxides, 19
nitrogen phosphorus, 87
N-nitrosamines, 45
No Observed Adverse Effect Level (NOAEL), 41, 42, 115, 116
nonbioaccumulative metals, 83
noncancer risk assessments, 201
noncancer risks, cumulative, 32
non-nutritive sweeteners (NNS), 43–44
nonpersistent chemicals, 82
postexposure fate, 88
theoretical, *82*
normal distribution, 214
norovirus, 49
notification procedure in EU, 321
numerical integration, 166
numerical stability, 220
Nurses' Health Study, 260

O

obesity, 4
O'Brien, Mary, 282, 287
occupational disease, 232, 235
occupational exposure assessment, 245
occupational exposures, 123, 233
occupational fatalities and non-fatalities by industry, *229, 230*
occupational health, study of, 226
occupational hygiene, 245
evolution of, 258
occupational illness, 226
occupational injuries, 226
occupational PELs, 247
occupational regulations, costs, 235
occupational risk, 226
occupational risk assessment,
mechanics of, 244–247
methodology, overview, 239, 241–242
occupational safety, 232
Occupational Safety and Health (OSH) Act, 26, 226, 236
Occupational Safety and Health Administration (OSHA), 16, 226, 233, 235–236, 239
regulations, 256
steps for transitioning to safer chemicals, *294*
occupational standards and ambient air quality standards, comparison, **233**
occupational studies, 99
ocean ecosystems across habitats, geographic and information landscapes, *328*
ocean microbiome, 336, 339
ochratoxin A (OTA), 48
Office of Science and Technology Policy, 20
omega-3 fatty acids, 47
omics,
approach, 9
technologies, 28

tools used in toxicology and risk assessment, **121**
oral presentations, 362
organophosphate pesticides (OPs), 51
organ-organ interactions, 118
organ toxicants, 123
organ toxicology studies, 118
Organisation of Economic Co-operation and Development (OECD), 30
authoritative lists, **299**, **311**
building blocks of an IATA, *306*
Outdoor Workers Exposed to Wildfire Smoke, 259
ozone, 70

P

P2OASys, 300
packaging, 42
paint, 10
removers, 11
Pandoravirus, 332
Paracelsus, 41, 111
paradigm, decision-making/risk management, 21
paralysis by analysis, 298
parameter uncertainty, 221
particles, 19
particulate matter, 70, 78–79, 116
partnering, 355–356
partnerships, building, 355
pathobiology, 26
pathways; *see also* adverse outcome pathways (AOPs)
human exposure assessment, 74
in occupational risk assessment, 245
PBPK, *see* physiologically based pharmacokinetic (PBPK) modeling
per- and polyfluoroalkyl substances (PFASs), 9, 21, 45, 81, 86, 97, 284–285
exposures, 206
long-chained, 88
toxicology of, 46
perchloroethene (PCE), *see* tetrachloroethylene
perfluorooctanoic acid (PFOA), 46
perfluorooctane sulfonate (PFOS), 46
permissible exposure limits (PELs), 234, 236
set by OSHA, **237**
persistent, bioaccumulative, and toxic chemicals (PBTs), 7
persistent organic pollutants (POPs), 6, 7, 60, 81, 82, 199–200
Review Committee (POPRC), 292
personalized health approaches, 348
personal protective equipment (PPE), 1, 256
pesticide products, regulation of, 7
pesticides, 7–8, 45, 50
current-use, 82
risk in the environment, 51
Pesticides in the Diets of Infants and Children, 268
PFASs, *see* per- and polyfluoroalkyl substances
pharmacokinetics, 28
Phase I and II metabolism, 131, 136
activation of amino acid, *139*
Phase II xenobiotic metabolism, example substrates, *138*
phenols, 82

photochemical oxidants, 19
phthalates, 82
physiologically based pharmacokinetic (PBPK)
        modeling, 28, *29*, *155*, 161–163, 168, 170–175,
        177–178, 250–251
    application in dichloromethane, *169*, 170
    biological relevance, 156–157
    chemical interactions in chemical mixtures,
        167–168
    data requirements for, 157–158
    data sets used for building and validation, 158
    definition, 154–155
    fundamentals of, 157
    guidance document, 158
    model code, written in Berkeley Madonna,
        160–162, 164–166
    numerical integration, 166
    OSHA's scientific criteria for, **251**
    overview, 154
    model structure, *159*
    simulation programs, 159
    software comparison, 158–159
physiological rates, and children's health, 271
pigmentation, 6
pinocytosis, 116
Pithovirus, 332
plague, 9
Plato, on alcohol, 133
point-of-contact approach, 68
points of entry, 59
poisons, use of, 112
Poisson distribution, 215
PolicyMap, 108
Pollution Prevention Act, 293
pollution prevention hierarchy, 293, *295*
polybrominated diphenyl ethers (PBDEs), 81
polychlorinated biphenyls (PCBs), 5, 45, 81
    co-planar, 28
    isomers, 45
    and polychlorinated dibenzofurans (PCDFs),
        health risks of, 10
polychlorinated dibenzo-p-dioxins, 81
polycyclic aromatic hydrocarbons (PAHs), 45, 78, 81
polyhalogenated aryl hydrocarbon receptor ligands, 5
polymorphisms, in genes, 142
polyvinylchloride, first official risk assessment, 1
population characteristics, and occupational risk
        assessment, 241
populations, susceptible, 1, 7
population size, and occupational risk assessment,
        239, 241
pork tapeworm, 49
portfolio approaches, importance of, 342
poverty, impact of, 143
precautionary principle, 34, 292, 350
predictability, 342
predictive causality networks, 337
pregnancy, 80, 82
preservatives in foods, 17
Presidential/Congressional Commission on Risk
        Assessment and Risk Management, 21, 286,
        348
Preventable Common Complex Diseases, **121**

probabilistic modeling
    critical issues in, 220–223
    fundamental approach for, 216
    scoping for, 215–216
probabilistic models, 209–211
    for exposure and risk assessment, 215–216
probability density function (PDF), 211–212
probability distributions, 211–212
    and probability density, **213**, **214**
probability mass function (PMF), 211–212
problem formulation, 2, 9, 21, 57, 65, 210
processing of foods, substances formed by, 45
prokaryotes, 333, 336
Protection of Children from Environmental Health
        Risks and Safety Risks (Executive Order
        13045), 268
proteins, alpha-2 mu globulin, 25
proteomics, 5, 28, 121, 124, 147
public awareness, 349
public health, 1
public health protection, 21st-century, 9
public health sciences, contributions to eco-genetics
        and risk assessment, 26
public involvement, 356
public perception of potential hazards and health
        risks, *16*
Pure Food and Drug Act (1906), 41

Q

QA/QC programs, 89
QGIS, 100
Q-Q plot, 215
qualitative assessments, 182
quantitative approach, 67
quantitative microbial risk assessment (QMRA), 49
quantitative risk assessment (QRA), 20, 200
    criticisms of, 281
    limitations of, 283
quantitative structure-activity relationships (QSAR),
        30, 155
questionnaires, 76–78

R

R programming, 158
R Studio, 100
random variable, probability distribution of, 211
raryl hydrocarbon receptor (AhR), 5
rashes, 10, 48
read across approach, 30
recommended exposure limits (RELs), 235
Red Book, 1, 2, *8*, 17–18, 23, 25, 49, 281, 347
Reference Dose (RfD), 118
Registration, Evaluation
    Authorisation, and Restriction of Chemicals
        (REACH) regulation, 9, 30, 318–320
    components, *8*
Risk Commission Report, 25
risk communication, 2, 348, 352
    approaches, **34**
    complex nature of, 363
risk comparisons, 364

risk evaluations, 17
risk indices, 351–352
risk levels, comparative, 69
risk management, 2
    approaches, **34**
    integration with risk assessment, 112
risk perception, 35, 360, 362
    importance of, 15
    primary factors, 361
risk reduction
    essential components for, **33**
    by orders of magnitude vs. linear, *34*
risk scales, 351
risk trade-offs, 20
    risk-risk trade-offs, 34
    in occupational health and safety, 252
risk transfer, from environment to workplace, 239
risks
    biotic, 9
    exotic, 361
    voluntary, 361
routes of exposure, 58, 61
Ruckelshaus, William, 23, 348, 356

S

SAAM II, 158
saccharin, 17, 43
Safe Drinking Water Act (SDWA), in relation to
        children, 268
Safer Choice Program, 294
Safety Data Sheet (SDS), 257
safety factors, 115
    use to adjust for uncertainties in risk, **115**
Saffir-Simpson Hurricane Wind Scale, 351
saliva, 82, 85, 88
salmon, 130
Salmonella enterica, 49
Sambavirus, 332
samples, collecting from infants and children, 86
sampling time frame, in exposure assessment, 86–87
SARS, 9
SARS-CoV-2, 1
SaTScan, 100
scenario evaluation, 67–68
scenario uncertainty, 221
Science and Decisions Advancing Risk Assessment, 9
Science and Judgment in Risk Assessment, 25
science of food safety, 40
scientists, *16*
SCoP, 158
scoping, 21, 65
seafood, 47
Sea Level Rise effects, minimization of, 333
selenium, 130
Selye, Hans, 70
sensitivity, of measurement method, 88
sensitivity analysis, 220, 222
    in PBPK modeling, 166–167
serum PFAS species levels, *207*
Shapiro-Wilk test, 215
shellfish, 48
Significant New Alternatives Policy (SNAP), 292

Significant New Use Rules (SNUR), 237
SimuSolv, 158
Sinclair, Upton, *The Jungle*, 41, 226
single chemical approach, 284
skin sensitization, assessment of,182–183
smog, deadly, 1
Snow, John, 143
    Cholera Map, *144*
snowballing, 356
SNP examples in various populations, **141**
social determinants of health, 143
Society of Risk Analysis (SRA), 348
socioeconomic status and toxic incidents, *105*
Socrates, 112
soft tissue sarcomas, 6
soil
    contaminated, 10
    oxidation, 333
source and fate models, 69
source-exposure-dose-effects continuum, *117*
source of exposure, 59
spatial autocorrelation, 100
spatial clustering, 100
specificity, of measurement method, 88
Sprawlwatch, 4
stakeholders
    engagement, 33
    identification, 359
    input, incorporating, 21
St. Anthony's Fire, 48
steady-state excretion with exposure to nonpersistent
        chemicals, *89*
Stockholm Convention on Persistent Organic
        Pollutants, 10, 292
    list, 7
Stockholm Declaration on the Human Environment, 6
storm surge hazards, 351
Strategic Approach to International Chemicals
        Management (SAICM), 292
stress, 70
stressors, 59, 180
stress response, 70
Structure-Activity Relation (SAR), *114*
Study of Asian Women and their Offspring's
        Development and Environmental
        Exposures (SAWASDEE), 85
study population, identifying, 99
S. typhi, 49
subjective probability distributions, 222
subpopulations, potentially exposed or susceptible,
        238
substitution
    in hazard control, 253–254
    of hazards in workplace, 293
Substitution and Alternatives Assessment Toolbox,
        296
substitution principle, 291–292
sucralose, 43
sulfur dioxide, 70
sulfur oxides, 19
Superfund Amendments and Reauthorization Act
        (SARA), 349
    Title III, 349

Superfund legislation, 348
survival analysis, 215
susceptibility
    variation in, 20, 26
sustainable solutions agenda, 287
Swedish Act on Chemical Products, 291
Swinomish Indigenous Health Indicators, 357
systematic review, 18
systems, endocrine, 11
systems toxicology, 111, 119–120, **121**, 145

T

tap water consumption, 31
TCDD, *see* 2,3,7,8-tetrachlorodibenzo-p-dioxin
TCE, health effects of, 11
technological change, and occupational health risk,
    261
temporal variability, in urine and blood samples, 87
terminology, 33
tetrachloroethylene, 11, 168, 173–174
    biodegradation of, 11
thalidomide, 116
threat maps, 144
three-step process, 21
threshold hypothesis, 41–42
threshold limit values (TLVs), 118
thyroid function, 10
time-activity diary, 79
time-resolution inaccuracies, 79
Times Beach contamination, 172
Tissue Chip Consortium, 118
tissue chips, 118
Tobler, Waldo, 100
Tolerable Daily Intake (TDI), 118
Total Diet Study, 47
toxicants, 112, 116
Toxic Equivalence Quotient (TEQ), 32
toxicity, chronic, 112
"Toxicity Testing in the 21st Century: A Vision and a
    Strategy", 9, 180
toxicodynamics, and children's health, 270
toxicokinetics, 28
    and children's health, 269–270
Toxicological Risk Assessment Study, data issues, **118**
toxicology, 111
    evolution of, 118
    genetic, 26
    modern, 121
    science of, 112
Toxic Substances Control Act (TSCA), 16, 46, 121, 237
    in relation to children, 268
Toxin-Toxin-Target Database (T3DB), 121
trade-offs, 291
traditional engineering approach, 34
training and education on hazardous substances, 349
transparency, 291, 348
Triangle Shirtwaist Fire, 226
triangular distribution, 215
trichloroethylene (TCE), 5
truncated distribution, 220

trust, 348
trustworthiness
    perceived, 355
    of sources, 361
two-way communication, importance of, 15

U

uncertainties, limited consideration of, 282–283
uncertainty, 220–221
    addressing, in NAMs and IATAs, 307
    and data gaps, 182
    definition, 167
uncertainty analysis, 221
    of cyrene's eye damage and irritation potential,
        310
    example, 307
    limitations of current forms, 283
    in PBPK modeling, 167
uncertainty assessment, 66
uncertainty reduction steps, **308**
uniform distribution, 215
United Nations Environment Program (UNEP), 6
unleaded gasoline extract, 25
unpredictability, 342
uptake, 61
Urban Sprawl and Public Health, 4
urinary leukotriene E4, 83
urine, 79, 82
    in exposure assessment, 84–85
US Census Bureau, 109, 265
US Environmental Protection Agency (US EPA), *see*
        Environmental Protection Agency (EPA)
US Food Quality Protection Act, *see* Food Quality
        Protection Act (FQPA)
Use Cluster Scoring System, 293
*Using 21st Century Science to Improve Risk-Related
        Evaluations*, 9, 18
US NRC framework, 297
US Superfund Regulation, 32
US Supreme Court, 19
UV absorbance detection, 87–88

V

variability and uncertainty, 25, 211, 222
vehicle-related deaths, 3
Venter, Craig, 120
ventilation, 1
    in hazard control, 255
veterinary drug residues, 45
videotaping, 77
Vietnam, *3*
    Operation Ranch Hand, 6
vinyl chloride, 11, 19
viral shunt, 340
    pathway, 333
viruses, 340
    in marine ecosystems, 341
volatile organic compounds (VOCs), 81–82
vomiting, 48

W

Waddington, Conrad, 187
Walmart, 296
Walsh-Healey Public Contracts Act, 236
Warner, John, 294
warnings, emergency, 351
water pollution, 3, 16
Weibull distribution, 215
wetlands, 333
Wetterhahn, Karen, 130
wheezing, 48
Wild, Christopher, 31, 106
workplace fatalities, 227, 229, 232
    since the passage of the OSH Act, **228**, **229**
workplace population risk, assessing trends in, 227
work-related fatal and non-fatal events, *230*
World Health Organization (WHO), 25
World Trade Center (WTC); *see also* biomarkers: and
        9/11 terrorist attacks
    exposure, *103*

Health Program, 227
Health Registry, 107
research, 103–104
World War II, Italian campaign and DDT, 6
Worth, Andrew, 31

X

xenobiotic absorption, 116
xenobiotic uptake, 123
xenobiotics, 116
    common groups, **125**

Y

Youth Risk Behavior Survey, 107

Z

zearalenone, 48
Zero Discharge of Hazardous Chemicals (ZDHC), 299

...UK
...oup UK Ltd.
...21223
...00013B/146